Handbook of Reward and Decision Making

Handbook of Reward and Decision Making

Edited by

Dr. Jean-Claude Dreher and Léon Tremblay

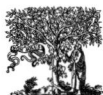

AMSTERDAM • BOSTON • HEIDELBERG • LONDON • NEW YORK • OXFORD
PARIS • SAN DIEGO • SAN FRANCISCO • SINGAPORE • SYDNEY • TOKYO

Academic Press is an imprint of Elsevier

ELSEVIER

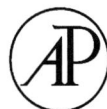

Academic Press is an imprint of Elsevier
30 Corporate Drive, Suite 400, Burlington, MA 01803, USA
525 B Street, Suite 1900, San Diego, CA 92101-4495, USA
32 Jamestown Road, London, NW1 7BY, UK
360 Park Avenue South, New York, NY 10010-1710, USA

First edition 2009

Library of Congress Cataloging-in-Publication Data
A catalog record for this book is available from the Library of Congress

British Library Cataloguing in Publication Data
A catalogue record for this book is available from the British Library

ISBN: 978-0-12-374620-7

For information on all Academic Press publications
visit our website at www.elsevierdirect.com

Typeset by Macmillan Publishing Solutions
www.macmillansolutions.com

Printed and bound in the United States of America

09 10 11 12 13   9 8 7 6 5 4 3 2 1

Contents

Visit the Handbook of *Reward and Decision Making* website at:

http://www.elsevierdirect.com/companions/9780123746207

The *Handbook of Reward and Decision Making* website features color images from the book, mathematical appendices, as well as computer programs implementing some of the algorithms described in the computational modelling chapter of the book.

Preface

Our behavior is motivated by rewards of different nature among which we frequently need to choose. Because there is no single sense organ transducing rewards of different types, our brain must integrate and compare them to choose the options with the highest subjective value. Neuroimaging, electrophysiological, behavioral, and pharmacological techniques, in combination with molecular and genetic tools have begun to elucidate the neuronal mechanisms underlying reward processing and decision-making. This book highlights some of these advancements that have led to the current understanding of the brain's involvement on reward and decision-making processes. The book addresses one fundamental question about the nature of behavior: how does the brain process reward and makes decisions when facing multiple options?

A reward is an object that generates approach behavior and consumption, produces learning, and represents a basis for decision-making. Reward is fundamental to motivation, learning, cognition, and the organization of behavior. It is also often a goal for behavior, allowing appropriate selection of sequences of responses and decisions in order to reach that goal. The brain has developed a network, known as the reward system, whose major components include dopaminergic midbrain neurons, the ventral striatum, the prefrontal cortex (especially its orbitofrontal part), and the amygdala. Dysfunction of this system is observed in several neurological and psychiatric disorders as schizophrenia, Parkinson's disease, eating disorders, and drug addiction.

Although the capacity to predict reward information is essential for cognitive functions, such as learning and motivation, the reward system is also involved in more complex cognitive functions. For example, brain dopamine circuitry underlies a number of behavioral functions that depend on sequential ordering, such as sequential choice behavior. Moreover, dopamine reward signals influence processes in both cortical and sub-cortical structures that modulate cognitive functions, such as economic decision-making and working memory. Because the reward system is involved in these different aspects, ranging from motivation to the organization of behavior, a number of researches have started to combine brain imaging and computational approaches to address problems related to classical conditioning, decision making under risk or uncertainty and weighting between costs and benefits.

It is still unclear whether specific functions can be ascribed to particular structures of the reward system. Such functions include computing the value signals of cues announcing potentially rewarded outcomes or of rewarded outcomes (incentive and hedonic values), holding them in working memory to plan and organize behavior toward an outcome, comparing actual and potential outcomes, determining how well the outcome satisfies current needs and evaluating the overall action schemes assessing the trade-offs between cost/efforts and benefits. A general framework remains to be developed to integrate these functions and to explain how specific brain regions ensure our behavior to be most efficient in satisfying our needs.

The neural bases of reward and decision-making processes are of great interest to a broad readership because of the fundamental role of reward in a number of behavioral processes (such as motivation, learning, and cognition) and because of their theoretical and clinical implications for understanding dysfunctions of the dopaminergic system and pathologies of reward processing. Findings in this research field are also important to basic neuroscientists interested in the reward system, cognitive psychologists working on conditioning/reinforcement, as well as computational neuroscientists studying probabilistic models of brain functions. Reward and decision-making cover a wide range of topics and levels of analysis, from molecular mechanisms to neural systems dynamics and to computational models. The contributions to this book are forward-looking assessments of the current and future issues faced by researchers. We were fortunate to assemble an outstanding collection of experts who addressed different aspects of reward and decision-making processes. Five current topics are specifically addressed.

Part One is devoted to basic monkey anatomical and electrophysiological data. In their natural environment, animals face a multitude of stimuli, very few of which are likely to be useful as predictors of reward. It is thus crucial that the brain learns to predict rewards, providing a critical evolutionary advantage for survival. This first part of the book offers a comprehensive view on the specific contributions of different brain structures as the dopaminergic midbrain neurons, the ventral striatum, and the prefrontal cortex, including the lateral prefrontal cortex and the orbitofrontal cortex, to the component processes underlying reinforcement-guided decision-making, such as the representation of instructions, expectations, and outcomes, the updating of action values and the evaluation process guiding choices between prospective rewards. Special emphasize is made on the neuroanatomy of the reward system and the fundamental roles of dopaminergic neurons in learning stimuli–reward associations. In particular, recent electrophysiological data in monkeys are reviewed showing that the activity of dopaminergic neurons carries information about two statistical parameters of reward: a transient reward prediction error signal that codes a discrepancy between the reward actually delivered and the anticipated reward, and a sustained signal covarying with reward uncertainty.

Part Two broadly covers brain imaging studies on reward and decision-making. There is a current explosion of fMRI studies on reward and decision-making. This area of research encompasses a broad range of issues, such as the neural substrates of different value-related signals involved when processing and deciding between rewards of different nature, such as prediction error, uncertainty, subjective value of each option, goal, and decision-value. This part of the book also addresses the study of the neural correlates of perceptual decision-making in humans using non-invasive methods such as fMRI and EEG and investigate the neural substrates underlying processes described by psychological theories, such as instrumental versus Pavlovian conditioning, goals, habits, and learning with different discount factors. Another question addressed in this part of the book is to know whether similar neural substrates underlie rewards of different types. In particular, primary (such as drink, food, and sex) and secondary rewards (such as money, power, ...) may both be processed by similar and distinct neural substrates and may also share neurobiological mechanisms subserved by non-natural (drug) rewards. Finally, the relationships between the two fields of neuroscience and economics is addressed in a number of fMRI studies investigating the neural substrates of different cognitive biases demonstrating that individuals do not operate as optimal decision-makers in maximizing utility (direct violation of the assumptions of the "standard economic model"). For example, people generally overestimate the loss they will derive from anticipated future events and discount future rewards relative to immediate ones.

Part Three of the book focuses on pathophysiology (lesion data and neuroimaging findings) involving disorders of decision-making and of the reward system that link together basic research areas, including systems, cognitive, and clinical neuroscience. Dysfunction of the reward system and decision-making is present in a number of neurological and psychiatric disorders, such as Parkinson's disease, schizophrenia, drug addiction, and focal brain lesions. In particular, the study of patients with Parkinson's disease and models of this disease in non-human primates indicate that dopamine depletion impair reward-based learning, but not punishment avoidance. Moreover, patients with Parkinson's disease treated with dopamine receptor agonists, may develop impulsive behavior such as pathological gambling, compulsive shopping or hypersexuality, providing a window in understanding how dopamine treatment influences reward mechanisms leading to impulsivity.

Part Four is devoted to the roles of hormones and different genes involved in dopamine transmission on the reward system and on decision-making processes. The combination of molecular genetic, endocrinology and neuroimaging has provided a considerable amount of data that helps understanding the biological mechanisms influencing reward processing. These studies have demonstrated that genetic and hormonal variations affecting dopaminergic transmission have an impact on the physiological response of the reward system and on its associated cognitive functions. These variations may account for some of the inter- and intra-individual behavioral differences observed in reward processing and social cognition. These findings are important because they point to the neural influence of genes conferring vulnerability to develop neuropathologies related to compulsive behavior.

Finally, *Part Five* presents computational models on decision-making, including Bayesian models of decision-making, models of decision under risk and uncertainty taking into account the roles of social learning, regret, and disappointments and models of the basal ganglia. New bridges have recently been made between animal neurophysiology, human neuroimaging, and behavior and theoretical models that provide a formal and quantitative account of reward and decision-making. For example, computational approaches have linked learning mechanisms with the underlying neurophysiology of reinforcements, using temporal difference learning approaches. Other types of models have shown how decisions based on uncertain information may benefit from an accumulation of information over time. These models show how neurons may compute the time integral of sensory signals as evidence for or against a proposition and propose that the decision is made when the integrated evidence reaches a certain threshold. These types of models explain a variety of behavioral and physiological measurements obtained from monkey electrophysiological data.

We anticipate that while some readers may read the volume from the first to the last chapter, other readers may read only one or more chapters at a time, and not necessarily in the order presented in this book. This is why we encouraged an organization of this volume whereby each chapter can stand alone, while making references to others and minimizing redundancies across the volume. Given the consistent acceleration of advances in the different approaches described in this book on reward and decision-making, you are about to be dazzled by a first-look at the new stages of an exciting era in brain research. Enjoy!

Dr Jean-Claude Dreher
CNRS
Reward and decision making team
Cognitive Neuroscience Center
67 Bd Pinel 69675 Bron
France

List of contributors

Céline Amiez, Montreal Neurological Institute, McGill University, 3801 University Street, Montreal, Quebec H3A 2B4, Canada.

Rafal Bogacz, Department of Computer Science University of Bristol, Bristol BS8 1UB, United Kingdom.

Peter Bossaerts, Laboratory for Decision-Making Under Uncertainty, Ecole Polytechnique Fédérale de Lausanne, Odyssea, Station 5, CH-1015 Lausanne, Switzerland.

Christian Büchel, NeuroImage Nord, Department of Systems Neuroscience, University Medical Center Hamburg-Eppendorf, Martinistr. 52, 20246 Hamburg, Germany.

Xavier Caldú, Reward and Decision Making Group, Cognitive Neuroscience Center, CNRS–Lyon 1 University, 67 Bd Pinel 69675 Bron, France.

Giorgio Coricelli, Institute of Cognitive Neuroscience, Cognitive Neuroscience Center, CNRS UMR5229, Lyon 1 University, 67 Bd Pinel 69675 Bron, France.

Mathieu d'Acremont, Laboratory for Decision-Making under Uncertainty, Ecole Polytechnique Fédérale de Lausanne, Odyssea, Station 5, CH-1015 Lausanne, Switzerland.

Kimberlee D'Ardenne, Department of Neuroscience, Baylor College of Medicine, Houston, TX 77030.

Mauricio R. Delgado, Department of Psychology, Rutgers University, 101 Warren St., Newark, NJ 07102.

Natalie L. Denburg, Department of Neurology, University of Iowa Hospitals and Clinics, 200 Hawkins Drive, Iowa City, IA 52242.

Sophie Deneve, Group for Neural Theory, Département d'Etudes Cognitives, Ecole Normale Supérieure, 29, rue d'Ulm and Groupe de Neuroscience Théorique, Collège de France, 3, rue d'Ulm, 75005 Paris, France.

Bradley B. Doll, Department of Cognitive and Linguistic Science and Department of Psychology, Brown University, 190 Thayer St., Providence, RI 02912-1978.

Jean-Claude Dreher, Reward and Decision Making Group, Cognitive Neuroscience Center, CNRS–Lyon 1 University, 67 Bd Pinel 69675 Bron, France.

P.C. Fletcher, Department of Psychiatry, Box 189, University of Cambridge, Addenbrooke's Hospital, Cambridge CB2 2QQ, United Kingdom.

Michael J. Frank, Department of Cognitive and Linguistic Science and Department of Psychology, Brown University, 190 Thayer St., Providence, RI 02912-1978.

Manfred Gilli, Department of Econometrics, University of Geneva, Uni Mail, CH-1205 Geneva, Switzerland.

Suzanne Haber, Department of Pharmacology and Physiology, University of Rochester School of Medicine, 601 Elmwood Avenue, Rochester, New York 14642.

Hauke R. Heekeren, Neurocognition of Decision Making Group, Max Planck Institute for Human Development, Lentzeallee 94, 14195 Berlin, Germany.

Andreas Heinz, Department of Psychiatry and Psychotherapy, Charité Campus Mitte, Charité – University Medical Center, Schumannstr. 20–21, 10117 Berlin, Germany.

Michael Hernandez, Department of Neurology, University of Iowa Hospitals and Clinics, 200 Hawkins Drive, Iowa City, IA 52242.

Jeffrey Hollerman, Psychology Department and Neuroscience Program, Allegheny College, 520 N. Main St., Meadville, PA 16335.

Shunsuke Kobayashi, Department of Physiology, Development and Neuroscience, University of Cambridge, Downing Street, Cambridge CB2 3DY, United Kingdom.

Samuel M. McClure, Department of Psychology, Stanford University, Stanford, CA 94305.

G.K. Murray, Department of Psychiatry, Box 189, University of Cambridge, Addenbrooke's Hospital, Cambridge CB2 2QQ, United Kingdom.

Mathias Pessiglione, Laboratoire INSERM U610, Institut Fédératif de Recherches en Neurosciences, Site Pitié-Salpêtrière, F-75013 Paris, France.

Michael Petrides, Montreal Neurological Institute, McGill University, 3801 University Street, Montreal, Quebec H3A 2B4, Canada.

Donald Pfaff, Laboratory of Neurobiology and Behavior, The Rockefeller University, 1230 York Avenue, New York 10065.

Marios G. Philiastides, Neurocognition of Decision Making Group, Max Planck Institute for Human Development, Lentzeallee 94, 14195 Berlin, Germany.

Anthony J. Porcelli, Department of Psychology, Rutgers University, 101 Warren St., Newark, NJ 07102.

Imke Puls, Department of Psychiatry and Psychotherapy, Charité Campus Mitte, Charité – University Medical Center, Schumannstr. 20–21, 10117 Berlin, Germany.

Edmund T. Rolls, Department of Experimental Psychology, Oxford Centre for Computational Neuroscience, South Parks Road, Oxford OX1 3UD, United Kingdom. www.oxcns.org

Aldo Rustichini, Department of Economics, University of Minnesota, 271 19th Avenue South, Minneapolis, MN 55455.

Justine Schober, Laboratory of Neurobiology and Behavior, The Rockefeller University, 1230 York Avenue, New York 10065 and Hamot Medical Center, 201 State Street, Erie, PA 16550.

Mihaela Stavarache, Laboratory of Neurobiology and Behavior, The Rockefeller University, 1230 York Avenue, New York 10065.

Philippe N. Tobler, Department of Physiology, Development and Neuroscience, University of Cambridge, Downing Street, Cambridge CB2 3DY, United Kingdom.

Daniel Tranel, Department of Neurology, University of Iowa Hospitals and Clinics, 200 Hawkins Drive, Iowa City, IA 52242.

Léon Tremblay, Institute of Cognitive Neuroscience, CNRS-5229-University Lyon 1, 67 Bd Pinel 69675 Bron, France.

Masataka Watanabe, Department of Psychology, Tokyo Metropolitan Institute for Neuroscience, 2-6 Musashidai, Fuchu, Tokyo 183-8526, Japan.

Yulia Worbe, Institute of Cognitive Neuroscience, CNRS-5229-University Lyon 1, 67 Bd Pinel 69675 Bron, France.

Juliana Yacubian, NeuroImage Nord, Department of Systems Neuroscience, University Medical Center Hamburg-Eppendorf, Martinistr. 52, 20246 Hamburg, Germany.

Part One

Monkey Anatomical and Electrophysiological Studies on Reward and Decision Making

1 Anatomy and connectivity of the reward circuit

Suzanne N. Haber

Department of Pharmacology and Physiology, University of Rochester School of Medicine, 601 Elmwood Avenue, Rochester, New York 14642

Abstract

While cells in many brain regions cells are responsive to reward, the cortical-basal ganglia circuit is at the heart of the reward system. The key structures in this network are: the anterior cingulate cortex, the orbital prefrontal cortex, the ventral striatum, the ventral pallidum, and the midbrain dopamine neurons. In addition, other structures including the dorsal prefrontal cortex, amygdala, hippocampus, thalamus, lateral habenular n., and specific brainstem structures, such as the pedunculopontine n. and the raphe n., are key components in regulating the reward circuit. Connectivity between these areas forms a complex neural network that is topographically organized, thus maintaining functional continuity through the cortico-basal ganglia pathway. However, the reward circuit does not work in isolation. The network also contains specific regions in which convergent pathways provide an anatomical substrate for integration across functional domains.

Key points

1. The cortico-basal ganglia network is at the center of the reward circuit that underlies the ability to make complex choices and accurately evaluate reward value, predictability, and risk.
2. The key structures are the anterior cingulate cortex, the ventral striatum, the ventral pallidum, and the dopamine neurons of the ventral tegmental area and the substantia nigra, pars compacta. The amygdala, hippocampus, thalamus, lateral habenular n., and specific brainstem structures, such as the pedunculopontine n., and the raphe n., are key components in regulating the reward circuit.
3. While pathways from the cortex through the striatum, pallidum, thalamus, and back to the cortex are generally topographically organized, there are key areas of convergence of between different functional regions, which provides an important substrate for integration between functional domains.
4. Through these integrative networks, the reward circuit impacts on cognition and motor control, allowing information about reward to be channeled through cognitive and motor control circuits to mediate the development of appropriate action plans.

1.1 Introduction

The reward circuit is a complex neural network that underlies the ability to effectively assess the likely outcomes from different choices. A key component to good decision-making and appropriate goal-directed behaviors is the ability to accurately evaluate reward value, predictability, and risk. While the hypothalamus is central for processing information about basic or primary rewards, higher cortical and subcortical forebrain structures are engaged when complex choices about these fundamental needs are required. Moreover, choices often involve secondary rewards, such as money, power, challenge, and so on that are more abstract (compared to primary needs), and not as dependent on direct sensory stimulation. Although cells that respond to different aspects of reward, such as anticipation or value, are found throughout the brain, at the center of this neural network is the ventral cortico-basal ganglia ((BG) circuit). The BG are traditionally considered to process information in parallel and segregated functional streams consisting of reward processing, cognition, and motor control areas [1]. Moreover, within the ventral BG, there are microcircuits thought to be associated with different aspects of reward processing. However, a key component for learning and adaptation of goal-directed behaviors is the ability not only to evaluate different aspects of reward but also to develop appropriate action plans and inhibit maladaptive choices on the basis of previous experience. This requires integration between different aspects of reward processing as well as interaction between reward circuits and brain regions involved in cognition. Thus, while parallel processing provides throughput channels by which specific actions can be expressed while others are inhibited, the BG also plays a key role in learning new procedures and associations, implying the necessity for integrative processing across circuits. Indeed, an emerging literature demonstrates the complexity of the cortico-BG network showing a dual organizational system, permitting both parallel and integrative processing [2–6]. Therefore, while the ventral BG network is at the heart of reward processing, it does not work in isolation. This chapter addresses not only the connectivities within this circuit, but also how this circuit anatomically interfaces with other BG circuits.

The frontal-BG network, in general, mediates all aspects of action planning, including reward and motivation, cognition, and motor control. However, specific regions within this network play a unique role in different aspects of reward processing and evaluation of outcomes, including reward value, anticipation, predictability, and risk. The key structures are: prefrontal areas (anterior cingulate cortex – ACC and orbital prefrontal cortex – OFC), the ventral striatum (VS), the ventral pallidum (VP), and the midbrain dopamine (DA) neurons. The ACC and OFC prefrontal areas mediate different aspects of reward-based behaviors, error prediction, value, and the choice between short- and long-term gains. Cells in the VS and VP respond to anticipation of reward and reward detection. Reward prediction and error detection signals are generated, in part from the midbrain DA cells. While the VS and the ventral tegmental area (VTA) DA neurons are the BG areas most commonly associated with reward, reward-responsive activation is not restricted to these, but found throughout the striatum and substantia nigra, pars compacta (SNc). In addition, other structures, including the dorsal prefrontal cortex (DPFC), amygdala, hippocampus, thalamus, lateral habenular n., and specific brainstem structures, such as the pedunculopontine n. and the raphe n., are key components in regulating the reward circuit (Fig. 1.1).

1.2 Prefrontal cortex

Although cells throughout the cortex fire in response to various aspects of reward processing, the main components of evaluating reward value and outcome are the anterior cingulate and orbital prefrontal cortices. Each of these regions is comprised of several specific cortical areas: The ACC is divided into areas 24, 25, and 32; the orbital cortex is divided into areas 11, 12, 13, 14, and caudal regions referred to as either parts of insular cortex

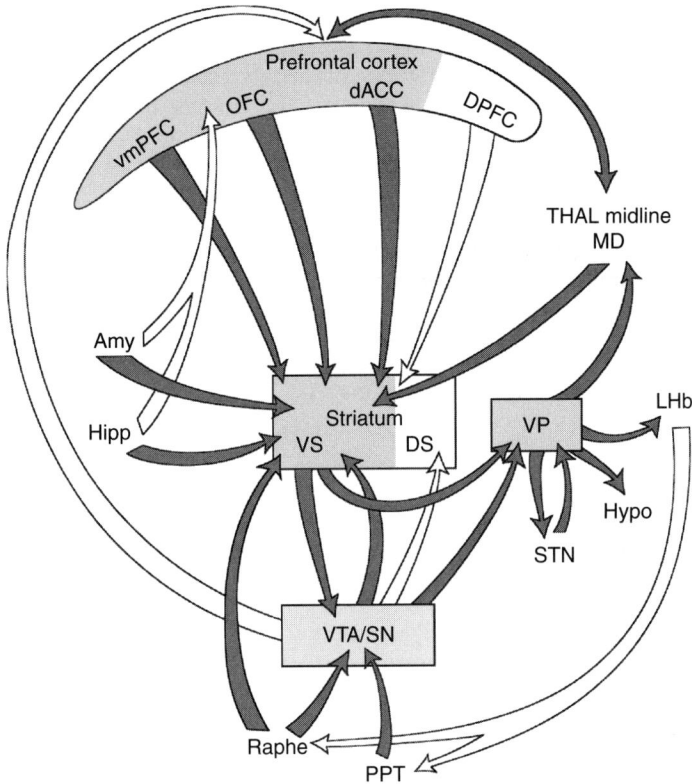

Figure 1.1 Schematic illustrating key structures and pathways of the reward circuit. Shaded areas and gray arrows represent the basic ventral cortico-BG structures and connections. Amy, amygdala; dACC, dorsal anterior cingulate cortex; DPFC, dorsal prefrontal cortex; DS, dorsal striatum; Hipp, hippocampus; hypo, hypothalamus; LHb, lateral habenula; OFC, orbital frontal cortex; PPT, pedunculopontine nucleus; SNc, substantia nigra, pars compacta; STN, subthalamic n.; Thal, thalamus; VP, ventral pallidum; VS, ventral striatum; VTA, ventral tegmental area; vmPFC, ventral medial prefrontal cortex.

or periallo- and proiso-cortical areas [7,8]. Based on specific roles for mediating different aspects of reward processing and emotional regulation, these regions can be functionally grouped into: (1) the dorsal anterior cingulate cortex (dACC), which includes parts of area 24 and 32; (2) the ventral, medial prefrontal cortex (vmPFC), which includes areas 25, 14, and subgenual area 32; (3) OFC, which includes areas 11, 13, and 12; and (4) caudal OFC, which includes parts of the insula cortex. The vmPFC plays a role in monitoring correct responses based on previous experience and the internal milieu, and is engaged when previously learned responses are no longer appropriate and need to be suppressed. This region is a key player in the ability to extinguish previous negative associations and is positively correlated with the magnitude of extinction memory [9]. The OFC plays a central role in evaluation of reward value [10–13]. The caudal parts are associated with sensory systems. The dACC is a unique part of frontal cortex, in that it contains within in it a representation of many diverse frontal lobe functions, including motivation (areas 24a and b), cognition (area 24b), and motor control (area 24c), which is reflected in its widespread connections with other limbic, cognitive, and motor cortical areas. This is a complex area, but the overall role of the ACC appears to be involved in monitoring these functions in conflict situations [14–16]. In addition to the dACC, OFC, and vmPFC, the DPFC, in particular areas 9 and 46, are engaged when working memory is required for monitoring incentive based behavioral responses. The DPFC also encodes reward amount and becomes active when anticipated rewards signal future outcomes [13,17].

Anatomical relationships both within and between different PFC regions are complex. Several organizational schemes have been proposed based on combinations of cortical architecture and connectivity [6–8,18]. In general, cortical areas within each prefrontal group are highly interconnected. However, these connections are quite specific in that a circumscribed region within each area projects to specific regions of other areas, but not throughout. For example, a given part of area 25 of the vmPFC projects to only specific parts of area 14. Overall, the vmPFC is primarily connected to other medial subgenual regions and to areas 24a and 12, with few connections to the dACC or areas 9 and 46. Area 24b of the dACC is interconnected with the different regions of the dACC areas, including 24c (motor cingulate cortex). It is also tightly linked to area 9. Different OFC regions are highly interconnected, but as with the vmPFC, these are specific connections. For example, not all of area 11 projects throughout area 13. Regions of the OFC are also connected to areas 9 and 46. Areas 9 and 46 are interconnected and also project to the dACC (areas 24b and 24c) lateral OFC, area 8, and rostral premotor regions. Fibers leave limbic cortex (vmPFC, OFC, and dACC) and take different pathways to reach their cortical targets. Axons travel in a dorsal route via the cingulate bundle to target cingulate cortical areas, a ventral route via the uncinate fasciculus to reach different areas of temporal cortex [19], or travel along the ventral amygdalofugal pathway to the amygdala. Descending fibers traveling to subcortical areas, such as the thalamus and brainstem, pass through the anterior, ventral limb of the internal capsule (IC) and the fiber bundles embedded within the VS. There is a clear topography to the organization of these fibers. Both the vmPFC and OFC fibers enter the capsule ventrally and maintain their position throughout, the vmPFC fibers traveling ventral to those from the OFC. In contrast, dACC enter the capsule dorsally and move to a more ventral position as they travel caudally (Haber, unpublished observations).

In addition, both the vmPFC and OFC are connected to the hippocampus, parahippocampus, and the amygdala [20–22]. The hippocampus projects most densely to the medial PFC regions, including the more caudal area. These projections are derived from the CA1 fields rostrally and the subicular fields more caudally. Hippocampal projections to the OFC are also substantial, but less prominent compared to medial regions. In contrast, there are few projections to the dorsal and lateral PFC areas (dACC, areas 9 and 46). Amygdala projections to the PFC terminate primarily in different regions of the OFC, dACC, and vmPFC. Like the hippocampal projections, and in contrast to the medial and orbital cortices, there are few amygdala connections with more lateral parts of the PFC. The amygdalo-cortical projections are bidirectional. The primary target of these cortical areas is the basal and lateral nuclear complex. Here, the OFC-amygdalo projections target the intercalated masses, whereas terminals from the vmPFC and dACC are more diffuse. Sensory systems play a key role in initiating and developing reward responses. The OFC, particularly the caudal parts, receive primary and multimodal sensory input from high-order association cortical areas, while more rostral areas receive input from auditory cortices [23,24]. PFC projects to multiple brain subcortical regions, but their largest output is to the thalamus and striatum. Cortical connections to ventral BG output nuclei of the thalamus are bidirectional and primarily target the mediodorsal n (see Section 1.6.1). The second largest subcortical PFC output is to the striatum.

1.3 The ventral striatum

The link between the n. accumbens and reward was first demonstrated as part of the self-stimulation circuit originally described by Olds and Milner [25]. Since then, the nucleus accumbens (and the VS in general) has been a central site for studying reward and drug reinforcement and for the transition between drug use as a reward and habit [26,27]. The term VS, coined by Heimer, includes the nucleus accumbens and the broad continuity between the caudate n. and putamen ventral to the rostral IC, the olfactory tubercle, and the rostrolateral portion of the anterior perforated space adjacent to the lateral olfactory tract in primates [28]. From a connectional perspective, it also includes the medial caudate n., rostral to the anterior commissure [29] (see below).

Human imaging studies demonstrate the involvement of the VS in reward prediction and reward prediction errors [30,31] and, consistent with physiological in nonhuman primate studies, the region is activated during reward anticipation [32]. Collectively, these studies demonstrate its key role in the acquisition and development of reward-based behaviors and its involvement in drug addiction and drug-seeking behaviors. However, it has been recognized for some time now that cells in the primate dorsal striatum (DS) as well as the VS respond to the anticipation, magnitude, and delivery of reward [33,34]. The striatum, as a whole, is the main input structure of the BG and receives a massive and topographic input from cerebral cortex (and thalamus). These afferent projections to the striatum terminate in a general topographic manner, such that the ventromedial striatum receives input from the vmPFC, OFC, and dACC, while the central striatum receives input from the DPFC, including areas 9 and 46. Indeed, the different prefrontal cortical areas have corresponding striatal regions that are involved in various aspects of reward evaluation and incentive-based learning [31,35,36], and are associated with pathological risk-taking and addictive behaviors [37,38].

1.3.1 Special features of the ventral striatum

While the VS is similar to the DS in most respects, there are also some unique features. The VS contains a subterritory, called the shell, which plays a particularly important role in the circuitry underlying goal-directed behaviors, behavioral sensitization, and changes in affective states [39,40]. While several transmitter and receptor distribution patterns distinguish the shell/core subterritories, calbindin is the most consistent marker for the shell across species [41]. Although a calbindin-poor region marks the subterritory of the shell, staining intensities of other histochemical markers in the shell distinguish it from the rest of the VS. In general, GluR1, GAP-43, acetylcholinesterase, serotonin, and Substance P are particularly rich in the shell, while the μ receptor is relatively low in the shell compared to the rest of the striatum [42–45] (Fig. 1.2). Finally, the shell has some unique connectivities compared to the rest of the VS. These are indicated below.

In addition to the shell compartment, several other characteristics are unique to the VS. The DA transporter is relatively low throughout the VS, including the core. This pattern is consistent with the fact that the dorsal tier DA neurons express relatively low levels of mRNA for the DA transporter compared to the ventral tier [46] (see discussion on *substantia nigra* elsewhere in this chapter). The VS has a greater frequency of smaller and more densely packed neurons than the more homogenous DS. In addition, unlike the DS, the VS contains numerous cell islands, including the islands of Calleja, which are thought to contain quiescent immature cells that remain in the adult brain [47–49]. The VS also contains many pallidal elements that invade this ventral territory (see Section 1.4). While

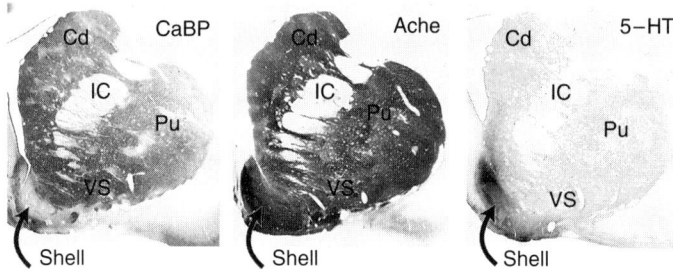

Figure 1.2 Photomicrographs of the rostral striatum stained for different histochemical markers to illustrate the shell. Ache, acetylcholinesterase; C, caudate nucleus; CaBP, calbindin; IC, internal capsule; Pu, Putamen; SERT, serotonin transporter.

collectively these are important distinguishing features of the VS, its dorsal and lateral border is continuous with the rest of the striatum and neither cytoarchitectonic nor histochemical distinctions mark a clear boundary between it and the DS. Moreover, of particular importance is the fact that, while both the dorsal and VS receive input from the cortex, thalamus, and brainstem, the VS alone also receives a dense projection from the amygdala and hippocampus. The best way, therefore, to define the VS is by its afferent projections from cortical areas that mediate different aspects of reward processing, the vmPFC, OFC, dACC, and the medial temporal lobe.

1.3.2   Connections of the ventral striatum

The VS is the main input structure of the ventral BG (Fig. 1.3). Like the DS, afferent projections to the VS are derived from three major sources: a massive, generally topographic input from cerebral cortex; a large input from the thalamus; and a smaller but critical input from the brainstem, primarily from the midbrain dopaminergic cells. The overall organization of inputs to the striatum projections terminate in a general functional topographic manner: The ventromedial striatum receives input from limbic areas, the central striatum receives input from associative cortical areas, and the dorsolateral striatum receives cortical input from sensory-motor areas [29,50]. While this section focuses on the connections of the VS, some attention is given to the DS, especially the caudate n., as it is also involved in reward-based learning and receives input from the DPFC.

Cortical projections to the ventral striatum

Cortico-striatal terminals are organized in two projection patterns: focal projection fields and diffuse projections [6,51] (Fig. 1.4). Focal projection fields consist of dense clusters of terminals forming the well-known dense patches that can be visualized at relatively low magnification. The diffuse projections consist of clusters of terminal fibers that are widely distributed throughout the striatum, both expanding the borders of the focal terminal fields and also extending widely throughout other regions of the striatum.

It is the general distribution of the focal terminal fields that give rise to the topography ascribed to the cortico-striatal projections. This organization is the foundation for the concept of parallel and segregated cortico-BG circuits. The volume occupied by the collective focal terminal fields from the vmPFC, dACC, and OFC is approximately 22% of the striatum. Together, these projections terminate primarily in the rostral, medial, and

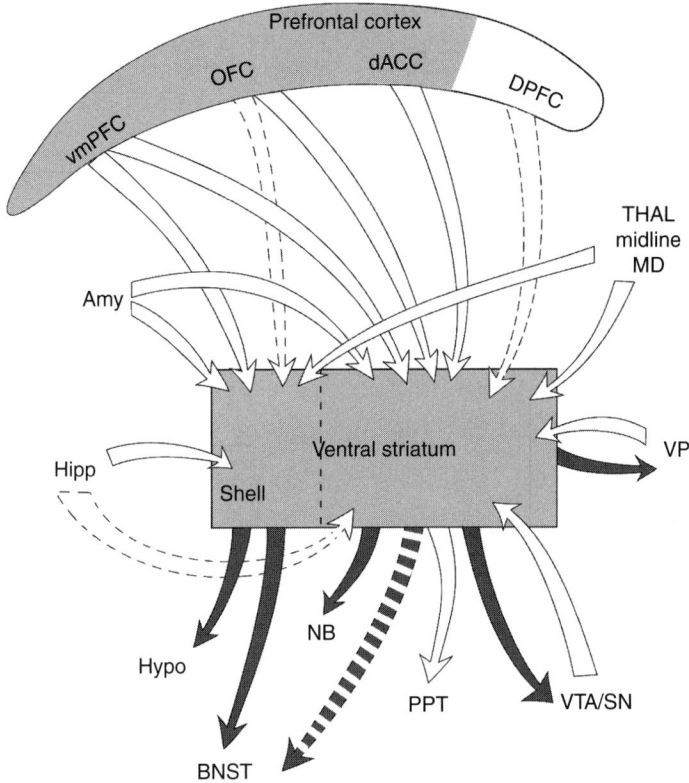

Figure 1.3 Schematic illustrating the connections of the ventral striatum. White arrows, inputs; gray arrows, outputs; weaker projections are indicated with dashed arrows; Amy, amygdala; BNST, bed n. stria terminalis; dACC, dorsal anterior cingulate cortex; DS, dorsal striatum; Hipp, hippocampus; hypo, hypothalamus; MD, mediodorsal n. of the thalamus; OFC, orbital frontal cortex; PPT N., pedunculopontine nucleus; SNc, substantia nigra, pars compacta; STN, subthalamic n.; Thal, thalamus; VP, ventral pallidum; VS, ventral striatum; VTA, ventral tegmental area; vmPFC, ventral medial prefrontal cortex.

ventral parts of the striatum and define the ventral striatal territory [6,52,53]. The large extent of this region is consistent with the findings that diverse striatal areas are activated following reward-related behavioral paradigms [38,54,55]. The focal projection field from the vmPFC is the most limited (particularly from area 25), and is concentrated within and just lateral to the shell (Fig. 1.4A). The innervation of the shell receives the densest input from area 25, although fibers from areas 14, 32, and from agranular insular cortex also terminate here. The vmPFC also projects to the medial wall of the caudate n., adjacent to the ventricle. In contrast, the central and lateral parts of the VS (including the ventral caudate n. and putamen) receive inputs from the OFC (Fig. 1.4B). These terminals also extend dorsally, along the medial caudate n., but lateral to those from the vmPFC. There is some medial to lateral and rostral to caudal topographic organization of the OFC terminal fields. For example, projections from area 11 terminate rostral to those from area 13 and those from area 12 terminate laterally. Despite this general topography, overlap between the OFC terminals is significant. Projections from the dACC (area 24b)

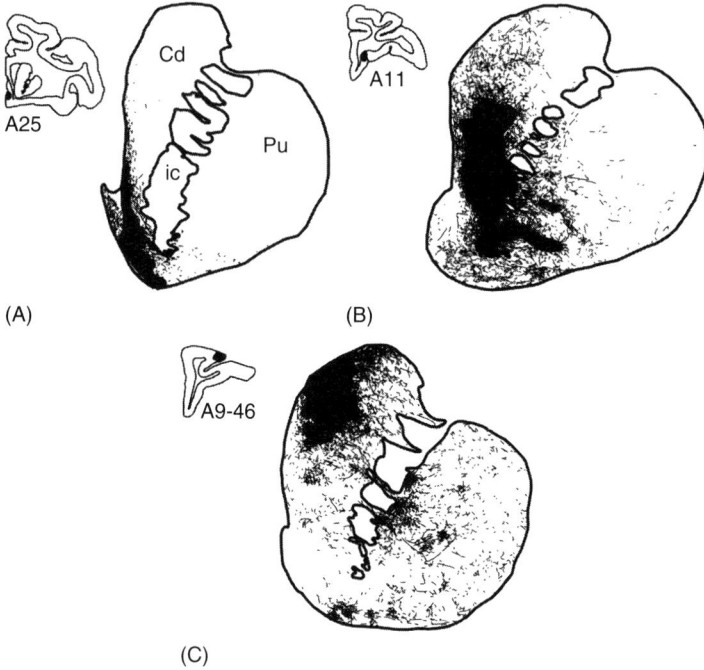

Figure 1.4 Schematic chartings of labeled fibers following injections into different prefrontal regions. (A) vmPFC injection site (area 25); (B) OFC injection site (area 11); (C) DLPFC injection site (area 9-46). The focal projection fields are indicated in solid black. Note the diffuse projection fibers outside of the focal projection fields.

extend from the rostral pole of the striatum to the anterior commissure and are located in both the central caudate n. and putamen. They primarily avoid the shell region. These fibers terminate somewhat lateral to those from the OFC. Thus, the OFC terminal fields are positioned between the vmPFC and dACC. In contrast, the DPFC projects primarily in the head of the caudate and part of the rostral putamen (Fig. 1.5C). Terminals from the areas 9 and 46 are somewhat topographically organized, extending from the rostral pole, through the rostral, central putamen and much of the length of the caudate n. [6,56].

Despite the general topography described above, focal terminal fields from the vmPFC, OFC, and dACC show a complex interweaving and convergence, providing an anatomical substrate for modulation between circuits [6] (Fig. 1.5A). Focal projections from the dACC and OFC regions do not occupy completely separate territories in any part of the striatum, but converge most extensively at rostral levels. By contrast, there is greater separation of projections between terminals from the vmPFC and the dACC/OFC, particularly at caudal levels. In addition to convergence between vmPFC, dACC, and OFC focal terminals, projections from dACC and OFC also converge with inputs from the DPFC, demonstrating that functionally diverse PFC projections also converge in the striatum. At rostral levels, DPFC terminals converge with those from both the dACC and OFC, although each cortical projection also occupies its own territory. Here, projections from all PFC areas occupy a central region, the different cortical projection extending into non-overlapping zones. Convergence is less prominent caudally, with almost complete

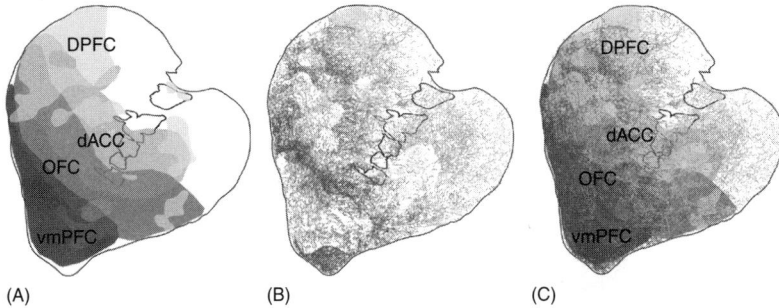

Figure 1.5 Schematics demonstrating convergence of cortical projections from different reward-related regions and dorsal prefrontal areas. (A) Convergence between focal projections from different prefrontal regions. (B) Distribution of diffuse fibers from different prefrontal regions. (C) Combination of focal and the diffuse fibers. ACC, dorsal anterior cingulate cortex; DPFC, dorsal lateral prefrontal cortex; OFC, orbital prefrontal cortex; vmPFC, ventral medial prefrontal cortex. Red, inputs from vmPFC; dark orange, inputs from OFC; light orange, inputs from dACC; yellow, inputs from DPFC. See Plate 1 of Color Plate section.

separation of the dense terminals from the DPFC and dACC/OFC just rostral to the anterior commissure. Since medium spiny neurons have a dendritic field spanning 0.5 mm [57], the area of convergence is likely to be larger than estimated, based solely on the relationship between the afferent projections. These regions of convergence between the focal terminal fields of the vmPFC, OFC, and dACC provide an anatomical substrate for integration between different reward processing circuits within specific striatal areas and may represent "hot spots" of plasticity for integrating reward value, predictability, and salience. Moreover, a coordinated activation of DPFC, dACC, and/or OFC terminals in the striatum would produce a unique combinatorial activation at the specific sites, suggesting specific subregions for reward-based incentive drive to impact on long-term strategic planning and habit formation.

In addition to the focal projections, each cortical region sends a diffuse fiber projection that extends outside of its focal terminal field [6] (Fig. 1.5B; see also Fig. 1.4). These axons can travel some distance, invading striatal regions that receive their focal input from other PFC areas. Diffuse diffuse projections are extensive. For example, the diffuse projection from the OFC extends deep into the dorsal, central caudate and putamen, with extensive convergence with the focal and diffuse projections from both the dACC and the DPFC. Likewise, the diffuse projections from dACC overlap with focal projections from the vmPFC, OFC, and DPFC. Moreover, clusters of fibers are found in the dorsal lateral caudate n. and in the caudal ventral putamen, areas that do not receive a focal input from other prefrontal regions. Finally, clusters of DPFC fibers terminate throughout the rostral striatum, including the VS and lateral putamen. Although the focal projections do not reach into the ventro-medial region, clusters of labeled fibers are located here.

Significant and extensive diffuse projection from each PFC region is consistent with the demonstration that a single cortico-striatal axon can innervate 14% of the striatum [58]. However, activation of medium spiny neuron requires a large coordinated glutamatergic input from many cortical cells [57]. Therefore, the invasions of relatively small fiber clusters from other functional regions are not considered to have much relevance for cortico-striatal information processing and, as a result, anatomical studies have focused on the large, dense focal projections [56,59]. While under normal conditions in which a routine behavior is executed, these fibers may have little impact, this diffuse projection may serve a separate integrative function. Collectively, these projections represent a large population of axons invading each focal projection field, and, under certain conditions, if collectively activated, they may provide the recruitment strength necessary to modulate the focal signal. This would serve to broadly disseminate cortical activity to a wide striatal region, thus providing an anatomical substrate for cross-encoding cortical information to influence the future firing of medium spiny neurons [4]. Taken together, the combination of focal and diffuse projections from the DPFC occupies much of the rostral striatum and continues caudally through the caudate n. (Fig. 1.5C). The fronto-striatal network, therefore, constitutes a dual system comprising topographically organized terminal fields along with subregions that contain convergent pathways derived from functionally discrete cortical areas [6,60].

The amygdala and hippocampal projections to the ventral striatum

The amygdala is a prominent limbic structure that plays a key role in emotional coding of environmental stimuli and provides contextual information used for adjusting motivational level that is based on immediate goals. It comprises the basolateral nuclear group (BLNG), the corticomedial region, and the central amygdaloid complex. The BLNG, the primary source of amygdaloid input to the VS outside the shell, processes higher-order sensory inputs in all modalities except olfactory, and responds to highly palatable foods and "multimodal" cues. Overall, the basal nucleus and the magnocellular division of the accessory basal nucleus are the main source of inputs to the VS [61,62]. The lateral nucleus has a relatively minor input to the VS. The amygdala has few inputs to the DS in primates. The basal and accessory basal nuclei innervate both the shell and ventromedial striatum outside the shell. Moreover, there is a topographic organization to that innervation, such that inputs from basal nucleus subdivisions target different regions of the VS. The shell is set apart from the rest of the VS by a specific set of connections derived from the medial part of the central nucleus (CeM), periamygdaloid cortex, and the medial nucleus of the amygdala. Thus, much like the topography of prefrontal inputs to the VS, nuclei of the amygdala that mediate various functions target subterritories of the ventromedial striatum. In contrast to the amygdala, the hippocampal formation projects to a more limited region of the VS. The main terminal field is located in the most medial and ventral parts of the VS, essentially confined to the shell region. However, addition fibers do extend outside the boundary of the shell. The subiculum appears to provide the main source of this input. Moreover, some afferent fibers are also derived from the parasubiculum, the parasubiculum, and part of CA1 [63]. Inputs from both the hippocampus and amygdala terminate in overlapping regions of the shell [63,64].

Thalamic projections to the ventral striatum

The midline and medial intralaminar thalamic nuclei project to medial prefrontal areas, the amygdale, and hippocampus, and, as such, are considered the limbic-related thalamic nuclear groups. The VS receive dense projections from the midline thalamic nuclei and from the medial parafascicular nucleus [65,66]. The midline nuclei include the anterior and posterior paraventricular, paratenial, rhomboid, and reuniens thalamic nuclei. The shell of the nucleus accumbens receives the most limited projection. The medial shell is innervated almost exclusively by the anterior and posterior paraventricular nuclei and the medial parafascicular nucleus. The ventral shell receives input from these nuclei as well as from the paratenial, rhomboid, and reuniens midline groups. The medial wall of the caudate nucleus receives projections, not only from the midline and the medial intralaminar nuclei, but also from the central superior lateral nucleus. In contrast, the central part of the VS receives a limited projection from the midline thalamic nuclei, predominantly from the rhomboid nucleus. It also receives input from the parafascicular nucleus and the central superior lateral nucleus. In addition to the midline and intralaminar thalamo-striatal projections, in primates there is a large input from the "specific" thalamic BG relay nuclei, the medial dorsalis (MD) nucleus, ventral anterior (VA), and ventral lateral (VL) nuclei [67,68]. The VS also receives these direct afferent projections, which are derived primarily from the medial MD n. and a limited input from the magnocellular subdivision of the ventral anterior nucleus.

Efferent projections from the ventral striatum

Efferent projections from the ventral striatal (Fig. 1.3), like those from the DS, project primarily to the pallidum and substantia nigra/VTA [69,70]. Specifically, they terminate topographically in the subcommissural part of the globus pallidus (classically defined as the VP), the rostral pole of the external segment, and the rostromedial portion of the internal segment. The more central and caudal portions of the globus pallidus do not receive this input. Fibers from the VS projecting to the substantia nigra are not as confined to a specific region as those projecting to the globus pallidus. Although the densest terminal fields occur in the medial portion, numerous fibers also extend laterally to innervate the dorsal tier of the midbrain dopaminergic neurons (see Section 1.5.3). This projection extends throughout the rostral-caudal extent of the substantia nigra. Projections from the medial part of the VS also project more caudally, terminating in the pedunculopontine n. and, to some extent, in the medial central gray. In addition to projections to the typical BG output structures, the VS also projects to non-BG regions. The shell sends fibers caudal and medially into the lateral hypothalamus. Axons from the medial VS (including the shell) travel to and terminate in the bed nucleus of the stria terminals and parts of the ventral regions of the VS terminate in the nucleus basalis [69]. A projection to the nucleus basalis in the basal forebrain is of particular interest, since this is the main source of cholinergic fibers to the cerebral cortex and the amygdala. These data indicate that the VS may influence cortex directly, without going through the pallidal, thalamic circuit. Potential connection between ventral striatal fibers and cholinergic neurons in the basal forebrain has been demonstrated at the light microscopic levels, in several species including primates, and verified at the EM level in rodents [71–75]. Likewise, the projection to the bed n. of the stria terminalis indicates direct striatal influence on the extended amygdala.

1.4 Ventral pallidum

The VP (Fig. 1.6) is an important component of the reward circuit in that cells in this forebrain region respond specifically during the learning and performance of reward-incentive behaviors and is an area of focus in the study of addictive behaviors [76,77]. The term VP was first used in rats to describe the region below the anterior commissure, extending into the anterior perforated space, based both on histological criteria and its input from the then defined VS [78]. However, in primates, it is best defined by its input from the entire input from reward-related VS. As indicated above, that would include

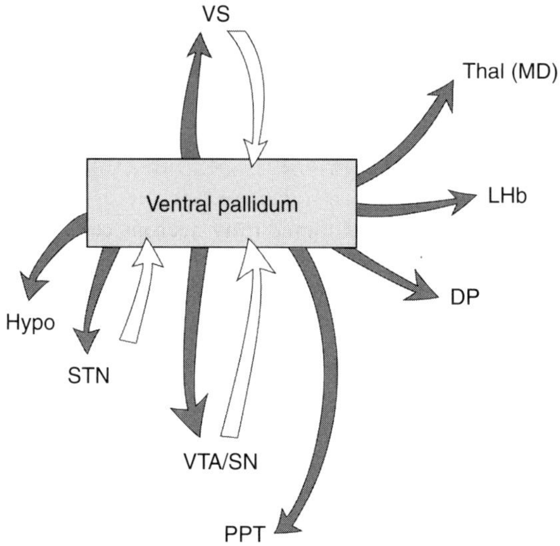

Figure 1.6 Schematic illustrating the connections of the ventral pallidum. DP, dorsal pallidum; hypo, hypothalamus; LHb, lateral habenula; MD n., mediodorsal n. of the thalamus; PPT, pedunculopontine nucleus; SN, substantia nigra; STN, subthalamic n.; Thal, thalamus; VTA, ventral tegmental area.

not only the subcommissural regions, but also the rostral pole of the external segment and the medial rostral internal segment of the globus pallidus. Like the dorsal pallidum, the VP contains two parts: a substance-P-positive and a enkephalin-positive component which project to the thalamus and STN, respectively [79–82]. Pallidal neurons have a distinct morphology that is outlined with immunoreactivity for these peptides, making these stains particularly useful for determining the boundaries and extent of the VP [82–86]. These fibers, which appear as tubular-like structures, referred to as "wooly fibers," demonstrate the extent of the VP and its continuity with the dorsal pallidum [85]. The VP reaches not only ventrally, but also rostrally to invade the rostral and ventral portions of the VS, sending finger-like extensions into the anterior perforated space. In the human brain, the VP extends far into the anterior perforated space, where the structure appears to be rapidly broken up into an interconnected lacework of pallidal areas, interdigitating with striatal cell islands and microcellular islands, including possibly deep islands of Calleja. The identification of the VP and VS simplified the structural analysis of ventral forebrain, demonstrating that a large part of the area referred to as "substantia innominata" is actually an extension of the reward-related striatopallidal complex [42]. In addition to the GABAergic ventral striatal input, there is a glutamatergic input from the STN nucleus and a dopaminergic input from the midbrain [87,88].

Descending efferent projection from the VP terminates primarily in the medial subthalamic nucleus, extending into the adjacent lateral hypothalamus [79,89,90]. Axons continue into the substantia nigra, terminating medially in the SNc, SNr, and VTA. Projections from the VP to the subthalamic nucleus and the lateral hypothalamus are topographically arranged. This arrangement demonstrates that pathways from distinct pallidal regions that receive specific striatal input terminate in specific subthalamic/hypothalamic regions, thus maintaining a topographic arrangement. In contrast, terminating fibers from the VP in the substantia nigra overlap extensively, suggesting convergence of terminals from different ventral pallidal regions. Fibers continue caudally to innervate the pedunculopontine n. As with the dorsal pallidum, components of the VP project to the thalamus, terminating in the midline nuclei and medial MD n. Pallidal fibers entering the thalamus give off several collaterals that form branches that terminate primarily onto the soma and proximal dendrites of thalamic projection cells. In addition, some synaptic contact is also made with local circuit neurons. This terminal organization indicates that, while pallidal projections to the thalamus are primarily inhibitory on thalamic relay neurons cells, they may also function to disinhibit projection cells via the local circuit neurons [91,92]. In addition, the VP also projects to both the internal and external segments of the dorsal pallidum. This is a unique projection, in that the dorsal pallidum does not seem to project ventrally.

Parts of the VP (along with the dorsal pallidum) project to the lateral habenular n. Most cells that project here are located in the region that circumvents the internal segment and, in particular, are embedded within accessory medullary lamina that divides the lateral and medial portions of the dorsal internal segment project [93,94]. Finally, part of the ventral pallidal (as with the GPe) also projects to the striatum [95]. This pallidostriatal pathway is extensive in the monkey and is organized in a topographic manner preserving a general, but not strict, medial to lateral and ventral to dorsal organization. The terminal field is widespread and non-adjacent pallidal regions send fibers to the striatum that overlap considerably, indicating convergence of terminals from different pallidal regions. Thus, the pallidostriatal pathway contains both a reciprocal and also a non-reciprocal pathway. The non-reciprocal component suggests that this feedback projection may play an additional role in integrating information between different ventral striatal subcircuits.

1.5   The midbrain DA neurons

Dopamine neurons play a central role in the reward circuit [96,97]. While behavioral and pharmacological studies of DA pathways have led to the association of the mesolimbic pathway and nigrostriatal pathway with reward and motor activity, respectively, more recently, both of these cell groups have been associated with reward. The midbrain DA neurons project widely throughout the brain. However, studies of the rapid signaling that is associated with incentive learning and habit formation focus on the DA striatal pathways. Before turning to its projections, it is important to understand the organization of the midbrain DA cells.

The midbrain DA neurons are divided into the VTA and the substantia nigra, pars compacta (SNc). Based on projection and chemical signatures, these cells are also referred to as the dorsal and ventral tier neurons [46] (Fig. 1.7A). The dorsal tier includes the VTA and the dorsal part of the SNc (also referred to as the retrorubral cell group). The cells of the dorsal tier are calbindin-positive and contain relatively low levels of mRNA for the DA transporter and D2 receptor subtype. They project to the VS, cortex, hypothalamus, and amygdala. The ventral tier of DA cells are calbindin-negative, have relatively high levels of mRNA for the DA transporter and D2 receptor and project primarily to the DS. Ventral tier cells (calbindin poor, DAT and D2 receptor rich) are more vulnerable to degeneration in Parkinson's disease and to N-methyl-4-phenyl-1,2,3,6-tetrahydropyridine (MPTP)-induced toxicity, while the dorsal tier cells are selectively spared [98]. As mentioned above, despite these distinctions, both cell groups respond to unexpected rewards.

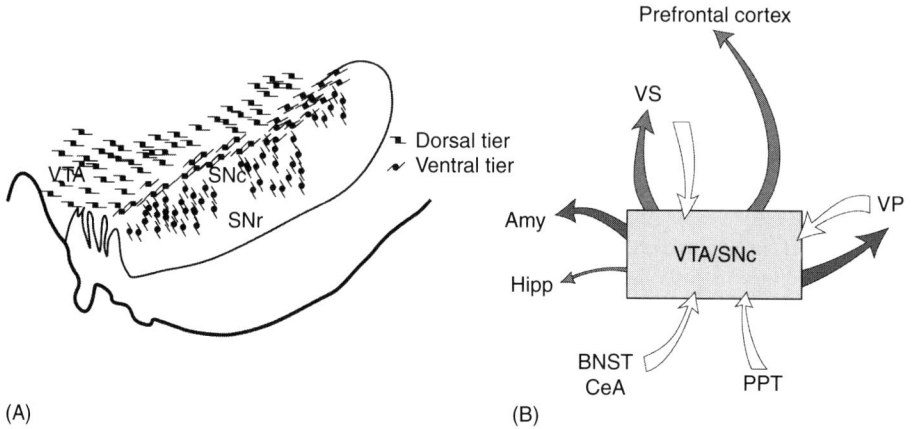

Figure 1.7 Schematic illustrating the organization (A) and connections (B) of the midbrain DA cells. Amy, amygdala; BNST, bed n. stria terminalis; CeA, central amygdala n.; Hipp, hippocampus; PPT, pedunculopontine nucleus; SNc, substantia nigra, pars compacta; VP, ventral pallidum; VTA, ventral tegmental area.

1.5.1   Afferent projections

Input to the midbrain DA neurons is primarily from the striatum, from both the external segment of the globus pallidus and the VP, and from the brainstem (Fig. 1.7B). In addition, there are projections to the dorsal tier from the bed nucleus of the stria terminalis, from the sublenticular substantia innominata and the extended amygdala (the bed nucleus of the stria terminalis and the central amygdala n.).

As described above, the striatonigral projection is the most massive projection to the SN and terminates in both the VTA/SNc and the substantia nigra, pars reticulate [99–101]. The ventral (like the dorsal) striatonigral connection terminates throughout the rostrocaudal extent of the substantia nigra. There is an inverse ventral/dorsal topography to the striatonigral projections. The dorsolateral striatonigral inputs are concentrated in the ventrolateral SN. These striatal cells project primarily to the SNr, but also terminate on the cell columns of DA neurons that penetrate deep into the SNr. In contrast, the ventral striatonigral inputs terminate in the VTA, the dorsal part of the ventral tier, and in the medial and dorsal SNr. Thus, the VS not only projects throughout the rostrocaudal extent of the substantia nigra but also covers a wide mediolateral range [5].

Descending projections from the central nucleus of the amygdala also terminate in a wide mediolateral region, but are limited primarily to the dorsal tier cells. In addition, there are projections to the dorsal tier from the bed nucleus of the stria terminalis and from the sublenticular substantia innominata that travel together with those from the amygdale [102,103]. Both the GPe and the VP project to the substantia nigra. The pallidal projection follows a similar inverse dorsal/ventral organization as the striatonigral projection. Thus, the VP projects dorsally, primarily to the dorsal tier and dorsal SNc. The pedunculopontine n. sends a major glutamatergic input to the dopaminergic cells bodies. In addition, there is a serotonergic innervation from the dorsal raphe nucleus, though there is disagreement regarding whether fibers terminate primarily in the pars compacta or the pars reticulata. Other brain stem inputs to the DA neurons include those from the superior colliculus, parabrachial nucleus, and locus coeruleus. These inputs raise the interesting possibility that DA cells receive a direct sensory input. The collicular input, in particular, has been suggested to be responsible for the short latency, burst-firing activity of the DA cells in response to a salient or rewarding stimuli [53]. Finally, in primates, there is a small and limited projection from the PFC to the midbrain DA neurons, to both the VTA and SNc. While considerable attention has been given to this projection, relative to the density of its other inputs, this projection is weak in primates [104].

1.5.2 Efferent projections

The largest efferent projection from the midbrain DA neurons is to the striatum [100,101,105] (Fig. 1.7B). As with the descending striatonigral pathway, there is a mediolateral and an inverse dorsoventral topography arrangement to the projection. The ventral pars compacta neurons project to the DS and the dorsally located DA neurons project to the VS. The shell region receives the most limited input, primarily derived from the medial VTA [106]. The rest of the VS receives input from the entire dorsal tier. In addition, there are some afferent projections from the medial region and dorsal part SNc. In contrast to the VS, the central striatal area (the region innervated by the DPFC) receives input from a wide region of the SNc. The dorsolateral (motor-related) striatum receives the largest midbrain projection from cells throughout the ventral tier. In contrast to the dorsolateral region of the striatum, the VS receives the most limited DA cell input. Thus, in addition to an inverse topography, there is also a differential ratio of DA projections to the different striatal areas [5].

The dorsal tier cells also project widely throughout the primate cortex and are found not only in granular areas but also in agranular frontal regions, parietal cortex, temporal cortex, and (albeit sparsely) in occipital cortex [107,108]. The majority of DA cortical projections are from the parabrachial pigmented nucleus of the VTA and the dorsal part of the SNc. The VTA also projects to the hippocampus, albeit to a lesser extent than in neocortex. The DA cells that project to functionally different cortical regions are intermingled with each other, in that individual neurons send collateral axons to different cortical regions. Thus nigrocortical projection is a more diffuse system compared to the nigrostriatal system and can modulate cortical activity at several levels. DA fibers are located in superficial layers, including a prominent projection throughout layer I. This input provides a general modulation of cortico cells at the distal apical dendrites. DA fibers are also found in the deep layers in specific cortical areas [109,110]. Projections to the amygdala arise primarily from the dorsal tier. These terminals form symmetric synapses primarily with spiny cells of specific subpopulations in the amygdale [111]. As indicated above, DA fibers also project to the VP.

1.5.3 The striato-nigro-striatal network

While the role of DA and reward is well established, the latency between the presentation of the reward stimuli and the activity of the DA cells is too short to reflect higher cortical processing necessary for linking a stimulus with its rewarding properties. The fast, burst-firing activity is likely, therefore, to be generated from other input such as in brainstem glutamatergic nuclei [53]. An interesting issue is, then, how do the DA cells receive information concerning reward value? The largest forebrain input to the DA neurons is from the striatum. However, this is a relatively slow GABAergic inhibitory projection, unlikely to result in the immediate, fast burst-firing activity. Nonetheless, the collective complex network of PFC, amygdala, and hippocampal inputs to the VS integrate information related to reward processing and memory to modulate striatal activity. These striatal cells then impact directly on a subset of medial DA neurons, which, through a series of connections, described below, influences the DS.

As mentioned above, projections from the striatum to the midbrain are arranged in an inverse dorsal-ventral topography and there is also an inverse dorsal-ventral topographic organization to the midbrain striatal projection. When considered separately, each limb of the system creates a loose topographic organization, the VTA and medial SN being associated with the limbic system, and the central and ventral SN with the associative and motor striatal regions, respectively. However, each functional region differs in its proportional projections that significantly alter their relationship to each other. The VS receives a limited midbrain input but projects to a large region. In contrast, the dorsolateral striatum receives a wide input but projects to a limited region. In other words, the VS influences a wide range of DA neurons, but is itself influenced by a relatively limited group of DA cells. On the other hand, the dorsolateral striatum influences a limited midbrain region, but is affected by a relatively large midbrain region.

With this arrangement, while the VS receives input from the vmPFC, OFC, dACC, and amygdala, its efferent projection to the midbrain extends beyond the tight VS/dorsal tier DA/VS circuit. It terminates also in the ventral tier, to influence the DS. Moreover, this part of the ventral tier is reciprocally connected to the central (or associative) striatum. The central striatum also projects to a more ventral region than it receives input from. This region, in turn, projects to the dorsolateral (or motor) striatum. Taken together, the interface between different striatal regions via the midbrain DA cells is organized in an ascending spiral interconnecting different functional regions of the striatum and creating a feed-forward organization, from reward-related regions of the striatum to cognitive and motor areas (Fig. 1.8). Thus, although the short latency, burst-firing activity of DA that signals immediate reinforcement is likely to be triggered from brainstem nuclei, the cortico-striato-midbrain pathway is in a position to influence DA cells to distinguish rewards and modify responses to incoming salient stimuli over time. This pathway is further reinforced via the nigro-striatal pathway, placing the striato-nigro-striatal pathway in a pivotal position for transferring from the VS to the DS during learning and habit formation. Indeed, cells in the DS are progressively recruited during different types of learning, from simple motor tasks to drug self administration [112–116]. Moreover, when the striato-nigro-striatal circuit is interrupted, information transfer from Pavlovian to instrumental learning does not take place [117].

1.6   Completing the cortico-BG reward circuit

In addition to the PFC, VS, VP, amygdala, and hippocampus, other key components of the circuit include the thalamus, the lateral habenula, the raphe nuclei, and the pedunculopontine tegmental n. Each of these structures has complex connectivities with multiple brain regions and their direct associations with the cortico-BG reward system have been discussed. However, below we add a few additional important points on their role in the reward circuitry.

1.6.1   The thalamus

The MD and midline thalamic n. are a critical piece of the frontal-BG circuit that mediate reward, motivation, and emotional drive. As noted above, each PFC region of the frontal cortex is connected with specific areas of striatum, pallidum, and thalamus. The

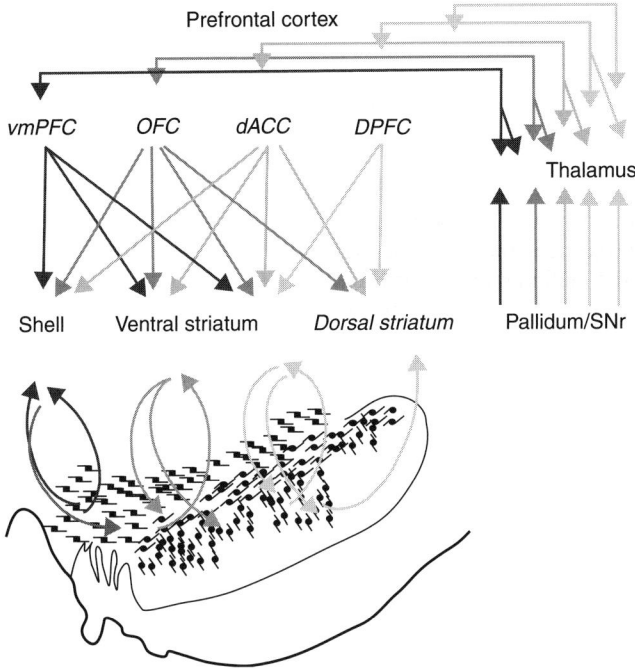

Figure 1.8 Three networks of integration through cortico-BG pathways. (1) Fibers from different prefrontal areas converge within subregions of the striatum. (2) Through the organization of striato-nigro-striatal (SNS) projections, the ventral striatum can influence the dorsal striatum [5]. Midbrain projections from the shell target both the VTA and ventromedial SNc. Projections from the VTA to the shell form a "closed," reciprocal loop, but also project more laterally to impact on DA cells projecting the rest of the ventral striatum, forming the first part of a feed-forward loop (or spiral). The spiral continues through the SNS projections, through which the ventral striatum impacts on cognitive and motor striatal areas via the midbrain DA cells. (3) The non-reciprocal cortico-thalamic projection carries information from reward-related regions, through cognitive and motor controls. dACC, dorsal anterior cingulate cortex; DPFC, dorsal prefrontal cortex; OFC, orbital prefrontal cortex; vmPFC, ventral medial prefrontal cortex. Red, vmPFC pathways; dark orange, OFC pathways; light orange, dACC pathways; yellow, DPFC pathways; green, output to motor control areas. See Plate 2 of Color Plate section.

thalamus represents the final BG link and is often treated as a simple "one-way relay" back to cortex. The medial MD n. projects to the PFC, and is the final link in the reward circuit [79,118,119]. However, these connections are bidirectional. Moreover, while corticothalamic projections of the specific thalamic relay nuclei follow a general rule of reciprocity, the corticothalamic projections the MD (as seen in other thalamocortical systems) are more extensive than its thalamocortical projections [119–121]. Importantly, they are, in part, derived from areas not innervated by the same thalamic region, indicating a non-reciprocal corticothalamic component. In particular, within the reward circuit, while the MD completes the reward cortico-BG circuit, its non-reciprocal input is derived from functionally distinct frontal cortical areas. For example, within the reward circuit, the central MD has reciprocal projections with the OFC, but also a non-reciprocal input from vmPFC. More lateral MD areas are reciprocally connected to the DPFC, but also have a non-reciprocal connection to from the OFC [119].

1.6.2   The lateral habenula, pedunculopontine tegmental n., and the raphe serotonergic systems

Recent studies have emphasized the potential importance of the lateral habenula (LHb) in regulating the DA reward signal. In particular, experiments show that stimulation of the lateral habenular nuclei in primates results in a negative reward-related signal in SNc by inhibiting DA activity when an expected reward does not occur [122]. These LHb cells are inhibited by a reward-predicting stimulus, but fire following a non-reward signal. Stimulation of the LHb inhibits DA cells, suggesting that it plays a key role in regulating the DA reward signal. Interestingly, few fibers from the LHb directly reach the SNc in primates, indicating an indirect regulation of the DA signal. There are several possible routes by which the lateral habenular might impact on the DA cell. Connections described in rats, in addition to those to BG structures, include the basal forebrain, preoptic area of hypothalamus, interpeduncular nucleus, pedunculopontine n., raphe n., superior colliculus, pretectal area, central gray, VTA, and reticular formation [79,123,124]. The pedunculopontine tegmental n. is connected to multiple BG structures and provides one of the strongest excitatory inputs to the midbrain DA cells [125,126]. Moreover, the cells in this brainstem area receive input from the lateral habenula. Anatomical and physiological studies, coupled with the central role of DA for reward prediction error, led to studies that support the hypothesis that PPT may play a role in this reward signal [127]. The brainstem serotonergic system plays an important role in reinforcement behaviors by encoding expected and received rewards [128]. This reward signal could arise from a number of brain regions, but perhaps the strongest might arise from inputs derived from the OFC and vmPFC, the amygdala, the substantia nigra, and the lateral habenula [129].

1.7   Complex network features of the reward circuit

The reward circuit is comprised of several cortical and subcortical regions that form a complex network to mediate different aspects of incentive learning, leading to adaptive behaviors and good decision-making. The cortical-BG network is at the center of this circuit. This complex network involves a system in which PFC exploits the BG for additional processing of reward to effectively modulate learning that leads to the development of goal-directed behaviors and action plans. To develop an appropriate behavioral response to external environmental stimuli, information about motivation and reward needs to be combined with a strategy and an action plan for obtaining the goal. In other words, it is not sufficient to desire or want to, for example, win at a card game. One has to understand the rules of the game, remember the cards played, and so on before executing the play. In addition, there is a complex interaction between the desire to put cards in play and the inhibition of impulse to play them too early. Thus, action plans developed toward obtaining a goal require a combination of reward processing, cognition, and motor control. Yet theories related to cortico-BG processing have emphasized the separation between functions (including different reward circuits), highlighting separate and parallel pathways [130–132]. The pathways and connections reviewed in this chapter clearly show that there are dual cortico-BG systems permitting both parallel and integrative processing.

Thus, the reward circuit does not work in isolation. Instead, this complex circuitry interfaces with pathways that mediate cognitive function and motor planning (Fig. 1.8). Within each of the cortico-BG structures, there are regions of convergence linking up areas that are associated with different functional domains. Convergence between terminals derived from different cortical areas in the striatum permits cortical information to be disseminated across multiple functional regions. In addition, there are several interconnections in the system that contain reciprocal-non-reciprocal networks. The two major ones are the striato-nigro-striatal pathway and the cortico-thalamo-cortical network. In addition, the VP-VS-VP also has a non-reciprocal component. Through these networks, the reward circuit impacts on cognition and motor control through several different interactive routes, allowing information about reward to be channeled through cognitive and motor control circuits to mediate the development of appropriate action plans.

References

[1] G.E. Alexander, M.D. Crutcher, M.R. DeLong, Basal ganglia-thalamocortical circuits: parallel substrates for motor, oculomotor, "prefrontal" and "limbic" functions, Prog. Brain Res. 85 (1990) 119–146.

[2] M.D. Bevan, A.D. Smith, J.P. Bolam, The substantia nigra as a site of synaptic integration of functionally diverse information arising from the ventral pallidum and the globus pallidus in the rat, Neuroscience 75 (1996) 5–12.

[3] L.L. Brown, D.M. Smith, L.M. Goldbloom, Organizing principles of cortical integration in the rat neostriatum: corticostriate map of the body surface is an ordered lattice of curved laminae and radial points, J. Comp. Neurol. 392 (1998) 468–488.

[4] F. Kasanetz, L.A. Riquelme, V. Della-Maggiore, P. O'Donnell, M.G. Murer, Functional integration across a gradient of corticostriatal channels controls UP state transitions in the dorsal striatum, Proc. Natl. Acad. Sci. USA 105 (2008) 8124–8129.

[5] S.N. Haber, J.L. Fudge, N.R. McFarland, Striatonigrostriatal pathways in primates form an ascending spiral from the shell to the dorsolateral striatum, J. Neurosci. 20 (2000) 2369–2382.

[6] S.N. Haber, K.S. Kim, P. Mailly, R. Calzavara, Reward-related cortical inputs define a large striatal region in primates that interface with associative cortical inputs, providing a substrate for incentive-based learning, J. Neurosci. 26 (2006) 8368–8376.

[7] S.T. Carmichael, J.L. Price, Architectonic subdivision of the orbital and medial prefrontal cortex in the macaque monkey, J. Comp. Neurol. 346 (1994) 366–402.

[8] H. Barbas, Architecture and cortical connections of the prefrontal cortex in the rhesus monkey, in: P. Chauvel, A.V. Delgado-Escueta (Eds.), Advances in Neurology, Raven Press, Ltd., New York, 1992, pp. 91–115.

[9] M.R. Milad, C.I. Wright, S.P. Orr, R.K. Pitman, G.J. Quirk, S.L. Rauch, Recall of fear extinction in humans activates the ventromedial prefrontal cortex and hippocampus in concert, Biol. Psychiatry 62 (2007) 446–454.

[10] C. Padoa-Schioppa, J.A. Assad, Neurons in the orbitofrontal cortex encode economic value, Nature 441 (2006) 223–226.

[11] L. Tremblay, W. Schultz, Reward-related neuronal activity during go-nogo task performance in primate orbitofrontal cortex, J. Neurophysiol. 83 (2000) 1864–1876.

[12] M.R. Roesch, C.R. Olson, Neuronal activity related to reward value and motivation in primate frontal cortex, Science 304 (2004) 307–310.

[13] J.D. Wallis, E.K. Miller, Neuronal activity in primate dorsolateral and orbital prefrontal cortex during performance of a reward preference task, Eur. J. Neurosci. 18 (2003) 2069–2081.

[14] M.E. Walton, D.M. Bannerman, K. Alterescu, M.F. Rushworth, Functional specialization within medial frontal cortex of the anterior cingulate for evaluating effort-related decisions, J. Neurosci. 23 (2003) 6475–6479.

[15] T. Paus, Primate anterior cingulate cortex: where motor control, drive and cognition interface, Nat. Rev. Neurosci. 2 (2001) 417–424.

[16] B.A. Vogt, L. Vogt, N.B. Farber, G. Bush, Architecture and neurocytology of monkey cingulate gyrus, J. Comp. Neurol. 485 (2005) 218–239.

[17] P.S. Goldman-Rakic, S. Funahashi, C.J. Bruce, Neocortical memory circuits, Cold Spring Harb. Symp. Quant. Biol. 55 (1990) 1025–1038.

[18] S.T. Carmichael, J.L. Price, Connectional networks within the orbital and medial prefrontal cortex of Macaque monkeys, J. Comp. Neurol. 371 (1996) 179–207.

[19] M. Petrides, D.N. Pandya, Efferent association pathways from the rostral prefrontal cortex in the macaque monkey, J. Neurosci. 27 (2007) 11573–11586.

[20] S.T. Carmichael, J.L. Price, Limbic connections of the orbital and medial prefrontal cortex in macaque monkeys, J. Comp. Neurol. 363 (1995) 615–641.

[21] H. Barbas, G.J. Blatt, Topographically specific hippocampal projections target functionally distinct prefrontal areas in the rhesus monkey, Hippocampus 5 (1995) 511–533.

[22] H.T. Ghashghaei, H. Barbas, Pathways for emotion: interactions of prefrontal and anterior temporal pathways in the amygdala of the rhesus monkey, Neuroscience 115 (2002) 1261–1279.

[23] S.T. Carmichael, J.L. Price, Sensory and premotor connections of the orbital and medial prefrontal cortex of macaque monkeys, J. Comp. Neurol. 363 (1996) 642–664.

[24] H. Barbas, H. Ghashghaei, S.M. Dombrowski, N.L. Rempel-Clower, Medial prefrontal cortices are unified by common connections with superior temporal cortices and distinguished by input from memory-related areas in the rhesus monkey, J. Comp. Neurol. 410 (1999) 343–367.

[25] J. Olds, P. Milner, Positive reinforcement produced by electrical stimulation of septal area and other regions of rat brain, J. Comp. Physiol. Psychol. 47 (1954) 419–427.

[26] S.A. Taha, H.L. Fields, Inhibitions of nucleus accumbens neurons encode a gating signal for reward-directed behavior, J. Neurosci. 26 (2006) 217–222.

[27] P.W. Kalivas, N. Volkow, J. Seamans, Unmanageable motivation in addiction: a pathology in prefrontal-accumbens glutamate transmission, Neuron 45 (2005) 647–650.

[28] L. Heimer, J.S. De Olmos, G.F. Alheid, J. Person, N. Sakamoto, K. Shinoda, J. Marksteiner, R.C. Switzer, The human basal forebrain. Part II, in: F.E. Bloom, A. Bjorkland, T. Hokfelt (Eds.), Handbook of Chemical Neuroanatomy, in: The Primate Nervous System, Part III, vol. 15, Elsevier, Amsterdam, 1999, pp. 57–226.

[29] S.N. Haber, N.R. McFarland, The concept of the ventral striatum in nonhuman primates, in: J.F. McGinty (Ed.), Advancing from the ventral striatum to the extended amygdala, vol. 877, The New York Academy of Sciences, New York, 1999, pp. 33–48.

[30] G. Pagnoni, C.F. Zink, P.R. Montague, G.S. Berns, Activity in human ventral striatum locked to errors of reward prediction, Nat. Neurosci. 5 (2002) 97–98.

[31] B. Knutson, C.M. Adams, G.W. Fong, D. Hommer, Anticipation of increasing monetary reward selectively recruits nucleus accumbens, J. Neurosci. 21 (2001) RC159.

[32] W. Schultz, Multiple reward signals in the brain, Nat. Rev. Neurosci. 1 (2000) 199–207.

[33] H.C. Cromwell, W. Schultz, Effects of expectations for different reward magnitudes on neuronal activity in primate striatum, J. Neurophysiol. 89 (2003) 2823–2838.

[34] K. Watanabe, O. Hikosaka, Immediate changes in anticipatory activity of caudate neurons associated with reversal of position-reward contingency, J. Neurophysiol. 94 (2005) 1879–1887.

[35] R. Elliott, J.L. Newman, O.A. Longe, J.F. Deakin, Differential response patterns in the stria-
      tum and orbitofrontal cortex to financial reward in humans: a parametric functional mag-
      netic resonance imaging study, J. Neurosci. 23 (2003) 303–307.

[36] W. Schultz, L. Tremblay, J.R. Hollerman, Reward processing in primate orbitofrontal cortex
      and basal ganglia, Cereb. Cortex 10 (2000) 272–284.

[37] N.D. Volkow, G.J. Wang, Y. Ma, J.S. Fowler, C. Wong, Y.S. Ding, R. Hitzemann,
      J.M. Swanson, P. Kalivas, Activation of orbital and medial prefrontal cortex by methylpheni-
      date in cocaine-addicted subjects but not in controls: relevance to addiction, J. Neurosci. 25
      (2005) 3932–3939.

[38] C.M. Kuhnen, B. Knutson, The neural basis of financial risk taking, Neuron 47 (2005)
      763–770.

[39] R. Ito, T.W. Robbins, B.J. Everitt, Differential control over cocaine-seeking behavior by
      nucleus accumbens core and shell, Nat. Neurosci. 7 (2004) 389–397.

[40] W.A. Carlezon, R.A. Wise, Rewarding actions of phencyclidine and related drugs in nucleus
      accumbens shell and frontal cortex, J. Neurosci. 16 (1996) 3112–3122.

[41] G.E. Meredith, A. Pattiselanno, H.J. Groenewegen, S.N. Haber, Shell and core in monkey and
      human nucleus accumbens identified with antibodies to calbindin-D28k, J. Comp. Neurol.
      365 (1996) 628–639.

[42] G.F. Alheid, L. Heimer, New perspectives in basal forebrain organization of special relevance
      for neuropsychiatric disorders: the striatopallidal, amygdaloid, and corticopetal components
      of substantia innominata, Neuroscience 27 (1988) 1–39.

[43] K. Ikemoto, K. Satoh, T. Maeda, H.C. Fibiger, Neurochemical heterogeneity of the primate
      nucleus accumbens, Exp. Brain Res. 104 (1995) 177–190.

[44] K. Sato, H. Kiyama, M. Tohyama, The differential expression patterns of messenger RNAs
      encoding non-N-methyl-D-aspartate glutamate receptor subunits (GluR1-4) in the rat brain,
      Neuroscience 52 (1993) 515–539.

[45] L.J. Martin, C.D. Blackstone, A.I. Levey, R.L. Huganir, D.L. Price, AMPA glutamate receptor
      subunits are differentially distributed in rat brain, Neuroscience 53 (1993) 327–338.

[46] S.N. Haber, H. Ryoo, C. Cox, W. Lu, Subsets of midbrain dopaminergic neurons in mon-
      keys are distinguished by different levels of mRNA for the dopamine transporter: comparison
      with the mRNA for the D2 receptor, tyrosine hydroxylase and calbindin immunoreactivity,
      J. Comp. Neurol. 362 (1995) 400–410.

[47] R.B. Chronister, R.W. Sikes, T.W. Trow, J.F. DeFrance, The organization of the nucleus
      accumbens, in: R.B. Chronister, J.F. DeFrance (Eds.), The Neurobiology of the Nucleus
      Accumbens, Haer Institute, Brunswick, ME, 1981, pp. 97–146.

[48] G. Meyer, T. Gonzalez-Hernandez, F. Carrillo-Padilla, R. Ferres-Torres, Aggregations of gran-
      ule cells in the basal forebrain (islands of Calleja): golgi and cytoarchitectonic study in differ-
      ent mammals, including man, J. Comp. Neurol. 284 (1989) 405–428.

[49] S.A. Bayer, Neurogenesis in the olfactory tubercle and islands of calleja in the rat, Int. J. Dev.
      Neurosci. 3 (1985) 135–147.

[50] A. Parent, Comparative Neurobiology of the Basal Ganglia, John Wiley and Sons, New York,
      1986.

[51] R. Calzavara, P. Mailly, S.N. Haber, Relationship between the corticostriatal terminals from
      areas 9 and 46, and those from area 8A, dorsal and rostral premotor cortex and area 24c: an
      anatomical substrate for cognition to action, Eur. J. Neurosci. 26 (2007) 2005–2024.

[52] S.N. Haber, K. Kunishio, M. Mizobuchi, E. Lynd-Balta, The orbital and medial prefrontal
      circuit through the primate basal ganglia, J. Neurosci. 15 (1995) 4851–4867.

[53] E. Dommett, V. Coizet, C.D. Blaha, J. Martindale, V. Lefebvre, N. Walton, J.E. Mayhew,
      P.G. Overton, P. Redgrave, How visual stimuli activate dopaminergic neurons at short latency,
      Science 307 (2005) 1476–1479.

[54] S.C. Tanaka, K. Doya, G. Okada, K. Ueda, Y. Okamoto, S. Yamawaki, Prediction of immediate and future rewards differentially recruits cortico-basal ganglia loops, Nat. Neurosci. 7 (2004) 887–893.

[55] P.R. Corlett, M.R. Aitken, A. Dickinson, D.R. Shanks, G.D. Honey, R.A. Honey, T.W. Robbins, E.T. Bullmore, P.C. Fletcher, Prediction error during retrospective revaluation of causal associations in humans: fMRI evidence in favor of an associative model of learning, Neuron 44 (2004) 877–888.

[56] L.D. Selemon, P.S. Goldman-Rakic, Longitudinal topography and interdigitation of corticostriatal projections in the rhesus monkey, J. Neurosci. 5 (1985) 776–794.

[57] C.J. Wilson, The basal ganglia, in: G.M. Shepherd (Ed.), Synaptic Organization of the Brain, fifth ed, Oxford University Press, New York, 2004, pp. 361–413.

[58] T. Zheng, C.J. Wilson, Corticostriatal combinatorics: the implications of corticostriatal axonal arborizations, J. Neurophysiol. 87 (2002) 1007–1017.

[59] A.T. Ferry, D. Ongur, X. An, J.L. Price, Prefrontal cortical projections to the striatum in macaque monkeys: evidence for an organization related to prefrontal networks, J. Comp. Neurol. 425 (2000) 447–470.

[60] B. Draganski, F. Kherif, S. Kloppel, P.A. Cook, D.C. Alexander, G.J. Parker, R. Deichmann, J. Ashburner, R.S. Frackowiak, Evidence for segregated and integrative connectivity patterns in the human Basal Ganglia, J. Neurosci. 28 (2008) 7143–7152.

[61] F.T. Russchen, I. Bakst, D.G. Amaral, J.L. Price, The amygdalostriatal projections in the monkey. An anterograde tracing study, Brain Res. 329 (1985) 241–257.

[62] J.L. Fudge, K. Kunishio, C. Walsh, D. Richard, S.N. Haber, Amygdaloid projections to ventromedial striatal subterritories in the primate, Neuroscience 110 (2002) 257–275.

[63] D.P. Friedman, J.P. Aggleton, R.C. Saunders, Comparison of hippocampal, amygdala, and perirhinal projections to the nucleus accumbens: combined anterograde and retrograde tracing study in the Macaque brain, J. Comp. Neurol. 450 (2002) 345–365.

[64] H.W. Berendse, H.J. Groenewegen, A.H.M. Lohman, Compartmental distribution of ventral striatal neurons projecting to the mesencephalon in the rat, J. Neurosci. 12 (1992) 2079–2103.

[65] J.M. Giménez-Amaya, N.R. McFarland, S. de las Heras, S.N. Haber, Organization of thalamic projections to the ventral striatum in the primate, J. Comp. Neurol. 354 (1995) 127–149.

[66] H.W. Berendse, H.J. Groenewegen, The organization of the thalamostriatal projections in the rat, with special emphasis on the ventral striatum, J. Comp. Neurol. 299 (1990) 187–228.

[67] N.R. McFarland, S.N. Haber, Convergent inputs from thalamic motor nuclei and frontal cortical areas to the dorsal striatum in the primate, J. Neurosci. 20 (2000) 3798–3813.

[68] N.R. McFarland, S.N. Haber, Organization of thalamostriatal terminals from the ventral motor nuclei in the macaque, J. Comp. Neurol. 429 (2001) 321–336.

[69] S.N. Haber, E. Lynd, C. Klein, H.J. Groenewegen, Topographic organization of the ventral striatal efferent projections in the rhesus monkey: an anterograde tracing study, J. Comp. Neurol. 293 (1990) 282–298.

[70] D.S. Zahm, L. Heimer, Two transpallidal pathways originating in the rat nucleus accumbens, J. Comp. Neurol. 302 (1990) 437–446.

[71] R. Martinez-Murillo, I. Blasco, F.J. Alvarez, R. Villalba, M.L. Solano, M.I. Montero-Caballero, J. Rodrigo, Distribution of enkephalin-immunoreactive nerve fibers and terminals in the region of the nucleus basalis magnocellularis of the rat: a light and electron microscopic study, J. Neurocytol. 17 (1988) 361–376.

[72] H.T. Chang, G.R. Penny, S.T. Kitai, Enkephalinergic-cholinergic interaction in the rat globus pallidus: a pre-embedding double-labeling immunocytochemistry study, Brain Res. 426 (1987) 197–203.

[73] T.G. Beach, H. Tago, E.G. McGeer, Light microscopic evidence for a substance P-containing innervation of the human nucleus basalis of Meynert, Brain Res. 408 (1987) 251–257.

[74] S.N. Haber, Anatomical relationship between the basal ganglia and the basal nucleus of Maynert in human and monkey forebrain, Proc. Natl. Acad. Sci. USA 84 (1987) 1408–1412.

[75] L. Zaborszky, W.E. Cullinan, Projections from the nucleus accumbens to cholinergic neurons of the ventral pallidum: a correlated light and electron microscopic double-immunolabeling study in rat, Brain Res. 570 (1992) 92–101.

[76] K.S. Smith, K.C. Berridge, Opioid limbic circuit for reward: interaction between hedonic hotspots of nucleus accumbens and ventral pallidum, J. Neurosci. 27 (2007) 1594–1605.

[77] A.J. Tindell, K.S. Smith, S. Pecina, K.C. Berridge, J.W. Aldridge, Ventral pallidum firing codes hedonic reward: when a bad taste turns good, J. Neurophysiol. 96 (2006) 2399–2409.

[78] L. Heimer, The olfactory cortex and the ventral striatum, in: K.E. Livingston, O. Hornykiewicz (Eds.), Limbic Mechanisms, Plenum Press, New York, 1978, pp. 95–187.

[79] S.N. Haber, E. Lynd-Balta, S.J. Mitchell, The organization of the descending ventral pallidal projections in the monkey, J. Comp. Neurol. 329 (1993) 111–129.

[80] S.N. Haber, D.P. Wolfe, H.J. Groenewegen, The relationship between ventral striatal efferent fibers and the distribution of peptide-positive woolly fibers in the forebrain of the rhesus monkey, Neuroscience 39 (1990) 323–338.

[81] F.T. Russchen, D.G. Amaral, J.L. Price, The afferent input to the magnocellular division of the mediodorsal thalamic nucleus in the monkey, *Macaca fascicularis*, J. Comp. Neurol. 256 (1987) 175–210.

[82] J.K. Mai, P.H. Stephens, A. Hopf, A.C. Cuello, Substance P in the human brain, Neuroscience 17 (1986) 709–739.

[83] M. DiFiglia, N. Aronin, J.B. Martin, Light and electron microscopic localization of immunoreactive leu-enkephalin in the monkey basal ganglia, J. Neurosci. 2 (1982) 303–320.

[84] S.N. Haber, S.J. Watson, The comparative distribution of enkephalin, dynorphin and substance P in the human globus pallidus and basal forebrain, Neuroscience 4 (1985) 1011–1024.

[85] S.N. Haber, W.J.H. Nauta, Ramifications of the globus pallidus in the rat as indicated by patterns of immunohistochemistry, Neuroscience 9 (1983) 245–260.

[86] C.H. Fox, H.N. Andrade, I.J. Du Qui, J.A. Rafols, The primate globus pallidus: a Golgi and electron microscope study, J. R. Hirnforschung 15 (1974) 75–93.

[87] M.S. Turner, A. Lavin, A.A. Grace, T.C. Napier, Regulation of limbic information outflow by the subthalamic nucleus: excitatory amino acid projections to the ventral pallidum, J. Neurosci. 21 (2001) 2820–2832.

[88] M.A. Klitenick, A.Y. Deutch, L. Churchill, P.W. Kalivas, Topography and functional role of dopaminergic projections from the ventral mesencephalic tegmentum to the ventral pallidum, Neuroscience 50 (1992) 371–386.

[89] S.N. Haber, H.J. Groenewegen, E.A. Grove, W.J. Nauta, Efferent connections of the ventral pallidum: evidence of a dual striato pallidofugal pathway, J. Comp. Neurol. 235 (1985) 322–335.

[90] D.S. Zahm, The ventral striatopallidal parts of the basal ganglia in the rat. II. Compartmentation of ventral pallidal efferents, Neuroscience 30 (1989) 33–50.

[91] I.A. Ilinsky, H. Yi, K. Kultas-Ilinsky, Mode of termination of pallidal afferents to the thalamus: a light and electron microscopic study with anterograde tracers and immunocytochemistry in *Macaca mulatta*, J. Comp. Neurol. 386 (1997) 601–612.

[92] P. Arecchi-Bouchhioua, J. Yelnik, C. Francois, G. Percheron, D. Tande, Three-dimensional morphology and distribution of pallidal axons projecting to both the lateral region of the thalamus and the central complex in primates, Brain Res. 754 (1997) 311–314.

[93] S.N. Haber, H.J. Groenewegen, E.A. Grove, W.J.H. Nauta, Efferent connections of the ventral pallidum. Evidence of a dual striatopallidofugal pathway, J. Comp. Neurol. 235 (1985) 322–335.

[94] A. Parent, L. De Bellefeuille, Organization of efferent projections from the internal segment of the globus pallidus in the primate as revealed by fluorescence retrograde labeling method, Brain Res. 245 (1982) 201–213.

[95] W.P.J.M. Spooren, E. Lynd-Balta, S. Mitchell, S.N. Haber, Ventral pallidostriatal pathway in the monkey: evidence for modulation of basal ganglia circuits, J. Comp. Neurol. 370 (1996) 295–312.

[96] R.A. Wise, Brain reward circuitry: insights from unsensed incentives, Neuron 36 (2002) 229–240.

[97] W. Schultz, Getting formal with dopamine and reward, Neuron 36 (2002) 241–263.

[98] B. Lavoie, A. Parent, Dopaminergic neurons expressing calbindin in normal and Parkinsonian monkeys, Neuroreport 2 (1991) 601–604.

[99] E. Lynd-Balta, S.N. Haber, Primate striatonigral projections: a comparison of the sensorimotor-related striatum and the ventral striatum, J. Comp. Neurol. 345 (1994) 562–578.

[100] J. Szabo, Strionigral and nigrostriatal connections. Anatomical studies, Appl. Neurophysiol. 42 (1979) 9–12.

[101] J.C. Hedreen, M.R. DeLong, Organization of striatopallidal, striatonigral, and nigrostriatal projections in the macaque, J. Comp. Neurol. 304 (1991) 569–595.

[102] J.L. Fudge, S.N. Haber, The central nucleus of the amygdala projection to dopamine subpopulations in primates, Neuroscience 97 (2000) 479–494.

[103] J.L. Fudge, S.N. Haber, Bed nucleus of the stria terminalis and extended amygdala inputs to dopamine subpopulations in primates, Neuroscience 104 (2001) 807–827.

[104] W.G. Frankle, M. Laruelle, S.N. Haber, Prefrontal cortical projections to the midbrain in primates: evidence for a sparse connection, Neuropsychopharmacology 31 (2006) 1627–1636.

[105] E. Lynd-Balta, S.N. Haber, The organization of midbrain projections to the striatum in the primate: Sensorimotor-related striatum versus ventral striatum, Neuroscience 59 (1994) 625–640.

[106] E. Lynd-Balta, S.N. Haber, The organization of midbrain projections to the ventral striatum in the primate, Neuroscience 59 (1994) 609–623.

[107] P. Gaspar, I. Stepneiwska, J.H. Kaas, Topography and collateralization of the dopaminergic projections to motor and lateral prefrontal cortex in owl monkeys, J. Comp. Neurol. 325 (1992) 1–21.

[108] M.S. Lidow, P.S. Goldman-Rakic, D.W. Gallager, P. Rakic, Distribution of dopaminergic receptors in the primate cerebral cortex: quantitative autoradiographic analysis using [3H] raclopride, [3H] spiperone and [3H]sch23390, Neuroscience 40 (1991) 657–671.

[109] D.A. Lewis, The catecholaminergic innervation of primate prefrontal cortex, J. Neural Transm. Suppl. 36 (1992) 179–200.

[110] P.S. Goldman-Rakic, C. Bergson, L.S. Krimer, M.S. Lidow, S.M. Williams, G.V. Williams, The primate mesocortical dopamine system, in: F.E. Bloom, A. Bjorklund, T. Hokfelt (Eds.), Handbook of Chemical Neuroanatomy, vol. 15, Elsevier Science, Amsterdam, (1999) 403–428.

[111] M. Brinley-Reed, A.J. McDonald, Evidence that dopaminergic axons provide a dense innervation of specific neuronal subpopulations in the rat basolateral amygdale, Brain Res. 850 (1999) 127–135.

[112] N.D. Volkow, G.J. Wang, F. Telang, J.S. Fowler, J. Logan, A.R. Childress, M. Jayne, Y. Ma, C. Wong, Cocaine cues and dopamine in dorsal striatum: mechanism of craving in cocaine addiction, J. Neurosci. 26 (2006) 6583–6588.

[113] L.J. Porrino, D. Lyons, H.R. Smith, J.B. Daunais, M.A. Nader, Cocaine self-administration produces a progressive involvement of limbic, association, and sensorimotor striatal domains, J. Neurosci. 24 (2004) 3554–3562.

[114] S. Lehericy, H. Benali, P.F. Van de Moortele, M. Pelegrini-Issac, T. Waechter, K. Ugurbil, J. Doyon, Distinct basal ganglia territories are engaged in early and advanced motor sequence learning, Proc. Natl. Acad. Sci. USA 102 (2005) 12566–12571.

[115] A. Pasupathy, E.K. Miller, Different time courses of learning-related activity in the prefrontal cortex and striatum, Nature 433 (2005) 873–876.

[116] B.J. Everitt, T.W. Robbins, Neural systems of reinforcement for drug addiction: from actions to habits to compulsion, Nat. Neurosci. 8 (2005) 1481–1489.

[117] D. Belin, B.J. Everitt, Cocaine seeking habits depend upon dopamine-dependent serial connectivity linking the ventral with the dorsal striatum, Neuron 57 (2008) 432–441.

[118] J.P. Ray, J.L. Price, The organization of projections from the mediodorsal nucleus of the thalamus to orbital and medial prefrontal cortex in macaque monkeys, J. Comp. Neurol. 337 (1993) 1–31.

[119] N.R. McFarland, S.N. Haber, Thalamic relay nuclei of the basal ganglia form both reciprocal and nonreciprocal cortical connections, linking multiple frontal cortical areas, J. Neurosci. 22 (2002) 8117–8132.

[120] C. Darian-Smith, A. Tan, S. Edwards, Comparing thalamocortical and corticothalamic microstructure and spatial reciprocity in the macaque ventral posterolateral nucleus (VPLc) and medial pulvinar, J. Comp. Neurol. 410 (1999) 211–234.

[121] S.M. Sherman, R.W. Guillery, Functional organization of thalamocortical relays, J. Neurophysiol. 76 (1996) 1367–1395.

[122] M. Matsumoto, O. Hikosaka, Lateral habenula as a source of negative reward signals in dopamine neurons, Nature 447 (2007) 1111–1115.

[123] M. Herkenham, W.J.H. Nauta, Afferent connections of the habenular nuclei in the rat: a horseradish peroxidase study, with a note on the fiber-of-passage problem, J. Comp. Neurol. 173 (1977) 123–146.

[124] M. Araki, P.L. McGeer, H. Kimura, The efferent projections of the rat lateral habenular nucleus revealed by the PHA-L anterograde tracing method, Brain Res. 441 (1988) 319–330.

[125] B. Lavoie, A. Parent, Pedunculopontine nucleus in the squirrel monkey: projections to the basal ganglia as revealed by anterograde tract-tracing methods, J. Comp. Neurol. 344 (1994) 210–231.

[126] C.D. Blaha, L.F. Allen, S. Das, W.L. Inglis, M.P. Latimer, S.R. Vincent, P. Winn, Modulation of dopamine efflux in the nucleus accumbens after cholinergic stimulation of the ventral tegmental area in intact, pedunculopontine tegmental nucleus-lesioned, and laterodorsal tegmental nucleus-lesioned rats, J. Neurosci. 16 (1996) 714–722.

[127] Y. Kobayashi, K. Okada, Reward prediction error computation in the pedunculopontine tegmental nucleus neurons, Ann. NY Acad. Sci. 1104 (2007) 310–323.

[128] K. Nakamura, M. Matsumoto, O. Hikosaka, Reward-dependent modulation of neuronal activity in the primate dorsal raphe nucleus, J. Neurosci. 28 (2008) 5331–5343.

[129] C. Peyron, J.M. Petit, C. Rampon, M. Jouvet, P.H. Luppi, Forebrain afferents to the rat dorsal raphe nucleus demonstrated by retrograde and anterograde tracing methods, Neuroscience 82 (1998) 443–468.

[130] G.E. Alexander, M.D. Crutcher, Functional architecture of basal ganglia circuits: neural substrates of parallel processing, Trends Neurosci. 13 (1990) 266–271.

[131] F.A. Middleton, P.L. Strick, Basal-ganglia 'projections' to the prefrontal cortex of the primate, Cereb. Cortex 12 (2002) 926–935.

[132] J.L. Price, S.T. Carmichael, W.C. Drevets, Networks related to the orbital and medial prefrontal cortex: a substrate for emotional behavior? Prog. Brain Res. 107 (1996) 523–536.

2 Electrophysiological correlates of reward processing in dopamine neurons

Philippe N. Tobler and Shunsuke Kobayashi

Department of Physiology, Development and Neuroscience, University of Cambridge, Downing Street, Cambridge CB2 3DY, United Kingdom

Abstract

Animal behavior is influenced by salient, arousing, aversive, and appetitive events. Models of reinforcement learning capture how animals come to predict such events. Models of microeconomic decision-making define the value of those events with multiple factors including magnitude, probability, delay, and risk. Electrophysiological studies on dopamine neurons of the primate midbrain found that appetitive (rewarding), salient, and novel stimuli evoke burst firing, whereas aversive stimuli, such as tail pinch and air-puff, suppress spontaneous firing. More specifically, rewards elicit phasic bursting of dopamine neurons in proportion to the degree of mismatch between expected and received reward. This mismatch, called reward prediction error, appears to provide a teaching signal similar to that of formal learning models. Dopamine responses also show parallels with models from behavioral economics. They code reward value and risk in phasic and sustained components, respectively. These parallels with psychological and microeconomic theories suggest a fundamental role of the dopamine system in the control of reward-related behavior.

Key points

1. Rewards are stimuli for which individuals are willing to work, which are approached, elicit learning, and influence decisions.
2. The blocking paradigm suggests that learning occurs only when rewards are not fully predicted (elicit a prediction error); blocking finds a straightforward explanation in formal learning models such as the Rescorla–Wagner model or its real-time extension, the temporal-difference model.
3. Microeconomic theories have identified reward magnitude, probability, risk, and delay as crucial decision parameters.
4. Testing the phasic activity of dopamine neurons with a blocking paradigm reveals that this activity processes prediction errors as proposed by formal learning rules.
5. Stimulus-induced phasic activity increases with increasing magnitude and probability of reward and decreases with longer reward delay; a more sustained activation building up toward the time of the reward reflects reward risk; thus, the activity of dopamine neurons reflects a variety of distinct reward parameters introduced by learning and microeconomic theories.

2.1   Introduction

Why do we act as we do? Attaining present and future rewards (and avoiding current and future punishments) is an obvious answer. Examples of rewards include food, liquid, an increase in the rate at which one's genes or ideas propagate (inclusive fitness), happiness, or wealth. We often have to trade off several reward attributes, such as reward magnitude, delay, and probability to choose the course of action with the highest value. Predictions of reward occurrence or omission may help us in preparing our actions early in time, which can give us an adaptive advantage over competitors. Learning of predictions corresponds to reducing the discrepancies between current predictions and actual reward outcomes (reducing errors in the prediction of reward). In addition to eliciting learning, rewards also fulfill other functions. For example, they induce subjective feelings of pleasure and they attract attention. Individuals explore potential sources of reward and orient to reward-predicting, salient, and novel stimuli. Midbrain dopamine neurons constitute one of the major reward processing regions of the brain. Specifically, they appear to contribute to reward learning by coding reward prediction errors and combining reward magnitude, delay, and probability. In the present review, we introduce basic concepts from learning (Sections 2.2.1–2.2.3) and economic (Section 2.2.4) theory, including prediction error, reward probability, magnitude, delay, and risk. In Section 2.2.2 we also summarize critical paradigms testing the importance of prediction errors for learning (blocking and conditioned inhibition). In Section 2.3, we show that by coding prediction errors and microeconomic reward parameters, the activity of dopamine neurons closely reflects core concepts of formal theories of reward function.

2.2   Conditioning and its explanations

2.2.1   Definitions and foundations

To start, we introduce basic terms and concepts. Because dopamine neurons are preferentially involved in reward processing, we focus primarily on reward learning. The events occurring in typical conditioning experiments include stimuli and responses or actions. The stimuli may somewhat arbitrarily fall into one of two categories: "unconditioned" and "conditioned." "Unconditioned" stimuli have motivational significance and are capable of eliciting responses on their own. Unconditioned stimuli can be appetitive and elicit approach behavior or aversive and elicit avoidance behavior. Rewards provide instances of appetitive unconditioned stimuli, such as palatable food or liquid and attractive sexual partners. What constitutes a reward can be inferred only from behavior: Rewards are stimuli for which individuals are willing to work and which are approached. Examples of aversive unconditioned stimuli include predators, pain, and illness-inducing stimuli; for their avoidance, individuals are equally willing to work. In contradistinction to unconditioned stimuli, "conditioned" stimuli have only little behavioral significance on their own. Such motivationally more neutral stimuli elicit (conditioned) responses similar to those elicited by unconditioned stimuli only after pairing with an unconditioned stimulus. As a result of learning, conditioned stimuli paired with rewards will acquire appetitive properties and elicit approach behavior, whereas stimuli associated with punishments will become aversive and elicit avoidance behavior. "Excitatory" conditioned stimuli increase the probability of a conditioned response; "inhibitory" conditioned stimuli reduce it (but see ref. [1]). When a conditioned stimulus predicts another conditioned stimulus, it enters a "second-order association" with the reward. If the delivery of the reward occurs irrespective of the individual's behavior, "classical" or "Pavlovian" conditioning arises; if it is dependent on some behavioral reaction, "instrumental" or "operant" conditioning arises. "Reinforcers" are stimuli, both conditioned and unconditioned, which change the strength of operant responses. "Positive" reinforcers increase response strength; "negative" ones decrease it. Learning corresponds to the formation of an association between (representations of) stimuli and responses or other stimuli, may depend on the relations (contingencies) between those stimuli (and responses), and is expressed in behavioral changes measured by the experimenter (for a more elaborate introduction, see ref. [2]).

In the history of learning psychology, the question of what individuals learn during conditioning has received several answers. Due to its simplicity and foundation in the observable, the idea that animals form associations between stimuli and responses appealed to many theorists since Thorndike [3] such as Watson [4] or Hull [5]. Because learning can be behaviorally silent, as may happen in inhibitory conditioning or sensory preconditioning, very strict versions of stimulus–response theories are no longer taken (for review, see ref. [6]). As an alternative, Pavlov [7] introduced the idea that individuals form associations between stimuli or their representations, and Tolman [8,9] and Konorski [10,11] followed him. Such associations allow for the possibility that individuals anticipate stimuli, and this laid the foundation for a cognitive turn in learning psychology. However, very strict versions of stimulus–stimulus theories have difficulty explaining how such associations cause changes in behavior. Current theories propose that animals form stimulus–stimulus, stimulus–outcome, stimulus–response, and response–outcome associations on the background of motivational states and knowledge of the causal relations between actions and outcome [12] (for a non-associationist view, see ref. [13]).

2.2.2   Causes

What elicits learning? The tradition of associationism has proposed a variety of factors eliciting or facilitating learning, conceived of as the formation of associations [14]. Modern learning theories singled out causality, in the form of an error in the prediction of an event, as a necessary and sufficient condition for the formation of an association. Resemblance and contiguity in time and space can have a facilitatory effect on association formation but might not be actual causes for learning.

Resemblance

Resemblance plays a role for generalization and as facilitator of association formation. The resemblance between two stimuli may correspond to the number of elements they have in common. Configurational theories of learning regard the entire stimulation pattern that the individual confronts during training as a unique, undividable conditioned stimulus [15]. The formation and expression of an association depends on the resemblance between the training configuration and the test configuration. The higher the resemblance between training and test configuration, the more will individuals generalize (not discriminate) between the two, and thus display behavior indicative of learning. With generalization controlled for, resemblance may further facilitate learning, for example, during the formation of second-order associations [16] and discrimination learning [17].

Temporal contiguity

The temporal relation of conditioned and unconditioned stimuli or response and outcome determines the speed with which they are associated, and individuals in general learn less contiguous relations less quickly. However, relative is more important for learning than absolute contiguity (relative contiguity as ratio of stimulus–outcome interval to outcome–outcome interval [18,19]). The optimal stimulus–outcome intervals vary with the type of conditioned response under study [20], and simultaneous or backward pairing may result in a weaker [21] or even an inhibitory [22,23] association. Note that simultaneous presentation of stimulus and outcome corresponds to the highest possible contiguity. The fact that the same contiguity can result in different types of learning depending on whether presentation of stimulus and outcome is forward or backward suggests that learning may follow a non-monotonic function of contiguity. In the sections on contingency and prediction error it will become apparent that temporal contiguity alone is not sufficient for learning to occur.

Contingency

In an attempt to determine the proper control procedure for simple conditioning experiments, Rescorla suggested a (truly random) condition in which the probability of the reward occurring in the presence of the conditioned stimulus is the same as the probability of it occurring in the absence of the conditioned stimulus [24]. He found that the more positive the difference between the first and the second probability is (positive contingency), the stronger will the excitatory conditioning be [25]. Conversely, stronger inhibitory conditioning will result from more negative differences (negative contingencies) [26]. With no difference (zero contingency), no conditioning will result, although conditioned and unconditioned stimuli may occur in temporal contiguity, indicating that contiguity is not sufficient for association formation (still, individuals might learn that the two stimuli are unrelated; see ref. [2] for review).

Prediction error

Current learning theories capture learning as the building up of predictions and expectations. Whenever events occur unexpectedly, corresponding to errors in predictions of unconditioned stimuli, individuals have reason to learn. For example, assume that an individual observes a stimulus it has never seen before. A short time period later, a reward occurs. Reward occurrence is unexpected and elicits a positive prediction error. After repeated pairing of the stimulus with the reward, the individual comes to expect the reward more and more, the reward elicits a smaller and smaller prediction error until it is fully predicted (Fig. 2.1).

Two paradigms showing the importance of prediction errors for learning: blocking and conditioned inhibition

The crucial role of prediction errors for learning can be shown formally in blocking experiments. Assume an individual has formed an association between a stimulus and a reward. Now, if another conditioned stimulus is presented in compound with the pretrained stimulus, and the reward occurs just as predicted, there is no reason to learn anything about the newly added stimulus. The reward occurs just as predicted and elicits no prediction error [27,28]. In other words, the pretrained association "blocks" the formation of a new association in these "blocking" experiments. This occurs even though the reward is contiguous and contingent with the newly added conditioned stimulus. Thus, the formation of an association crucially requires an additional factor, that is, surprise [27], or an error in the prediction of reward. In the case of a pre-established association, the reward is already predicted by the pretrained stimulus, and its occurrence therefore is not surprising. The idea that the amount of what an individual learns depends on the size of a prediction error became the cornerstone of many models of association formation (see below).

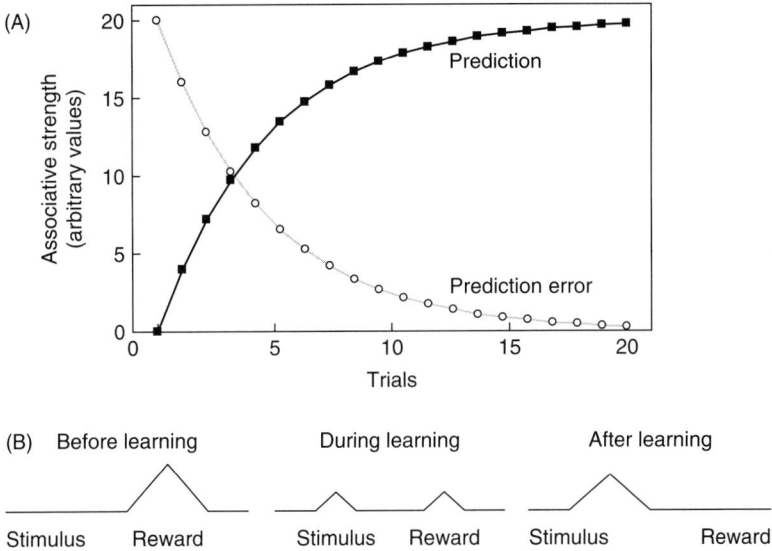

Figure 2.1 Learning according to the Rescorla–Wagner model and schematic dopamine responses. (A) Change of prediction and prediction error over the course of learning. At the beginning of learning, reward prediction (measured as associative strength, black line) is low. The occurrence of a reward elicits a large prediction error (gray line). With repeated pairing of stimulus and reward, the prediction becomes more accurate and the prediction error decreases. When learning is complete, the reward occurs just as predicted and elicits no prediction error. For this plot, Eq. 2.1 was used with learning rates $\alpha = \beta = 0.2$ and reward magnitude $\lambda = 20$. (B) Schematic dopamine responses. Unpredicted rewards elicit a strong phasic burst, which, over the course of learning, gradually decreases while bursting to the conditioned stimulus increases. After learning, dopamine neurons respond to conditioned stimulus but not to reward occurring as predicted.

Modern learning theories explain not only excitatory but also inhibitory conditioning with prediction errors. In a standard paradigm [7], individuals form an association between a stimulus and a reward. Subsequently, a second stimulus is added and the reward is withheld. Here, reward omission is surprising, and it elicits a negative prediction error. After repeated experience, the newly added stimulus becomes a conditioned inhibitor: The negative prediction error moves from the time of reward omission to the time of the stimulus. Individuals learn to inhibit responding upon presentation of the conditioned inhibitor because it predicts reward omission. Thus, a conditioned inhibitor is a behaviorally relevant, attention-inducing stimulus. It can inhibit the behavior that the pretrained excitor would elicit in the standard version of the task only if the individual attends it. And because it is paired with attention but not with reward, it allows experimental separation of these functions. In the conditioned inhibition paradigm, the unconditioned stimulus and the conditioned inhibitor correlate negatively (negative contingency); greater negative correlation between the two results in stronger conditioned inhibition [26,29]. However, the repeated presentation of an untrained stimulus on its own does not result in conditioned inhibition [30,31]. Thus, it is necessary to explicitly set up a negative correlation between the unconditioned stimulus and a conditioned stimulus for the conditioned stimulus to become an inhibitor.

To sum up, most of the various potential causes of association formation combine in the hypothesis that individuals will form an association between events that are or are not in a (experienced) relation of cause (conditioned stimulus) and effect (reward). Prediction errors persist and learning continues as long as the effects predicted upon occurrence of a cause fail to correspond with the occurring effects. Causes and effects are necessarily correlated and thus contingent, often co-localize (or then the cause is inferred at the location of the effect) and normally occur one after the other and at typical time intervals, explaining the contributions of contingency and spatial and temporal contiguity to association formation. Resemblance integrates less easily into the scheme of cause and effect but could reflect the notion that similar causes often tend to have similar effects such that similar stimuli might become associated through an effect associated with one of them.

2.2.3 Models

Modern learning theories (for review, see ref. [2]) describe association formation as a function of the degree to which individuals process the conditioned and unconditioned stimuli. According to Rescorla and Wagner [32], learning of an association between stimulus and reward depends upon the extent of processing of the reward alone. This in turn depends upon the extent to which the reward is surprising or elicits a prediction error. Learning is captured as changes in reward prediction or in the "associative strength" between stimuli and reward:

$$\Delta V_A = \alpha\beta(\lambda - \Sigma V), \tag{2.1}$$

where ΔV_A denotes the change in associative strength of conditioned stimulus A in a trial; α and β are learning rate parameters and denote the salience or intensity of the stimulus and the reward, respectively; λ corresponds to the asymptotic processing of the reward when it is completely unpredicted; and ΣV denotes the sum of the associative strengths of all the conditioned stimuli present for the reward. $\lambda - \Sigma V$ corresponds to the error in prediction of the reward and can assume positive or negative values in a bidirectional fashion (Fig. 2.1A). Less formally, learning is a function of the difference between the value of unpredicted reward and how well it is predicted. This difference is weighted by learning parameters, which determine the speed of learning.

Occurrence of the reward causes a greater prediction error and thus a greater change in associative strength if the summed current associative strength of all stimuli present for the reward is low. In other words, an unpredicted reward will cause a greater prediction error than a predicted reward. Once the reward no longer elicits a prediction error, learning stops and the maximum associative strength for that reward is achieved. According to the model, reward occurring after a stimulus previously not paired with reward will elicit a prediction error. Thus, reward will be processed sufficiently to enter an association with the added stimulus in the control condition of the blocking paradigm. Conversely, the model explains blocking as follows: When reward occurs after a previously trained stimulus, ΣV will be high and $\lambda - \Sigma V$ therefore low when the experimenter introduces the to-be-blocked stimulus. Thus, little prediction error will occur, the reward will be processed insufficiently, and the added stimulus will be blocked from learning.

Rescorla and Wagner regard an error in the prediction of reward as the only necessary factor for the formation of an association [32]. However, not all phenomena can be explained with this scheme. For example, the latent inhibition effect suggests that learning depends also on processing of conditioned stimuli. The latent inhibition effect refers to the observation that, compared to a novel stimulus, repeated presentation of a stimulus on its own reduces the capability of this stimulus to enter into an association with an unconditioned stimulus. As a consequence, models that focus more on attention and the processing of conditioned stimuli have been proposed [33–35]. For example, attention may be driven by how uncertain reward occurrence is; in particular, stimuli about which we are unsure what they entail may capture our attention [35]. All these models, including the Rescorla–Wagner model, however, suffer from a lack of temporal precision because updating of predictions and attention occurs only on a trial-to-trial basis. Sutton and Barto [36–38] developed a machine-learning–based model as a real-time extension of the Rescorla–Wagner learning rule [32]. In their temporal-difference (TD) model of reinforcement, learning is a function of prediction errors across successive time steps:

$$\delta(t) = r(t) + \gamma V(t + 1) - V(t), \tag{2.2}$$

where $r(t)$ corresponds to reward at time (t), γ is a discount factor that weighs future rewards less than sooner rewards, $V(t)$ is the prediction reward at time t. $\delta(t)$ is the TD error and serves as a real-time prediction error (see chapter 10 for more detail on the TD model).

2.2.4 Views from microeconomic theory

Full reward learning should include a complete characterization of how much reward will occur and with what probability upon presentation of a conditioned stimulus. In agreement with this notion, behavior depends on a variety of parameters characterizing reward and the predictive relation between conditioned stimuli and reward. For example, both higher magnitude and probability of reward facilitate learning and performance in a variety of individuals (for review, see ref. [39]). Rats run faster down an alleyway for more reward [40]; a group of ducks distributes itself between two bread-throwing experimenters according to the probability and morsel magnitude with which each of them throws [41]; and monkeys perform more accurately, lick longer, and react more quickly for larger rewards [42]. Learning theorists disagree on whether individuals learn probability and magnitude separately [39] or combined as associative strength (traditional learning theory) and expected value (EV) (see below).

Modern microeconomic theory starts from preferences as revealed in decision-making and overt choice. Making a decision involves picking one out of several options in situations of uncertainty. Uncertain situations are "risky" when probabilities are known and "ambiguous" when probabilities are unknown. Risk is often measured as variance (or its square root, standard deviation). It can be formally dissociated from reward value (Fig. 2.2, see chapter 22 for detailed theoretical arguments on this issue). In binary probability distributions, reward value increases monotonically with reward probability and is highest at $P = 1.0$. By contrast, reward risk is highest at $P = 0.5$, when individuals are most uncertain whether they will get reward or not. With increasing and decreasing reward probability, individuals are more certain that reward will occur or not, respectively. While individuals are often risk averse but can also be risk seeking, increasing reward probability makes an option more valuable for all. Both probability and magnitude of reward associated with each option should influence choice and somehow be combined to pick the best option. Historically, Blaise Pascal invented probability theory to determine how the gains at stake in a game between two gentlemen should be distributed (for overview, see ref. [43]). He proposed that the probability of outcomes should be multiplied with the gains in order to determine the best possible outcome in a choice situation and thereby laid the foundation to EV theory.

$$EV = \Sigma(P \times m), \tag{2.3}$$

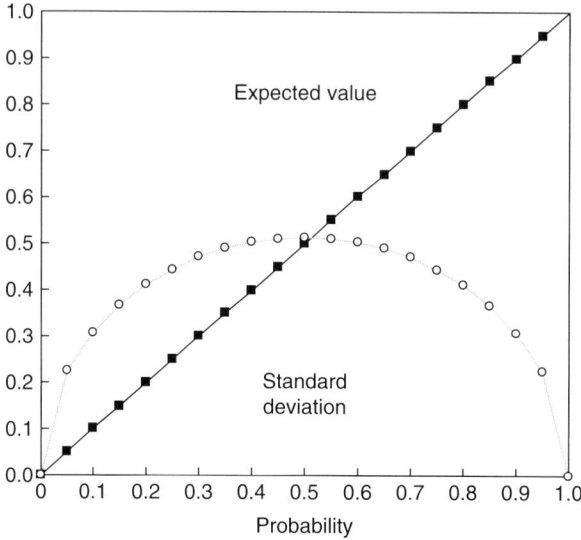

Figure 2.2 Dissociation of value and uncertainty. With increasing reward probability, the value of an option increases (black line), whereas the uncertainty or risk, measured here as standard deviation, increases from 0 at $P = 0.0$ to maximal values at $P = 0.5$ and then decreases again to reach 0 at $P = 1.0$ (gray line).

where the EV of an option corresponds to the sum of probability (P)-weighted magnitude (m) of possible outcomes. EV theory is a normative theory. It subsequently became clear that it fails to precisely describe actual human behavior. Obvious reasons could be distortions in magnitude or probability processing. Such distortions have been proposed by Daniel Bernoulli [44] for magnitude and Kahneman and Tversky [45] for probability.

Daniel Bernoulli suggested that the subjective value people assign to an outcome depends on the wealth of the assigning person and grows more slowly than its magnitude [44]. For example, $100 is worth more to us when we are poor than when we are rich. In this view, "utility" is a formal measure of subjective value and follows a concave (more specifically, Bernoulli suggested a logarithmic) function of reward magnitude. Probability-weighted utility (u) corresponds to expected utility (EU), which provides an alternative to EV for determining the best possible outcome in a risky situation [46]:

$$EU = \Sigma[P \times u(m)]. \tag{2.4}$$

The concave shape of the utility function explains why individuals often are averse to taking risks: The utilities of two equiprobable outcomes on average yield less utility than the utility of the average of those outcomes.

Kahneman and Tversky investigated and confirmed Bernoulli's notion of utility further but suggested that only the utility of gains follows a concave function of objective magnitude, whereas the utility of losses follows a convex function [45]. In other words, individuals often are risk seeking in the domain of losses, as opposed to being risk averse in the domain of gains. In addition, the utility function is steeper for losses than for gains, implying that individuals are usually unwilling to accept gambles with an equiprobable gain or loss of equal magnitude; the utility of the potential loss is larger than that of the gain (loss aversion). This entails that human subjects choose differently depending on whether possible choices or outcomes are presented (framed) in terms of gains or losses [47]. The research of Kahneman and Tversky also suggests that not only the perception of magnitude but also the perception of probability fails to live up to what EV theory prescribes [45]. They found that small probabilities are often overweighted, whereas intermediate and high probabilities are underweighted. However, with increasing experience of probabilistic outcomes, the opposite pattern becomes more prevalent: underweighting of small and overweighting of large probabilities [48]. Combining distortions in magnitude and probability gives rise to prospect theory:

$$\text{Prospect} = \Sigma[w(P) \times u(m)]. \tag{2.5}$$

When individuals face a choice between a small reward delivered immediately and a larger reward delivered later, they often prefer the small immediate reward. Thus, future rewards are subjectively less valuable than immediate rewards. Microeconomic theory and behavioral economics capture this basic observation by discounting future rewards with a decay function. These decay functions come in two flavors, exponential [49] and hyperbolic [50–52]. Behavioral findings suggest that value decays more rapidly in the near than in the far future. Such a pattern of discounting is well captured by hyperbolic discounting functions:

$$V = A/(1 + kD), \tag{2.6}$$

where V is the discounted value, A corresponds to the immediate amount, k to the discount factor, and D to the delay to reward.

2.3   Neurophysiology of the dopamine system

Many earlier dopamine studies were prompted by movement disorders caused by impairments of dopamine transmission, but subsequent electrophysiological studies revealed that impulse activity of dopamine neurons are profoundly influenced by behaviorally salient events, rather than body movements [53]. Although physically salient stimuli can activate dopamine neurons, reward most efficiently shifts dopamine activity from irregular spontaneous firing to stimulus-induced phasic bursting. A series of studies by Schultz and colleagues demonstrated that the phasic activity of dopamine neurons can serve as a teaching signal in association learning and found many parallels with psychological learning theories. These studies used single-neuron extracellular recording techniques in behaving monkeys.

2.3.1   Electrophysiological characteristics of dopamine neurons and afferent inputs

The electrophysiological study of dopamine neurons is facilitated by the fact that dopamine neurons can be identified by their unique electrophysiological signatures. This makes it possible to observe extracellular potentials of dopamine neurons while animals perform various behavioral tasks. Conventionally, dopamine discharges show (1) polyphasic initially positive or negative waveforms followed by a prolonged positive component, (2) relatively long durations (1.8–3.6 ms, measured at 100 Hz high-pass filter), and (3) irregular firing at low baseline frequencies (0.5–8.5 spikes/s) in contrast to the high-frequency firing of neurons in the substantia nigra pars reticulata [54,55].

A recent *in vitro* study suggested a degree of cellular diversity in physiological properties of dopamine neurons [56]. In perforated-patch-clamp recordings, subtypes of dopamine neurons show faster spiking (10–15 Hz) than conventional dopamine neurons upon injection of hyperpolarizing currents. Those relatively fast-spiking dopamine neurons lack somatodendritic dopamine inhibition and possess lower mRNA expression of dopamine active transporter compared to other dopamine subtypes, which reduces dopamine reuptake capacity and contributes to slower decay of extracellular dopamine concentrations in the target areas. These fast-firing dopamine neurons selectively project to medial prefrontal cortex, basolateral amygdala, and the core and the medial shell of nucleus accumbens (NAc).

In response to behaviorally salient stimuli, dopamine neurons shift their irregular slow firing to stimulus-induced phasic bursting. The burst firing is modulated by glutamatergic and cholinergic inputs. Glutamatergic modulation is mediated by *N*-methyl d-aspartate (NMDA) receptors, and potential input sources include the prefrontal cortex [57], pedunculopontine tegmentum (PPTg) [58], bed nucleus of the stria terminalis [59,60], superior colliculus [61,62], lateral preoptic-rostral hypothalamic area [61] and the lateral habenula [63]. Glutamate alone is insufficient to elicit bursting. It has been proposed that there is a gating mechanism from the laterodorsal tegmentum (LDTg) that regulates the ability of dopamine neurons to respond to glutamate and initiate burst firing [64,65].

A substantial fraction of dopamine neurons seem to be held at a constant hyperpolarized inactive state, presumably owing to constant GABA-mediated inhibitory postsynaptic potentials. Only neurons not under GABA-mediated hyperpolarization seem to be capable of entering a burst-firing mode in response to a glutamatergic input. The ventral pallidum, a GABA-producing region known to exhibit high levels of spontaneous activity, may provide such an inhibitory input [64,66].

2.3.2 Mechanisms of dopamine transmission

The cell bodies of midbrain dopamine neurons are in the dorsal sector of the SNc (group A9) and the more medially located VTA (group A10). Dopamine neurons in the SNc primarily project to the dorsal striatum, and the projection is called nigrostriatal pathway. Dopamine neurons in the VTA primarily project to the ventral striatum (NAc and olfactory tubercle) as part of the so-called mesolimbic pathway, and to the prefrontal cortex (the mesocortical pathway) (see chapter 1 for anatomy of cortico-basal ganglia circuit and ref. [67] for review on anatomy of the dopamine system).

Activation of dopamine neurons could influence neuronal processing in their projecting areas in several ways. Phasic bursting of dopamine neurons results in rapid increase of intrasynaptic dopamine concentrations estimated to reach a low millimolar range (e.g., 1.6 mM in the NAc). Phasic release of dopamine will affect a relatively restricted number of postsynaptic neurons within and around the synapses, because diffusion to extrasynaptic sites is heavily restricted by the powerful dopamine reuptake mechanisms [68,69]. Activation of D_1 receptors located within striatal synapses enhances the excitatory action of glutamate at NMDA receptors, whereas activation of dopamine D_2 receptors, which are predominantly at extrasynaptic sites, is associated with depression of postsynaptic activity [70,71]. Thus, rapid increase of dopamine concentration at intrasynaptic regions creates zones of enhanced corticostriatal transmission.

In contrast to the phasic firing, tonic firing of dopamine neurons results in dopamine trickling into the extrasynaptic space, which has low steady state levels (5–40 nM) and changes on a slow time course, on the order of seconds to minutes. Such low concentration of dopamine is insufficient to trigger intrasynaptic receptors, but sufficient to stimulate presynaptic D_2 receptors to downregulate neurotransmitter release.

2.3.3 Novel and physically salient stimuli

Novel or physically intense stimuli induce substantial activations often followed by depressions in dopamine neurons [72,73]. It has been suggested that direct visual input from the superior colliculus may provide short-latency phasic response of dopamine neurons; inactivation of the superior colliculus by microinjection of bicuculline potentiates visual response of dopamine neurons in anesthetized rats [74,75]. The PPTg may also be a source of short-latency sensory input to dopamine neurons. The PPTg is a mesopontine nucleus that receives input from the superior colliculus [76] and provides a dense glutamatergic and cholinergic input to the VTA and SNc [58,77–80]. The majority of PPTg neurons show phasic activation to the onset of salient sensory stimuli at significantly shorter latency than dopamine neurons [81,82]. The sensory response is observed independent of whether the stimuli are associated with reward or not [81], but it appears to be modulated by the motivational state of the animal [82]. Electrical stimulation of the PPTg induces a time-locked burst in dopamine neurons in the rat [83]. Inactivation of the PPTg by microinfusion of lidocaine results in suppression of conditioned sensory responses of dopamine neurons [81]. Reward learning is impaired following excitotoxic lesions of the PPTg [84,85]. The PPTg may relay sensory and reward signals from the lateral hypothalamus and the limbic cortex to dopamine neurons [82].

2.3.4 Aversive events

Aversive events, which have motivationally opposite effects to rewards, generally produce depressions of dopamine activity in contrast to activations produced by rewarding events [86,87]. Only a small fraction of dopamine neurons show phasic activations to primary aversive stimuli, such as an air puff to the hand or hypertonic saline to the mouth, and most of the activated neurons also respond to rewards [88]. The juxtacellular labeling technique in anesthetized rats confirmed phasic excitation of dopaminergic neurons, especially in the ventral VTA, by footshocks [89].

Although aversive events generally suppress single-unit dopamine response, microdialysis studies have shown elevated dopamine release in response to unconditioned and conditioned stimuli for foot shock [90,91]. Several explanations are possible for the different directions of dopamine response to aversive events across the two methods. The microdialysis results may reflect a subgroup of dopamine neurons that show phasic excitation to aversive events. The difference findings may also be due to differences in sensitivity and temporal resolution between the two techniques. A third hypothesis is that aversive events might enhance dopamine release through presynaptic inputs on terminals of dopamine axons, rather than through dopamine impulse activity. It has been shown that glutamate and other excitatory amino acid inputs to the striatum are capable of enhancing presynaptic dopamine release [92]. In tail pinch experiments, however, local infusion of glutamate receptor antagonists did not attenuate dopamine elevations in the striatum measured by *in vivo* microdialysis. In contrast, tetrodotoxin infusion, which blocks action potential propagation along dopamine axons, abolished dopamine release [93]. Further research is needed to reconcile the inconsistent findings on dopamine response to aversive events.

2.3.5   Primary rewards and reward-predicting stimuli

The majority of dopamine neurons (60–80%) in the SNc and VTA show a phasic burst following primary food and liquid rewards (i.e., unconditioned stimulus). Burst activity is typically in the order of 10–50 spikes/s with latencies of 80–110 ms and durations of less than 300 ms. The response to a reward, however, does not occur when reward is predicted by conditioned stimuli in Pavlovian and instrumental conditioning paradigms [94–96]. While animals learn the stimulus–reward associations, initially present dopamine activations to primary reward disappear and responses to conditioned stimuli emerge (Fig. 2.3). About 55–70% of dopamine neurons respond to conditioned visual and auditory stimuli in various Pavlovian and instrumental tasks [95–101]. If a predicted reward is omitted or smaller than predicted, dopamine neurons show phasic depression (negative prediction error). If unpredicted reward occurs or reward is larger than predicted, dopamine neurons show burst activation (positive prediction error). Phasic dopamine release to unpredicted reward and reward-predicting visual stimuli was also confirmed in the NAc, a target of the mesolimbic dopamine pathway, by using fast-scan cyclic voltammetry while rats formed a Pavlovian stimulus–reward association [102].

Dopamine responses during learning suggest that dopamine neurons signal the difference between the values of received and predicted reward in a graded manner, parametrically reflecting reward prediction error. The prediction error coding resembles the crucial learning term $(\lambda - \Sigma V)$ of the Rescorla–Wagner learning rule (Eq. 2.1), in which positive or negative prediction errors increase or decrease the association strength, respectively, and learning progresses until prediction errors reach zero. The Rescorla–Wagner model, however, has inherent limitations as a trial-level model. The model may predict by how much synaptic weights change on a trial-by-trial basis, but it cannot predict how neurons will fire during the course of a trial. The TD model updates associative strength continuously, based on the real-time reward prediction error between successive time steps (Eq. 2.2). The TD model accurately replicates real-time activity of dopamine neurons in learning paradigms [103].

Reward-predicting stimuli and physically salient stimuli appear to have separate underlying mechanisms in activating dopamine neurons. Physically salient and novel stimuli can activate dopamine neurons without reward association, whereas visual stimuli, which are physically not salient enough to activate dopamine neurons, can efficiently evoke burst firing if they are associated with reward. Dopamine neurons discriminate between rewarding and neutral stimuli if they are physically sufficiently dissimilar [95], but they show progressively more generalizing, activation–depression responses to unrewarded stimuli with increasing resemblance to reward-predicting stimuli [89,104].

A recent study showed that neurons in the primate lateral habenula, part of the structure called the epithalamus, emit prediction error signals similar to those emitted by dopamine

No prediction
Reward occurs

(No CS)   R

Reward predicted
Reward occurs

CS   R

Reward predicted
No reward occurs

−1   0   1   2 s
CS   (No R)

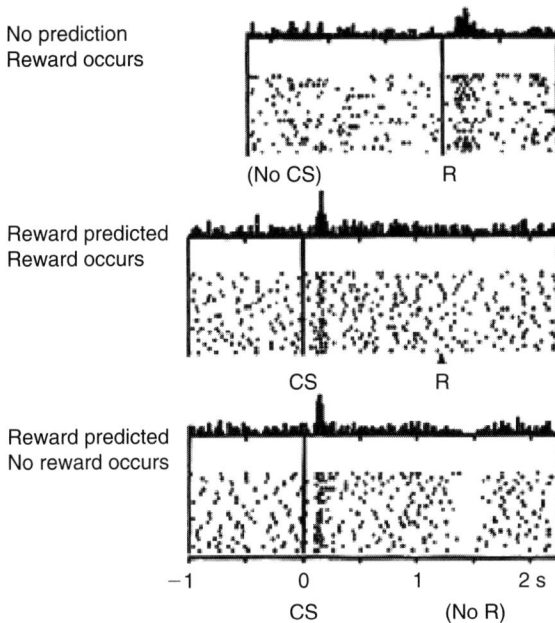

Figure 2.3 Changes in dopamine neurons' output code for an error in the prediction of appetitive events. (Top) Before learning, a drop of appetitive fruit juice occurs in the absence of prediction – hence a positive error in the prediction of reward. The dopamine neuron is activated by this unpredicted occurrence of juice. (Middle) After learning, the conditioned stimulus predicts reward, and the reward occurs according to the prediction – hence no error in the prediction of reward. The dopamine neuron is activated by the reward-predicting stimulus but fails to be activated by the predicted reward (right). (Bottom) After learning, the conditioned stimulus predicts a reward, but the reward fails to occur because of a mistake in the behavioral response of the monkey. The activity of the dopamine neuron is depressed exactly at the time when the reward would have occurred. The depression occurs more than 1 s after the conditioned stimulus without any intervening stimuli, revealing an internal representation of the time of the predicted reward. Neuronal activity is aligned on the electronic pulse that drives the solenoid valve delivering the reward liquid (top) or the onset of the conditioned visual stimulus (middle and bottom). Each panel shows the peri-event time histogram and raster of impulses from the same neuron. Horizontal distances of dots correspond to real-time intervals. Each line of dots shows one trial. Original sequence of trials is plotted from top to bottom. CS = conditioned, reward-predicting stimulus; R = primary reward. *Source*: Schultz et al. (1997) [103]. Reprinted with permission from *Science*.

neurons, but in the opposite direction: Habenula neurons are activated by a cue that predicts no reward and suppressed by a cue that predicts reward. In addition, they are activated when the expected reward is omitted, and suppressed when a reward is given unexpectedly [105]. The lateral habenula neurons send presumably glutamatergic projections not only to (interneurons of) the dopamine system (the VTA and SNc), but also to serotonergic (dorsal and median raphe), cholinergic (PPTg, LDTg), and noradrenergic (locus coeruleus) systems. Thus, the lateral habenula appears to send a formal reward prediction error signal to all major neuromodulatory systems.

2.3.6 Temporal coding

The prediction error signal of dopamine neurons is sensitive to timing of the reward. If reward is delivered 500 ms earlier than expected, dopamine neurons show activation to the unexpectedly early reward, even though reward occurs at the expected amount. If reward delivery is delayed, dopamine neurons show depression at the expected time [101]. Even if reward is delivered at the predicted time, long intervals between prediction and reward evoke large dopamine activation on reward delivery [106,107]. The time sensitivity of dopamine neurons may relate to the role of temporal contiguity in behavioral learning theories. Behaviorally, long and variable intervals between a stimulus and reward make learning slow and association weak. It is also known that behavioral timing measures become increasingly imprecise with longer delays (scalar expectancy theory) [108]. Thus, long delays between conditioned stimulus and reward may make the reward expectation spread out in time and generate prediction error due to temporal uncertainty.

2.3.7 Psychological learning paradigms

The blocking paradigm shows the crucial role of prediction errors for learning. Accordingly, only stimuli paired with prediction errors will be learned, whereas stimuli paired with no prediction error will be blocked from learning (see 2.2.2 and 2.2.3). In agreement with this notion, monkeys show considerably less conditioned licking to stimuli that are blocked from learning than to control stimuli that are learned and paired with a reward prediction error [104]. Similarly, dopamine neurons respond less to blocked than to control stimuli. Thus, the reward prediction error signal of dopamine neurons appears to be ideally suited to learn stimulus–reward associations according to the mechanisms suggested by formal learning theories.

In the conditioned inhibition task, animals first acquire a behavioral response to a normal conditioned stimulus. Then they learn to inhibit these behavioral responses when a stimulus occurs that predicts explicitly the omission of the reward that would have occurred otherwise [7,109]. To inhibit behavior, the second, added, stimulus has to attract the animal's attention, although the stimulus itself is associated with reward absence. Dopamine neurons are primarily depressed rather than activated by conditioned inhibitors [110]. Thus, dopamine neurons appear to reflect primarily the reward omission–predicting properties rather than the attention-inducing properties of conditioned inhibitors.

2.3.8 Value coding

The responses of dopamine neurons are influenced by multiple factors that determine the value of reward. When different visual stimuli specify both magnitude and probability of reward in a Pavlovian conditioning paradigm, the phasic responses of dopamine neurons to the visual stimuli monotonically increase with larger magnitude and probability [111,112]. The responses reflect products of the magnitude and probability of reward, which could form the basis for a value term such as EV or EU (Eqs 2.3–2.5). Another study used an instrumental conditioning task, in which reward probability varied depending on the subject's past choices [113]. In this task, the monkey has to learn the order in which to press three buttons by trial and error. After making an error, the probability of success in the next step is higher because the correct button is limited to the button(s) not yet selected. Dopamine responses to a conditioned stimulus increase in proportion to the reward probability. These findings suggest that the value coding of dopamine neurons does not depend on whether it is a Pavlovian or instrumental conditioning paradigm, nor does it depend on whether value is predicted by an explicit cue or implicit learning.

Delay is another factor that determines reward value. Consistent with the psychological and microeconomic theories of temporal discounting, reward delay reduces the dopamine responses to delay-predicting stimuli in both Pavlovian conditioning [107] and intertemporal choice [114]. More specifically, it is consistent with a hyperbolic discounting model (Eq. 2.6); the population response of dopamine neurons decreases more steeply for predictions of earlier than later rewards. When both magnitude and delay of reward vary, phasic responses to the reward-predicting stimuli increase with larger reward magnitudes and decrease with longer reward delay. Thus, dopamine responses appear to reflect the discounting of subjective reward value by imposed delay.

Dopamine responses to primary reward appear to reflect differences in value between expected and received rewards. When a reward occurs exactly at the predicted value, dopamine neurons show no response. However, when liquid volume is smaller or larger than predicted, dopamine neurons are suppressed or activated, respectively. Accordingly, when three visual stimuli are presented with probabilistic reward outcomes ($P = 0.5$) at different volumes (0 or 0.05 ml, 0 or 0.15 ml, and 0 or 0.5 ml), reward occurrence always elicits dopamine activation at the time of reward. Interestingly, the activation is nearly identical in each case, despite the fact that the absolute difference between actual and expected volume varied over a 10-fold range. Thus, prediction error signals of dopamine neurons may not be scaled with the absolute value but appear to be rescaled (normalized) by the range of available reward values in each situation [111].

In sum, dopamine neurons reflect prediction errors, combining multiple factors that determine subjective reward value, including magnitude, probability, and delay. Yet value coding of dopamine neurons is relative, not absolute, shifting references to the expected reward value and adjusting gain to the variance of reward value.

2.3.9   Reward uncertainty

The effects of reward uncertainty can be tested with dopamine responses by manipulating reward probability in a Pavlovian conditioning paradigm. When different visual stimuli indicate a fixed amount of reward at different probability ($P = 0.0, 0.25,$ 0.5, 0.75, 1.0), more than one-third of dopamine neurons show a relatively sustained and gradually increasing activation between reward-predicting stimulus and reward (Fig. 2.4) [112]. This activation is highest for conditioned stimuli predicting reward at $P = 0.5$, and progressively lower for probabilities farther away from $P = 0.5$ in either direction. The uncertainty-related response is separate from the earlier phasic response that monotonically increases with larger probability and higher value. The results suggest that dopamine neurons distinctly encode reward value and uncertainty.

Uncertainty influences individual preferences for rewards. According to EU theory, the curvature of the utility function reflects an individual's risk attitude: Risk-neutral individuals have linear utility functions, while risk-seeking and risk-averse individuals have convex and concave utility functions (Eq. 2.4) [46]. If dopamine neurons signal EU, the level of uncertainty might influence the initial phasic response separate from the direct uncertainty coding in the sustained activity. However, dissociation between EV and EU has not yet been made for dopamine signals.

The uncertainty signal can be interpreted as reflecting attention processes, as psychologists have proposed that the level of attention is proportional to uncertainty about reinforcers [35]. As described above, attention-driving stimuli have limited effects on the phasic

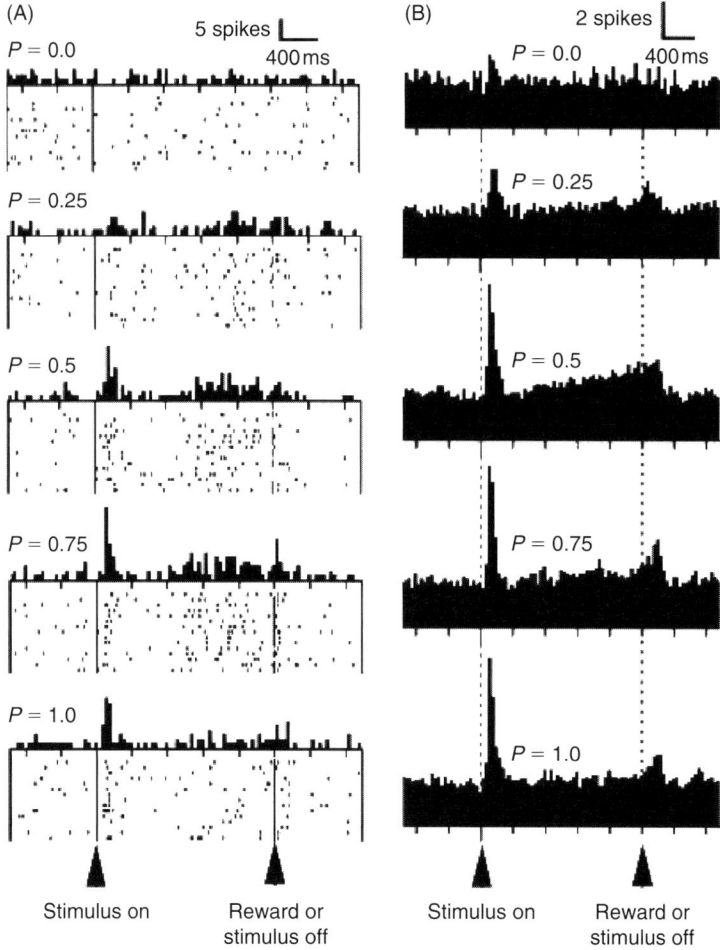

Figure 2.4 Sustained activation of dopamine neurons precedes uncertain rewards. Rasters (A) and histograms (B) of activity in a single cell with reward probabilities ranging from 0.0 (top) to 1.0 (bottom). Both rewarded and unrewarded trials are included at intermediate probabilities. (A) This neuron showed sustained activation before potential reward at all three intermediate probabilities. The longer vertical marks in the rasters indicate the occurrence of reward. Bin = 20 ms. (B) At $P = 0.5$, the mean ($\pm$SD) rate of basal activity in this population was 2.5 ± 1.4 impulses/s before stimulus onset and 3.9 ± 2.7 in the 500 ms before potential reward. *Source*: Fiorillo et al. (2003) [112]. Reprinted with permission from *Science*.

component of dopamine responses as compared to profound effects of appetitive rewards. However, it is possible that attentional states do affect dopamine response in their sustained component. If this is the case, the two distinct types of dopamine responses might embody two fundamental principles of learning: reinforcement and attention. Postsynaptic neurons might be able to discriminate the dual dopamine signals, as the value signal is encoded in the phasic burst that increases intrasynaptic dopamine concentration in a short time scale and the uncertainty signal is encoded in the tonic firing that affects extrasynaptic dopamine concentration in a long time scale.

2.3.10 Decision-making

Little is known about the role of dopamine neurons in decision-making. When an individual chooses among many options with different properties (e.g., different reward probabilities and different delays), would dopamine neurons reflect the value of the to-be-chosen option, the average value of all options presented, or the highest value of all? According to a recent study, dopamine responses reflect the value of the option to be chosen, even if it is the less valuable of two options with different reward probabilities [115]. However, another study showed that dopamine neurons signal the higher value of two options regardless of the choice itself [114]. Although it is possible that the difference is due to anatomical differences (the former study sampled from the SNc and the latter from the VTA), future investigation is needed to clarify the role of the dopamine system in economic decision-making.

2.4   Conclusion

Animal behavior is influenced by various factors, including salient, novel, arousing, aversive, and appetitive events. Most of these events have some impact on dopamine neurons, usually activation except suppression by aversive events. However, rewards have the greatest impact on dopamine responses. Reward processing is very specific in dopamine neurons, in that they process reward prediction errors. Such prediction errors play a fundamental role in psychological learning models such as the one proposed by Rescorla and Wagner.

The value of rewards can be decomposed into separate parameters including magnitude, probability, and delay. Systematic tests of these value components have revealed that dopamine neurons reflect and integrate all of these reward parameters. It currently remains unclear how the value coding of dopamine neurons relates to theories of microeconomics, such as EU and prospect theories. Future studies need to test neural responses that correspond to value and probability weighting functions in EU and prospect theories. Also, it is important to know how individual risk attitudes influence neural value signals. It could be demanding to examine the concavity/convexity of neural correlates of utility curves because of the noise and nonlinearity inherent in neural signal processing. For example, loss aversion creates asymmetry of the value function between gain and loss. It is, however, difficult to test the asymmetry with responses of dopamine neurons, because their low baseline firing rate limits the dynamic range for suppression and creates intrinsic asymmetry on the encoding scale (see refs. [116] and [117]). Besides testing parallels between microeconomic theories and dopamine responses, future research needs to tackle the questions of how the neural system constructs value representation and how it influences behavioral decision.

Acknowledgements

We thank Wolfram Schultz, the Wellcome Trust, and the Cambridge Medical Research Council – Wellcome Behavioral and Clinical Neuroscience Institute for support.

References

[1] J.D. Batson, M.R. Best, Single-element assessment of conditioned inhibition, Bull. Psychon. Soc. 18 (1981) 328–330.

[2] A. Dickinson, Contemporary animal learning theory, Cambridge, Cambridge University Press, 1980.

[3] E.L. Thorndike, Animal intelligence: experimental studies, Macmillan, New York, 1911.

[4] J.B. Watson, Behavior: an introduction to comparative psychology, Holt, Rinehart and Winston, New York, 1914.

[5] C.L. Hull, Principles of behavior, Appleton-Century-Crofts, New York, 1943.

[6] N.J. Mackintosh, Conditioning and associative learning, Oxford University Press, Oxford, 1983.

[7] I.P. Pavlov, Conditional Reflexes, Dover Publications, New York, 1927/1960 (the 1960 edition is an unaltered republication of the 1927 translation by Oxford University Press).

[8] E.C. Tolman, Purposive behavior in animals and men, Century, New York, 1932.

[9] E.C. Tolman, There is more than one kind of learning, Psychol. Rev. 56 (1949) 144–155.

[10] J. Konorski, Conditioned reflexes and neuron organization, Hafner Publishing, London, 1948/1968 (the edition of 1968 is a facsimile reprint of the 1948 edition by Cambridge University Press).

[11] J. Konorski, Integrative action of the brain, University of Chicago Press, Chicago, IL, 1967.

[12] A. Dickinson, B. Balleine, Motivational control of goal-directed action, Anim. Learn. Behav. 22 (1994) 1–18.

[13] C.R. Gallistel, J. Gibbon, Time, rate, and conditioning, Psychol. Rev. 107 (2000) 289–344.

[14] D. Hume, A treatise of human nature, John Noon, London, 1739/2000 (edited in 2000 by D. F. Norton & M. J. Norton. Oxford: Oxford University Press).

[15] J.M. Pearce, A model for stimulus generalization in Pavlovian conditioning, Psychol. Rev. 94 (1987) 61–73.

[16] R.A. Rescorla, D.R. Furrow, Stimulus similarity as a determinant of Pavlovian conditioning, J. Exp. Psychol. Anim. Behav. Process. 3 (1977) 203–215.

[17] J.B. Trobalon, D. Miguelez, I.P. McLaren, N.J. Mackintosh, Intradimensional and extradimensional shifts in spatial learning, J. Exp. Psychol. Anim. Behav. Process. 29 (2003) 143–152.

[18] J. Gibbon, M.D. Baldock, C. Locurto, L. Gold, H.S. Terrace, Trial and intertrial durations in autoshaping, J. Exp. Psychol. Anim. Behav. Process. 3 (1977) 264–284.

[19] B.A. Williams, Information effects on the response-reinforcer association, Anim. Learn. Behav. 6 (1978) 371–379.

[20] N. Schneiderman, Response system divergencies in aversive classical conditioning, in: A. Black, W.F. Prokasy (Eds.), Classical conditioning II: current research and theory, Appleton-Century-Crofts, New York, 1972, pp. 341–376.

[21] C.D. Heth, R.A. Rescorla, Simultaneous and backward fear conditioning in the rat, J. Comp. Physiol. Psychol. 82 (1973) 434–443.

[22] F. Hellstern, R. Malaka, M. Hammer, Backward inhibitory learning in honeybees: a behavioral analysis of reinforcement processing, Learn. Mem. 4 (1998) 429–444.

[23] H.C. Plotkin, D.A. Oakley, Backward conditioning in the rabbit (*Oryctolagus cuniculus*), J. Comp. Physiol. Psychol. 88 (1975) 586–590.

[24] R.A. Rescorla, Pavlovian conditioning and its proper control procedures, Psychol. Rev. 74 (1967) 71–80.

[25] R.A. Rescorla, Probability of shock in the presence and absence of CS in fear conditioning, J. Comp. Physiol. Psychol. 66 (1968) 1–5.

[26] R.A. Rescorla, Conditioned inhibition of fear resulting from negative CS-US contingencies, J. Comp. Physiol. Psychol. 67 (1969) 504–509.

[27] L.J. Kamin, Predictability, surprise, attention and conditioning, in: B.A. Campbell, R.M. Church (Eds.), Punishment and aversive behavior, Appleton-Century-Crofts, New York, 1969, pp. 279–296.

[28] R.A. Rescorla, Variation in the effectiveness of reinforcement and nonreinforcement following prior inhibitory conditioning, Learn. Motiv. 2 (1971) 113–123.

[29] R.A. Rescorla, Establishment of a positive reinforcer through contrast with shock, J. Comp. Physiol. Psychol. 67 (1969) 260–263.

[30] S. Reiss, A.R. Wagner, CS habituation produces a "latent inhibition effect" but no active "conditioned inhibition", Learn. Motiv. 3 (1972) 237–245.

[31] R.A. Rescorla, Summation and retardation tests of latent inhibition, J. Comp. Physiol. Psychol. 75 (1971) 77–81.

[32] R.A. Rescorla, A.R. Wagner, A theory of Pavlovian conditioning: variations in the effectiveness of reinforcement and nonreinforcement, in: A. Black, W.F. Prokasy (Eds.), Classical conditioning II: current research and theory, Appleton-Century-Crofts, New York, 1972, pp. 64–99.

[33] N.J. Mackintosh, A theory of attention: variations in the associability of stimuli with reinforcement, Psychol. Rev. 82 (1975) 276–298.

[34] A.R. Wagner, Expectancies and the priming of STM, in: S.H. Hulse, H. Fowler, W.K. Honig (Eds.), Cognitive processes in animal behavior, Lawrence Erlbaum, Hillsdale, NJ, 1978, pp. 177–209.

[35] J.M. Pearce, G. Hall, A model of Pavlovian learning: variations in the effectiveness of conditioned but not of unconditioned stimuli, Psychol. Rev. 87 (1980) 532–552.

[36] R.S. Sutton, A.G. Barto, Toward a modern theory of adaptive networks: expectation and prediction, Psychol. Rev. 88 (1981) 135–170.

[37] R.S. Sutton, A.G. Barto, Time-derivative models of Pavlovian reinforcement, in: M. Gabriel, J. Moore (Eds.), Learning and computational neuroscience: foundations of adaptive networks, MIT Press, Boston, MA, 1990, pp. 497–537.

[38] R.S. Sutton, Learning to predict by the method of temporal difference, Mach. Learn. 3 (1988) 9–44.

[39] C.R. Gallistel, The organization of learning, MIT Press, Boston, MA, 1990.

[40] G.H. Bower, A contrast effect in differential conditioning, J. Exp. Psychol. 62 (1961) 196–199.

[41] D.G.C. Harper, Competitive foraging in mallards: ideal free ducks, Anim. Behav. 30 (1982) 575–584.

[42] H.C. Cromwell, W. Schultz, Effects of expectations for different reward magnitudes on neuronal activity in primate striatum, J. Neurophysiol. 89 (2003) 2823–2838.

[43] P.W. Glimcher, Decisions, uncertainty, and the brain: the science of neuroeconomics, MIT Press, Boston, MA, 2003.

[44] D. Bernoulli, Exposition of a new theory on the measurement of risk, Econometrica 22 (1738/1954) 23–36 (translated from Latin).

[45] D. Kahneman, A. Tversky, Prospect theory: an analysis of decision under risk, Econometrica 47 (1979) 263–291.

[46] J. von Neumann, O. Morgenstern, Theory of games and economic behavior, Princeton University Press, Princeton, NJ, 1944.

[47] A. Tversky, D. Kahneman, The framing of decisions and the psychology of choice, Science 211 (1981) 453–458.

[48] R. Hertwig, G. Barron, E.U. Weber, I. Erev, Decisions from experience and the effect of rare events, Psychol. Sci. 15 (2004) 534–539.

[49] P.A. Samuelson, Some aspects of the pure theory of capital, Q. J. Economics 51 (1937) 469–496.

[50] G. Ainslie, Specious rewards: a behavioral theory of impulsiveness and impulse control, Psychol. Bull. 82 (1975) 463–496.

[51] J.E. Mazur, An adjusting procedure for studying delayed reinforcement, in: M.L. Commons, J.E. Mazur, J.A. Nevin, H. Rachlin (Eds.), Quantitative analyses of behavior, vol. 5, Erlbaum, Hillsdale, NJ, 1987, pp. 55–73.

[52] J.B. Richards, S.H. Mitchell, H. de Wit, L.S. Seiden, Determination of discount functions in rats with an adjusting-amount procedure, J. Exp. Anal. Behav. 67 (1997) 353–366.

[53] M.R. DeLong, M.D. Crutcher, A.P. Georgopoulos, Relations between movement and single cell discharge in the substantia nigra of the behaving monkey, J. Neurosci. 3 (1983) 1599–1606.

[54] A.A. Grace, B.S. Bunney, Nigral dopamine neurons: intracellular recording and identification with L-dopa injection and histofluorescence, Science 210 (1980) 654–656.

[55] W. Schultz, R. Romo, Responses of nigrostriatal dopamine neurons to high-intensity somato-sensory stimulation in the anesthetized monkey, J. Neurophysiol. 57 (1987) 201–217.

[56] S. Lammel, A. Hetzel, O. Häckel, I. Jones, B. Liss, J. Roeper, Unique properties of mesoprefron-tal neurons within a dual mesocorticolimbic dopamine system, Neuron 57 (2008) 760–773.

[57] S.R. Sesack, V.M. Pickel, Prefrontal cortical efferents in the rat synapse on unlabeled neuronal targets of catecholamine terminals in the nucleus accumbens septi and on dopamine neurons in the ventral tegmental area, J. Comp. Neurol. 320 (1992) 145–160.

[58] T. Futami, K. Takakusaki, S.T. Kitai, Glutamatergic and cholinergic inputs from the pedun-culopontine tegmental nucleus to dopamine neurons in the substantia nigra pars compacta, Neurosci. Res. 21 (1995) 331–342.

[59] J.L. Fudge, S.N. Haber, Bed nucleus of the stria terminalis and extended amygdala inputs to dopamine subpopulations in primates, Neuroscience 104 (2001) 807–827.

[60] F. Georges, G. Aston-Jones, Activation of ventral tegmental area cells by the bed nucleus of the stria terminalis: a novel excitatory amino acid input to midbrain dopamine neurons, J. Neurosci. 22 (2002) 5173–5187.

[61] S. Geisler, D.S. Zahm, Afferents of the ventral tegmental area in the rat-anatomical substratum for integrative functions, J. Comp. Neurol. 490 (2005) 270–294.

[62] J.G. McHaffie, H. Jiang, P.J. May, V. Coizet, P.G. Overton, B.E. Stein, P. Redgrave, A direct projection from superior colliculus to substantia nigra pars compacta in the cat, Neuroscience 138 (2006) 221–234.

[63] M. Araki, P.L. McGeer, H. Kimura, The efferent projections of the rat lateral habenular nucleus revealed by the PHA-L anterograde tracing method, Brain Res. 441 (1988) 319–330.

[64] S.B. Floresco, A.R. West, B. Ash, H. Moore, A.A. Grace, Afferent modulation of dopamine neuron firing differentially regulates tonic and phasic dopamine transmission, Nat. Neurosci. 6 (2003) 968–973.

[65] D.J. Lodge, A.A. Grace, The laterodorsal tegmentum is essential for burst firing of ventral teg-mental area dopamine neurons, Proc. Natl. Acad. Sci. USA 103 (2006) 5167–5172.

[66] M. Wu, A.W. Hrycyshyn, S.M. Brudzynski, Subpallidal outputs to the nucleus accumbens and ven-tral tegmental area: anatomical and electrophysiological studies, Brain Res. 740 (1996) 151–161.

[67] S.N. Haber, J.L. Fudge, The primate substantia nigra and VTA: integrative circuitry and func-tion, Crit. Rev. Neurobiol. 11 (1997) 323–342.

[68] F. Gonon, Nonlinear relationship between impulse flow and dopamine released by rat midbrain dopaminergic neurons as studied by *in vivo* electrochemistry, Neuroscience 24 (1988) 19–28.

[69] K.T. Kawagoe, P.A. Garris, D.J. Wiedemann, R.M. Wightman, Regulation of transient dopamine concentration gradients in the microenvironment surrounding nerve terminals in the rat striatum, Neuroscience 51 (1992) 55–64.

[70] C. Cepeda, N.A. Buchwald, M.S. Levine, Neuromodulatory actions of dopamine in the neos-triatum are dependent upon the excitatory amino acid receptor subtypes activated, Proc. Natl. Acad. Sci. USA 90 (1993) 9576–9580.

[71] F. Gonon, L. Sundstrom, Excitatory effects of dopamine released by impulse flow in the rat nucleus accumbens *in vivo*, Neuroscience 75 (1996) 13–18.

[72] G.F. Steinfels, H. Heym, B.L. Jacobs, Single unit activity of dopaminergic neurons in freely moving animals, Life Sci. 29 (1981) 1435–1442.

[73] J.C. Horvitz, T. Stewart, B.L. Jacobs, Burst activity of ventral tegmental dopamine neurons is elicited by sensory stimuli in the awake cat, Brain Res. 759 (1997) 251–258.

[74] E. Comoli, V. Coizet, J. Boyes, J.P. Bolam, N.S. Canteras, R.H. Quirk, P.G. Overton, P. Redgrave, A direct projection from superior colliculus to substantia nigra for detecting salient visual events, Nat. Neurosci. 6 (2003) 974–980.

[75] E. Dommett, V. Coizet, C.D. Blaha, J. Martindale, V. Lefebvre, N. Walton, J.E. Mayhew, P.G. Overton, P. Redgrave, How visual stimuli activate dopaminergic neurons at short latency, Science 307 (2005) 1476–1479.

[76] P. Redgrave, I.J. Mitchell, P. Dean, Descending projections from the superior colliculus in rat: a study using orthograde transport of wheatgerm-agglutinin conjugated horseradish peroxidase, Exp. Brain Res. 68 (1987) 147–167.

[77] M. Beninato, R.F. Spencer, A cholinergic projection to the rat substantia nigra from the pedunculopontine tegmental nucleus, Brain Res. 412 (1987) 169–174.

[78] M. Beninato, R.F. Spencer, The cholinergic innervation of the rat substantia nigra: a light and electron microscopic immunohistochemical study, Exp. Brain Res. 72 (1988) 178–184.

[79] J.P. Bolam, C.M. Francis, Z. Henderson, Cholinergic input to dopaminergic neurons in the substantia nigra: a double immunocytochemical study, Neuroscience 41 (1991) 483–494.

[80] S.A. Oakman, P.L. Faris, P.E. Kerr, C. Cozzari, B.K. Hartman, Distribution of pontomesencephalic cholinergic neurons projecting to substantia nigra differs significantly from those projecting to ventral tegmental area, J. Neurosci. 15 (1995) 5859–5869.

[81] W.X. Pan, B.I. Hyland, Pedunculopontine tegmental nucleus controls conditioned responses of midbrain dopamine neurons in behaving rats, J. Neurosci. 25 (2005) 4725–4732.

[82] Y. Kobayashi, K. Okada, Reward prediction error computation in the pedunculopontine tegmental nucleus neurons, Ann. NY Acad. Sci. 1104 (2007) 310–323.

[83] S.J. Lokwan, P.G. Overton, M.S. Berry, D. Clark, Stimulation of the pedunculopontine tegmental nucleus in the rat produces burst firing in A9 dopaminergic neurons, Neuroscience 92 (1999) 245–254.

[84] W.L. Inglis, M.C. Olmstead, T.W. Robbins, Pedunculopontine tegmental nucleus lesions impair stimulus-reward learning in autoshaping and conditioned reinforcement paradigms, Behav. Neurosci. 114 (2000) 285–294.

[85] H.L. Alderson, V.J. Brown, M.P. Latimer, P.J. Brasted, A.H. Robertson, P. Winn, The effect of excitotoxic lesions of the pedunculopontine tegmental nucleus on performance of a progressive ratio schedule of reinforcement, Neuroscience 112 (2002) 417–425.

[86] C.T. Tsai, S. Nakamura, K. Iwama, Inhibition of neuronal activity of the substantia nigra by noxious stimuli and its modification by the caudate nucleus, Brain Res. 195 (1980) 299–311.

[87] H. Maeda, G.J. Mogenson, Effects of peripheral stimulation on the activity of neurons in the ventral tegmental area, substantia nigra and midbrain reticular formation of rats, Brain Res. Bull. 8 (1982) 7–14.

[88] J. Mirenowicz, W. Schultz, Preferential activation of midbrain dopamine neurons by appetitive rather than aversive stimuli, Nature 379 (1996) 449–451.

[89] F. Brischoux, S. Chakraborty, D.I. Brierley, M.A. Ungless, Phasic excitation of dopamine neurons in ventral VTA by noxious stimuli, Proc. Natl. Acad. Sci. U. S. A. 106 (2009) 4894–4899.

[90] B.A. Sorg, P.W. Kalivas, Effects of cocaine and footshock stress on extracellular dopamine levels in the ventral striatum, Brain Res. 559 (1991) 29–36.

[91] A.M. Young, M.H. Joseph, J.A. Gray, Latent inhibition of conditioned dopamine release in rat nucleus accumbens, Neuroscience 54 (1993) 5–9.

[92] R. Romo, A. Chéramy, G. Godeheu, J. Glowinski, In vivo presynaptic control of dopamine release in the cat caudate nucleus – III. Further evidence for the implication of corticostriatal glutamatergic neurons, Neuroscience 19 (1986) 1091–1099.

[93] K.A. Keefe, A.F. Sved, M.J. Zigmond, E.D. Abercrombie, Stress-induced dopamine release in the neostriatum: evaluation of the role of action potentials in nigrostriatal dopamine neurons or local initiation by local excitatory amino acids, J. Neurochem. 61 (1993) 1943–1952.

 [94] R. Romo, W. Schultz, Dopamine neurons of the monkey midbrain: contingencies of responses to active touch during self-initiated arm movements, J. Neurophysiol. 63 (1990) 592–606.

 [95] T. Ljungberg, P. Apicella, W. Schultz, Responses of monkey dopamine neurons during learning of behavioral reactions, J. Neurophysiol. 67 (1992) 145–163.

 [96] J. Mirenowicz, W. Schultz, Importance of unpredictability for reward responses in primate dopamine neurons, J. Neurophysiol. 72 (1994) 1024–1027.

 [97] J.D. Miller, M.K. Sanghera, D.C. German, Mesencephalic dopaminergic unit activity in the behaviorally conditioned rat, Life Sci. 29 (1981) 1255–1263.

 [98] W. Schultz, Responses of midbrain dopamine neurons to behavioral trigger stimuli in the monkey, J. Neurophysiol. 56 (1986) 1439–1461.

 [99] W. Schultz, R. Romo, Dopamine neurons of the monkey midbrain: contingencies of responses to stimuli eliciting immediate behavioral reactions, J. Neurophysiol. 63 (1990) 607–624.

[100] T. Ljungberg, P. Apicella, W. Schultz, Responses of monkey midbrain dopamine neurons during delayed alternation performance, Brain Res. 567 (1991) 337–341.

[101] J.R. Hollerman, W. Schultz, Dopamine neurons report an error in the temporal prediction of reward during learning, Nat. Neurosci. 1 (1998) 304–309.

[102] J.J. Day, M.F. Roitman, R.M. Wightman, R.M. Carelli, Associative learning mediates dynamic shifts in dopamine signalling in the nucleus accumbens, Nat. Neurosci. 10 (2007) 1020–1028.

[103] W. Schultz, P. Dayan, P.R. Montague, A neural substrate of prediction and reward, Science 275 (1997) 1593–1599.

[104] P. Waelti, A. Dickinson, W. Schultz, Dopamine responses comply with basic assumptions of formal learning theory, Nature 412 (2001) 43–48.

[105] M. Matsumoto, O. Hikosaka, Lateral habenula as a source of negative reward signals in dopamine neurons, Nature 447 (2007) 1111–1115.

[106] C.D. Fiorillo, W.T. Newsome, W. Schultz, The temporal precision of reward prediction in dopamine neurons, Nat. Neurosci. 11 (2008) 966–973.

[107] S. Kobayashi, W. Schultz, Influence of reward delays on responses of dopamine neurons, J. Neurosci. 28 (2008) 7837–7846.

[108] R.M. Church, J. Gibbon, Temporal generalization, J. Exp. Psychol. Anim. Behav. Process. 8 (1982) 165–186.

[109] R.A. Rescorla, Pavlovian conditioned inhibition, Psychol. Bull. 72 (1969) 77–94.

[110] P.N. Tobler, A. Dickinson, W. Schultz, Coding of predicted reward omission by dopamine neurons in a conditioned inhibition paradigm, J. Neurosci. 23 (2003) 10402–10410.

[111] P.N. Tobler, C.D. Fiorillo, W. Schultz, Adaptive coding of reward value by dopamine neurons, Science 307 (2005) 1642–1645.

[112] C.D. Fiorillo, P.N. Tobler, W. Schultz, Discrete coding of reward probability and uncertainty by dopamine neurons, Science 299 (2003) 1898–1902.

[113] T. Satoh, S. Nakai, T. Sato, M. Kimura, Correlated coding of motivation and outcome of decision by dopamine neurons, J. Neurosci. 23 (2003) 9913–9923.

[114] M.R. Roesch, D.J. Calu, G. Schoenbaum, Dopamine neurons encode the better option in rats deciding between differently delayed or sized rewards, Nat. Neurosci. 10 (2007) 1615–1624.

[115] G. Morris, A. Nevet, D. Arkadir, E. Vaadia, H. Bergman, Midbrain dopamine neurons encode decisions for future action, Nat. Neurosci. 9 (2006) 1057–1063.

[116] H.M. Bayer, P.W. Glimcher, Midbrain dopamine neurons encode a quantitative reward prediction error signal, Neuron 47 (2005) 129–141.

[117] H.M. Bayer, B. Lau, P.W. Glimcher, Statistics of midbrain dopamine neuron spike trains in the awake primate, J. Neurophysiol. 98 (2007) 1428–1439.

3 The ventral striatum: a heterogeneous structure involved in reward processing, motivation, and decision-making

Léon Tremblay[1], Yulia Worbe[1] and Jeffrey R. Hollerman[2]

[1]CNRS-5229-University Lyon 1, Institute of Cognitive Neuroscience, 67 Bd Pinel 69675 Bron, France
[2]Psychology Department and Neuroscience Program, Allegheny College, 520 N. Main St., Meadville, PA 16335

Abstract

This chapter reviews the evidence for the involvement of the ventral striatum in the processes of reward, motivation, and decision-making based on three principal approaches used in non-human primates. The anatomical approach has shown that the ventral striatum receives information from cortical areas implicated in the processes of reward and motivation and could take part in a heterogeneous aspect in these functions by their different ways of projections. Neuronal recordings in monkeys performing delay tasks confirmed the role of ventral striatum in the processes of reward and motivation while revealing a remarkable heterogeneity in the manner in which neuronal activity reflected these variables. Finally, the local activation of the neuronal activity clearly identified sub-territories inside ventral striatum that appear to be devoted specifically to different aspects of motivation. The convergence of these results derived from different approaches provides strong evidence of the importance of ventral striatum in the treatment of reward, motivation, and decision-making.

Key points

1. The ventral striatum is at the crossroads of neural networks that treat various aspects of reward processes and motivation.
2. Separate neuronal populations in ventral striatum, closely linked with the dopamine neurons or the orbitofrontal cortex, respectively, treat information relating to the reinforcing aspect of reward and the determination of the goal of a particular action.
3. Basic types of neuronal activity in the ventral striatum reflect the different populations in the anticipation of versus the detection of a reward or a stimulus predicting reward.

4. The role of ventral striatum in anticipation and detection of a rewarding goal for action make it important for preparing, directing, and adapting the decision-making process in a variety of contexts (e.g., familiar, novel, choice contexts).
5. Selective disturbances of subregions of ventral striatum could be at the origin of disorders of different forms of motivation (e.g., relating to food intake, sexual behavior, or avoidance-behavior).

3.1   Introduction

The role of ventral striatum in the processes of reward, motivation, and decision-making is now generally accepted based on a broad range of results coming from neuroimaging studies in humans and from local pharmacological disturbances studies in animals, mostly rats. In the rat, it was shown that the disturbance of the dopaminergic and opioid transmission in the nucleus accumbens induced compulsive behaviors such that decision-making and motivation are strictly directed towards food or drug-taking, two stimuli with strong reward properties [1–3]. This type of result has suggested to some authors that the accumbens functions largely as a hedonic structure. For others, it is a structure dedicated to processing the reinforcing aspect of reward, underlying the establishment stimulus–response or context–habit associations via procedural or instrumental learning. Finally, others regard ventral striatum as being a structure primarily implicated in the determination of the goal of an action; the "thing" that we want to obtain (food, water, sex, or "positive emotion") or to avoid (pain or "negative emotion"), as well as selecting among alternative goals and actions. In this last conception, the nucleus accumbens seems to function as an interface between motivation and action [4]. Over the past several years, a large number of neuroimaging studies have appeared, further highlighting these concepts and expanding the range of domains of reward and motivation processed by ventral striatum from variables such as food [5] and sex [6,7] to financial [8] and social [9] domains. However, while results such as these may provide additional insight into the types of variables treated by the ventral striatum, they do not show how the neurons of ventral striatum contribute to these functions. How is the basic information represented in the neuronal activity in this structure? How is this modified in a specific context of choice or decision-making? What could be the relative contribution of ventral striatum in comparison with other cerebral structures implicated in the same network and how does the ventral striatum interact with these structures?

In this chapter, we will concentrate on results from studies carried out in monkeys that enable us to understand how the ventral striatum could be involved in these various functions. We will draw primarily on results obtained from three technical approaches: (1) the study of the anatomical pathways traced by injection of classical and viral tracers, (2) the recording of neuronal activity in monkeys engaged in different behavioral tasks, and (3) the studies of behavioral effects produced by local perturbation of neuronal function within the ventral striatum. Each of these fields of research provides a complementary point of view regarding the functional position of ventral striatum relative to other structures, the kind of information processed by its neurons, and the relative implication of their activity in different domains of motivation. These results will be described in the next sections and discussed relative to the concepts mentioned previously in this introduction.

3.2   The complex anatomical organization of the ventral striatum

The anatomical approach has permitted the detailed study of afferent and efferent projections, as well as neuronal organization and neuronal connectivity within given anatomical structures. Indeed, most of our knowledge of brain connectivity has been assessed in anatomical studies on monkeys with "classic" antero- and retrograde neuronal tracers such as biotinylated dextran amine (BDA) or horseradish peroxidase (HRP) [10], complemented by recent methods of neuronal tracing with herpes simplex [11] or rabies viruses [12,13]. The main difference between these methods of neuronal tracing consists in the possibility of tracing neuronal connections across several synapses for viral tracing, whereas for the classic methods trans-synaptic transmission does not occur. Such methods have been crucial in determining the constitution of the functional neural networks involved in motor as well as non-motor brain functions such as motivation, decision-making, and reward processing.

3.2.1   The relation between the cortex and the basal ganglia: input and output

Within the basal ganglia, and in particular within the striatum, the processing of motor and non-motor information arises from the massive, topographically and functionally organized cortical projections [14–16] that provide anatomical evidence for the functional subdivision into sensorimotor, associative, and limbic territories within the basal ganglia. Some years ago, the basal ganglia was largely considered to be a motor complex in which different inputs converged to produce an output specific to the control of motor execution. At that time, the anatomical approach with classic tracers had shown that cortical regions projected to the striatum with a topographical organization in which regions could be indentified based on different functional properties, that is, the ventral striatum (limbic territory), the caudate nucleus (associative territory) and the posterior putamen (sensorimotor territory) [15–17]. However, the reduction in the number of neurons from the striatum to the output structures of basal ganglia, the internal segment of globus pallidus (GPi) and the substantia nigra pars reticulata (SNr), and the large dendrites of the neurons in these output nuclei [18,19] strongly suggested that a large functional convergence could occur at these levels of the basal ganglia circuit before the information returned to the cortex via the thalamic relay. In addition, only the basal ganglia return projections to the motor and the supplementary motor area were well described at this time, thus strengthening the view that basal ganglia was influencing exclusively motor function. It is from this viewpoint that Mogenson and collaborators [4] first suggested that the ventral striatum or nucleus accumbens is a perfect candidate to be the interface between motivation and action. The specific afferents of ventral striatum come from limbic structures such as the amygdala, the medial prefrontal, and the orbitofrontal cortex, areas well known to be involved in motivational and emotional processing. Combined with the prevailing view that the principal if not exclusive output of basal ganglia was through the motor cortex, the idea of motivation and action being integrated in the basal ganglia via the ventral striatum was compelling, and this concept continues to be expressed frequently in the literature. Nevertheless, it was never clearly demonstrated that this concept of interface between motivation and action assigned to the ventral striatum is accurate!

An alternative view of basal ganglia circuitry can be seen to have arisen from the specific investigation of the basal ganglia output pathway(s) using rabies virus (a retro-grade trans-synaptic tracer) injections inside different frontal areas. This work, done by the team of Peter Strick, provided two major new pieces of information: (1) the output of basal ganglia could go not only to the motor cortex but also to more anterior areas inside the prefrontal cortex dedicated to non-motor functions [20,21], and (2) the output pathways to the cortex are organized in different parallel circuits where different func-tional domains could be processed independently [20,22]. Although Strick's team did not study the basal ganglia projections to the orbitofrontal or the anterior cingulate cortex, their conclusions from data on other prefrontal territories strongly suggested the exist-ence of similar closed loops in which information relative to motivation originating from the orbitofrontal and/or anterior cingulate cortex would return to the same cortical areas after passing through the basal ganglia. In this way, as illustrated in Fig. 3.1A, the ventral striatum and the return pathways to these structures could specifically process motiva-tional variables without necessarily exerting a direct influence on the selection or execu-tion of action. As will be developed in the following section, this circuit could process

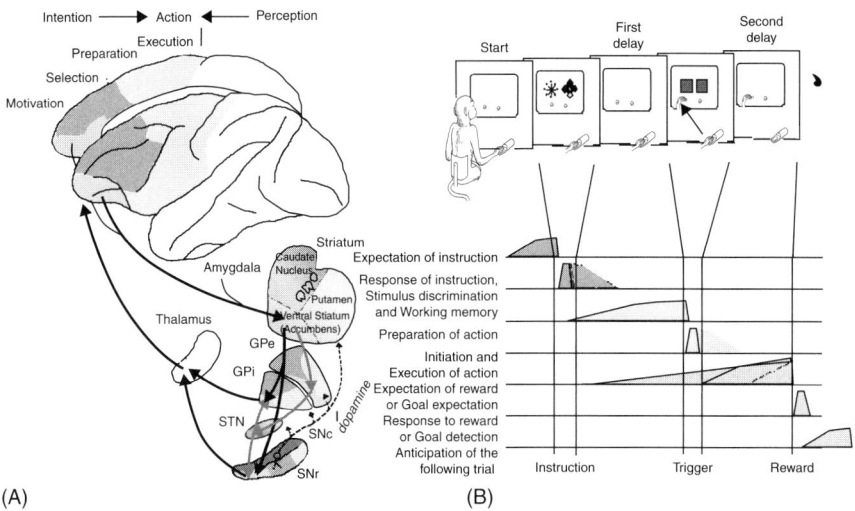

Figure 3.1 Schematic representation of the anatomical circuits of the striatum (A) and a schematic overview of the main forms of activity (B) that could be observed in the striatum when monkeys perform a delayed response and reward task. The colors purple, green, and yellow delineate ter-ritories and activities that reflect motivation, cognitive, and motor processes, respectively. Inside the striatum the territories have been characterized based on anatomical and electrophysiological inves-tigations, whereas the territories inside the two segments of the globus pallidus (internal GPi and external GPe) as well as the substantia nigra pars reticulata (SNr) are based only on anatomical investigation. Return projections to cortex are illustrated only for the limbic circuit that is presumed to be dedicated to motivation processes. The direct and indirect pathways from the ventral striatum to the output structure of basal ganglia are indicated in black and red arrows, respectively. In order not to overload the picture, some basal ganglia projections are not illustrated. All type of neuronal activities illustrated in B could be found in the striatum with a gradient that respects the striatal ter-ritories illustrated in A. See Plate 3 of Color Plate section.

only the goal aspect of the action (what do I want?) without determining the appropriate action (which action do I have to perform to obtain what I want?). As illustrated in Fig. 3.1A, a second circuit (in green in Fig. 3.1A) involving the dorsolateral prefrontal cortex and the caudate nucleus could be involved in cognitive processes for the selection of action, and a third separate circuit (in yellow in Fig. 3.1A) involving the premotor and motor cortices together with the putamen appears to be more specifically dedicated to the preparation and execution of action. In this view, at least three cortico-basal ganglia loops are implicated in the different functional processes (motivation, selection, and execution of action) involved in going from an intention to an action. The interaction between these different loops could happen at the cortical level or at the thalamic level. Indeed, the hierarchical projection from the anterior prefrontal areas to premotor and motor cortex is well known [23], and these cortico-cortical projections could provide the link between the parallel cortico-basal ganglia circuits. The other anatomical site for convergence between these different circuits would at the thalamic level. McFarland and Haber [24] had shown in monkeys that the thalamic relay nuclei that transmit basal ganglia output (the VA/VL and MD nucleus) to the frontal cortex provide not only a feedback closed loop projection, but also initiate feed-forward, open loop projections to the cortical areas involved in the different functional circuits. In this way, the circuit that passes through the ventral striatum and then returns to the cortex could specifically process the motivational variables (via return projections to the orbitofrontal and/or anterior cingulate cortex) and also indirectly influence the processes of action selection (by projection to the dorsolateral prefrontal cortex).

3.2.2   The heterogeneous projections of the ventral striatum

The ventral striatum in primates encompasses a large region including, in addition to nucleus accumbens ("classic" ventral striatum), the ventromedial caudate nucleus, and ventromedial putamen. The ventral striatum has been thus defined by the cortical projections from the medial prefrontal and orbitofrontal networks, the entorhinal cortex, and the projections from the amygdala and the hippocampus, all considered to be limbic brain areas involved in motivational and emotional processing [25–28]. Nevertheless, in monkeys, the delimitation between the dorsal and ventral striatum is not sharply defined. Although it is often assumed that the ventral striatum represents the ventral third of the anterior striatum, it is in fact not limited to the anterior striatum, but rather continues caudally to include the ventral posterior putamen. Whereas in rats there had been some difficulty in differentiating the nucleus accumbens into two distinct parts, the core and the shell [29], in monkeys, the shell is clearly distinguished from the ventral striatum (including the classically defined core) by its lack of calbindin-positive staining and its efferent projections, which further indicate that it lies outside the basal ganglia network [30].

As illustrated in Fig. 3.2 by the example of BDA injection into the monkey ventral striatum, the ventral striatum projects to the pallidal and nigral complexes. The different targets of these projections provide the means by which the ventral striatum could be engaged in different processes that pass through different pathways within the basal ganglia. The three principal targets considered here are: (1) a direct pathway projection to the medial, limbic, part of the both output structures of basal ganglia, the GPi, and the SNr; (2) an indirect pathway to the ventral part of the external segment of the globus pallidus (GPe); and (3) a specific projection to the dopaminergic neurons of the substantia nigra pars compacta (SNc).

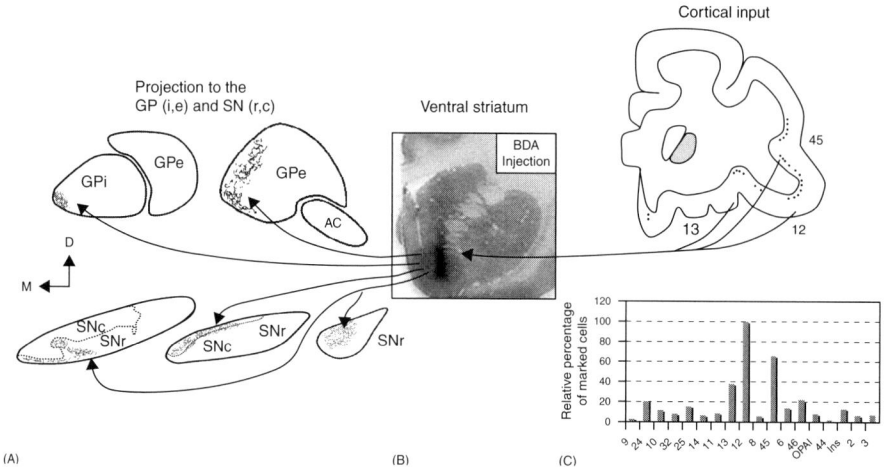

Figure 3.2 Example of BDA injection in the ventral striatum (B) that illustrate preferential afferents from areas 13, 12, and 45 of the orbitofrontal cortex (C) and the diverse targets upon which ventral striatum neurons could exert their influence (A). Terminal projections are found in both segments of globus pallidus, internal (GPi) and external segment (GPe), and in both parts of the substantia nigra pars compacta (SNc) and pars reticulata (SNr). The SNc is a structure containing primarily dopamine neurons. The SNr and GPi are the two output structures of the basal ganglia. In SNr and GPi, the labeled terminal fibers are in both cases in what is defined as limbic territory. The histogram represents the relative number of retrograde labeled cell bodies in different cortical areas.

3.2.3 The dopamine pathway

In light of the great interest in the dopaminergic neurons due to their role in Parkinson's disease, schizophrenia, drug addiction, and reward processes, this projection has received more attention than the two other projections. It is known that the ventral striatum has a direct and reciprocal connection with the dopaminergic neurons located in the substantia nigra pars compacta (SNc) and the ventral tegmental area (VTA). As showed by the team of Suzan Haber, this striatonigral projection comes mainly from the ventral striatum in primate (see review from Haber, 2003 [16], and chapter 1 in this book). In return, dopaminergic neurons project to the ventral striatum. Although this reciprocal anatomical relation between ventral striatum and the DA neurons is frequently used to attribute similar functions to these structures, it is important to note that the DA projections are not restricted to the ventral striatum, but rather target widespread regions of the striatum [16] and other basal ganglia structures [31,32].

The role of dopamine in reward processes has been and continues to be the object of the numerous studies, and the results of these studies will be specifically addressed by Tobler and Kobayashi in Chapter 2 of this book. In parallel, the impact of the loss of dopamine on the function of the basal ganglia, as seen in Parkinson's disease, has also been an important field of research for more than 20 years, a topic reviewed in a further chapter 2 of this book, by Pessiglione and Tremblay. These disparate lines of research, regarding motivation and reward on the one hand and motor function on the other, can be taken to symbolize the presumed role of dopamine in the selection of information that passes through the basal ganglia. If we could summarize one of the central principles arising from these two large domains of research concerning the DA function in the striatum, we could say that the dopamine influences striatal activity by two distinct modes of release: a tonic and a phasic mode. The tonic mode of dopamine release appears to be implicated in the passage of information through the basal ganglia, influencing the selectivity in relation to ongoing processes [33,34], whereas the phasic dopamine release is crucial for modification of functional synaptic connections and consequently for building stimulus–response or context–habit associations by procedural or instrumental learning [35–37].

Although afferent control of the dopamine neurons arises from various structures [38], the striatum is believed to be a major source. The precise function of this striatal projection to the DA neurons is not known, but some interesting ideas were proposed from computational approaches. In a context of actor–critic models that were developed to study the role of basal ganglia in the selection of action and the role of DA in reinforcement learning, it was proposed that the striatonigral projection to the DA neurons could be engaged in the regulation of the DA neuronal activity and responses to the reward signal. The neurons that project to the DA neurons are inhibitory GABAergic neurons, and thus these neurons could modulate the DA neurons' response to a reward signal in relation to the predictability of this reward signal. This supposes that the striatal neurons have reward-specific activity and that they have temporal and probabilistic information regarding the occurrence of the reward signal. We will see in the following section that some neurons within the ventral striatum effectively have these proprieties. (For more information about the actor–critic model and other hypotheses about the role of this projection, see the review by Joel et al. [39].)

A last point relative to this projection that we could mention here is relative to the organization of the striatum in the striosome (also call patch)/matrix compartment that is frequently used in the literature of computational models of the basal ganglia. In this nomenclature, the striatal neurons that compose the striatonigral projection appear to be localized in the patch compartments (striosomes), surrounded by the matrix compartment containing neurons projecting to the other basal ganglia structures (the SNr, the GPi, and the GPe) that compose the two other pathways previously mentioned, the direct and indirect pathways [40,41]. However, this organization into striosome-matrix compartments that has been described in the dorsal striatum is not consensually accepted to be characteristic of the ventral part of the striatum in monkeys [42]. Two factors in particular make it difficult to determine the presence and nature of a patch-matrix system in this part of the striatum: first, it is difficult with classic anatomical tracers to distinguish projections to the SNc from those to the SNr because these two parts of the SN are not only immediately adjacent to one another, but are interdigitated (see schematic in Fig. 3.2A, for example). Second, the histological markers originally used to characterize the patch/matrix compartments are not consistently in register and have different interrelationships in ventral versus dorsal parts of the striatum [43,44]. Further complicating the issue has been the fact that the function of these compartments is still poorly understood more than 20 years after their initial description. However, recent reports suggest that in both rodents and non-human primates, striosomes are preferentially activated in response to drug treatments that induce repetitive stereotyped behavior, suggesting a possible implication in some types of motivation disorders [45,46]. Similarly, in human patients with Huntington's disease (a neuropsychiatric disease characterized by progressive degeneration of striatal projection neurons), a significant association between pronounced mood dysfunction and differential loss of the GABA(A) receptor marker in striosomes of the striatum has been reported [47].

3.2.4   The direct and indirect pathways of the ventral striatum

As for the dorsal striatum, the neurons in the ventral striatum could project directly to the output structures of basal ganglia, the SNr, and the GPi, or indirectly via a projection to the GPe, which in turn projects to those output structures or to the subthalamic nucleus (STN), which also has projections to the output structures (see Fig. 3.1A). The existence of these direct and indirect pathways provides a form of functional organization of the basal ganglia that helps greatly to explain the hypo- and hyperkinetic symptoms of Parkinson's disease [48,49]. Substantial evidence suggests that the two pathways exert opposite control on movement, and an imbalance between the activity in the two pathways could induce the opposite motor states observed in Parkinsonian patients both with and without medication [49].

It well known that the neurons of the output structures, the GPi and the SNr, have high levels of spontaneous activity (means around 60 spikes/s) and thereby exert an constant inhibitory (GABAergic) tone on their ascending targets (thalamic neurons projecting to the cortex) or their descending targets pedunculopontine nucleus (PPN) for the GPi and Superior Colliculus (SC) for the SNr). Hikosaka and Wurtz [50] have well demonstrated in a series of elegant experiments using microinjections of GABA agonists and antagonists in monkeys trained to perform memory eye saccade tasks that the inhibitory tone of the SNr has a direct suppressive effect on the production of saccadic eye movements. Complementary results indicate that when this inhibitory tone is suppressed or inhibited, the production of saccade is facilitated. In another series of experiments performed in rats using single unit recording, Deniau and Chevalier [51,52] demonstrated that when the striatal neurons are activated, they can directly inhibit neurons in the SNr and thereby disinhibit the thalamic neurons under the tonic inhibitory influence of these SNr neurons. This disinhibition mechanism, in which a series of two inhibitions have an activating effect on the target, is particularly prominent in processing within the basal ganglia. In the case of the striatal neurons involved in the direct pathway, their activation results in a "permissive" effect on their thalamic targets by this disinhibition mechanism. In contrast, activation of the striatal neurons that project to the GPe (i.e., the indirect pathway) would lead to disinhibition of the basal ganglia output structures, producing a suppressive effect on the target neurons in the thalamus. Several authors have suggested that these dual and opposing pathways could be the substrate for the role of basal ganglia in a selection of movement [53,54]. In the motor domain attributed to the dorsal striatum, it has been suggested that activation of the direct pathway permits (via disinhibition) the execution of a desired motor program, while activation of the indirect pathway has a suppressing effect on other competing motor programs. If the same mechanism could be attributed to the ventral striatum in the domain of reward processing or motivation, the direct pathway could be engaged in the selection of a specific goal of action, while the indirect pathway suppresses other competing goals (e.g., those that are not appropriate to the current need, situation, or context). This hypothesis, based on our knowledge about the physiology and physiopathology of the dorsal striatum, is supported by studies involving local perturbations of function in the ventral striatum of behaving monkeys, as will be reviewed in the final section of this chapter.

The role of the DA neurons in reward processes has been well described, in large part due to the work of the team of Wolfram Schultz. His extensive work recording neuronal activity in behaving monkeys provides a foundation for understanding the processing of reward in the basal ganglia. On the other hand, the functional role in reward processes and motivation of the other targets of the ventral striatum (GPi, SNr , GPe, and STN) is much less well understood. Few if any researchers have performed neuronal recording in these structures in monkeys trained to perform tasks designed to study these functions. In order to determine the roles of these structures and understand their real contributions to the cortico-basal ganglia circuit, it will be necessary to record neuronal activity in those structures that received afferents from the ventral striatum and are believed to be specifically dedicated to reward and motivational function. To date, it appears that only associative and sensorimotor territories of the GPi and SNr [55–57] have been studied by neuronal recording in monkey. Within the STN, a recent study in monkeys described activity reflecting a reward signal but did not localize the neurons that express this activity in relation to the different cortico-basal ganglia circuits [58]. In the absence of any neuronal recording study in monkeys in the limbic part of the GPe, it is worth noting here that perturbation of neuronal activity in limbic GPe by microinjection of an antagonist of GABA (bicuculline) has been performed in monkeys. This study showed that abnormal behavioral activity could be induced by such perturbation, and the main manifestation of this effect was the abnormal production of licking and biting fingers, an anxiety-like behavior [59]. In rats, neuronal recording inside the ventral pallidum have indicated reward-related activity, and in this context it was suggested that the interaction between the ventral pallidum and the accumbens is important in the hedonic aspect of the food intake [60,61].

In summary, anatomical studies have placed the ventral striatum in monkeys within an organization clearly implicated in reward processes and motivation. The cortical afferents this striatal territory receives provide information that specifically concerns reward and motivational processes and, via the multiple pathways inside the basal ganglia, the neurons of the ventral striatum could direct this information to several different mechanisms linking reward processes and motivation to behavior.

3.3   Neuronal recording in monkeys

3.3.1   A tool to study the neuronal basis of reward processes, motivation, and decision-making

Most of our decisions and actions are driven by the combination of immediate or delayed expectation of reward and corresponding internal motivational factors. Numerous neuroimaging studies in human have contributed in recent years to identifying brain areas and neural networks that could be involved in specific functional processes that drive decisions and actions in both healthy subjects and in pathological contexts. Several chapters in the second part of this book will be dedicated specifically to reviewing these studies and their implications. One aspect of neuronal processing not accessible in neuroimaging studies, however, involves how information is represented at the neuronal level in the various brain areas identified by imaging, and thus what role each area plays in its functional networks. Knowledge about processing at the neuronal level comes primarily from animal studies using electrophysiological single unit neuronal recording or local pharmacological modulation of cerebral circuits. This part of the chapter is dedicated to the description of the electrophysiological studies performed in the ventral striatum of monkeys, and the following part to the recent data obtained in monkeys by local perturbation of neuronal activity in the ventral striatum. In both sections the results are discussed relative to the complementary results obtained from neuroimaging studies on humans.

Recording the activity of single neurons in identified brain structures of awake monkeys using inserted microelectrodes has been a classic approach for acquiring knowledge in diverse areas of sensory, motor, and cognitive neuroscience. In spite of tremendous advancements in the field of functional neuroimaging, electrophysiological neuronal recording retains the advantage of being a direct measure of neuronal activity with a notably better temporal definition (1 ms compared to 1 s for the most advanced functional magnetic resonance imaging [fMRI]), a crucial factor when attempting to determine relationships to transient sensory, motor, and cognitive events. Recording single neurons is, however, a time-consuming approach, as it takes time to accumulate data from sufficient numbers of neurons to have confidence that a representative sample of the structure being studied has been obtained. Even at that point, it can be argued that what the sample represents is restricted to a relatively small proportion of neurons in the structure, and that proportion could be biased by the experimental conditions. In contrast, with fMRI the entire brain can be measured virtually simultaneously in a single session, although the small size and relatively deep location in the brain of the basal ganglia has meant that these structures have frequently been omitted from analysis, especially in earlier fMRI studies.

Studies involving either recording neuronal activity in awake animals or functional neuroimaging generally are crucially dependent on the tasks used. The task is the tool for asking the neurons or the structures about their functions. Most of the initial studies of neuronal activity in the basal ganglia of monkeys focused on motor processes and used tasks designed to differentiate variables of motor behavior. In order to study processes such as reward, motivation, or decision-making, it is important to use tasks adapted to these processes, differentiating variables in these dimensions. Moreover, when studying a structure such as the striatum, where there is the suspicion that it could integrate different domains of function, it is important to account for all of these domains (motivation, cognition, and motor control) in the task to maximize interpretation of results. One classic technique that is used for isolating different variables (across or within a domain) is the insertion of a delay between different task components. This isolation of variables over time helps prevent the association of activity with one variable from confounding the interpretation of the activity as related to another variable, and to dissociate activity related to different variables.

In considering the task used to study the ventral striatum, it is important to define clearly how we are using the terms motivation, reward, and decision-making. Motivation here is defined as a driving force of goal-directed actions that translates an expectation of reward into action. Reward is then defined as an appetitive environmental event that serves as a goal for voluntary, intentional action. In this context, food, liquid, and sexual activity are considered as primary rewards. In learning processes, rewards generally function as positive reinforcers, producing an increase in the frequency of a preceding action. In addition, during learning, a stimulus that is consistently paired with an action and a primary reward can become a conditioned stimulus for the action and a predictor of the reward, as well as a potential conditioned reinforcer. This perspective on reward highlights two somewhat distinct functions: (1) reward as a goal for action and (2) reward as a learning signal – a positive reinforcer in the learning process for stimulus–reward and stimulus–response associations. Finally, decision-making is defined here as processing in which one option is selected among different competing choices.

For a simple example, consider my intention to drink water when I am working at my desk and become thirsty. There are various stimuli present in my environment that function as conditioned stimuli for a variety of actions and outcomes. From amongst those stimuli I need to select one that I know to be associated with obtaining water (if I perform the appropriate action). In this situation, the bottle of water on my desk is a more appropriate stimulus to select than my cup of coffee, or the apple also present in my desk. In other words, the bottle is the conditioned stimulus with the best predictor for obtaining water and thus reducing thirst. Having identified the bottle as the most appropriate stimulus for my desired goal, I now proceed to the selection of the appropriate actions associated with that stimulus for attaining the end goal in the past, and adapting those actions to the details of the current situation. For example, past experience has involved grasping the bottle with one hand, removing the cap with the other hand, bringing the bottle opening to my mouth, and pouring the contents in. Past experience may not have involved the precise spatial arrangement of the current environment, which would require some adaptation of the details of prior motor acts (although similar adaptations may have been necessary in similar situations in the context of other goals). Thirst provides the motivation to translate the expectation of reward (drinking water) into the actions needed to obtain and consume the water. Finally, as this action or series of actions concludes, I compare the results of my action to my expectations. If my expectations are met, that is, my thirst is sufficiently reduced, my actions will be directed toward other objects and goals. If the result of my action does not correspond to my expectations, that is, my thirst is not reduced sufficiently, I would need to identify other stimuli and actions that would produce the desired outcome. This last step would be a decision-making step involving a behavioral adaptation process at a broader level than the adaptation of the motor act mentioned above. The experience described could result in strengthening a set of associations between stimulus, action, and outcome (especially if expectations are met) or possibly weakening them (if expectation are not met, for example). Hopefully, this example with a natural, familiar context clarifies how we are conceiving reward, motivation, and the decision-making processes and also provides a framework for discussion of the task used in monkeys to explore the relationship of ventral striatal neuronal activity to these different functional domains.

The motivational domain is generally represented in tasks for monkeys by thirst or hunger, produced via mild water or food deprivation and/or the use of particularly palatable items. Delivery of liquid or food thus normally functions as the goal of actions the monkey performs. Specific stimulus–action–outcome relationships are established via training in the particular behavioral task employed. Two types of visual discrimination tasks proved to be of particular use in investigations of the ventral striatum by the team of Wolfram Schultz. In the first, a conditioned stimulus (instruction) was displayed on a computer screen and, following a delay, another stimulus (trigger, identical for all trial types) was presented, at which time the monkey had to select the action associated with the conditioned stimulus in order to obtain, after another delay, the outcome associated with that stimulus (see Fig. 3.1B). Conditioned stimuli in this task could have one of three sets of associations: (1) make a reaching action and receive a liquid reward (rewarded movement trial), (2) refrain from taking any overt action and receive a liquid reward (rewarded non-movement trials), or (3) make a reaching action as in #1 to produce an auditory stimulus and proceed to a different trial type (unrewarded movement trials).

Thus, as illustrated in the Fig. 3.1B, all trials in this task consisted of a sequence of three events (instruction, trigger, and reward) separated by two delay periods. The first period of delay helped to dissociate neuronal activity related to the discrimination and memory processes associated with the conditioned stimulus (illustrated in green in Fig. 3.1B) from activity related to executive processes engaged in the selection, preparation, and execution of the motor response (illustrated in yellow in Fig. 3.1B). This activity related to motor functions was in turn dissociated from that related to reward processes by the second delay (between the action and the outcome). The outcome, delivery of reward presentation of the auditory signal, or the absence of either (when the action was incorrect for the given instruction) was the third and last event of each trial. Trials were separated by an inter-trial delay, which proved useful in isolating reward responses from anticipatory activity for the instruction signal of the upcoming trial.

In order to assess the ways in which neurons in both dorsal and ventral striatum represented the variables involved in performing this task, monkeys were trained with a standard set of three instruction stimuli, one for each trial type, until their performance had reached a plateau [62]. In this version of the task, the monkey did not have true choice with regard to the action he would perform (if he had motivation for the associated outcome). Any decision-making about which action to execute and for which outcome presumably arose from the learned associations between stimulus, action, and outcome. In a second version of this task, a learning set version, sets of novel instruction stimuli were introduced to examine how the striatal neuronal activity was modified in a context in which the monkey was learning new associations. In this context, the behavioral and reward associations of the new instruction stimuli were unknown, and during the initial trials with new stimuli the monkey selected actions in a "trial and error" learning fashion based on the known alternatives. The learning set context thus provides a clearer decision-making context in which it was possible to study how the neurons of the ventral striatum react in context and how the neurons modify their activity as new associations are established [63,64].

A separate task was utilized to further enhance the choice, and thus decision-making, aspect of the task. In this task, two instruction stimuli were displayed simultaneously, with each stimulus associated via extensive training with a different type of liquid reward. The appropriate action for obtaining the desired reward was to reach and press a lever on the side of the screen on which the associated stimulus was presented. Thus, the monkey could receive a reward for either of two actions on any given trial, although the nature of the reward would differ depending on the action chosen. This task, initially developed to study the orbitofrontal cortex, allowed the study of neuronal activity in a context in which the monkey was engaged in a specific decision-making process guided by reward preferences [65].

3.3.2   The neuronal activity in the striatum

Generally, two main types of neurons have been identified in the striatum on the basis of their spontaneous electrophysiological activity: (1) low-activity neurons that are believed to be the medium spiny cells that compose more than 95% of all striatal neurons and (2) tonically active neurons (TANs), presumed to be the striatal cholinergic interneurons that represent around 1% of the striatal neurons. This review focuses on only the first type of neurons, which presumably represents the striatal projection neurons communicating to the targets outlined previously. Specific information relative to the role of TANs in reward processes could be found in a recent review by Apicella [66].

Recordings obtained from the low-activity neurons during performance of the standard version of the three-trial type task described above were remarkable, first, in the extensive heterogeneity of the task-related activity and, second, in their strong dependence on the reward context throughout the anterior striatum [62]. In fact, each of the events in the task could be seen to be coded by specific neurons in the anterior striatum.

As summarized in Fig. 3.1B, some neurons had activity relative to the instruction stimulus, coding action or reward associations, or both. Other neurons had activity related to the trigger signal and could relate to the action by contributing to movement preparation and execution. Finally, some neurons had activity directly related to the reward event or reinforcer, the last signal of the task. Although it was possible to observe neurons specific to each of these different events in each of the different parts of the anterior striatum studied, the distribution of neurons dedicated to different events was uneven. Neurons with activity related to the instruction signal were mainly observed in the caudate nucleus, with an increasing proportion of neurons expressing anticipatory activity in the most anterior levels. Neurons with activity related to the trigger signal, and thus potentially involved in movement preparation and execution, were more frequently observed in putamen (see also [67,68]). Finally, neurons with a direct relation to the reward, or reinforcer, signal were mainly localized in the ventral striatum (see also [69]). This functional distribution of neuronal activity matches well with fMRI studies that have shown a specific role of the ventral striatum in reward processes [70–74], the caudate nucleus in cognitive processes involved during performance of complex task [75], and the role of various territories inside the putamen in the preparation and execution of actions [76]. Moreover, we observed a larger proportion of neurons with specific activity relative to the unrewarded movement trial in the central and ventral parts of the caudate nucleus [62], which fits well with imaging studies showing a region inside the ventral striatum with an increase of signal during anticipation of aversive stimuli in humans [77].

A second general observation made of striatal activity during the performance of the standard version of the task involved the presence of two types of temporal relationships of activity to events in the task. One type was a response activity following the event and the second an anticipatory activity beginning before an event, but not time-locked to a preceding event, and continuing or even increasing until the occurrence of the anticipated event (see Fig. 3.1B). Of the population of neurons recorded [62], we observed that around one-third of neurons had only anticipatory activity, another third had only responses to events, and the final third had a combination of anticipatory activity and response to a specific event. An example of this last category of neurons is shown in Fig. 3.3A. This neuron had an anticipatory activity before the instruction and a specific response to the instruction indicating to the monkey that the current trial that his was performing required a movement that would not be rewarded. In the trials on which the instruction indicated to the monkey that a liquid reward was available (rewarded movement and non-movement trials), the anticipatory activity stopped at the appearance of the instruction and there was no response to the instruction. By separating trials based on the preceding trial type, it is apparent that this form of anticipation activity appears only after trials where the monkey was rewarded. The activity of this neuron appears to reflect what the monkey anticipated for the upcoming trial, dependent on the trial that the monkey had just performed. This is a particularly strong example of how activity that is not directly related to the reward event (i.e., anticipatory of or response to the reward) is nevertheless highly dependent on the reward context, a characteristic observed for the majority of neurons recorded in the anterior striatum, both dorsal and ventral.

3.3.3   Reward processing in ventral striatum: goal of action and reinforcer

Anticipation and detection of a predictable event in a learned context seem to be among the main functions of the striatal neurons, with the specific contribution of the ventral

(A) Expectation and response to instruction

Rewarded trial   Non-reward trial   Rewarded trial   Non-reward trial
Current trial   Trial after

Instruction trigger reward   Instruction trigger reward   Instruction trigger reward   Instruction trigger reward

(B) Modification of expectation rewardon uncertain context

Familiar

Rewarded movement   Rewarded non-movement   Unrewarded movement

Learning

23   22   21   0   1   2   23   22   21   0   1   2   23   22   21   0   1   2s

Trigger   Reward   Return   Trigger   Reward   Trigger
                     to key   return to key

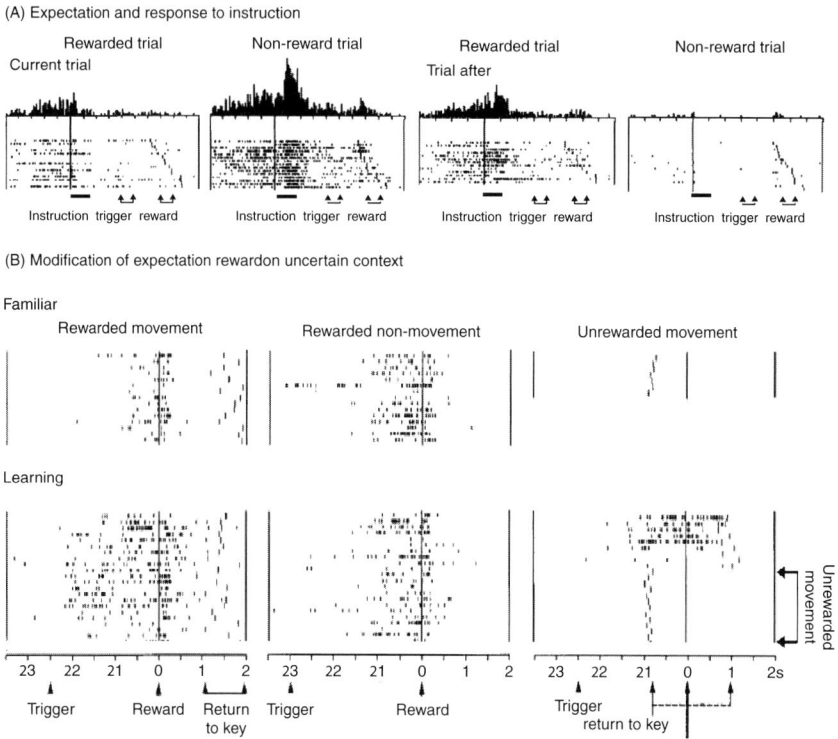

Figure 3.3 Example of ventral striatal neurons that express anticipatory activity preceding and response activity following the instruction (A) and a second ventral striatal neuron that expresses anticipatory activity preceding reward both in a familiar context and a learning context (B). In A, the neuron that responds selectively to the instruction for non-rewarded trial (see Current trial panels), also has an anticipatory activity before the instruction that is specifically expressed after trials in which the monkey received a liquid reward (see Trial after panels). In B, during a block of trials in which familiar instruction stimuli were used, activations of another striatal neuron occurred preceding reward delivery in both rewarded movement and non-movement trial types, but not preceding the auditory reinforcer in unrewarded movement trials. In a separate block of trial using novel instruction stimuli, this neuron continued to exhibit activations in rewarded movement and non-movement trials. Activations were also observed in initial unrewarded movement trials and disappeared some three trials before the animal's behavior reflected the unrewarded nature of the trial type (arrows on right indicating trials in which movement parameters differed from that on rewarded movement trials). *Source*: From Tremblay et al. (1998) [63].

striatum involving the anticipation and detection of primary rewards and conditioned stimuli associated with rewards. Indeed, within the ventral striatum, many neurons exhibit anticipatory activity preceding or response activity following food and liquid reward. An example of anticipatory activity before delivery of liquid reward is shown in Fig. 3.3B. This activity was observed in trials in which liquid reward was expected independent of whether the action required was a reaching movement or the inhibition of movement. No such activation was observed during unrewarded trials in which the monkey performed a reaching movement with the only immediate outcome being an auditory stimulus functioning as a reinforcer, albeit with potential aversive associations. This observation indicates that the activity of the ventral striatal neurons does not represent a general reinforcer signal (regardless of association) or a generic "end of trial" signal. Rather, this reward anticipatory and response activity in the ventral striatum appears to code for appetitive rewards. As stated previously, an appetitive reward could influence behavior in at least two distinct ways: it could serve as a goal for action or serve a positive reinforcement function in learning. Does the neuronal activity in the ventral striatum reflect processes for one of these functions or for both? It seems reasonable to say that the ventral striatum is involved in both processes through the action of at least two different populations of neurons; one population working in conjunction with the orbitofrontal cortex could process reward as the outcome of an action (the goal) and another one working in conjunction with the midbrain dopamine neurons could be involved in the function of reward as a reinforcer.

It is in the context of this question that the second behavioral task described above, using conditioned stimuli associated with different appetitive rewards, becomes particularly important. While the different appetitive rewards represent different specific goals of action, they both can serve the function of a positive reinforcer. As such, a neuron encoding a specific goal signal would be expected to express selective activity with regard to the different rewards, whereas a neuron providing a general reinforcer signal would presumably exhibit nonselective activity in relation to different appetitive rewards. In results paralleling those in orbitofrontal cortex [65], a subpopulation of neurons inside the ventral striatum exhibited task-related activity that discriminated between different rewards, and other neurons, as for the dopamine neurons' response, in a similar way for different reward [78,79]. Moreover, a neuron providing a reinforcer signal should be sensitive to the predictability of reward, a property clearly demonstrated for the dopamine neurons [78,79]. Although some neurons inside the ventral striatum appear to be sensitive to the predictability of reward and thus could participate in the processing of a reinforcer signal, the contribution of these striatal neurons is probably different from that of dopamine neurons. Dopamine neurons exhibit their greatest phasic responses to primary reward when reward occurrence is not predicted, and this response diminishes as reward occurrence becomes more predictable [79]. Some authors have suggested that striatal neurons projecting to the DA neurons could participate in this phasic DA response to unpredicted reward via a disinhibitory action involving interneurons in SN [80]. However, it seems more plausible that striatonigral neurons would be involved in the suppression of the DA neuron response in a predictable reward context. In this case, the striatal neurons that express anticipatory activity preceding and/or responses following predictable reward delivery could produce direct inhibitory actions on the dopamine neurons under conditions in which those neurons lose their responses to rewards. The idea that an active inhibitory process is involved in blocking these responses is consistent with reports of a depression in DA neuron activity when a predicted reward is omitted [79]. The function of these striatal neurons could be to regulate the DA response to rewards based on predictability, and thus play a crucial role in the function of rewards as reinforcers.

3.3.4   Motivation in ventral striatum: from expectation to the goal determination

As mentioned above, in addition to neurons anticipating or responding to rewards and reinforcers, other groups of neurons in the ventral and anterior striatum have activations preceding or responses to conditioned stimuli. The majority of these neurons have activity specific to the action and/or outcome associated with the stimulus in question. The example above (Fig. 3.3A) was of one such neuron that expresses specific expectation for and response to a conditioned stimulus that indicated the unrewarded trial (reaching action followed by auditory signal but no liquid reward). Again, selectivity is evident in the presence of anticipatory activity in trials following a rewarded trial and its absence in trials following a successful unrewarded trial. The latter condition was, in fact, an effective predictor of a subsequent reward associated conditioned stimulus: an unrewarded trial *never* followed a successful unrewarded trial, a restriction placed in the software controlling the task to prevent excessive frustration on the part of the monkey performing the task. As might be expected given this restriction, another group of neurons exhibited a complementary selectivity, expressing expectation for a rewarded trial after successful completion of an unrewarded trial. Because the instruction stimulus was the first stimulus presented in a trial, this anticipatory activity prior to the instruction stimulus had to be based on events in the preceding trial. Nevertheless, some neurons had expectation activity preceding instructions that appeared to be independent of the previous trial (although perhaps sensitive to other restrictions in trial sequence, such as the limit to three consecutive trials of either rewarded trial type). In any case, there are neurons in the ventral striatum that are engaged in active expectation processing, even between the researcher-defined trials. It is possible that this anticipatory activity could be an expression of the monkey's motivation. As we previously defined motivation, it is the driving force that translates an expectation into action. Indeed, this anticipatory activity could prime the system for rapidly identifying the available goal and the appropriate action for obtaining that goal. This would be consistent with the fact that a large proportion of neurons expressing anticipatory activity for conditioned stimuli also exhibit responses to the corresponding conditioned stimuli and thus could aid in their identification. Another interpretation of anticipatory activity preceding conditioned stimuli is that it is an expression of attentional processes, but it is difficult to dissociate motivation from attention, as these two processes are strongly intertwined. Motivation can act via attentional processes to increase the processing of some stimuli and/or decrease the processing of others. Unselective responses of striatal neurons to conditioned stimuli could play a role in a general increase of attention, representing an arousal signal, for example. The selective responses of other striatal neurons to conditioned stimuli, with or without selective anticipatory activity, could then be implicated in selective attention. Dissociating the relationship between striatal neuronal activity and motivation versus attention does not appear to be possible with existing data, and may not be possible using this technique. If this is at the limit of what the neuronal recording techniques can ask about processing in the ventral striatum, application of a different approach may be more useful in addressing these questions. We will return to this in the last section of this chapter, where we describe the behavioral effects on attention and motivation induced by reversible perturbation of the neuronal activity inside the ventral and dorsal components of the anterior striatum, indicating that ventral striatum appears to subserve a more motivational and the dorsal striatum a more attentional function [81].

3.3.5   *Decision-making in ventral striatum: guiding choice and building new associations*

In the standard version of the three-trial type task described above, the instruction stimuli used were well learned and the monkey simply needed to identify and execute the action appropriate to the instruction stimulus in order to obtain the associated reward or rein-forcer. The monkey did not have true choice in this context: any decision-making about the action to perform and the outcome to be obtained was based on previously learned associations. In this condition, we have seen that the ventral striatum contains neurons with specific activity related to the conditioned stimuli and to the outcomes resulting from specific behavioral actions. These neurons in the ventral striatum can be considered to anticipate and identify the goal of action, the appropriate action, and the occurrence of the associated outcome when confronted with familiar stimuli.

In the second version of this task, sets of novel instruction stimuli were introduced to examine how striatal activity was modified when the context was altered and the monkey had to learn new associations. In this learning set paradigm, the monkey was confronted with unfamiliar stimuli, albeit in a familiar context. Thus, although the potential appro-priate actions and potential outcomes were already defined, the monkey did not know which action and outcome combination was associated with which of the new instruc-tion stimuli. In this context, monkeys initially engaged in basic trial and error behavior in which the action executed and outcome anticipated could not be dictated by learned associations with the instruction stimulus. As can be seen in the example of Fig. 3.3B, during these initial trials neuronal activity reflecting expectation of liquid reward was present, as it was with the standard stimuli, although in this case it was evident in trials with each of the three novel instruction stimuli (Fig. 3.3B). This would indicate that in this uncertain context the monkey expected to receive a liquid reward for the behav-ior performed on all initial trials with new instruction stimuli. This was confirmed by the parameters of the movements executed in initial trials in comparison to trials with standard stimuli and later trials with the novel stimuli (see marker for "return to key" in movement trials in Fig. 3.3B). As the new associations were learned, reward anticipa-tory activity disappeared in the unrewarded movement trials and the behavioral marker shifted to reflect the monkey's treatment of the trial as unrewarded, although reinforced by the auditory stimulus (see Fig. 3.3B). Similar patterns of altered activity were observed for striatal neurons, with selective activity related to the conditioned stimuli [63,64]. For example, some neurons responded to all novel stimuli on initial trials, and selective activ-ity was apparent only after the monkey learned the new associations. In comparison with responses to the instruction stimuli, expectation activity preceding the conditioned stim-uli regained its selectivity more quickly. These results suggest that neurons that respond to conditioned stimuli may be more reflective of the creation of new associations for long-term memory, while the expectation activity appears to be more related to the ini-tiation of choice from amongst competing alternatives.

In the delay task involving simultaneous presentation of two instruction stimuli, each associated with a different liquid reward, the monkey could exert choice in the behavioral action based on preference. This task was used initially to study the orbitofrontal cortex, where neuronal activity could be seen to reflect reward preferences [65]. As in orbitof-rontal cortex, striatal neurons also exhibited selective activity for different rewards and the associated conditioned stimuli [78]. Some neurons coded for the preferred reward and others for the less preferred reward and, as in orbitofrontal cortex, these neurons expressed relative preference dependent on the context of the comparison [82]. Thus, neurons of the ventral striatum can provide information regarding reward preference in the context of choosing goals and actions. Moreover, in this context, where alterna-tives are simultaneously present in the two instruction signals, the activity of neurons that exhibit anticipatory activity before instructions appear would seem to be of particu-lar importance with regard to preparing and facilitating the decision-making process. In this way, selective anticipatory activity could clearly facilitate the choice by directing the monkey's action toward the preferred, or away from the non-preferred, outcome. Such expectation activity selective for conditioned stimuli was also observed in the orbitofrontal cortex [83], suggesting that this information is shared between orbitofrontal cortex and the ventral striatum.

As somewhat of an aside, the information reviewed above makes it clear that the implications of activity preceding the initial stimulus in a trial can be immense. Because it has generally been assumed that the "slate is wiped clear" between trials in a behavioral task, few studies have analyzed this type of activity in detail. A closer look at this inter-trial activity could be very beneficial in determining the role of this early anticipatory activity in preparation not only for motor action but also in preparation, or priming, of a decision-making process.

In summarizing this neuronal recording section, we could say that results from the electrophysiological approach applied in monkeys strongly support multiple roles for the ventral striatum in reward processes, motivation, and decision-making. The basic types of activity observed in ventral striatum were anticipatory activity preceding and responses following reward, or conditioned stimuli associated with reward. It is suggested that some of these neurons, working with neurons in orbitofrontal cortex, play a greater role in the identification of the goal of action, whereas other neurons are more implicated in the reinforcer role of reward through interactions with midbrain dopamine neurons. Both populations of neurons potentially could be involved in decision-making processes engaged in the face of novel conditions encountered in familiar contexts as well as in well a context in which different alternatives and preferences (or non-preferences) guide decision-making.

3.4   Dysfunction in ventral striatum and perturbation of different motivational domains

As previously defined, motivation is a driving force of goal-directed behaviors that translates an expectation of a goal into action. In this sense, motivation could be specific for initiating approach behavior for a specific kind of appetitive reward, such as food, liquid, or sex, and could be also specific for initiating avoidance behavior for specific kinds of aversive stimuli. From the standpoint of behavior, the level of motivation could be measured by different parameters, including the number of initiated actions, the speed with which the actions are performed, and the level of accuracy of the performance. As food is a highly salient appetitive stimulus with biological relevance and is an easy variable to manipulate in an experimental context, motivation for food has been a classic paradigm for studying motivation [84]. One way in which the neural basis for this form of motivation is studied is by local intracerebral pharmacological perturbation, an approach previously applied mostly in rats. Generally, a cannula is chronically implanted into the brain and fixed to the skull, enabling injection of pharmacological agents directly into the chosen anatomical structure or substructure. Observation of behavior following injections is used to draw inferences about the role of the specific target region in the behaviors based upon the specific mechanism of pharmacological perturbation. This approach has a considerable advantage over the classic lesion approach in that the perturbation produced can be of different types and can be reversible. The latter characteristic can be particularly advantageous in allowing replication of results obtained at a single site as well as comparison of effects of perturbation of different sites or using different agents in the same animal. This approach has been applied to investigation of the role of the ventral striatum (or nucleus accumbens) in food motivation using a variety of pharmacological agents (see [2,85,86]). A portion of these investigations in rodents were designed to test the hypothesis that the nucleus accumbens contains distinct ensembles of neurons that function as segregated microcircuits involved in distinct processes [87,88]. In this way, the nucleus accumbens of rats was shown to play a specific role in food motivation in addition to specific roles in food seeking and food intake [2,89]. Moreover, some studies have indicated a rostrocaudal segregation of food, or appetitive, motivation versus fear, or aversive motivation, suggesting that different territories of the ventral striatum are engaged in positive versus negative motivational factors [85,90].

Despite the potential power of such microinjection approaches to address questions regarding the role of specific cerebral regions in behavior, this approach has not been frequently utilized in non-human primates. Given the extent of cerebral evolution between rodent and primate, it seems crucial to assess the conclusions drawn from the data obtained in rodents using non-human primates in order to better understand their potential relevance to human neural function and dysfunction. Therefore, we applied this approach of intracerebral microinjection to produce a local neuronal activation (induced by bicuculline, an antagonist of GABA receptors) in different regions of the anterior and ventral striatum to determine the behavioral effects in monkeys [81]. The specificity of effects produced by microinjection into the ventral striatum was assessed using similar modification of neuronal activity induced in the dorsal striatum. The central hypothesis, drawn from the data described above, was that dorsal striatum perturbation would produce greater effects in the selection of action to execute, whereas the ventral striatum perturbation would produce its effects via motivational processes. In fact, a striking difference between the effects of microinjections in the dorsal striatum versus the ventral part of the striatum was observed. In dorsal striatum, the effects observed generally involved the production of abnormal movements or a hyperactivity state, which could suggest that this striatal territory participates in selection and preparation of movement acts. Effects of microinjection in the ventral striatum could be grouped into three different classes of abnormal behaviors, each associated with different anatomical subregions of the ventral striatum.

One class of abnormal behavior was induced after microinjections into the ventrolateral putamen on the anterior level. We have called this a hypoactivity state as it was characterized by diminished global behavioral activity and corresponding changes in behavior while performing a food retrieval task (Fig. 3.4C). These changes involved a decrease in frequency of food retrieval associated with an increase in latency to initiate choices, both parameters previously described as behavioral markers of motivational processes in Parkinsonian monkeys [91]. In contrast to Parkinsonian monkeys, the development of the hypoactivity state in our studies was associated neither with executive disorders, such as freezing or hesitation, nor with motor slowness as in bradykinesia. The association of diminished food motivation with global behavioral hypoactivity in monkeys could be compared to the apathy that has been characterized as the quantitative reduction of self-generated voluntary and purposeful behaviors [92]. Interestingly, in a recent positron emission tomography (PET) study in Parkinsonian patients with markers of both dopamine and noradrenaline transporters, binding in the ventrolateral part of the striatum was inversely correlated with apathy [93]. Moreover, in a PET study on patients with bipolar II type depression, the glucose metabolism was shown to be abnormally increased in the anteroventral putamen [94], a region similar to the one where we produced the hypoactive state in monkeys. The fact that we frequently observed in our monkeys an association between this hypoactivity state and vomiting strongly suggest a specific loss in the domain of food motivation.

Changes in behavior characterized by the arrest of food retrieval were observed after bicuculline microinjections in the most medial part of the ventral striatum, and were associated with sexual manifestations characterized by erection and ejaculation, comprising the second class of behavioral effects observed after microinjections onto the ventral striatum (Fig. 3.4A). Anatomical data in monkeys indicate that the most medial part of the head of the caudate receives projections from the medial prefrontal network, which appears to function as a sensory-visceromotor link and to be critical for guidance of reward-related behaviors and mood setting [95,96]. Thus, our data suggest that the ventromedial striatum, as a part of this medial prefrontal network, could be a node linking motivational and emotional components of sexual behavior with the peripheral autonomic component. In addition, neuroimaging studies in humans have enabled the neuronal correlates of human sexual behavior to be investigated, and in particular have demonstrated its association with limbic brain areas in general and the ventromedial striatum in particular [6,7]. This latter observation was made in a subregion of the striatum in humans similar to the one where we observed the expression of sexual behavior in our monkey model.

Finally, the third class of behaviors affected was observed after bicuculline microinjections in the central part of the ventral striatum and presented as persistent and abnormal repetition of one type of behavior, and we therefore called this class stereotyped behavior (Fig. 3.4B). It has been suggested that stereotyped behavior in monkeys could reflect a state of anxiety [97]. Moreover, the ventral striatum and especially the nucleus accumbens have been shown to be implicated in the expression and the contextual regulation of anxiety in monkeys [98]. In humans, dysfunction of the head of caudate nucleus has also been demonstrated in anxiety spectrum disorders, and particularly in obsessive-compulsive disorder (OCD) [99]. From neurobehavioral point of view, the anticipation of a negative event is a key component of anxiety and can lead to behavioral, emotional, and physiological adjustment in preparation for or prevention of aversive outcomes. The role of the ventral striatum and particularly that of the nucleus accumbens in the processing of aversive events such as pain or injections of anxiogenic drugs has been evidenced not only in animal studies [100,101], but also in human functional imaging studies [77,102,103]. Taken together, these data provide strong evidence that a part of the ventral striatum is engaged in the emotional anticipation of an aversive event and its behavioral regulation.

In conclusion, our data using local microinjections clearly confirmed the functional heterogeneity of the ventral striatum in primates, as was anticipated from rodent results. These results from monkeys implicate the ventral striatum in regulation of different aspects of motivation, from behavioral initiation – motivation to move and take food to specific sexual motivation, as well as aspects of negative motivation in contextual regulation of aversion (Fig. 3.4E). Interestingly, in contrast to data obtained in rodents, all of the different classes of effects on motivated behaviors observed in monkeys were apparent using injections at the same antero-posterior level of the ventral striatum, suggesting a mediolateral gradient for positive and negative motivation in primate, rather than the anteroposterior gradient described in rodents. This is obviously of importance when trying to apply results from these studies to humans. Future fMRI studies taking into account the potential difference in distribution of the heterogeneous striatal circuits could shed light on this issue. In addition, given what has been learned in non-human primates using the microinjection approach, it appears important now to use the two other approaches reviewed here, neuronal recording and anatomical tracing, to further

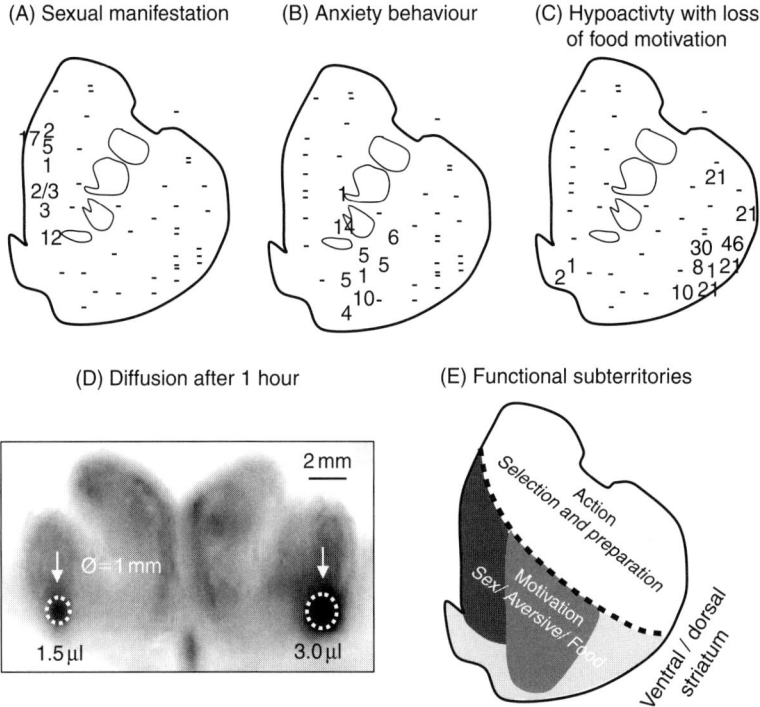

Figure 3.4 Summary of the three main effects produced by local activity perturbation induced by bicuculline injection into different locations inside the anterior ventral striatum in monkeys (A–C). Sexual manifestation (erection and ejaculation), anxiety behaviors (stereotypy), and hypoactivity with loss of food motivation were, respectively, produced with short latencies from injections in the medial, central, and lateral part of the ventral striatum. The numbers represent the latency of the effect for each injection and the dashes indicate the sites where the same effect was not observed (from Worbe et al., 2008 [81]). D shows the diffusion areas of two dye injections made into the lateral part of the ventral striatum performed 1 h before sacrifice and fixation of the brain. This gives an approximation of the bicuculline diffusion for the two volumes used in this study (1.5 μl in left and 3.0 μl in right). Neuronal recording in this zone of diffusion during bicuculline injection confirmed that the increase of local activity inside the striatum is limited to an area of 2 mm diameter around the injection side after 30 min (see Worbe et al., 2008 [81]). All injections with a behavioral effect that appeared with a latency less than 30 min were considered as local striatal effects induced by specific perturbation in the specified territory. In E, we illustrate a hypothetical representation of the anterior striatum that integrates the results of this last study in which the ventral striatum appears to be implicated in three different domains of motivation (sex, aversion, and food motivation) from the most medial to the lateral part. Similar perturbations produced by bicuculline injections inside the dorsal striatum induced mainly abnormal movements. Thus, the results of this study also clearly dissociated the role of ventral striatum in motivation processes from the role of the adjacent dorsal striatum in the selection of and preparation for action. *Source*: For A–C, from Worbe et al. (2008) [81].

characterize the specific neuronal activity within and the specific anatomical connections of these sub-territories of the ventral striatum. These future investigations will help to elucidate the role of the ventral striatum in the multiple facets of reward processing, motivation, and decision-making.

Acknowledgement

This work was supported by the Agency of National Research (ANR, France).

References

[1] R.N. Cardinal, N. Daw, T.W. Robbins, B.J. Everitt, Local analysis of behaviour in the adjusting-delay task for assessing choice of delayed reinforcement, Neural Netw. 15 (4–6) (2002) 617–634.

[2] A.E. Kelley, B.A. Baldo, W.E. Pratt, M.J. Will, Corticostriatal-hypothalamic circuitry and food motivation: integration of energy, action and reward, Physiol. Behav. 86 (5) (2005) 773–795.

[3] M. Le Moal, G.F. Koob, Drug addiction: pathways to the disease and pathophysiological perspectives, Eur. Neuropsychopharmacol. 17 (6–7) (2007) 377–393.

[4] G.J. Mogenson, D.L. Jones, C.Y. Yim, From motivation to action: functional interface between the limbic system and the motor system, Prog. Neurobiol. 14 (2–3) (1980) 69–97.

[5] J.P. O'Doherty, T.W. Buchanan, B. Seymour, R.J. Dolan, Predictive neural coding of reward preference involves dissociable responses in human ventral midbrain and ventral striatum, Neuron 49 (1) (2006) 157–166.

[6] J. Ponseti, H.A. Bosinski, S. Wolff, M. Peller, O. Jansen, H.M. Mehdorn, C. Buchel, H.R. Siebner, A functional endophenotype for sexual orientation in humans, Neuroimage 33 (3) (2006) 825–833.

[7] S. Bray, J. O'Doherty, Neural coding of reward-prediction error signals during classical conditioning with attractive faces, J. Neurophysiol. 97 (4) (2007) 3036–3045.

[8] B. Knutson, P. Bossaerts, Neural antecedents of financial decisions, J. Neurosci. 27 (31) (2007) 8174–8177.

[9] K. Izuma, D.N. Saito, N. Sadato, Processing of social and monetary rewards in the human striatum, Neuron 58 (2) (2008) 284–294.

[10] Y. Smith, M.D. Bevan, E. Shink, J.P. Bolam, Microcircuitry of the direct and indirect pathways of the basal ganglia, Neuroscience 86 (2) (1998) 353–387.

[11] M.C. Zemanick, P.L. Strick, R.D. Dix, Direction of transneuronal transport of herpes simplex virus 1 in the primate motor system is strain-dependent, Proc. Natl. Acad. Sci. USA 88 (18) (1991) 8048–8051.

[12] K.H. Taber, P.L. Strick, R.A. Hurley, Rabies and the cerebellum: new methods for tracing circuits in the brain, J. Neuropsychiatry Clin. Neurosci. 17 (2) (2005) 133–139.

[13] R.M. Kelly, P.L. Strick, Rabies as a transneuronal tracer of circuits in the central nervous system, J. Neurosci. Methods 103 (1) (2000) 63–71.

[14] G.E. Alexander, M.R. DeLong, P.L. Strick, Parallel organization of functionally segregated circuits linking basal ganglia and cortex, Annu. Rev. Neurosci. 9 (1986) 357–381.

[15] A. Parent, L.N. Hazrati, Functional anatomy of the basal ganglia. I. The cortico-basal ganglia-thalamo-cortical loop, Brain Res. Brain Res. Rev. 20 (1) (1995) 91–127.

[16] S.N. Haber, The primate basal ganglia: parallel and integrative networks, J. Chem. Neuroanat. 26 (4) (2003) 317–330.

[17] L.D. Selemon, P.S. Goldman-Rakic, Longitudinal topography and interdigitation of corticostriatal projections in the rhesus monkey, J. Neurosci. 5 (3) (1985) 776–794.

[18] J. Yelnik, Functional anatomy of the basal ganglia, Mov. Disord. 17 (Suppl. 3) (2002) S15–S21.

[19] J. Yelnik, C. Francois, G. Percheron, Spatial relationships between striatal axonal endings and pallidal neurons in macaque monkeys, Adv. Neurol. 74 (1997) 45–56.

[20] F.A. Middleton, P.L. Strick, Basal ganglia output and cognition: evidence from anatomical, behavioral, and clinical studies, Brain Cogn. 42 (2) (2000) 183–200.

[21] F.A. Middleton, P.L. Strick, Basal-ganglia 'projections' to the prefrontal cortex of the primate, Cereb. Cortex 12 (9) (2002) 926–935.

[22] F.A. Middleton, P.L. Strick, New concepts about the organization of basal ganglia output, Adv. Neurol. 74 (1997) 57–68.

[23] J.M. Fuster, The prefrontal cortex – an update: time is of the essence, Neuron 30 (2) (2001) 319–333.

[24] N.R. McFarland, S.N. Haber, Thalamic relay nuclei of the basal ganglia form both reciprocal and nonreciprocal cortical connections, linking multiple frontal cortical areas, J. Neurosci. 22 (18) (2002) 8117–8132.

[25] S.N. Haber, K. Kunishio, M. Mizobuchi, E. Lynd-Balta, The orbital and medial prefrontal circuit through the primate basal ganglia, J. Neurosci. 15 (7 Pt. 1) (1995) 4851–4867.

[26] M. Chikama, N.R. McFarland, D.G. Amaral, S.N. Haber, Insular cortical projections to functional regions of the striatum correlate with cortical cytoarchitectonic organization in the primate, J. Neurosci. 17 (24) (1997) 9686–9705.

[27] J.L. Fudge, K. Kunishio, P. Walsh, C. Richard, S.N. Haber, Amygdaloid projections to ventromedial striatal subterritories in the primate, Neuroscience 110 (2) (2002) 257–275.

[28] K. Kunishio, S.N. Haber, Primate cingulostriatal projection: limbic striatal versus sensorimotor striatal input, J. Comp. Neurol. 350 (3) (1994) 337–356.

[29] H.J. Groenewegen, C.I. Wright, A.V. Beijer, P. Voorn, Convergence and segregation of ventral striatal inputs and outputs, Ann. NY Acad. Sci. 877 (1999) 49–63.

[30] G.E. Meredith, A. Pattiselanno, H.J. Groenewegen, S.N. Haber, Shell and core in monkey and human nucleus accumbens identified with antibodies to calbindin-D28k, J. Comp. Neurol. 365 (4) (1996) 628–639.

[31] C. Francois, C. Savy, C. Jan, D. Tande, E.C. Hirsch, J. Yelnik, Dopaminergic innervation of the subthalamic nucleus in the normal state, in MPTP-treated monkeys, and in Parkinson's disease patients, J. Comp. Neurol. 425 (1) (2000) 121–129.

[32] C. Jan, C. Francois, D. Tande, J. Yelnik, L. Tremblay, Y. Agid, E. Hirsch, Dopaminergic innervation of the pallidum in the normal state, in MPTP-treated monkeys and in Parkinsonian patients, Eur. J. Neurosci. 12 (12) (2000) 4525–4535.

[33] L. Tremblay, M. Filion, P.J. Bedard, Responses of pallidal neurons to striatal stimulation in monkeys with MPTP-induced Parkinsonism, Brain Res. 498 (1) (1989) 17–33.

[34] M. Pessiglione, D. Guehl, A.S. Rolland, C. Francois, E.C. Hirsch, J. Feger, L. Tremblay, Thalamic neuronal activity in dopamine-depleted primates: evidence for a loss of functional segregation within basal ganglia circuits, J. Neurosci. 25 (6) (2005) 1523–1531.

[35] W. Schultz, Neural coding of basic reward terms of animal learning theory, game theory, microeconomics and behavioural ecology, Curr. Opin. Neurobiol. 14 (2) (2004) 139–147.

[36] A.M. Graybiel, Habits, rituals, and the evaluative brain, Annu. Rev. Neurosci. 31 (2008) 359–387.

[37] M.S. Jog, Y. Kubota, C.I. Connolly, V. Hillegaart, A.M. Graybiel, Building neural representations of habits, Science 286 (5445) (1999) 1745–1749.

[38] I.D. Smith, A.A. Grace, Role of the subthalamic nucleus in the regulation of nigral dopamine neuron activity, Synapse 12 (4) (1992) 287–303.

[39] D. Joel, Y. Niv, E. Ruppin, Actor-critic models of the basal ganglia: new anatomical and computational perspectives, Neural. Netw. 15 (4–6) (2002) 535–547.

[40] A.M. Graybiel, J.J. Canales, C. Capper-Loup, Levodopa-induced dyskinesias and dopamine-dependent stereotypies: a new hypothesis, Trends Neurosci. 23 (10 Suppl.) (2000) S71–S77.

[41] C.R. Gerfen, Molecular effects of dopamine on striatal-projection pathways, Trends Neurosci. 23 (10 Suppl.) (2000) S64–S70.

[42] S.N. Haber, N.R. McFarland, The concept of the ventral striatum in nonhuman primates, Ann. NY Acad. Sci. 877 (1999) 33–48.

[43] L.J. Martin, M.G. Hadfield, T.L. Dellovade, D.L. Price, The striatal mosaic in primates: patterns of neuropeptide immunoreactivity differentiate the ventral striatum from the dorsal striatum, Neuroscience 43 (2–3) (1991) 397–417.

[44] D.J. Holt, A.M. Graybiel, C.B. Saper, Neurochemical architecture of the human striatum, J. Comp. Neurol. 384 (1) (1997) 1–25.

[45] J.J. Canales, A.M. Graybiel, A measure of striatal function predicts motor stereotypy, Nat. Neurosci. 3 (4) (2000) 377–383.

[46] E. Saka, C. Goodrich, P. Harlan, B.K. Madras, A.M. Graybiel, Repetitive behaviors in monkeys are linked to specific striatal activation patterns, J. Neurosci. 24 (34) (2004) 7557–7565.

[47] L.J. Tippett, H.J. Waldvogel, S.J. Thomas, V.M. Hogg, W. van Roon-Mom, B.J. Synek, A.M. Graybiel, R.L. Faull, Striosomes and mood dysfunction in Huntington's disease, Brain 130 (Pt. 1) (2007) 206–221.

[48] R.L. Albin, A.B. Young, J.B. Penney, The functional anatomy of basal ganglia disorders, Trends Neurosci. 12 (10) (1989) 366–375.

[49] M.R. DeLong, Primate models of movement disorders of basal ganglia origin, Trends Neurosci. 13 (7) (1990) 281–285.

[50] O. Hikosaka, R.H. Wurtz, Modification of saccadic eye movements by GABA-related substances. I. Effect of muscimol and bicuculline in monkey superior colliculus, J. Neurophysiol. 53 (1) (1985) 266–291.

[51] J.M. Deniau, G. Chevalier, Disinhibition as a basic process in the expression of striatal functions. II. The striato-nigral influence on thalamocortical cells of the ventromedial thalamic nucleus, Brain Res. 334 (2) (1985) 227–233.

[52] G. Chevalier, S. Vacher, J.M. Deniau, M. Desban, Disinhibition as a basic process in the expression of striatal functions. I. The striato-nigral influence on tecto-spinal/tecto-diencephalic neurons, Brain Res. 334 (2) (1985) 215–226.

[53] J.W. Mink, The basal ganglia: focused selection and inhibition of competing motor programs, Prog. Neurobiol. 50 (4) (1996) 381–425.

[54] P. Redgrave, T.J. Prescott, K. Gurney, The basal ganglia: a vertebrate solution to the selection problem? Neuroscience 89 (4) (1999) 1009–1023.

[55] T. Wichmann, H. Bergman, P.A. Starr, T. Subramanian, R.L. Watts, M.R. DeLong, Comparison of MPTP-induced changes in spontaneous neuronal discharge in the internal pallidal segment and in the substantia nigra pars reticulata in primates, Exp. Brain Res. 125 (4) (1999) 397–409.

[56] O. Hikosaka, K. Nakamura, H. Nakahara, Basal ganglia orient eyes to reward, J. Neurophysiol. 95 (2) (2006) 567–584.

[57] M. Sato, O. Hikosaka, Role of primate substantia nigra pars reticulata in reward-oriented saccadic eye movement, J. Neurosci. 22 (6) (2002) 2363–2373.

[58] Y. Darbaky, C. Baunez, P. Arecchi, E. Legallet, P. Apicella, Reward-related neuronal activity in the subthalamic nucleus of the monkey, Neuroreport 16 (11) (2005) 1241–1244.

[59] D. Grabli, K. McCairn, E.C. Hirsch, Y. Agid, J. Feger, C. Francois, L. Tremblay, Behavioural disorders induced by external globus pallidus dysfunction in primates: I. Behavioural study, Brain 127 (Pt. 9) (2004) 2039–2054.

[60] A.J. Tindell, K.S. Smith, S. Pecina, K.C. Berridge, J.W. Aldridge, Ventral pallidum firing codes hedonic reward: when a bad taste turns good, J. Neurophysiol. 96 (5) (2006) 2399–2409.

[61] K.S. Smith, K.C. Berridge, Opioid limbic circuit for reward: interaction between hedonic hotspots of nucleus accumbens and ventral pallidum, J. Neurosci. 27 (7) (2007) 1594–1605.

[62] J.R. Hollerman, L. Tremblay, W. Schultz, Influence of reward expectation on behavior-related neuronal activity in primate striatum, J. Neurophysiol. 80 (2) (1998) 947–963.

[63] L. Tremblay, J.R. Hollerman, W. Schultz, Modifications of reward expectation-related neuronal activity during learning in primate striatum, J. Neurophysiol. 80 (2) (1998) 964–977.

[64] W. Schultz, L. Tremblay, J.R. Hollerman, Changes in behavior-related neuronal activity in the striatum during learning, Trends Neurosci. 26 (6) (2003) 321–328.

[65] L. Tremblay, W. Schultz, Relative reward preference in primate orbitofrontal cortex, Nature 398 (6729) (1999) 704–708.

[66] P. Apicella, Leading tonically active neurons of the striatum from reward detection to context recognition, Trends Neurosci. 30 (6) (2007) 299–306.

[67] R. Romo, E. Scarnati, W. Schultz, Role of primate basal ganglia and frontal cortex in the internal generation of movements. II. Movement-related activity in the anterior striatum, Exp. Brain Res. 91 (3) (1992) 385–395.

[68] W. Schultz, R. Romo, Role of primate basal ganglia and frontal cortex in the internal generation of movements. I. Preparatory activity in the anterior striatum, Exp. Brain Res. 91 (3) (1992) 363–384.

[69] W. Schultz, P. Apicella, E. Scarnati, T. Ljungberg, Neuronal activity in monkey ventral striatum related to the expectation of reward, J. Neurosci. 12 (12) (1992) 4595–4610.

[70] B. Knutson, G.W. Fong, C.M. Adams, J.L. Varner, D. Hommer, Dissociation of reward anticipation and outcome with event-related fMRI, Neuroreport 12 (17) (2001) 3683–3687.

[71] B. Knutson, J.C. Cooper, Functional magnetic resonance imaging of reward prediction, Curr. Opin. Neurol. 18 (4) (2005) 411–417.

[72] J.P. O'Doherty, R. Deichmann, H.D. Critchley, R.J. Dolan, Neural responses during anticipation of a primary taste reward, Neuron 33 (5) (2002) 815–826.

[73] M. Ernst, E.E. Nelson, E.B. McClure, C.S. Monk, S. Munson, N. Eshel, E. Zarahn, E. Leibenluft, A. Zametkin, K. Towbin, J. Blair, D. Charney, D.S. Pine, Choice selection and reward anticipation: an fMRI study, Neuropsychologia 42 (12) (2004) 1585–1597.

[74] R.A. Adcock, A. Thangavel, S. Whitfield-Gabrieli, B. Knutson, J.D. Gabrieli, Reward-motivated learning: mesolimbic activation precedes memory formation, Neuron 50 (3) (2006) 507–517.

[75] S. Lehericy, E. Bardinet, L. Tremblay, P.F. Van de Moortele, J.B. Pochon, D. Dormont, D.S. Kim, J. Yelnik, K. Ugurbil, Motor control in basal ganglia circuits using fMRI and brain atlas approaches, Cereb. Cortex 16 (2) (2006) 149–161.

[76] E. Gerardin, J.B. Pochon, J.B. Poline, L. Tremblay, P.F. Van de Moortele, R. Levy, B. Dubois, D. Le Bihan, S. Lehericy, Distinct striatal regions support movement selection, preparation and execution, Neuroreport 15 (15) (2004) 2327–2331.

[77] J. Jensen, A.R McIntosh, A.P. Crawley, D.J. Mikulis, G. Remington, S. Kapur, Direct activation of the ventral striatum in anticipation of aversive stimuli, Neuron 40 (6) (2003) 1251–1257.

[78] O.K. Hassani, H.C. Cromwell, W. Schultz, Influence of expectation of different rewards on behavior-related neuronal activity in the striatum, J. Neurophysiol. 85 (6) (2001) 2477–2489.

[79] J.R. Hollerman, L. Tremblay, W. Schultz, Involvement of basal ganglia and orbitofrontal cortex in goal-directed behavior, Prog. Brain Res. 126 (2000) 193–215.

[80] W. Schultz, Predictive reward signal of dopamine neurons, J. Neurophysiol. 80 (1) (1998) 1–27.

[81] Y. Worbe, N. Baup, D. Grabli, M. Chaigneau, S. Mounayar, K. McCairn, J. Feger, L. Tremblay, Behavioral and movement disorders induced by local inhibitory dysfunction in primate striatum, Cereb. Cortex (2008) Published December 9.

[82] H.C. Cromwell, O.K. Hassani, W. Schultz, Relative reward processing in primate striatum, Exp. Brain Res. 162 (4) (2005) 520–525.

[83] L. Tremblay, W. Schultz, Reward-related neuronal activity during go-nogo task performance in primate orbitofrontal cortex, J. Neurophysiol. 83 (4) (2000) 1864–1876.

[84] J.S. Morris, R.J. Dolan, Involvement of human amygdala and orbitofrontal cortex in hunger-enhanced memory for food stimuli, J. Neurosci. 21 (14) (2001) 5304–5310.

[85] K.C. Berridge, Motivation concepts in behavioral neuroscience, Physiol. Behav. 81 (2) (2004) 179–209.

[86] A. Jean, G. Conductier, C. Manrique, C. Bouras, P. Berta, R. Hen, Y. Charnay, J. Bockaert, V. Compan, Anorexia induced by activation of serotonin 5-HT4 receptors is mediated by increases in CART in the nucleus accumbens, Proc. Natl. Acad. Sci. USA 104 (41) (2007) 16335–16340.

[87] C.M. Pennartz, H.J. Groenewegen, F.H. Lopes da Silva, The nucleus accumbens as a complex of functionally distinct neuronal ensembles: an integration of behavioural, electrophysiological and anatomical data, Prog. Neurobiol. 42 (6) (1994) 719–761.

[88] P. O'Donnell, et al., Modulation of cell firing in the nucleus accumbens, Ann. NY Acad. Sci. 877 (1999) 157–175.

[89] A.E. Kelley, Ventral striatal control of appetitive motivation: role in ingestive behavior and reward-related learning, Neurosci. Biobehav. Rev. 27 (8) (2004) 765–776.

[90] S.M. Reynolds, K.C. Berridge, Fear and feeding in the nucleus accumbens shell: rostrocaudal segregation of GABA-elicited defensive behavior versus eating behavior, J. Neurosci. 21 (9) (2001) 3261–3270.

[91] M. Pessiglione, D. Guehl, C. Jan, C. Francois, E.C. Hirsch, J. Feger, L. Tremblay, Disruption of self-organized actions in monkeys with progressive MPTP-induced Parkinsonism: II. Effects of reward preference, Eur. J. Neurosci. 19 (2) (2004) 437–446.

[92] R. Levy, B. Dubois, Apathy and the functional anatomy of the prefrontal cortex-basal ganglia circuits, Cereb. Cortex 16 (7) (2006) 916–928.

[93] P. Remy, M. Doder, A. Lees, N. Turjanski, D. Brooks, Depression in Parkinson's disease: loss of dopamine and noradrenaline innervation in the limbic system, Brain 128 (Pt. 6) (2005) 1314–1322.

[94] L. Mah, C.A. Jr. Zarate, J. Singh, Y.F. Duan, D.A. Luckenbaugh, H.K. Manji, W.C. Drevets, Regional cerebral glucose metabolic abnormalities in bipolar II depression, Biol. Psychiatry 61 (6) (2007) 765–775.

[95] D. Ongur, J.L. Price, The organization of networks within the orbital and medial prefrontal cortex of rats, monkeys and humans, Cereb. Cortex 10 (3) (2000) 206–219.

[96] H. Barbas, S. Saha, N. Rempel-Clower, T. Ghashghaei, Serial pathways from primate prefrontal cortex to autonomic areas may influence emotional expression, BMC Neurosci. 4 (2003) 25.

[97] C. Lutz, A. Well, M. Novak, Stereotypic and self-injurious behavior in rhesus macaques: a survey and retrospective analysis of environment and early experience, Am. J. Primatol. 60 (1) (2003) 1–15.

[98] N.H. Kalin, S.E. Shelton, A.S. Fox, T.R. Oakes, R.J. Davidson, Brain regions associated with the expression and contextual regulation of anxiety in primates, Biol. Psychiatry 58 (10) (2005) 796–804.

[99] J. Riffkin, M. Yucel, P. Maruff, S.J. Wood, B. Soulsby, J. Olver, M. Kyrios, D. Velakoulis, C. Pantelis, A manual and automated MRI study of anterior cingulate and orbito-frontal cortices, and caudate nucleus in obsessive-compulsive disorder: comparison with healthy controls and patients with schizophrenia, Psychiatry Res. 138 (2) (2005) 99–113.

[100] G. Schoenbaum, B. Setlow, Lesions of nucleus accumbens disrupt learning about aversive outcomes, J. Neurosci. 23 (30) (2003) 9833–9841.

[101] K. Yanagimoto, H. Maeda, The nucleus accumbens unit activities related to the emotional significance of complex environmental stimuli in freely moving cats, Neurosci. Res. 46 (2) (2003) 183–189.

[102] L. Becerra, H.C. Breiter, R. Wise, R.G. Gonzalez, D. Borsook, Reward circuitry activation by noxious thermal stimuli, Neuron 32 (5) (2001) 927–946.

[103] S.M. Tom, C.R Fox, C. Trepel, R.A. Poldrack, The neural basis of loss aversion in decision-making under risk, Science 315 (5811) (2007) 515–518.

4 Role of the primate lateral prefrontal cortex in integrating decision-making and motivational information

Masataka Watanabe

Department of Psychology, Tokyo Metropolitan Institute for Neuroscience, 2-6 Musashidai, Fuchu, Tokyo 183-8526, Japan

Abstract

The lateral prefrontal cortex (LPFC) plays important roles in both cognition and motivation. The LPFC appears to receive reward information regarding the reward prediction error, stimulus value, and action value, from the midbrain, limbic, and striatum as well as orbital and medial prefrontal areas; it also appears to play important roles in integrating reward information with task-related cognitive information for adaptive goal-directed behavior. When a monkey expects a more preferred reward, cognitive-control–related LPFC neuronal activity is enhanced, and the animal is led to correctly and efficiently perform the task. Monkey LPFC neurons are also concerned with integrating information regarding the previous response with its outcome (reward or no reward), and this integration is considered to lead the monkey to make decisions that would be advantageous in obtaining future rewards, and to learn the stimulus–response contingencies more efficiently.

Key points

1. Primate lateral prefrontal cortex (LPFC) neurons show reward (and/or absence of reward) expectancy-related as well as reward-dependent tonic baseline activity.
2. The LPFC neurons show post-trial outcome (reward and no-reward)-related activity.
3. The LPFC is concerned with the integration of motivational and cognitive information.
4. The LPFC plays important roles in outcome-dependent explicit decision-making.
5. The LPFC is also concerned with reward-related implicit decision-making.

4.1 Introduction

The lateral prefrontal cortex [LPFC, consisting of lateral aspects of Brodman's area (BA) 8, 9, 10, 44, 45, and 46 in the human] plays important roles in higher-order cognitive control, such as planning, behavioral inhibition, set shifting, and decision-making [1–4].

However, this area of the brain is also important for motivational operations, such as processing reward information [2,5,6]. Recently, there has been considerable interest in the interaction between cognition and motivation. The accuracy of performance increases and the reaction time (RT) decreases when a more preferred reward is expected as a response outcome during cognitive tasks. Primate LPFC neurons demonstrate reward-related activities as well as reward-induced modulation of activities concerned with cognitive control [7].

In this chapter, I will describe neuronal bases of motivational operations in primate LPFC (consisting of lateral parts of Walker's [8] areas 8, 9, 10, 12, and 46) and then will discuss the interaction between cognition and motivation, focusing on neuronal mechanisms of the interaction between decision-making and reward. Thus, I will first describe (1) neuronal activity related to the anticipation of the presence or absence of reward during the waiting delay period as well as reward-dependent tonic baseline activity, and then describe (2) post-trial outcome-related neuronal activity. Then I will discuss (3) the roles of the LPFC in the integration of motivational and cognitive information. Thereafter, I will focus on neuronal mechanisms of interaction between decision-making and reward. There, I will first describe (4) LPFC neuronal activity related to perceptual decision-making and forced choice discrimination, and then describe (5) LPFC neuronal activity related to outcome-dependent decision-making and (6) reward-related implicit decision-making and possible roles of the LPFC in this process. Finally, I will describe (7) multiple brain areas that are concerned with processing the reward, and discuss functional relationships between the LPFC and other reward-related areas in reward processing and decision-making.

4.2   Reward-related sustained neuronal activity in the LPFC

Here I first describe reward expectancy-related LPFC neuronal activity. Behavioral experiments indicate that the monkey expects not simply a reward in general, but rather a specific reward (or no reward) during the task performance [9]. We examined delay-related neuronal activity in the primate LPFC during a working memory (WM) task (spatial delayed-response task) [10] using several different rewards. In this task, the monkey sat facing a panel with right and left rectangular windows, right and left circular keys, and a holding lever below them (Fig. 4.1A).

The monkey initially depressed the lever for several seconds (*Pre-Inst*). Then an instructional red light was presented on the right or left key for 1 s (*Inst*). After a delay of 5 s (*Delay*), this was followed by a "go" signal (*Go Signal*) consisting of white lights on both keys, and the monkey was required to respond (*Resp*) to the cued side. Correct responses were rewarded with food, which was prepared behind the opaque window (*Reward*).

Figure 4.1 Reward expectancy-related LPFC neuronal activity and monkey's behavior during the delayed response task. (A) Sequence of events in the spatial delayed-response task. (B) An example of a reward expectancy-related LPFC delay neuron. (C) An example of a reward expectancy-related LPFC delay neuron with WM-related activity. (D) An example of reward expectancy and WM-related LPFC neuron that showed cue-related activity that differed in magnitude between the preferred (grape juice) and non-preferred (water) rewards. For B, C, and D, neuronal activity is shown separately for each reward block in raster and histogram displays, with left-sided displays for the left trials and right-sided displays for the right trials. For each display, the first two vertical lines from the left indicate the instruction onset and offset, and the third line indicates the end of the delay period. Each row indicates one trial. The reward used is indicated. The leftmost scale indicates impulses per second and the time scale at the bottom

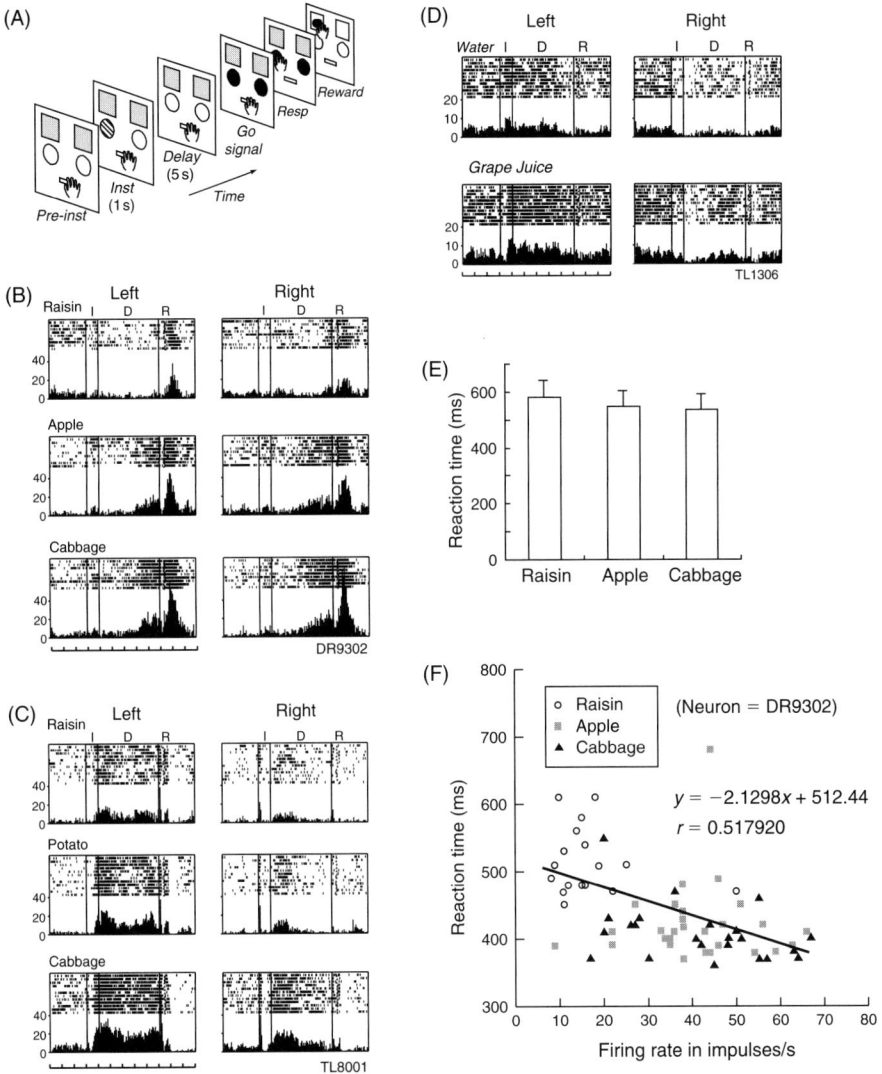

Figure 4.1 (*Continued*)
represents 1 s. Only data from correct trials are shown. Neuron numbers are indicated at the bottom right. (E) Reaction times in different reward blocks in one animal during performance of the spatial delayed response task. Error bars indicate quartile deviations. Statistical analyses indicated significant differences in RT between raisin and other reward trials, but there was no significant difference between apple and cabbage reward trials. (F) Scatter plots showing the relationship between the magnitude of delay-related firings (of both right and left trials) in a reward expectancy-related neuron (shown in Fig. 4.1B) and the animal's RT. Each symbol represents the data of each trial in each block of reward trials (raisin, apple, and cabbage). Abbreviations: (A) *Inst*, instruction; *Pre-Inst*, pre-instruction; *Resp*, response; (B, C, and D) D, delay; I, instruction; R, response. *Source*: For A–C, from Watanabe (1996) [10]; for D, from Watanabe et al. (2005) [33]; and for E, from Watanabe et al. (2001) [36].

Pieces (approximately 0.5 g) of raisin, sweet potato, cabbage, or apple were used as food rewards. The same reward was used for a block of about 50 trials, so the monkey would know the current reward after one or two trials. Figure 4.1B shows an example of an LPFC neuron with differential delay activity depending on the reward used in each block of trials; the highest firing rate was detected for cabbage (the most preferred reward) and the lowest firing rate was detected with raisins (the least preferred reward). As there was no external signal representing the reward information during the delay period, the differential delay activity in this neuron appeared to be related to the expectancy of different types of reward. Similar reward expectancy-related LPFC neuronal activities have been reported in the oculomotor-type delayed response task [11–15].

Monkeys in the wild are not always able to expect a reward and sometimes would anticipate the absence of reward as the response outcome. We also examined the delay-related neuronal activity in the primate LPFC in relation to the anticipation of the absence of reward during a non-WM task (delayed reaction task with reward and no reward) [16]. In this experiment, the monkey faced a panel on which a rectangular window, a circular key, and a holding lever were arranged vertically (Fig. 4.2A and 2B).

The monkey initially depressed the lever for several seconds (*Pre-Inst*). Then a 1-s color instruction (*Inst*) on the key indicated whether a reward would be delivered (red predicted a reward while green predicted no reward). After a delay of 5 s (*Delay*), a white light appeared on the key as a go signal (*Go Signal*). When the monkey pressed the key (*Resp*) after the go signal, the opaque window opened and the animal either collected the food reward (reward trials) or went unrewarded (no-reward trials), depending on the trial type (Fig. 4.2A). The same types of food reward were used as during the delayed-response task. Drops (approximately 0.3 ml) of water, sweet isotonic beverage, orange juice, or grape juice were also used as liquid rewards, which were delivered through a tube close to the mouth of the monkey (Fig. 4.2B). Reward and no-reward trials were alternated pseudo-randomly. The monkey was required to press the key even in no-reward trials in order to advance to the next trial. The same reward was used for a block of about 50 trials. The monkey was not required to perform any differential operant action related to differences between rewards.

In this experiment as well, many reward expectancy-related neurons were identified. Figure 4.2C shows an example of an LPFC neuron that showed a significantly higher firing rate during the delay period in reward compared to no-reward trials for any type of reward block. On reward trials, this neuron showed significantly different activity changes depending on the reward block, with increased firing rates when the more preferred reward was used. Figure 4.2D shows an example of an LPFC neuron that showed activity changes in relation to the anticipation of an absence of reward. Thus, this was active only during the delay period in no-reward trials. In this type of trial, despite the fact that the outcome of the

Figure 4.2 Reward and absence-of-reward expectancy-related LPFC neuronal activity and monkey's behavior during the delayed reaction task. (A and B) Sequence of events in the delayed reaction task with reward and no reward (A, food reward; B, liquid reward). (C) An example of a reward expectancy-related LPFC delay neuron that showed differential activity not only between reward and no-reward trials but also between different reward blocks. (D) An example of an absence-of-reward expectancy-related LPFC delay neuron that showed differential activity between different reward blocks in no-reward trials. (E) An example of an LPFC neuron showing differential activity depending on the reward block, not only during the instruction and delay periods, but also during the pre-instruction period. For C, D, and E, the upper panel indicates the reward trials while the lower panel indicates the no-reward trials. The first and second vertical lines indicate the onset and offset of the 1-s Instruction presentation,

(A)

Food reward

(B)

Liquid reward

Pre-inst | Inst | Delay signal (5 s) | Go signal | Resp | Reward (No reward)

Time

(F)

Reward
No reward

Reaction time (ms)

800
600
400
200
0

Water Isotonic Grape

(C)

Reward expectancy

Raisin | D Reward | Potato | D Reward | Cabbage | D Reward

20
10
0

No reward

20
10
0

TL4003

(G)

○ Water
▪ Isotonic
▲ Grape

(Neuron = SL8704)

Reaction time (ms)

1500
1200
900
600
300

$y = -0.6096x + 885.88$
$r = -0.04871$

0   10   20   30   40   50

Firing rate in impulses/s

(D)

Anticipation of the absence of reward

Water | D Reward | Isotonic | D Reward | Grape | D Reward

20
10
0

No reward

20
10
0

SL8704

(E)

Reward-dependent baseline activity

Raisin | D Reward | Potato | D Reward | Cabbage | D Reward

20
10
0

No reward

20
10
0

TL2701

(H)

After reward
After no-reward

Impulses/s

12
10
8
6
4
2
0

Raisin Potato Cabbage

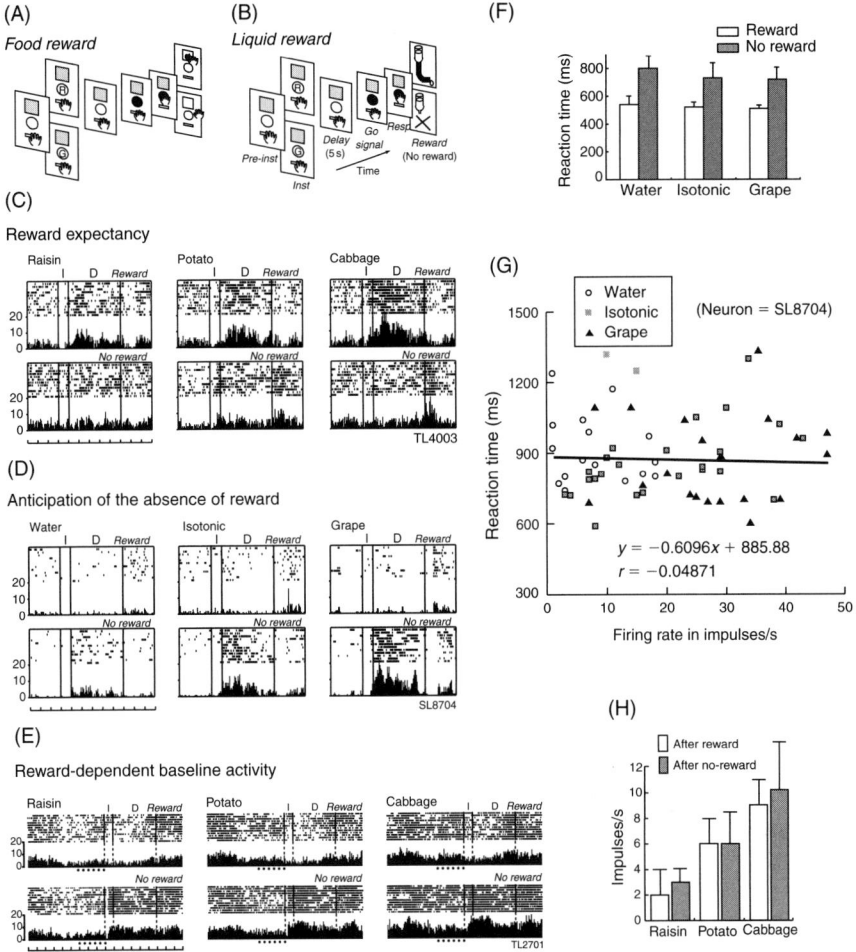

Figure 4.2 (Continued)

while the third vertical line indicates the time of the Go signal presentation. In E only, activity is shown from 9 s before the Instruction presentation to 3 s after the Go signal presentation. (F) Reaction times in different reward blocks in one animal during performance of the delayed reaction task with reward and no reward. Error bars indicate quartile deviations. Statistical analyses indicated significant differences in RT between reward and no-reward trials as well as between any two reward blocks on both reward and no-reward trials. (G) Scatter plots showing the relationship between the magnitude of firings during the delay period on no-reward trials for the neuron shown in Fig. 4.2D and the animal's RT. In this figure, each symbol represents the data of each trial in each block of reward trials (water, isotonic, and grape juice reward). Correlation coefficient within each block of reward trials was −0.20591, +0.22004, and −0.3051 for water, isotonic, and grape juice reward, respectively. (H) Magnitude of pre-instruction activity observed after reward and after no-reward trials for each reward block. Abbreviations: (A and B) G, green light cue; R, red light cue; (C, D and E) No reward, no-reward trials; Reward, reward trials. Neuron numbers are indicated at the bottom right. Other conventions are the same as in Fig. 4.1. Source: For A–E, from Watanabe et al. (2002) [16]; for F, from Watanabe et al. (2001) [36].

response by the monkey was the same (no reward), the LPFC neuron showed an increased firing rate when a more preferred reward was used; the highest firing rate occurred when the monkey anticipated an absence of grape juice (most preferred), and the lowest firing rate was seen when the monkey anticipated an absence of water (least preferred).

In order to correctly anticipate the response outcome, reward information should be monitored continuously during task performance. Our data show that LPFC neurons are involved in this process with their reward-discriminative tonic baseline activities [16]. Figure 4.2E shows an example of an LPFC neuron that showed differential pre-instruction baseline activity depending on the difference in the reward used in each block of trials. Thus, this neuron showed the highest firing on the cabbage reward block and the lowest firing on the raisin reward block during the pre-instruction period. (This neuron also showed absence-of-reward expectancy-related activity after the instruction cue presentation, despite the fact that the same color cues were used as the instruction on any reward block.) It should be noted that the magnitude of pre-instruction activity after reward trials did not significantly differ from that after no-reward trials, even though taste stimuli were different (Fig. 4.2H).

Baseline neuronal activity in the primate LPFC is reported to be modified by the monkey's arousal level [17]. Hasegawa et al. [18] reported LPFC neurons whose pre-cue activity reflected the monkey's performance level in the past trial, or predicted the performance level in the future trial, but not in the present trial. Such activity is considered to reflect the monkey's motivational or arousal level. The pre-instruction baseline activity observed in our experiment may also be related to the monkey's motivational level since the monkey may be more motivated on preferred than on non-preferred reward blocks (the monkey preferred cabbage to potato to raisin).

4.3   Coding the response outcome in prefrontal neurons

It is important for the monkey to code the outcome of the response, in order to make an appropriate decision concerning whether it should keep or change the current response strategies. In primate LPFC neurons, four kinds of post-trial activity change are observed: (1) non-selective reward-related, (2) reinforcement-related, (3) error-related, and (4) end-of-the-trial-related [19]. (1) Non-selective reward-related neurons show activity changes whenever the food or liquid reward is delivered to the subject irrespective of whether it is given during or outside the task situation. (2) Reinforcement-related neurons show activity changes only when the reward is given subsequent to the animal's correct response and do not show activity change to reward delivery outside the task situation. (3) Error-related neurons show activity changes when the animal commits an error and the reward is not given to the animal. (4) End-of-the-trial-related neurons show activity changes whenever the trial ends, irrespective of whether the animal responds correctly, and irrespective of whether the animal obtains the reward. This type of neuron is considered to be involved in coding the "termination of the trial."

Figure 4.3A shows an example of an error-related LPFC neuron observed during a delayed Go/No-go discrimination task. This neuron showed activation when the animal committed an error and could not obtain the reward. Reinforcement- and error-related neurons are considered to be concerned with coding the congruence with or deviation from the expectancy; reinforcement-related neurons may be involved in coding the congruence between expectancy and response outcome, whereas error-related neurons may be involved in coding the incongruence or mismatch between expectancy and outcome. Some neurons have combined characteristics of the second and the third types, showing a

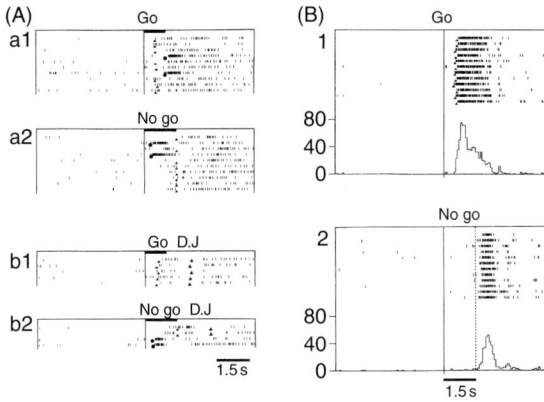

Figure 4.3 Reward- and error-related LPFC neuronal activities during the delayed Go/No-go task. (A) An example of an LPFC error-related neuron observed in the Go/No-go discrimination task. a1 and a2 denote the activity of the neuron when the reward was given immediately after the animal's correct response. b1 and b2 denote the activity of the same neuron when the reward was given 1.5 s after the animal's correct response ("D.J" indicates delayed juice delivery 1.5 s after the animal's correct response). The animal had to perform a key-release response within 1 s ("Go period") on Go trials, but had to continue depressing the hold lever for 1.5 s ("No-go period") on No-go trials after the end of the delay period. Neuronal activity is shown in raster display. a1 and b1 are for Go trials and a2 and b2 are for No-go trials. The center line indicates the end of the delay period when the imperative stimulus was presented, indicating the time when the animal should perform a Go or No-go response depending on the previously presented cue. The animal was informed of the correctness of the response by the turn-off time of the imperative stimulus, independent of the presence or absence of the reward. Horizontal black bars under headings of Go and No Go indicate 1 s of "Go period" and 1.5 s of "No-go period," respectively. Small, filled triangles indicate the time of the animal's Go correct response on Go trials and the end of the No-go period (1.5 s after the end of the delay period) on No-go correct trials. Large, filled triangles in b1 and b2 indicate the time of the delayed juiced reward delivery. Filled circles indicate the time when the animal committed an error, when the animal did not release the hold lever within 1 s of Go period, and when the animal released the hold lever too early, that is, within 1.5 s of the No-go period. This neuron showed activation when the animal committed an error, but did not show activation even when the reward was not given immediately after the correct response. (B) An example of an LPFC reward-related neuron that responded differently after Go and No-go correct responses despite the fact that the same amount of juice reward was given to the animal. The task situation is the same as explained above. Neuronal activity is shown in raster and histogram displays. The upper display (1) shows correct Go trials and the lower display (2) shows correct No-go trials. The center line indicates the end of the delay period. The dotted line on No-go trials indicates the time of the end of the No-go period. This neuron did not show any detectable activity change when the reward was omitted after the animal's correct Go response. Thus, the difference in post-trial activities after correct Go and No-go responses was not considered due to the simple summation of reward-related activity and response-related activity. *Source*: For A, from Watanabe (1989) [19]; for B, from Watanabe (2002) [7].

different magnitude of or reciprocal (increased versus decreased) activity changes between reinforced and error trials [19]. It was also found that most of these reinforcement- and/or error-related LPFC neurons did not respond to the delivery or omission of reward during the classical conditioning situation [20]; when a conditional stimulus (CS) of 1 s tone was associated with the unconditional stimulus (UCS) of a drop of juice, they did not respond to the delivery or omission of juice, indicating that their activity was dependent on the operant task situation.

Reinforcement- and error-related LPFC neurons have also been observed in other task situations [21–23]. The majority of error-related neurons show similar activity changes when the reward is omitted after the animal's correct response as well as when the animal commits an error and no reward is given. Such neurons may be called "error- and reinforcement omission-related neurons." However, in the task situation where the animal was informed of the correctness of the response, some error-related neurons showed activity changes only when the animal committed an error, and did not show activity change when the reward was omitted following the animal's correct response. The neuron shown in Fig. 4.3A showed clear activation when the animal recognized that it had committed an error in both the immediate reward delivery (a1 and a2) and delayed reward delivery (b1 and b2) situations. However, it did not show activation when the reward delivery was delayed by 1.5 s and the reward was not given immediately after the animal's correct response (b2), nor when the reward was omitted following the animal's correct response (not shown in the figure). Such correctness-related neurons may play especially important roles in guiding the animal during future behavior involving the decision as to whether current behavioral strategies should be maintained or not. Thus, there are two kinds of reinforcement- and/or error-related neurons; one kind is related to coding the reinforcement itself or its omission, and the other kind is apparently related to coding the correctness of the response.

4.4   Integration of motivational and cognitive information in prefrontal neurons

The LPFC receives not only sensory and cognitive information from the posterior association cortices, but also a variety of motivational information from the limbic system [1,2]. Thus, it is not surprising to find LPFC neurons where motivational and cognitive information interact. I have already described LPFC neurons that were related to reward expectancy (Fig. 4.1B). In the LPFC, there are also many neurons that show cognitive control-related activity [2,3]. Furthermore, there are neurons that are related to both

---

Figure 4.4 Modulation of WM-related LPFC activity by both positive and negative motivation. (A) Sequence of task situation. The monkey faced a video monitor. A trial was initiated when the animal fixated on a point presented at the center of the monitor. After 500 ms, a cue was presented at the center instructing the reinforcement condition. Then a peripheral target flashed (200 ms) at one of two possible positions, indicating the future location of the saccade. After a delay period (1–2 s), the central cue disappeared, which signaled the animal to make a saccade to the instructed position. Instruction regarding behavioral outcomes was given using one of two sets of cues (geometric figures/typographic characters) in one block of trials. In the rewarded trials, correct responses were followed by a liquid reward, but error responses were not followed by an air-puff. In the aversive trials, correct responses were not followed by a liquid reward, but error responses were followed by an air-puff. In sound-only trials, responses were followed by feedback sounds. The three trial types were given randomly, instructed by geometric figures or typographic characters. (B and C) Examples of LPFC neurons with WM-related activities (spatially differential activity) modulated by reward expectancy (B) and expectancy of the omission-of-aversive-stimulus (C). For B and C, raster and line-graph displays are shown for each target direction (right or left) and each reinforcement type (rewarded, sound only, and aversive). The schema on the left indicates the geometric figure and typographic character presented on the screen to denote the behavioral outcome. The vertical lines in the display indicate the time of target onset (left) and saccade onset (right). *Source*: From Kobayashi et al. (2006) [13].

(A)

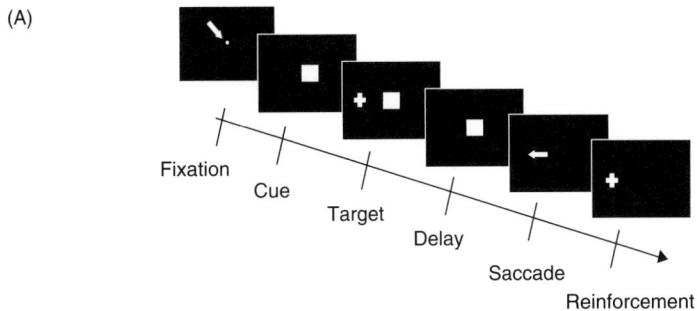

Fixation

Cue

Target

Delay

Saccade

Reinforcement

(B)

Left   Right

Target on   Sac on   Target on   Sac on

Rewarded

Sound only

Aversive

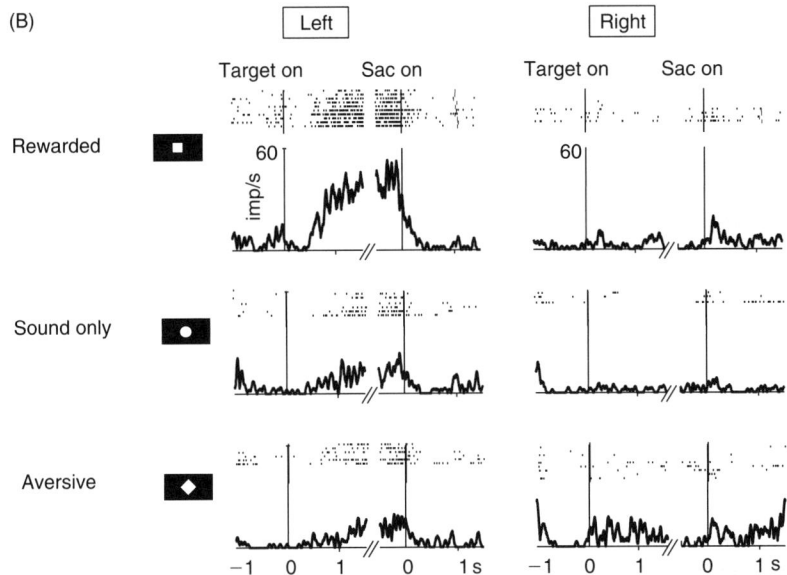

(C)

Target on   Sac on   Target on   Sac on

Rewarded

Sound only

Aversive

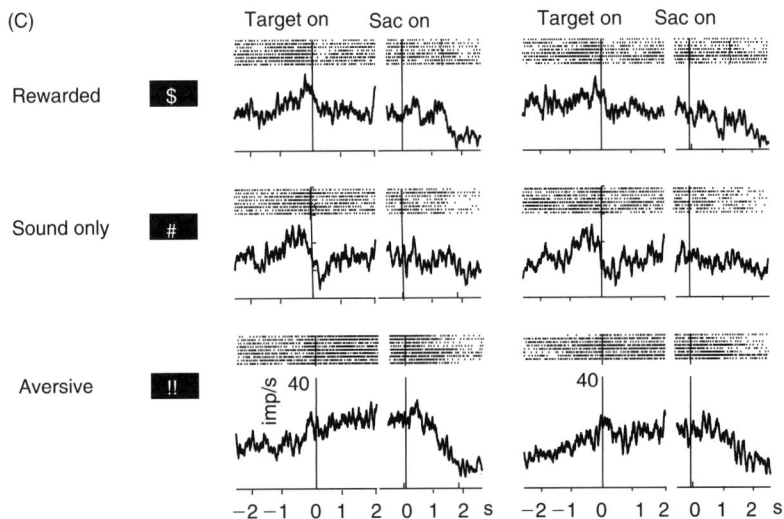

reward expectancy and cognitive control. In our study in the spatial delayed-response task, many LPFC neurons showed WM-related (spatially differential delay) activity. The majority of these showed modulation of WM-related activity depending on the different rewards. For example, the WM-related LPFC neuron pictured in Fig. 4.1C showed a higher firing rate during left, compared to right, trials and also showed increased firing for trials with more preferred, compared to less preferred, rewards [10]. Similarly, Leon and Shadlen [11] have indicated that a larger reward enhances WM-related activity in primate LPFC neurons during the oculomotor delayed response task. Such enhancement of neuronal activity induced by a larger reward may facilitate correct task performance in the discrimination task. Conversely, Kobayashi et al. [12] showed that anticipation of the absence of reward suppressed WM-related LPFC activity.

Although the effects of positive reinforcement on cognitive control have been investigated in several studies, the effects of negative reinforcement on cognitive control have rarely been examined at the neuronal level. In order to examine how LPFC neurons would process aversive information, and to compare the effects of reward and punishment in cognitive control-related LPFC neuronal activity, we trained monkeys on a memory-guided saccade task in three reinforcement conditions (reward, punishment, and sound only) (Fig. 4.4A) [13].

The monkey's performance was best in the reward condition, intermediate in the punishment condition, and worst in the sound-only condition. The majority of task-related neurons showed cue- and/or delay-related activity that was modulated only by reward (Fig. 4.4B), while activity of other neurons was modulated only by punishment (Fig. 4.4C), although the number of punishment-modulated neurons was much smaller than that of reward-modulated neurons. Activities of some neurons were modulated by both positive and negative reinforcers (that is, neurons reflecting general reinforcement or attention processes), but the number of such neurons was much smaller than that of reward-modulated neurons. The results suggest that information on reward and punishment is processed differentially in the LPFC, and the two kinds of information appear not to be integrated within the LPFC.

Interaction between cognition and motivation is observed not only during the delay period but also during the pre-cue and cue periods in primate LPFC neurons. In a study by Kobayashi et al. [24], monkeys were trained on an oculomotor-type delayed response task. In this task, one cue position was associated with reward delivery while the other cue position was not (monkeys were rewarded only when the eye movement response was directed to one predetermined position, but not when it was directed to the alternative position). The position that was associated with reward delivery was changed about every 60 trials without explicitly indicating the change to the monkey.

They found LPFC neurons that showed pre-cue baseline activity in relation to both the cognitive and motivational context. Thus, some neurons showed higher firing rates during the pre-cue period in the context of reward on the left, and other neurons, in the context of reward on the right. Furthermore, they found those LPFC neurons that coded the cue stimulus depending on both the cognitive and motivational context; these neurons showed differential activity to the same (directional) cue depending on the context of which direction (cognitive context) was associated with reward delivery (motivational context). Thus, some neurons showed higher firing rates to the same left cue presentation in the context of reward on the left than in the context of reward on the right.

Integration of cognitive and motivational information in LPFC neuronal activity is also observed after the response of the animal. For example, some reward- and reinforcement-related neurons showed differential activity to a reward delivery of the same kind and of the same magnitude after different responses (Go and No-go) (Fig. 4.3B). In such neurons, there was an interaction between motivational (presence or absence of reward) and cognitive (what task situation the animal was faced with or what behavioral response the animal had performed) information. Such neurons may be involved in coding the consequence of Go and No-go responses separately and thus may be involved in facilitating learning and performance of the discrimination task.

Similarly, during the oculomotor delayed response task, Tsujimoto and Sawaguchi [25] found LPFC neurons that showed post-response activity representing both the response outcome (reward or no reward) and the direction of the completed saccade response. Furthermore, in their subsequent study involving both memory- and sensory-guided saccade tasks [26], each of which had two outcome conditions (reward and no reward), they found that post-response activity of LPFC neurons was modulated by three factors: (1) the direction of the immediately preceding response, (2) its outcome (reward or non-reward), and (3) information type (memory or sensory) that guided the response. Such neuronal coding may play a role in associating response-outcome with information used to guide behavior – and these neurons may play important roles in guiding the monkey to acquire and perform the discrimination task more efficiently.

4.5 Prefrontal neurons related to perceptual decision-making and forced choice discrimination

Decision-making refers to a process of selecting a particular action from a set of alternatives. Perceptual decision-making is a situation where the subject is asked to make a decision in relation to whether the stimulus is presented or not, or whether the presented stimulus is A or B. Neuronal activity in relation to the monkey's perceptual decision-making has been examined in many brain areas such as middle temporal area (MT), medical superior temporal area (MST), lateral prefrontal, and posterior parietal areas [27–31]. Here I will introduce an experiment [32] in which LPFC neurons were examined in relation to perceptual decision-making.

The monkey was required to judge the direction (rightward or leftward) of random dot motion and to indicate its judgment of direction by making appropriate eye movements. The animal was required to make difficult judgments near the psychophysical threshold, and the neuronal response in the LPFC was found to be comprised of a mixture of high-level oculomotor signals and weaker visual sensory signals that reflected the strength and direction of motion. This combination of sensory integration and motor planning was interpreted to reflect the conversion of visual motion information into a categorical decision about the direction of motion. The neural response predicted the monkey's subsequent gaze shift – hence its judgment of direction – even when the motion strength was negligible, as in the 0% coherent motion condition. Although monkeys performed the task and made the decision in order to obtain the reward, the correct response was always reinforced with the same reward and the influence of reward information on perceptual decision-making-related neuronal activity was not examined.

The (two-alternative) forced-choice discrimination is another kind of decision-making situation. One example is the spatial delayed response task, in which the animal must decide whether it should respond to the right or to the left. In our study, we found that decision-related neuronal activity was modulated by the reward [33]. The neuron displayed in Fig. 4.1D showed more activity changes when the spatial cue was presented on the left side, regardless of the reward used. The magnitude of activity changes became larger when the reward was changed from less-preferred water to more-preferred grape juice. It appears that a more preferred reward facilitates discrimination task performance by enhancing decision-related LPFC activity.

4.6   Outcome-dependent decision-making and prefrontal neurons

Besides the above described (1) perceptual judgment situation and (2) two-alternative forced-choice discrimination situation, there are other kinds of decision-making situations, such as (3) the self-control situation (e.g., whether to respond immediately to obtain a small reward or to respond slowly to obtain a large reward), (4) the gambling game situation (e.g., whether to select a high probability–small or low probability–large alternative), and (5) a competitive zero-sum game between two participants.

In the former two situations (1) and (2), only one action is correct and the reward is usually set constant, while in the latter three situations, no unique action is correct and the organism is required to make a choice between or among the alternatives based on its own preference. Recently, neuronal activities have been examined in task situations where no unique response is correct and the subject makes a decision based on its preference. For example, Lee and his colleagues examined LPFC neuronal activity in relation to the monkey's outcome-dependent decision-making [34,35]. In their task, monkeys played a game analogous to matching pennies against a computer in an oculomotor choice task. The animal was rewarded when it selected the same target as the computer. Monkeys played the game under three different conditions depending on the algorithm the computer employed: algorithm 0, 1, and 2. In algorithm 0, the computer selected its targets randomly regardless of the animal's choice behaviors. Under this condition, the animal was rewarded in roughly 50% of the trials when responding mostly to one side (here the rightward target). In algorithms 1 and 2, the computer was programmed to minimize the animal's reward using statistical data reflecting the animal's choice behavior. In algorithm 1, the computer opponent analyzed the animal's choices in all the previous trials of a given session and tested whether the animal displayed any systematic biases in its choice sequence – for example, in relation to whether the animal tended to alternate between the two targets in successive trials. Here, the animal was required to choose the two targets equally often and independently across successive trials. In response, the animal was more likely to choose the same target as in the previous trial after it was rewarded and to switch to the other target otherwise (a win-stay, lose-shift strategy). When spontaneously employing this strategy, the animal was rewarded in roughly half of the trials.

In the more sophisticated algorithm 2, the computer considered the monkey's rewards on previous trials as well as its choices. This negated the win-stay, lose-shift strategy and caused the animals to choose in a truly random manner, as if choice was governed by the unpredictable toss of a weighted coin, and monkeys' average frequency of choosing the two targets resulted in a 50/50 split.

The authors recorded neuronal activity from the monkey LPFC while algorithm 2 was running. They identified those neurons that reflected (1) the monkey's choice on the preceding trial, (2) its outcome (reward or not), and (3) the conjunction between the two. These neurophysiological data are interpreted to indicate that the LPFC plays important roles in integrating the response and its outcome to lead the animal to make a decision that would be more advantageous to obtain the reward in future trials.

4.7   Implicit decision-making and prefrontal neuronal activity

Besides the decision-making situations described above, there are other situations where monkeys are induced to do some implicit decision-making, for example (1) between responding and not responding, (2) between responding correctly and responding incorrectly, and (3) between responding with a short RT and responding with a long RT. Here, I describe behavioral manifestations of the monkey's implicit decision-making and discuss the possible roles of reward-related LPFC neurons in such implicit decision-making.

In our experiments on the delayed response task as well as delayed reaction task with reward and no reward (Figs. 4.1 and 4.2), monkeys sometimes did not respond within the predetermined time limit of 2 s after the go signal presentation. This occurred predominantly when the monkey became satiated and the non-preferred reward or absence of reward was anticipated. For the animal to obtain the maximum amount of rewards within the limited time period during the daily experiment, the best strategy was to respond correctly on all (kind of reward or no-reward) trials. However, monkeys sometimes were inclined to refrain from responding when the outcome was not attractive. In the oculomotor delayed response task situation, the monkey must maintain eye fixation until the time of the eye movement response. In this task situation also, fixation breaks sometimes occur when the less preferable reward is expected. In the study by Tsujimoto and Sawaguchi [26] using the oculomotor delayed response task with large and small rewards, the proportion of fixation break was 5% in small reward trials while there was almost no fixation break in large reward trials. The high proportion of fixation breaks in small reward trials may be induced by the animal's reluctance to continue the trial, and thus by the animal's implicit decision-making of refraining from completing the trial.

The implicit decision-making is also demonstrated by the correct performance rate. In the oculomotor delayed response task with reward and no-reward trials, Kobayashi et al. [12] showed that the correct performance rate was 94.5% in reward-present and 88.8% in reward-absent condition, respectively. It should be noted that it is more advantageous for the monkey to respond correctly on both reward-present and reward-absent trials in order to obtain more rewards, since the next reward trial never comes when the monkey does not correctly complete the current no-reward trial. However, monkeys appear to have been induced to make implicit decisions not to eagerly perform the task correctly.

Furthermore, the implicit decision-making is demonstrated in the monkey's RT during both the delayed response task and delayed reaction task with reward and no-reward conditions. To obtain the reward much earlier and more often, the monkey should respond as fast as possible on all reward and no-reward trials. However, the monkey's RT was significantly shorter when the monkey could expect a more preferred reward than when it could expect a less preferred (including the absence of) reward (Figs. 4.1E and 4.2F) [36]. Interestingly, the RT on no-reward trials also differed depending on the reward block (which reward would be delivered on reward trials) although the monkey could not expect any reward in no-reward trials (Fig. 4.2F). Here again, anticipation of the seemingly less preferred outcome appears to have induced the animal's implicit decision-making to respond slowly.

When the more preferred reward was used during the delayed response task, the RT of the animal was shorter (Fig. 4.1E) and the majority of reward expectancy-related LPFC neurons showed greater activity changes (e.g., Fig. 4.1B and 4.1C). It appears that larger firings induce shorter RT. Indeed, in some LPFC neurons, weak but significant correlations were found between the monkey's RT and magnitude of firings during the delay period (e.g., Fig. 4.1F). However, even for the neuron shown in Fig. 4.1B, when the correlation coefficient was calculated between the firings and animal's RT within each block with a different reward, there was no or only a very weak correlation obtained ($r = -0.19363$, $+0.034864$ and -0.36535 for raisin, apple, and cabbage rewards, respectively). Therefore, it was not possible to predict the animal's RT in each trial from the delay-related firing within each block of reward trials, although mean firing was significantly larger (Fig. 4.1B) and mean RT was significantly shorter (Fig. 4.1E) when a more preferred reward was used in a block of trials. For other types of neurons, such as the absence-or-reward expectancy-related neuron shown in Fig. 4.2D, there was no correlation at all between delay-related firing and RT within no-reward trials, while mean firing was significantly larger (Fig. 4.2D) and mean RT was significantly shorter (Fig. 4.2F) in no-reward trials when a more preferred reward was used in a block of trials.

These findings indicated that there is no direct relationship between the LPFC neuronal activity and the animal's RT. Thus, different from explicit decision-making situations where the monkey's response (i.e., go right or go left) could be predicted almost perfectly from the LPFC activity during the waiting period, implicit decision-making is considered not to be directly supported by the LPFC. It may be that motivational factors from the limbic system play more significant roles in such implicit decision-making. If the short-term attractiveness of withholding the response or responding with a prolonged RT is much higher than the attractiveness of responding with a short RT for the monkey, such implicit decision-making may be supported by orbitofrontal cortex (OFC) neurons that reflect the relative outcome preference [37,38]. Further studies are needed to clarify which areas of the brain are more directly concerned with this process, and which role the LPFC plays in such implicit decision-making.

4.8   Decision-making and multiple reward signals in the primate brain

Information about rewards is processed in neurons of many brain areas. Neurons that detect the delivery of rewards are considered to provide information about the motivational value and identity of encountered objects. This information might be used to construct neuronal representations concerning the expectancy for future reward. And expected rewards may influence neuronal activities related to the behavior that leads to the rewards.

The midbrain dopamine neurons in the substantia nigra pars compacta and ventral tegmental area play key roles in the representation of reward by projecting axons to other reward-related brain areas, such as the ventral and dorsal striatum, limbic structures, and prefrontal cortex. Dopamine neurons report reward prediction error (mismatch between the reward expectancy and the actual outcome) and seem to emit alerting, enhancing, and plasticity-inducing effects on neurons in the striatum and prefrontal cortex [39]. Dopamine neurons are insensitive to the nature of the reward, which is coded by striatal and prefrontal neurons.

Neurons in the dorsal and ventral striatum are concerned with the detection of rewards as well as reward-predicting stimuli, and show activity changes during the expectation of rewards. They discriminate between reward and no reward as well as between different kinds or different magnitudes of rewards [40]. In striatal neurons, not only the reward but also the movement toward the reward are represented, and reward expectancy influences movement preparation [39]. For example, Hikosaka and his colleagues trained monkeys in the oculomotor type delayed response task, where the amount of reward was unequal among possible target positions, so that only one direction was associated with reward. Similar to LPFC neurons, striatal neurons had delay-related directional selectivity, and their selectivity was enhanced or depressed depending on the expected outcome. In some striatal neurons, the reward modulation was so strong that the neurons' original direction selectivity was shifted or even reversed [41]. These findings suggest that the striatum plays significant roles in representing the value of the action (action value) in relation to which action leads to certain reward.

Although the amygdala has been well documented to process aversive stimuli for survival [42], neurons of the primate amygdala are also indicated to show reward-related activity [43]. However, delay-related activity in this brain area is not directly concerned with cognitive control, but appears to be more concerned with arousal or attention [44].

In the anterior cingulate (ACC), OFC, and LPFC, there are also neurons that show activity changes in relation to the detection of reward and reward-predicting stimulus as well as in relation to the reward expectancy. These neurons also discriminate between reward and no reward as well as between different rewards [45]. The OFC is intimately connected with the amygdala [46] and is concerned with processing not only positive but also negative stimuli. A recent study has indicated the importance of the OFC in coding the value of good in a choice situation [47]. In this experiment, the subjective values of different rewards were determined by finding a balance point at which the monkey was faced with a choice between certain units of one kind of (i.e., preferred) reward and certain units of another kind of (i.e., non-preferred) reward so that the value of each reward could be assigned based on a kind of common currency. Some OFC neurons were found to code the value of the chosen item. This experiment indicates that the OFC plays important roles in value assignment underlying economic choice. The other experiment indicates that reward-predicting activity of the OFC is also modulated by the length of the delay until reward delivery, suggesting the role of this area in encoding the delay-discounted value for each target [48]. These results indicate that the OFC plays important roles in decision process by coding the value of the choice object, although the OFC has not been shown to be concerned with the action value.

The ACC neurons not only respond to post-trial events (reward and error) but also demonstrate reward expectancy-related activity [49]. There are neurons in the ACC that reflect not just expected reward but also progress through a course of actions toward the reward, as successive actions predict the same future reward but less future incurred cost [50]. The ACC is suggested to be involved in combining information about the costs and benefits associated with alternative actions, and thus in decision-making in relation to which action would lead to an economically more valuable reward [51]. Matsumoto et al. [52] recorded neurons from the monkey ACC and found activity changes in relation to both the object value and action value of the cue. Seo et al. [53] showed that some ACC neurons reflected information about the history of the monkey's past choices as well as the history of reinforcement for at least three previous trials. By integrating the animal's choice and reinforcement history with the current cue information, the ACC may play important roles in comparing values associated with different actions and in making more advantageous decision-making. Neurons in the cingulate motor area of the frontal cortex appear to play critical roles in internal decision processes for movements based on the assessment of reward value regarding the response outcome. These neurons are selectively active when monkeys switch to a different movement in situations where performing the current movement would lead to less reward [54]. These activities do not occur when movements switch after an explicit trigger, nor with reward reduction without movement switch. These data suggest a role for the cingulate motor area in transferring action value to actual movement.

Neurons in the posterior parietal area show stronger task-related activity when monkeys choose larger or more frequent rewards over smaller or less frequent rewards in situations involving a choice between different rewards [55]. Since parietal neurons are not responsive to reward *per se*, modulation of cognitive control-related activity in parietal neurons may be attained by receiving information from the ACC, where both object and action values are represented [52], as well as from the LPFC, where integration of cognitive and motivational information is attained [6].

In summary, different neuronal systems play different roles for adaptive behavior directed toward rewards. Midbrain dopamine neurons code reward prediction errors and may send an alert signal to allow rapid behavioral reactions toward rewarding events. OFC and striatal neurons are concerned with coding the object value and action value, respectively. ACC neurons appear to be involved in coding both the object and action value as well as being involved in the value-based selection of appropriate action. The LPFC is mutually interconnected with all of these three areas. In the LPFC, cognitive and motivational operations appear to be integrated, and the LPFC might use reward information to prepare, plan, sequence, and execute behavior directed toward the acquisition of more advantageous outcomes. Neuronal activity of the LPFC has only recently begun to be examined during the decision-making situation where no unique response is correct and the choice is determined by the animal's preference. Future studies will clarify how object and action values coded by the OFC, striatum, and ACC are used in the LPFC, where motivational and cognitive information is integrated for goal-directed behavior.

References

[1] D.T. Stuss, D.F. Benson, The Frontal Lobes, Raven Press, New York, 1986.

[2] J.M. Fuster, The Prefrontal Cortex Anatomy, Physiology and Neuropsychology of the Frontal Lobe, third ed., Lippincott-Raven, New York, 1997.

[3] E.K. Miller, J.D. Cohen, An integrative theory of prefrontal cortex function, Annu. Rev. Neurosci. 24 (2001) 167–202.

[4] P.S. Goldman-Rakic, H. Leung, Functional architecture of the dorsolateral prefrontal cortex in monkeys and humans, in: D.T. Stuss, R.T. Knight (Eds.), Principles of Frontal Lobe Function, Oxford University Press, New York, 2002, pp. 85–95.

[5] M. Watanabe, Cognitive and motivational operations in primate prefrontal neurons, Rev. Neurosci. 9 (1998) 225–241.

[6] M. Watanabe, M. Sakagami, Integration of cognitive and motivational context information in the primate prefrontal cortex, Cereb. Cortex 17 (2007) 101–109.

[7] M. Watanabe, Functional architecture of the dorsolateral prefrontal cortex in monkeys and humans, in: D.T. Stuss, R.T. Knight (Eds.), Principles of Frontal Lobe Function, Oxford University Press, New York, 2002, pp. 326–337.

[8] A.E. Walker, A cytoarchitectural study of the prefrontal area of the macaque monkey, J. Comp. Neurol. 73 (1940) 59–86.

[9] O.L. Tinklepaugh, An experimental study of representation factors in monkeys, J. Comp. Psychol. 8 (1928) 197–236.

[10] M. Watanabe, Reward expectancy in primate prefrontal neurons, Nature 383 (1996) 629–632.

[11] M.I. Leon, M.N. Shadlen, Effect of expected reward magnitude on the response of neurons in the dorsolateral prefrontal cortex of the macaque, Neuron 24 (1999) 415–425.

[12] S. Kobayashi, J. Lauwereyns, M. Koizumi, M. Sakagami, O. Hikosaka, Influence of reward expectation on visuospatial processing in macaque lateral prefrontal cortex, J. Neurophysiol. 87 (2002) 1488–1498.

[13] S. Kobayashi, K. Nomoto, M. Watanabe, O. Hikosaka, W. Schultz, M. Sakagami, Influences of rewarding and aversive outcomes on activity in macaque lateral prefrontal cortex, Neuron 51 (2006) 861–870.

[14] K. Amemori, T. Sawaguchi, Contrasting effects of reward expectation on sensory and motor memories in primate prefrontal neurons, Cereb. Cortex 16 (2006) 1002–1015.

[15] S. Ichihara-Takeda, S. Funahashi, Activity of primate orbitofrontal and dorsolateral prefrontal neurons: effect of reward schedule on task-related activity, J. Cogn. Neurosci. 20 (2008) 563–579.

[16] M. Watanabe, K. Hikosaka, M. Sakagami, S. Shirakawa, Coding and monitoring of motivational context in the primate prefrontal cortex, J. Neurosci. 22 (2002) 2391–2400.

[17] J.C. Lecas, Prefrontal neurons sensitive to increased visual attention in the monkey, NeuroReport 7 (1995) 305–309.

[18] R.P. Hasegawa, A.M. Blitz, N.L. Geller, M.E. Goldberg, Neurons in monkey prefrontal cortex that track past or predict future performance, Science 290 (2000) 1786–1789.

[19] M. Watanabe, The appropriateness of behavioral responses coded in post-trial activity of primate prefrontal units, Neurosci. Lett. 101 (1989) 113–117.

[20] H. Niki, Reward-related and error-related neurons in the primate frontal cortex, in: S. Saito, T. Yanagita (Eds.), Learning and Memory: Drugs as Reinforcer, Excerpta Med. 620 (1982) 22–34.

[21] C.E. Rosenkilde, R.H. Bauer, J.M. Fuster, Single cell activity in ventral prefrontal cortex of behaving monkeys, Brain Res. 209 (1981) 375–394.

[22] H. Niki, M. Watanabe, Prefrontal and cingulate unit activity during timing behavior in the monkey, Brain Res. 171 (1979) 213–224.

[23] S. Ichihara-Takeda, S. Funahashi, Reward-period activity in primate dorsolateral prefrontal and orbitofrontal neurons is affected by reward schedules, J. Cogn. Neurosci. 18 (2006) 212–226.

[24] S. Kobayashi, R. Kawagoe, Y. Takikawa, M. Koizumi, M. Sakagami, O. Hikosaka, Functional differences between macaque prefrontal cortex and caudate nucleus during eye movements with and without reward, Exp. Brain Res. 176 (2007) 341–355.

[25] S. Tsujimoto, T. Sawaguchi, Neuronal representation of response-outcome in the primate prefrontal cortex, Cereb. Cortex 14 (2004) 47–55.

[26] S. Tsujimoto, T. Sawaguchi, Context-dependent representation of response-outcome in monkey prefrontal neurons, Cereb. Cortex 15 (2005) 888–898.

[27] K.H. Britten, M.N. Shadlen, W.T. Newsome, J.A. Movshon, The analysis of visual motion: a comparison of neuronal and psychophysical performance, J. Neurosci. 12 (1992) 4745–4765.

[28] M.N. Shadlen, W.T. Newsome, Motion perception: seeing and deciding, Proc. Natl. Acad. Sci. USA 93 (1996) 628–633.

[29] M.N. Shadlen, K.H. Britten, W.T. Newsome, J.A. Movshon, A computational analysis of the relationship between neuronal and behavioral responses to visual motion, J. Neurosci. 16 (1996) 1486–1510.

[30] K.G. Thompson, N.P. Bichot, J.D. Schall, Dissociation of visual discrimination from saccade programming in macaque frontal eye field, J. Neurophysiol. 77 (1997) 1046–1050.

[31] K. Tsutsui, M. Jiang, H. Sakata, M. Taira, Short-term memory and perceptual decision for three-dimensional visual features in the caudal intraparietal sulcus (Area CIP), J. Neurosci. 23 (2003) 5486–5495.

[32] J.N. Kim, M.N. Shadlen, Neural correlates of a decision in the dorsolateral prefrontal cortex of the macaque, Nat. Neurosci. 2 (1999) 176–185.

[33] M. Watanabe, K. Hikosaka, M. Sakagami, S. Shirakawa, Functional significance of delay-period activity of primate prefrontal neurons in relation to spatial working memory and reward/omission-of-reward expectancy, Exp. Brain Res. 166 (2005) 263–276.

[34] D.J. Barraclough, M.L. Conroy, D. Lee, Prefrontal cortex and decision making in a mixed-strategy game, Nat. Neurosci. 7 (2004) 404–410.

[35] D. Lee, B.P. McGreevy, D.J. Barraclough, Learning and decision making in monkeys during a rock-paper-scissors game, Brain Res. Cogn. Brain Res. 25 (2005) 416–430.

[36] M. Watanabe, H.C. Cromwell, L. Tremblay, J.R. Hollerman, K. Hikosaka, W. Schultz, Behavioral reactions reflecting differential reward expectations in monkeys, Exp. Brain Res. 140 (2001) 511–518.

[37] L. Trembley, W. Schultz, Relative reward preference in primate orbitofrontal cortex, Nature 398 (1999) 704–708.

[38] T. Hosokawa, K. Kato, M. Inoue, A. Mikami, Neurons in the macaque orbitofrontal cortex code relative preference of both rewarding and aversive outcomes, Neurosci. Res. 57 (2007) 434–445.

[39] W. Schultz, Multiple dopamine functions at different time courses, Annu. Rev. Neurosci. 30 (2007) 259–288.

[40] W. Schultz, L. Tremblay, Involvement of primate orbitofrontal neurons in reward, uncertainty, and learning, in: D.H. Zald, S.L. Rauch (Eds.), The Orbitofrontal Cortex, Oxford University Press, Oxford, 2006, pp. 173–198.

[41] R. Kawagoe, Y. Takikawa, O. Hikosaka, Expectation of reward modulates cognitive signals in the basal ganglia, Nat. Neurosci. 1 (1998) 411–416.

[42] J. LeDoux, The emotional brain, fear, and the amygdale, Cell. Mol. Neurobiol. 23 (2003) 727–738.

[43] J.J. Paton, M.A. Belova, S.E. Morrison, C.D. Salzman, The primate amygdala represents the positive and negative value of visual stimuli during learning, Nature 439 (2006) 865–870.

[44] E.A. Murray, The amygdala, reward and emotion, Trends. Cogn. Sci. 11 (2007) 489–497.

[45] E.T. Rolls, Emotion Explained, Oxford University Press, Oxford, 2005.

[46] H.T. Ghashghaeia, H. Barbas, Pathways for emotion: interactions of prefrontal and anterior temporal pathways in the amygdala of the rhesus monkey, Neuroscience 115 (2002) 1261–1279.

[47] C. Padoa-Schioppa, J.A. Assad, Neurons in the orbitofrontal cortex encode economic value, Nature 441 (2006) 223–226.

[48] M.R. Roesch, C.R. Olson, Neuronal activity related to reward value and motivation in primate frontal cortex, Science 304 (2004) 307–310.

[49] M.F. Rushworth, T.E. Behrens, P.H. Rudebeck, M.E. Walton, Contrasting roles for cingulate and orbitofrontal cortex in decisions and social behaviour, Trends. Cogn. Sci. 11 (2007) 168–176.

[50] M. Shidara, B.J. Richmond, Anterior cingulate: single neuronal signals related to degree of reward expectancy, Science 296 (2002) 1709–1711.

[51] P.H. Rudebeck, M.E. Walton, A.N. Smyth, D.M. Bannerman, M.F. Rushworth, Separate neural pathways process different decision costs, Nat. Neurosci. 9 (2006) 1161–1168.

[52] K. Matsumoto, W. Suzuki, K. Tanaka, Neuronal correlates of goal-based motor selection in the prefrontal cortex, Science 301 (2003) 229–232.

[53] H. Seo, D.J. Barraclough, D. Lee, Dynamic signals related to choices and outcomes in the dorsolateral prefrontal cortex, Cereb. Cortex 17 (Suppl. 1) (2007) i110–i117.

[54] K. Shima, J. Tanji, Role for cingulate motor area cells in voluntary movement selection based on reward, Science 282 (1998) 1335–1338.

[55] M.L. Platt, P.W. Glimcher, Neural correlates of decision variables in parietal cortex, Nature 400 (1999) 233–238.

5 From reward value to decision-making: neuronal and computational principles

Edmund T. Rolls

Department of Experimental Psychology, Oxford Centre for Computational Neuroscience, Oxford, United Kingdom

Abstract

I consider where sensory representations are transformed into reward based representations in the brain; how associations are learned and reversed between stimuli (that thereby become secondary reinforcers) and primary reinforcers such as taste and touch; how these processes lead to representations of reward magnitude, expected reward value, and reward prediction error; how cognition and attention specifically modulate these processes; and then how decisions that involve a choice are made between different rewards.

Key Points

1. Taste, olfactory, flavour, oral texture, and visual rewards are made explicit in the firing of primate orbitofrontal cortex neurons, but not at earlier stages of cortical processing.
2. These rewards are also represented in areas to which the orbitofrontal cortex projects, including the anterior cingulate cortex and ventral striatum.
3. Predicted reward, and negative reward prediction error, are made explicit in the firing of orbitofrontal cortex neurons.
4. The results of human fMRI neuroimaging, and of the effects of damage to these regions in humans, are consistent with these findings, and show that cognition modulates reward processing in these areas.
5. Because of their roles in reinforcer evaluation, these brain areas are fundamental to emotion.
6. Decision-making in which a binary choice is made by attractor neuronal networks involves the next tier of processing in for example the medial prefrontal cortex.

5.1 Introduction

I start with some definitions [1]. A reward is anything for which an animal will work. A punisher is anything that an animal will work to escape or avoid, or that will suppress actions on which it is contingent. Rewards and punishers are instrumental reinforcing stimuli.

Instrumental reinforcers are stimuli that, if their occurrence, termination, or omission is made contingent upon the making of an action, alter the probability of the future emission of that action [2–6]. Some stimuli are primary (unlearned) reinforcers (e.g., the taste of food if the animal is hungry, or pain); while others may become reinforcing by learning, because of their association with such primary reinforcers, thereby becoming "secondary reinforcers." This type of learning may thus be called "stimulus–reinforcer association," and occurs via an associative learning process between two stimuli, for a reinforcer is a stimulus. A positive reinforcer (such as food) increases the probability of emission of a response on which it is contingent; the process is termed *positive reinforcement*, and the outcome is a reward (such as food). A negative reinforcer (such as a painful stimulus) increases the probability of emission of a response that causes the negative reinforcer to be omitted (as in active avoidance) or terminated (as in escape), and the procedure is termed *negative reinforcement*. In contrast, *punishment* refers to procedures in which the probability of an action is decreased. Punishment thus describes procedures in which an action decreases in probability if it is followed by a painful stimulus, as in passive avoidance. Punishment can also be used to refer to a procedure involving the omission or termination of a reward ("extinction" and "time out," respectively), both of which decrease the probability of responses [1].

Part of the adaptive, evolutionary, value of primary rewards and punishers is that they are gene-specified goals for action, and a genome that specifies the goals to obtain (e.g., food when hungry) is much more efficient than one that attempts to specify responses to stimuli, for specifying a set of stimuli that are reinforcers is much simpler for the genome than specifying particular responses to each stimulus, and in addition allows flexibility of the action that is performed to obtain the goal [1,7]. Reinforcers are for these reasons extremely important in behavior, and their importance is underlined by the fact that emotions, acknowledged to be important by most people, can be defined as states elicited by rewards and punishers, that is, by instrumental reinforcers [1,2,8].

The focus is on humans and macaques, because there are many topological, cytoarchitectural, and probably connectional similarities between macaques and humans with respect to the orbitofrontal cortex and related structures important in reward processing (Fig. 5.1; [9–14]). Moreover, the orbitofrontal cortex receives visual information in primates from the inferior temporal visual cortex, which is a highly developed area for primate vision enabling invariant visual object recognition [15–19], and which provides visual inputs used in the primate orbitofrontal cortex for one-trial object-reward association reversal learning, and for representing face expression and identity. Further, even the taste system of primates and rodents may be different, with obligatory processing from the nucleus of the solitary tract via the thalamus to the cortex in primates, but a subcortical pathway in rodents via a pontine taste area to the amygdala and hypothalamus [20], and differences in where satiety influences taste-responsive neurons in primates and rodents [1,21]. The implication is that the reward pathways and reward processing for primary reinforcers, even as fundamental as taste, may be different in rodents and primates. For these reasons, and to understand reward processing, emotion, and decision-making in humans, the majority of the studies described here were performed with macaques or with humans. Although the nature of the representation of information is understood best at the levels of how individual neurons and populations of neurons respond, as these are the computing elements of the brain and the level at which information is exchanged between the computing elements which are the neurons [17], these data are complemented in what follows by functional neuroimaging studies in humans, and then by computational studies that indicate how populations of neurons achieve computations such as making a decision.

5.2 A connectional and functional framework

A connectional overview of the sensory pathways that lead into reward decoding systems in structures such as the orbitofrontal cortex and amygdala, and the structures to which they connect such as the ventral striatum, anterior cingulate cortex, and hypothalamus, is shown in Fig. 5.1, based on much anatomical and related work [1,9–11,13,14,17,22–25]. Conceptually, the orbitofrontal cortex and amygdala can be thought of as receiving from the ends of each modality-specific "what" cortical pathway. These areas are represented by the column in Fig. 5.1 with inferior temporal visual cortex, primary taste cortex in the

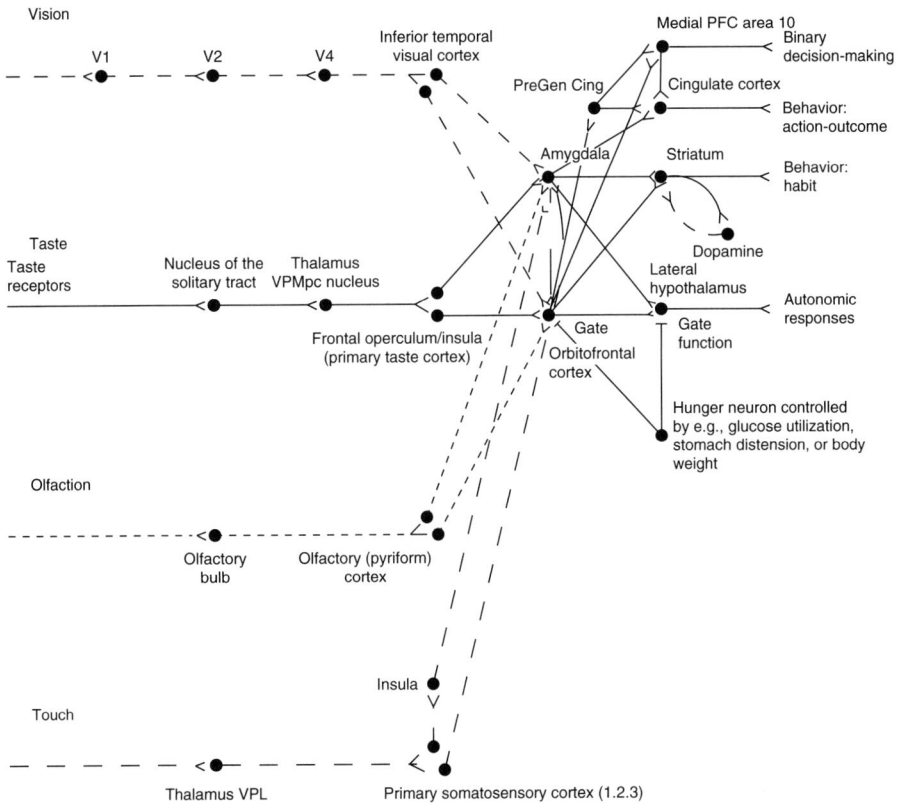

Figure 5.1 Schematic diagram showing some of the gustatory, olfactory, visual, and somatosensory pathways to the orbitofrontal cortex, and some of the outputs of the orbitofrontal cortex, in primates. The secondary taste cortex and the secondary olfactory cortex are within the orbitofrontal cortex (V1 – primary visual cortex; V4 – visual cortical area V4; PreGen Cing – pregenual cingulate cortex). "Gate" refers to the finding that inputs such as the taste, smell, and sight of food in some brain regions only produce effects when hunger is present [1]. The column of brain regions including and below the inferior temporal visual cortex represents brain regions in which what stimulus is present is made explicit in the neuronal representation, but not its reward or affective value, which are represented in the next tier of brain regions, the orbitofrontal cortex and amygdala, and in areas beyond these.

anterior insula, pyriform olfactory cortex, and somatosensory cortex, and reward is not made explicit in the representation in these areas. By made explicit in the representation, I mean reflected in the firing rates (and can be decoded from the firing rates of the neurons by a process that could be implemented by a receiving neuron, dot product decoding) [17]. Some of the evidence for this is described below, and in more detail elsewhere [1,17,25].

Figure 5.1 helps to set a functional framework in which neuronal activity in the inferior temporal cortex, and the primary taste, olfactory, and somatosensory cortices provides a representation of what stimulus is present, and its intensity, and in which reward value is represented at the next stages of processing, the orbitofrontal cortex and the amygdala. Part of the utility of this functional architecture is that there is a representation of what stimulus is present, independent of its reward value, so that learning to associate that stimulus with its spatial position, to recognize and name it, and to learn about its properties can occur independently of its current affective value [1,17]. A simple example is that we can learn about the location of a food even if we are not hungry and it has no reward value. At the subjective level, we can report on the properties and intensity of stimuli independently of whether they are currently pleasant. A computational principle is thus that there are separate representations of what a stimulus is, together with its intensity and its affective value. Some computational reasons for this segregation into different areas are described later.

5.3   Taste reward

Taste can act as a primary reinforcer, and given that taste reward is represented in the orbitofrontal cortex, we now have the start for a fundamental understanding of the function of the orbitofrontal cortex in stimulus–reinforcer association learning [1,7,17,26]. The representation (shown by analyzing the responses of single neurons in macaques) of taste in the orbitofrontal cortex includes robust representations of the prototypical tastes sweet, salt, bitter, and sour [27], but also separate representations of the "taste" of water [27], and of protein or umami as exemplified by monosodium glutamate (MSG) [28,29] and inosine monophosphate [30,31]. An example of an orbitofrontal cortex neuron with different responses to different taste stimuli is shown in Fig. 5.2B. As will be described below, some neurons have taste-only responses, and others respond to a variety of oral somatosensory stimuli, including, for some neurons, viscosity [32], fat texture [33,34], and for other neurons, astringency as exemplified by tannic acid [35]. There are analogous data for distributed coding in rats of oral sensory including gustatory stimuli [36].

The nature of the representation of taste in the orbitofrontal cortex is that for the majority of neurons the reward value of the taste is represented. The evidence for this is that the responses of orbitofrontal taste neurons are modulated by hunger (as is the reward value or palatability of a taste). In particular, it has been shown that orbitofrontal cortex taste neurons gradually stop responding to the taste of a food as the monkey is fed to satiety [30,37]. The example shown in Fig. 5.3 is of a single neuron with taste, olfactory, and visual responses to food, and the neuronal responses elicited through all these sensory modalities showed a decrease. Moreover, this type of neuronal responsiveness shows that it is the preference for different stimuli that is represented by these neurons, in that the neuronal response decreases in parallel with the decrease in the acceptability or reward value of the food being eaten to satiety, but the neuronal responses remain high (or even sometimes become a little larger) to foods not eaten in the meal (see, e.g., Fig. 5.3), but which remain acceptable, with a high reward value. Sensory-specific satiety, the decrease in the reward value of a food eaten

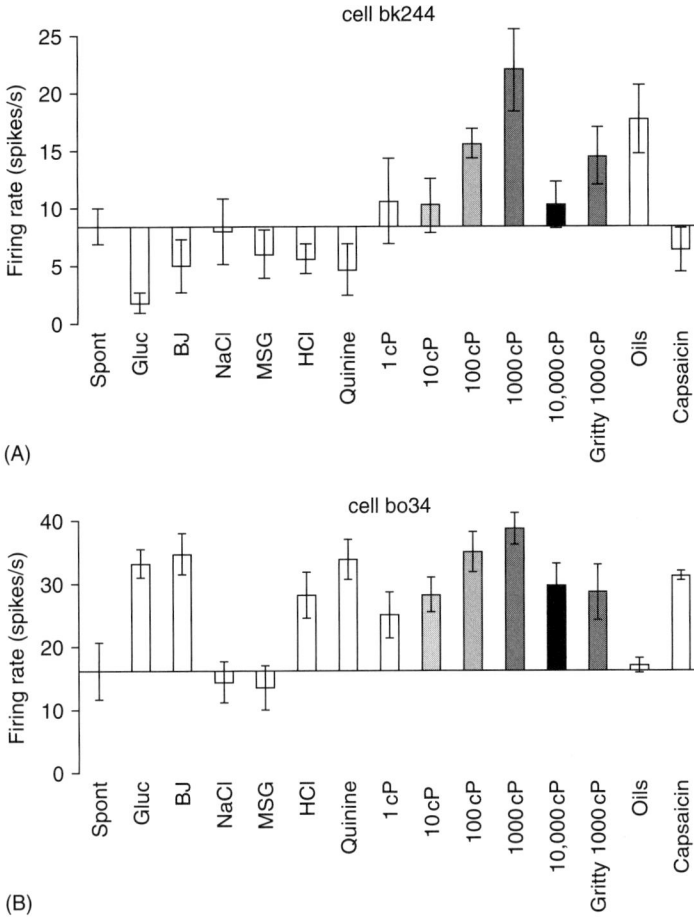

Figure 5.2 Oral somatosensory and taste inputs to orbitofrontal cortex neurons. (A) Firing rates (mean ± sem) of viscosity-sensitive neuron bk244, which did not have taste responses in that it did not respond differentially to the different taste stimuli. The firing rates are shown to the viscosity series, to the gritty stimulus (carboxymethylcellulose with Fillite microspheres), to the taste stimuli 1 M glucose (Gluc), 0.1 M NaCl, 0.1 M MSG, 0.01 M HCl, and 0.001 M QuinineHCl, and to fruit juice (BJ, blackcurrant juice; Spont, spontaneous firing rate). (B) Firing rates (mean ± sem) of viscosity-sensitive neuron bo34, which had no response to the oils (mineral oil, vegetable oil, safflower oil, and coconut oil, which have viscosities that are all close to 50 cP). The neuron did not respond to the gritty stimulus in a way that was unexpected given the viscosity of the stimulus, was taste tuned, and did respond to capsaicin. *Source*: After Rolls et al. (2003) [32].

to satiety relative to other foods not eaten to satiety, is thus implemented in the orbitofrontal cortex. Further, in humans, feeding to satiety decreases the activation of the orbitofrontal cortex to the food eaten to satiety in a sensory-specific way [38], and activations in the human orbitofrontal cortex are correlated with the pleasantness of taste [39]. Additional evidence that the reward value of food is represented in the orbitofrontal cortex is that

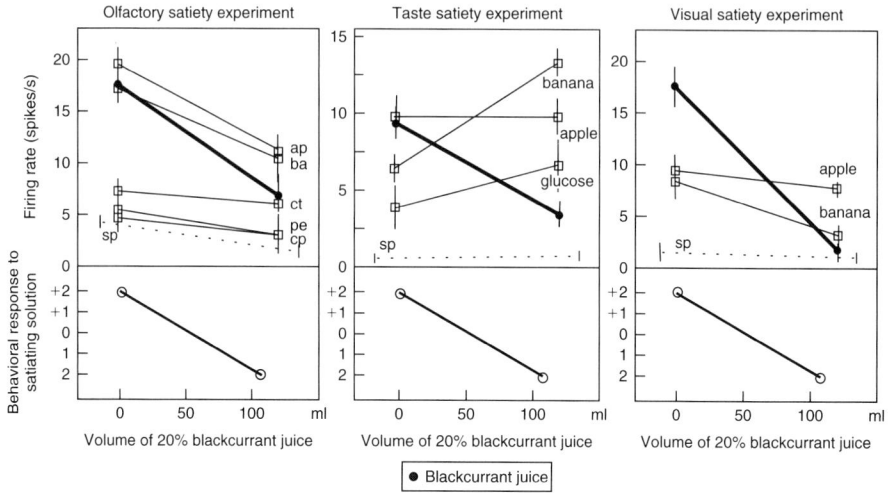

Figure 5.3 Multimodal orbitofrontal cortex neuron with sensory-specific satiety-related responses to visual, taste, and olfactory sensory inputs. The responses are shown before and after feeding to satiety with blackcurrant juice. The solid circles show the responses to blackcurrant juice. The olfactory stimuli included apple (ap), banana (ba), citral (ct), phenylethanol (pe), and caprylic acid (cp). The spontaneous firing rate of the neuron is shown (sp). *Source*: After Critchley and Rolls, 1996 [47].

monkeys work for electrical stimulation of this brain region if they are hungry, but not if they are satiated [1,40]. Further, neurons in the orbitofrontal cortex are activated from many brain-stimulation reward sites [41,42].

The computational basis for sensory-specific satiety is that each neuron in the orbitofrontal cortex responds to different combinations of taste, odor, fat texture, viscosity, astringency, roughness, temperature, capsaicin, and visual inputs (see examples in Fig. 5.2), and by making it a property that these neurons show adaptation after several minutes of stimulation, the reward value can decrease to the particular combination of sensory inputs, but much less to others. *Reward-specific satiety* is probably a property of all rewards, and facilitates the selection of a variety of different rewards, which is adaptive [1,17].

An interesting property of sensory-specific satiety is that after eating one food to satiety, the neuronal responses and subjective pleasantness of other foods can increase a little (see example in Fig. 5.3, middle). This is probably part of a mechanism to facilitate behavioral switching between different positive reinforcers, and in the case of food, may facilitate eating a varied diet with the consequent beneficial nutritional implications, but may contribute to overeating and obesity if too much variety is available [1,43].

The caudolateral part of the orbitofrontal cortex is secondary taste cortex, as defined anatomically (using horseradish peroxidase tracing from the site of the taste neurons) by major direct inputs from the primary taste cortex in the rostral insula and adjoining frontal operculum [44]. This region projects onto other regions in the orbitofrontal cortex [44], and neurons with taste responses (in what can be considered as a tertiary gustatory cortical area) can be found in many regions of the orbitofrontal cortex [27,45,46]. Although some taste neurons are found laterally in the orbitofrontal cortex (area 12o)

[27,45,46], others are found through the middle and even toward the medial part of the orbitofrontal cortex in areas 13m and 13l [25,30,35,46–50]. Most but not all of these area 13 neurons decrease their responses to zero to a taste with which the monkey is fed to satiety [30,35,47,51].

The primate amygdala contains neurons activated by taste and also by oral texture and temperature [52–55], but satiety has inconsistent effects on neuronal responses to taste and related stimuli, producing a mean suppression of 58% [56], indicating that reward is much less clearly represented here than in the orbitofrontal cortex (see above) and the hypothalamus [57], which receives inputs from the orbitofrontal cortex. The human amygdala is not specialized for taste stimuli that happen to be aversive, for pleasant stimuli such as the taste of glucose produce as much activation as salt [58].

The pregenual cingulate cortex also contains taste neurons, which respond to, for example, sweet taste if hunger is present and so represent reward value [50]. The pregenual cingulate cortex (which is clearly multimodal [59]) can be considered a tertiary taste cortical area, in that it receives inputs from the orbitofrontal cortex [50].

5.4   Olfactory reward

Although some odors (such as pheromones and perhaps some odors related to fruit/flowers or rotting/uncleanliness) are primary reinforcers; we learn about the reward value of most odors by association with a primary reinforcer such as taste [1].

A ventral frontal region has been implicated in olfactory processing in humans [60,61] and macaques [62]. For 35% of orbitofrontal cortex neurons with olfactory responses, Critchley and Rolls [63] showed that the odors to which a neuron responded were influenced by the taste (glucose or saline) with which the odor was associated. Thus the odor representation for 35% of orbitofrontal neurons appeared to be built by olfactory-to-taste association learning. This possibility was confirmed by reversing the taste with which an odor was associated in the reversal of an olfactory discrimination task. It was found that 68% of the sample of neurons analyzed altered the way in which they responded to an odor when the taste reinforcement association of the odor was reversed [45] (25% showed reversal, and 43% no longer discriminated after the reversal, so were conditional reward neurons as also found in rats [64]). The olfactory-to-taste reversal was quite slow, both neurophysiologically and behaviorally, often requiring 20–80 trials, consistent with the need for some stability of flavor representations. Thus the rule according to which the orbitofrontal olfactory representation was formed was, for some neurons, by association learning with taste, a primary reinforcer.

To analyze the nature of the olfactory representation in the orbitofrontal cortex, Critchley and Rolls [47] measured the responses of olfactory neurons that responded to food while they fed the monkey to satiety. They found that the majority of orbitofrontal olfactory neurons decreased their responses to the odor of the food with which the monkey was fed to satiety (see example in Fig. 5.3). Thus, for these neurons, the reward value of the odor is what is represented in the orbitofrontal cortex. We do not yet know whether this is the first stage of processing at which reward value is represented in the olfactory system in macaques (although in rodents the influence of reward association learning appears to be present in some neurons in the pyriform cortex [65]). However, an fMRI investigation in humans showed that whereas in the orbitofrontal cortex the pleasantness versus unpleasantness of odors is represented, this was not the case in primary olfactory cortical areas, where instead the activations reflected the intensity of the odors [66]. Further evidence that the pleasantness or reward value of odor is represented in the orbitofrontal cortex is that feeding humans to satiety decreases the activation found to the odor of the food, and this effect is relatively specific to the food eaten in the meal [67–69].

5.5   Flavor reward

In the orbitofrontal cortex, not only are there unimodal taste and unimodal olfactory neurons, but also some single neurons respond to both gustatory and olfactory stimuli, often with correspondence between the two modalities [46]. It is probably here in the orbitofrontal cortex of primates, including humans, that these two modalities converge to produce the representation of flavor [46,70], for neurons in the macaque primary taste cortex in the insular/frontal opercular cortex do not respond to olfactory (or visual) stimuli [71]. As noted above, these neurons may be formed by olfactory–gustatory association learning, an example of stimulus–reinforcer association learning.

   The importance of the combination of taste and smell for producing affectively pleasant and rewarding representations of sensory stimuli is exemplified by findings with umami, the delicious taste or flavor that is associated with combinations of components that include meat, fish, milk, tomatoes, and mushrooms, all of which are rich in umami-related substances such as glutamate or inosine 5′monophosphate. Umami taste is produced by glutamate acting on a fifth taste system [72–74]. Umami (protein) taste is not only represented by neurons in the primate orbitofrontal cortex [28,30], but also human fMRI studies show that umami taste is represented in the orbitofrontal cortex, with an anterior part responding supralinearly to a combination of MSG and inosine monophosphate [75]. Glutamate presented alone as a taste stimulus is not highly pleasant and does not act synergistically with other tastes (sweet, salt, bitter, and sour). However, when glutamate is given in combination with a consonant, savory odor (vegetable), the resulting flavor can be much more pleasant [76]. We showed, using functional brain imaging with fMRI, that this glutamate taste and savory odor combination produced much greater activation of the medial orbitofrontal cortex and pregenual cingulate cortex than the sum of the activations by the taste and olfactory components presented separately [76]. Supralinear effects were much less (and significantly less) evident for sodium chloride and vegetable odor. Further, activations in these brain regions were correlated with the pleasantness and fullness of the flavor, and with the consonance of the taste and olfactory components. Supralinear effects of glutamate taste and savory odor were not found in the insular primary taste cortex. We suggested that umami can be thought of as a rich and delicious flavor that is produced by a combination of glutamate taste and a consonant savory odor. Glutamate is thus a flavor enhancer because of the way that it can combine supra-linearly with consonant odors in cortical areas where the taste and olfactory pathways converge far beyond the receptors [76].

   A concept here is that combinations of sensory stimuli represented by neurons in the orbitofrontal cortex appear to contribute to the representation of the reward value of particular combinations of sensory stimuli, and these may involve nonlinear processing.

5.6   Oral texture and temperature reward

A population of orbitofrontal neurons responds when a fatty food such as cream is in the mouth. These neurons can also be activated by pure fat such as glyceryl trioleate, and by non-fat substances with a fat-like texture such as paraffin oil (hydrocarbon) and silicone oil $((Si(CH_3)_2O)_n)$. These neurons thus provide information by somatosensory pathways that a fatty food is in the mouth [33]. These inputs are perceived as pleasant when hungry, because of the utility of ingestion of foods that are likely to contain essential fatty acids and to have a high calorific value [1,77]. Satiety produced by eating a fatty food, cream, can decrease the responses of orbitofrontal cortex neurons to the texture of fat in the mouth [33], showing that they represent oral texture reward.

Some orbitofrontal cortex neurons encode fat texture independently of viscosity (by a physical parameter that varies with the slickness of fat) [34]; other orbitofrontal cortex neurons encode the viscosity of the texture in the mouth (with some neurons tuned to viscosity, and others showing increasing or decrease firing rates as viscosity increases) [32]; other neurons have responses that indicate the presence of texture stimuli (such as grittiness and capsaicin) in the mouth independently of viscosity and slickness [32]. The ensemble (i.e., population, distributed) encoding of all these variables is illustrated by the different tuning to the set of stimuli of the two neurons shown in Fig. 5.2. An overlapping population of orbitofrontal cortex neurons represents the temperature of what is in the mouth [78].

These single-neuron recording studies thus provide clear evidence of the rich sensory representation of oral stimuli, and of their reward value, that is provided in the primate orbitofrontal cortex, and how this differs from what is represented in the primary taste cortex and in the amygdala [54]. In a complementary human functional neuroimaging study, it has been shown that activation of parts of the orbitofrontal cortex, primary taste cortex, and mid-insular somatosensory region posterior to the insular taste cortex have activations that are related to the viscosity of what is in the mouth, and that there is in addition a medial prefrontal/cingulate area where the mouth feel of fat is represented [79]. Also, in humans, there is a representation of the temperature of what is in the mouth [80]. The oral temperature stimuli (cooled and warmed, 5, 20, and 50°C) activated the insular taste cortex (identified by glucose taste stimuli), a part of the somatosensory cortex, the orbitofrontal cortex, the anterior cingulate cortex, and the ventral striatum. Brain regions where activations correlated with the pleasantness ratings of the oral temperature stimuli included the orbitofrontal cortex and pregenual cingulate cortex.

Part of the advantage of having a representation of oral temperature in these regions is that neurons can then encode combinations of taste, texture, and oral temperature [71,78]. These combination-responsive neurons may provide the basis for particular combinations of temperature, taste, texture, and odor to be especially pleasant [1,81]; for sensory-specific satiety to apply to that combination, but not necessarily to the components; and more generally for learning and perception to apply to that combination and not necessarily to the components [17].

5.7 Somatosensory and temperature inputs to the orbitofrontal cortex, and affective value

In addition to these oral somatosensory inputs to the orbitofrontal cortex, there are also somatosensory inputs from other parts of the body, and indeed an fMRI investigation we have performed in humans indicates that pleasant and painful touch stimuli to the hand produce greater activation of the orbitofrontal cortex relative to the somatosensory cortex than do affectively neutral stimuli [67,82].

Non-glabrous skin, such as that on the forearm, contains C fiber tactile afferents that respond to light moving touch [83]. The orbitofrontal cortex is implicated in some of the affectively pleasant aspects of touch that may be mediated through C fiber tactile afferents, in that it is activated more by light touch to the forearm than by light touch to the gla-brous skin (palm) of the hand [84].

Warm and cold stimuli have affective components such as feeling pleasant or unpleasant, and these components may have survival value, for approach to warmth and avoidance of cold may be reinforcers or goals for action built into us during evolution to direct our behavior to stimuli that are appropriate for survival [1]. Understanding the brain processing that underlies these prototypical reinforcers provides a direct approach to understanding the brain mecha-nisms of emotion. In an fMRI investigation in humans, it was found that the mid-orbitofrontal and pregenual cingulate cortex and the ventral striatum have activations that are correlated with the subjective pleasantness ratings made to warm (41°C) and cold (12°C) stimuli, and combinations of warm and cold stimuli, applied to the hand [85]. Activations in the lateral and some more anterior parts of the orbitofrontal cortex were correlated with the unpleasant-ness of the stimuli. In contrast, activations in the somatosensory cortex and ventral posterior insula were correlated with the intensity but not the pleasantness of the thermal stimuli.

A principle thus appears to be that processing related to the affective value and associ-ated subjective emotional experience of thermal stimuli that are important for survival is performed in different brain areas than those where activations are related to sensory properties of the stimuli such as their intensity. This conclusion appears to be the case for processing in a number of sensory modalities, including taste [39,86] and olfaction [66,87,88], and the findings with such prototypical stimuli as warm and cold [85,89] provide strong support for this principle.

5.8   Visual inputs to the orbitofrontal cortex, and visual stimulus–reinforcement association learning and reversal

There is a major visual input to many neurons in the orbitofrontal cortex, and what is represented by these neurons is in many cases the reinforcement association of visual stimuli. The visual input is from the ventral, temporal lobe, visual stream concerned with "what" object is being seen [15–19,90]. Using this object-related and transform invari-ant information, orbitofrontal cortex visual neurons frequently respond differentially to objects or images depending on their reward association [45,91]. The primary reinforcer that has been used is taste, and correlates of visual to taste association learning have been demonstrated in the human orbitofrontal cortex with fMRI [92]. Many of these neurons show visual–taste reversal in one or a very few trials (see example in Fig. 5.4A). (In a visual discrimination task, they will reverse the stimulus to which they respond (from, e.g., a triangle to a square) in one trial when the taste delivered for a behavioral response to that stimulus is reversed [91]. This reversal learning probably occurs in the orbitofron-tal cortex, for it does not occur one synapse earlier in the visual inferior temporal cortex [93], and it is in the orbitofrontal cortex that there is convergence of visual and taste pathways onto the same single neurons [45,46,91].

The probable mechanism for this learning is an associative modification of synapses conveying visual input onto taste-responsive neurons, implementing a pattern association network [1,17,18,94] (see Section 5.16 and Fig. 5.6). When the reinforcement association of a visual stimulus is reversed, other "conditional reward" orbitofrontal cortex neurons stop responding, or stop responding differentially, to the visual discriminanda [91]. An example is a neuron in the orbitofrontal cortex that responded to a blue stimulus when it was rewarded (blue S+) and not to a green stimulus when it was associated with aversive

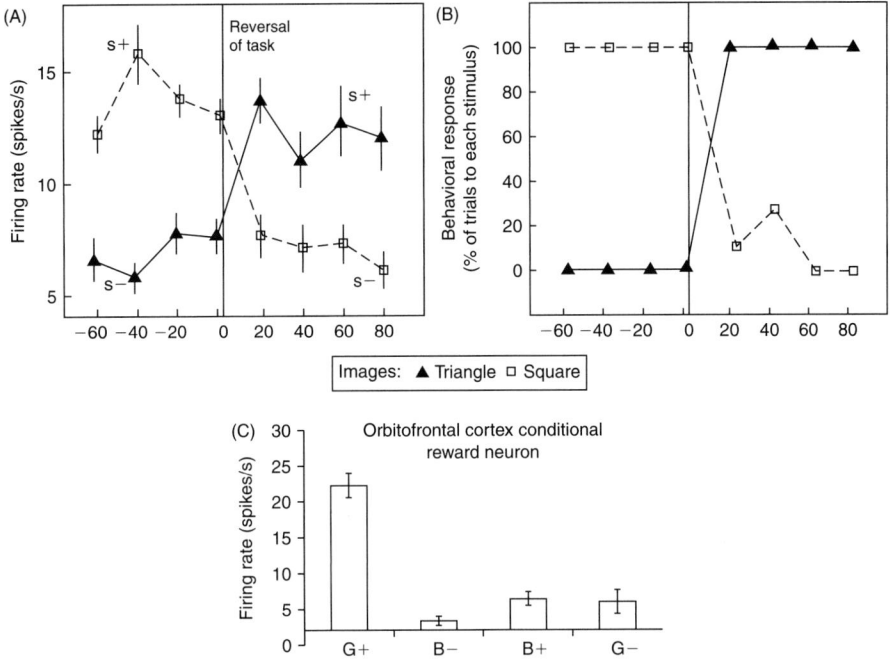

Figure 5.4 (A) Visual discrimination reversal of the responses of a single neuron in the macaque orbitofrontal cortex when the taste with which the two visual stimuli (a triangle and a square) were associated was reversed. Each point is the mean post-stimulus firing rate measured in a 0.5 s period over approximately 10 trials to each of the stimuli. Before reversal, the neuron fired most to the square when it indicated (S+) that the monkey could lick to obtain a taste of glucose. After reversal, the neuron responded most to the triangle when it indicated that the monkey could lick to obtain glucose. The response was low to the stimuli when they indicated (S−) that if the monkey licked then aversive saline would be obtained. (B) The behavioral response to the triangle and the square, indicating that the monkey reversed rapidly. (C) A conditional reward neuron recorded in the orbitofrontal cortex by Thorpe et al. [91] in a visual discrimination task which responded only to the green stimulus when it was associated with reward (G+), and not to the blue stimulus when it was associated with reward (B+), or to either stimulus when they were associated with a punisher, the taste of salt (G− and B−). *Source*: For B, after Rolls et al. (1996) [45].

saline (green S−). However, the neuron did not respond after reversal to the blue S− or to the green S+ (Fig. 5.4C). Similar conditional reward neurons are found not only for visual but also for olfactory stimuli [45]. Such conditional reward neurons convey information about the current reinforcement status of particular stimuli. They may be part of a system that can implement very rapid reversal, by being biased on by-rule neurons if that stimulus is currently associated with reward, and being biased off if that stimulus is currently not associated with reward [95], as described in Section 5.16. This theory provides an account of the utility of conditional reward neurons.

The visual and olfactory neurons in primates that respond to the sight or smell of stimuli that are primary reinforcers such as taste clearly signal an expectation of reward that is based on previous stimulus–reinforcement associations [45,91]. So do the conditional reward neurons [45,91]. Olfactory reward expectation and conditional reward neurons have also been found in rats in a region that may correspond to the orbitofrontal cortex, and some of these neurons can start to respond after a delay period as the expected taste becomes closer in time [96]. In primates the orbitofrontal cortex neurons that change their responses during olfactory to taste reversal learning do so sufficiently rapidly to play a role in the behavioral change [45], but in rodents it has been suggested that the amygdala may be more important in reflecting the changing association [64]. However, the situation is clear in the case of visual–taste association learning and reversal in primates, in which the orbitofrontal cortex neurons and the behavior can change in one trial [45,91], so that the changing responses of the orbitofrontal cortex neurons can contribute to the reversed behavior, a view supported by the impaired reversal learning produced in primates, including humans, by orbitofrontal cortex damage [97–99]. Indeed, in primates, visual-to-taste reversal is so rapid that after a punishment has been received to the negative discriminative stimulus (S−), the next time the previous S− is shown, the neurons respond to it as an S+ , and the monkey responds [45,91]. This is a non-associative process that involves a rule change, and this is a special contribution that the primate orbitofrontal cortex makes to reversal learning, and for which a computational theory that utilizes the conditional reward and error neurons has been produced [95] that is described in Section 5.16.

With respect to the primate amygdala, the evidence is that any reversal of neurons in a visual discrimination reversal is relatively slow if it occurs taking tens of trials [52,100], and so in primates the amygdala appears to make a less important contribution than the orbitofrontal cortex. This is in line with the hypothesis that the orbitofrontal cortex, as a cortical area versus the subcortical amygdala, becomes relatively more important in primates, including humans, than in rodents [1]. This is based not only on the neurophysiology described here, but also on the relative development in primates including humans versus rodents of the orbitofrontal cortex versus amygdala, and the more severe effects of damage to the primate including human orbitofrontal cortex than amygdala on emotion and reward-related processing referred to elsewhere in this chapter. The computational basis for the hypothesis is that because of the well-developed recurrent collateral excitatory connections of cortical areas, the orbitofrontal cortex can make especial contributions by its attractor dynamics when states must be remembered, as in rule-based reversal, and also in other operations where a short-term memory can facilitate reward-based processing, as described in Section 5.16. Indeed, attractor networks in cortical areas such as the orbitofrontal cortex and anterior cingulate cortex may contribute to the persistence of mood states, which is an adaptive function with respect to emotion in that, for example, after non-reward, the persistence of the state will keep behavior directed toward obtaining the goal. Cortical areas such as the orbitofrontal cortex may make a special contribution to the adaptive persistence of emotional states (which reflect rewards received) because of their attractor properties implemented by the local recurrent collaterals [1,17], as considered further in Section 5.16.

To analyze the nature of the visual representation of food-related stimuli in the orbitofrontal cortex, Critchley and Rolls [47] measured the responses of neurons that responded to the sight of food while they fed the monkey to satiety. They found that the majority of orbitofrontal visual food-related neurons decreased their responses to the sight of the food with which the monkey was fed to satiety (see example in Fig. 5.3). Thus, for these neurons, the reward value of the sight of food is what is represented in the orbitofrontal cortex. At a stage of visual processing one synapse earlier, in the inferior temporal visual cortex, neurons do not show visual discrimination reversal learning, nor are their responses modulated by feeding to satiety [93]. Thus, both of these functions are implemented for visual processing in the orbitofrontal cortex.

5.9 Reward prediction error neurons

In addition to these neurons that encode the reward association of visual stimuli, other, "error," neurons in the orbitofrontal cortex detect non-reward, in that they respond, for example, when an expected reward is not obtained when a visual discrimination task is reversed [91] (Fig. 5.5), or when reward is no longer made available in a visual discrimination task, that is, in extinction [25,91]. These may be called "negative reward prediction error neurons." Different populations of such neurons respond to other types of non-reward, including the removal of a formerly approaching taste reward, and the termination of a taste reward in the extinction of ad-lib licking for juice, or the substitution of juice reward by aversive tasting saline during ad-lib licking [17,25,91]. The presence of these neurons is fully consistent with the hypothesis that they are part of the mechanism by which the orbitofrontal cortex enables very rapid reversal of behavior by stimulus–reinforcement association relearning when the association of stimuli with reinforcers is altered or reversed [1,17,95]. The finding that different orbitofrontal cortex neurons respond to different types of non-reward (or negative reward prediction error) [91] may provide part of the brain's mechanism that enables task or context-specific reversal to occur [17,25].

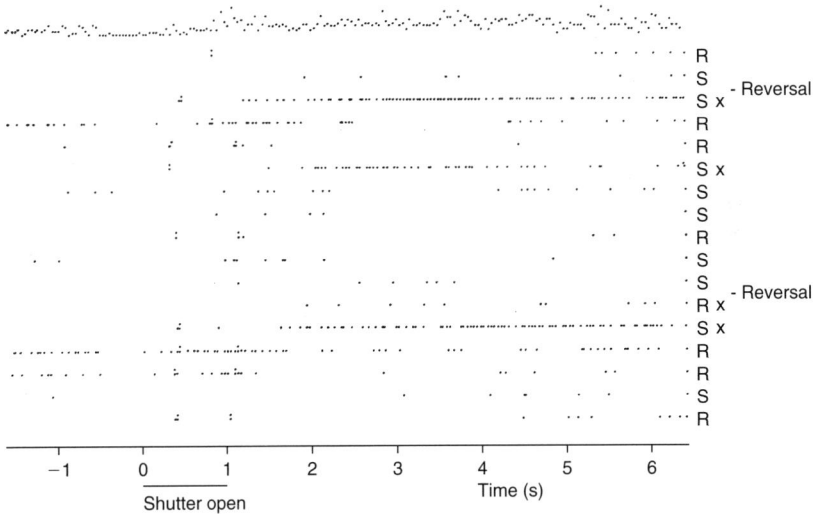

Figure 5.5 Negative reward prediction error neuron: responses of an orbitofrontal cortex neuron that responded only when the monkey licked to a visual stimulus during reversal, expecting to obtain fruit juice reward, but actually obtaining the taste of aversive saline because it was the first trial of reversal. Each single dot represents an action potential; each vertically arranged double dot represents a lick response. The visual stimulus was shown at time 0 for 1 s. The neuron did not respond on most reward (R) or saline (S) trials, but did respond on the trials marked x, which were the first trials after a reversal of the visual discrimination on which the monkey licked to obtain reward, but actually obtained saline because the task had been reversed. *Source*: After Thorpe et al. (1983) [91].

Evidence that there may be similar negative reward prediction error neurons in the human orbitofrontal cortex is that in a model of social learning, orbitofrontal cortex activation occurred in a visual discrimination reversal task at the time when the face of one person no longer was associated with a smile, but became associated with an angry expression, indicating on such error trials that reversal of choice to the other individual's face should occur [101].

The orbitofrontal cortex negative reward prediction error neurons respond to a mismatch between the reward expected ("expected value") and the reward that is obtained ("reward outcome") [17]. Both signals are represented in the orbitofrontal cortex, in the form of, for example, neurons that respond to the sight of a learned reinforcer such as the sight of a stimulus paired with taste, and neurons that respond to the primary reinforcer, the taste (or texture or temperature). Similarly, in a probabilistic monetary reward task, activations in the human orbitofrontal and pregenual cingulate cortex are related to both expected value and to reward outcome (the magnitude of the reward actually obtained on each trial) [102]. The orbitofrontal cortex is the probable brain region for the computation of negative reward prediction error, because both the signals required to compute negative reward prediction error are present in the orbitofrontal cortex, as are the negative reward prediction error neurons, and lesions of the orbitofrontal cortex impair tasks such as visual discrimination reversal in which this type of negative reward prediction error is needed (see above).

It may be noted that the dopamine neurons in the midbrain may not be able to provide a good representation of negative reward prediction error, because their spontaneous firing rates are so low [103] that much further reduction would provide only a small signal. In any case, the dopamine neurons would not appear to be in a position to compute a negative reward prediction error, as they are not known to receive inputs that signal expected reward (expected value), and the actual reward (outcome) that is obtained, and indeed do not represent the reward obtained (reward outcome), in that they stop responding to a taste reward outcome if it is predictable [103,104]. Although dopamine neurons do appear to represent a positive reward prediction error signal (responding if a greater than expected reward is obtained) [103,104], they do not appear to have the signals required to compute this, the expected reward, and the reward outcome obtained, so even this must be computed elsewhere. The orbitofrontal cortex does contain representations of these two signals, the expected reward value and the reward outcome, and has projections to the ventral striatum, which in turn projects to the region of the midbrain dopamine neurons, and so this is one possible pathway along which the firing of positive reward prediction error might be computed (see Fig. 5.1). Consistent with this, activations in parts of the human ventral striatum are related to positive reward prediction error (positive temporal difference error) [102,105]. Thus, the dopamine projections to the prefrontal cortex and other areas are not likely to convey information about reward to the prefrontal cortex, which instead is likely to be decoded by the neurons in the orbitofrontal cortex that represent primary reinforcers, and the orbitofrontal cortex neurons that learn associations of other stimuli to the primary reinforcers to represent expected value [17,45,91,102]. Although it has been suggested that the firing of dopamine neurons may reflect the earliest signal in a task that indicates reward and could be used as a positive reward prediction error signal during learning [104,106], it is likely, partly on the basis of the above evidence, though an interesting topic for future investigation, that any error information to which dopamine neurons fire originates from representations in the orbitofrontal cortex that encode expected value and reward outcome, and which connect to the ventral striatum [1,17,102].

In responding when the reward obtained is less than that expected, the orbitofrontal cortex negative reward prediction error neurons are working in a domain that is related to the sensory inputs being received (expected reward and reward obtained). There are also error neurons in the anterior cingulate cortex that respond when errors are made [107], or when rewards are reduced [108] (and in similar imaging studies [109]). Some of these neurons may be influenced by the projections from the orbitofrontal cortex, and reflect a mismatch between the reward expected and the reward that is obtained. However, some error neurons in the anterior cingulate cortex may reflect errors that arise when particular behavioral responses or actions are in error, and this type of error may be important in helping an action system to correct itself, rather than, as in the orbitofrontal cortex, when a reward prediction system needs to be corrected. Consistent with this, many studies provide evidence that errors made in many tasks activate the anterior/midcingulate cortex [110–113].

5.10   Social reinforcers such as face and voice expression

Another type of visual information represented in the orbitofrontal cortex is information about faces. There is a population of orbitofrontal cortex neurons that respond in many ways similarly to those in the temporal cortical visual areas [15–18,90,114–116]. The orbitofrontal face-responsive neurons, first observed by Thorpe et al. [91], then by Rolls et al. [117], tend to respond with longer latencies than temporal lobe neurons (140–200 ms typically, compared to 80–100 ms); they also convey information about which face is being seen, by having different responses to different faces; and they are typically rather harder to activate strongly than temporal cortical face-selective neurons, in that many of them respond much better to real faces than to two-dimensional images of faces on a video monitor (cf. [118]). Some of the orbitofrontal cortex face-selective neurons are responsive to face expression, gesture, or movement [117]. The findings are consistent with the likelihood that these neurons are activated via the inputs from the temporal cortical visual areas in which face-selective neurons are found (see Fig. 5.1).

The significance of these orbitofrontal cortex neurons is likely to be related to the fact that faces convey information that is important in social reinforcement in at least two ways that could be implemented by these neurons. The first is that some may encode face expression ([117]; cf. [119]), which can indicate reinforcement. The second way is that they encode information about which individual is present [117], which by stimulus–reinforcement association learning is important in evaluating and utilizing learned reinforcing inputs in social situations, for example, about the current reinforcement value as decoded by stimulus–reinforcement association to a particular individual.

This system has also been shown to be present in humans. For example, Kringelbach and Rolls [101] showed that activation of a part of the human orbitofrontal cortex occurs during a face discrimination reversal task. In the task, the faces of two different individuals are shown, and when the correct face is selected, the expression turns into a smile. (The expression turns to angry if the wrong face is selected.) After a period of correct performance, the contingencies reverse, and the other face must be selected to obtain a smile expression as a reinforcer. It was found that activation of a part of the orbitofrontal cortex occurred specifically in relation to the reversal, that is, when a formerly correct face was chosen, but an angry face expression was obtained. Thus in humans, there is a part of the orbitofrontal cortex that responds selectively in relation to face expression specifically when it indicates that behavior should change, and this activation is error-related [101] and occurs when the error neurons in the orbitofrontal cortex become active [91]. In addition, activations in the human orbitofrontal cortex are related to the attractiveness or beauty of a face [120].

Also prompted by the neuronal recording evidence of face and auditory neurons in the orbitofrontal cortex [117], it has further been shown that there are impairments in the identification of facial and vocal emotional expression in a group of patients with ventral frontal lobe damage who had socially inappropriate behavior [121]. The expression identification impairments could occur independently of perceptual impairments in facial recognition, voice discrimination, or environmental sound recognition. Poor performance on both expression tests was correlated with the degree of alteration of emotional experience reported by the patients. There was also a strong positive correlation between the degree of altered emotional experience and the severity of the behavioral problems (e.g., disinhibition) found in these patients [121]. A comparison group of patients with brain damage outside the ventral frontal lobe region, without these behavioral problems, was unimpaired on the face expression identification test, was significantly less impaired at vocal expression identification, and reported little subjective emotional change [121]. It has further been shown that patients with discrete surgical lesions of restricted parts of the orbitofrontal cortex may have face and/or voice expression identification impairments, and these are likely to contribute to their difficulties in social situations [122].

5.11   Top-down effects of cognition and attention on the reward value of affective stimuli

How does cognition influence affective value? How does cognition influence the way that we feel emotionally? Do cognition and emotion interact in regions that are high in the brain's hierarchy of processing, or do cognitive influences descend down to influence the first regions that represent the affective value of stimuli?

An fMRI study to address these fundamental issues in brain design has shown that cognitive effects can reach down into the human orbitofrontal cortex and influence activations produced by odors [123]. In this study, a standard test odor, isovaleric acid with a small amount of cheese flavor, was delivered through an olfactometer. (The odor alone, like the odor of brie, might have been interpreted as pleasant, or perhaps as unpleasant.) On some trials the test odor was accompanied with the visually presented word label "cheddar cheese," and on other trials with the word label "body odor." It was found that the activation in the medial orbitofrontal cortex to the standard test odor was much greater when the word label was cheddar cheese than when it was body odor. (Controls with clean air were run to show that the effect could not be accounted for by the word label alone.) Moreover, the word labels influenced the subjective pleasantness ratings to the test odor, and the changing pleasantness ratings were correlated with the activations in the human medial orbitofrontal cortex. Part of the interest and importance of this finding is that it shows that cognitive influences, originating here purely at the word level, can reach down and modulate activations in the first stage of cortical processing that represents the affective value of sensory stimuli [1,123].

Also important is how cognition influences the affective brain representations of the taste and flavor of a food. This is important not only for understanding top-down influences in the brain, but also in relation to the topical issues of appetite control and obesity [43,124]. In an fMRI study it was shown that activations related to the affective value of umami taste and flavor (as shown by correlations with pleasantness ratings) in the orbitofrontal cortex were modulated by word-level descriptors (e.g., "rich and delicious flavor") [86]. Affect-related activations to taste were modulated in a region that receives from the orbitofrontal cortex, the pregenual cingulate cortex, and to taste and flavor in another region that receives from the orbitofrontal cortex, the ventral striatum. Affect-related cognitive modulations were not found in the insular taste cortex, where the intensity but not the pleasantness of the taste was represented. Thus, the top-down language-level cognitive effects reach far down into the earliest cortical areas that represent the reward value of taste and flavor. This is an important way in which cognition influences the neural mechanisms that control reward and appetite.

When we see a person being touched, we may empathize the affective feelings being produced by the touch. Interestingly, cognitive modulation of this effect can be produced. When subjects were informed by word labels that a cream seen being rubbed onto the forearm was a "Rich moisturizing cream" versus "Basic cream," these cognitive labels influenced activations in the orbitofrontal/pregenual cingulate cortex and ventral striatum to the sight of touch and their correlations with the pleasantness ratings [84]. Some evidence for top-down cognitive modulation of the effects produced by the subject being rubbed with the cream was found in brain regions such as the orbitofrontal and pregenual cingulate cortex and ventral striatum, but some effects were found in other brain regions, perhaps reflecting backprojections from the orbitofrontal cortex [84].

What may be a fundamental principle of how top-down attention can influence affective versus non-affective processing has recently been discovered. For an identical taste stimulus, paying attention to pleasantness activated some brain systems, and paying attention to intensity, which reflected the physical and not the affective properties of the stimulus, activated other brain systems [39]. In an fMRI investigation, when subjects were instructed to remember and rate the pleasantness of a taste stimulus, 0.1 M MSG, activations were greater in the medial orbitofrontal and pregenual cingulate cortex than when subjects were instructed to remember and rate the intensity of the taste. When the subjects were instructed to remember and rate the intensity, activations were greater in the insular taste cortex. Thus, depending on the context in which tastes are presented and whether affect is relevant, the brain responds to a taste differently. These findings show that when attention is paid to affective value, the brain systems engaged to represent the sensory stimulus of taste are different from those engaged when attention is directed to the physical properties of a stimulus such as its intensity [39]. This differential biasing of brain regions engaged in processing a sensory stimulus depending on whether the attentional demand is for affect-related versus more sensory-related processing may be an important aspect of cognition and attention. This has many implications for understanding attentional effects to affective value not only on taste, but also on other sensory stimuli.

Indeed, the concept has been validated in the olfactory system too. In an fMRI investigation, when subjects were instructed to remember and rate the pleasantness of a jasmine odor, activations were greater in the medial orbitofrontal and pregenual cingulate cortex than when subjects were instructed to remember and rate the intensity of the odor [125]. When the subjects were instructed to remember and rate the intensity, activations were greater in the inferior frontal gyrus. These top-down effects occurred not only during odor delivery, but started in a preparation period after the instruction before odor delivery, and continued after termination of the odor in a short-term memory period. These findings show that when attention is paid to affective value, the brain systems engaged to prepare for, represent, and remember a sensory stimulus are different from those engaged when attention is directed to the physical properties of a stimulus such as its intensity.

The principle thus appears to be that top-down attentional and cognitive effects on reward or affective value influence representations selectively in cortical areas that process the affective value and associated subjective emotional experience of taste [39,86] and olfactory [66,87,88] stimuli in brain regions such as the orbitofrontal cortex, whereas top-down attentional and cognitive effects on intensity influence representations in brain areas that process the intensity and identity of the stimulus such as the primary taste and olfactory cortical areas [39,66,86–88]. This is computationally appropriate in top-down biased competition models of attention [17,18,126]. Indeed, the mechanisms that underlie these top-down attentional and cognitive effects include top-down biased competition of the bottom-up (sensory) effects, and are now starting to be elucidated computationally [17,18,127–129].

5.12 Emotion and reward

From earlier approaches [2,8,130], Rolls has developed the theory over a series of articles that emotions are states elicited by instrumental reinforcers [1,7,131–135]. Given that the evidence described above indicates that primary (unlearned) reinforcers, such as taste, touch, and oral texture, are made explicit in the representations in the orbitofrontal cortex, there is a basis for understanding part of the role of the orbitofrontal cortex in emotion.

Further, the evidence described above indicates that associations between previously neutral stimuli such as a visual stimulus with primary reinforcers are formed and rapidly reversed in the orbitofrontal cortex, and thus the orbitofrontal cortex is likely because of this to have important functions in emotions that are produced by these secondary (learned) reinforcers. For example, the ability to perform this learning very rapidly is probably very important in social situations in primates, in which reinforcing stimuli are continually being exchanged, and the reinforcement value of stimuli must be continually updated (relearned), based on the actual reinforcers received and given. This type of learning also allows the stimuli or events that give rise to emotions and are represented in the orbitofrontal cortex to be quite abstract and general, including, for example, working for "points" or for monetary reward, as shown by visual discrimination reversal deficits in patients with orbitofrontal cortex lesions working for these rewards [97–99,136–138], and activation of different parts of the human orbitofrontal cortex by monetary gain versus loss [139], and other reinforcers [12].

The changes in emotion produced by damage to the orbitofrontal cortex are large, as the evidence described above and elsewhere shows [1,17,25]. The importance of the orbitofrontal cortex in emotion in humans is emphasized by a comparison with the effects of bilateral amygdala damage in humans, which, although producing demonstrable deficits in face processing [140,141], decision-making with linked autonomic deficits [142,143], and autonomic conditioning [144], may not produce major changes in emotion that are readily apparent in everyday behavior [17,144,145].

Further evidence on the close relation between rewards (or, more generally, reinforcers, to include punishers) and emotion, including the subjective feelings of emotion, and the brain regions that implement this processing, such as the orbitofrontal cortex, pregenual cingulate cortex, and amygdala, is described elsewhere [1,17,25,146].

5.13 Individual differences in reward processing and emotion

Given that there are individual differences in emotion, can these individual differences be related to the functioning of brain systems involved in reward and affective behavior such as the orbitofrontal and pregenual cingulate cortex?

Some individuals, chocolate cravers, report that they crave chocolate more than non-cravers, and this is associated with increased liking of chocolate, increased wanting of chocolate, and eating chocolate more frequently than non-cravers [208]. In a test of whether these individual differences are reflected in the affective systems in the orbitofrontal cortex and pregenual cingulate cortex that are the subject of this chapter, Rolls and McCabe [147] used fMRI to measure the response to the flavor of chocolate, to the sight of chocolate, and to their combination, in chocolate cravers versus non-cravers. Statistical parametric mapping (SPM) analyses showed that the sight of chocolate produced more activation in chocolate cravers than in non-cravers in the medial orbitofrontal cortex and ventral striatum. For cravers versus non-cravers, a combination of a picture of chocolate with chocolate in the mouth produced a greater effect than the sum of the components (i.e., supralinearity) in the medial orbitofrontal cortex and pregenual cingulate cortex. Furthermore, the pleasantness ratings of the chocolate and chocolate-related stimuli had higher positive correlations with the fMRI Blood oxygenation-level dependent (BOLD) signals in the pregenual cingulate cortex and medial orbitofrontal cortex in the cravers than in the non-cravers.

An implication is that individual differences in brain responses to very pleasant foods help to understand the mechanisms that drive the liking for specific foods by indicating that some brain systems (but not others such as the insular taste cortex) respond more to the rewarding aspects of some foods, and thus influence and indeed even predict the intake of those foods (which was much higher in chocolate cravers than non-cravers) [147].

Investigating another difference between individuals, Beaver et al. [148] showed that reward sensitivity in different individuals (as measured by a behavioral activation scale) is correlated with activations in the orbitofrontal cortex and ventral striatum to pictures of appetizing versus disgusting food.

It is also becoming possible to relate the functions of the orbitofrontal cortex to some psychiatric symptoms that may reflect changes in behavioral responses to reinforcers, which may be different in different individuals. We compared the symptoms of patients with a personality disorder syndrome, borderline personality disorder (BPD), with those of patients with lesions of the orbitofrontal cortex [137,149,150]. The symptoms of the self-harming BPD patients include high impulsivity, affective instability, and emotionality, as well as low extroversion. It was found that orbitofrontal cortex and BPD patients performed similarly in that they were more impulsive, reported more inappropriate behaviors in the Frontal Behaviour Questionnaire, and had more BPD characteristics and anger, and less happiness, than control groups (either normals or patients with lesions outside the orbitofrontal cortex).

Another case in which it is possible to relate psychiatric types of symptom to the functions of the orbitofrontal cortex in processing reinforcers is frontotemporal dementia, which is a progressive neurodegenerative disorder attacking the frontal lobes and producing major and pervasive behavioral changes in personality and social conduct, some of which resemble those produced by orbitofrontal lesions [151,152]. Patients appear either socially disinhibited, with facetiousness and inappropriate jocularity, or apathetic and withdrawn. The dementia is accompanied by gradual withdrawal from all social interactions. These behaviors could reflect impaired processing of reinforcers. Interestingly, given the anatomy and physiology of the orbitofrontal cortex, frontotemporal dementia causes profound changes in eating habits, with escalating desire for sweet food coupled with reduced satiety, which is often followed by enormous weight gain.

The negative symptoms of schizophrenia include flattening of affect. As part of a dynamical attractor systems theory of schizophrenia, in which hypofunction of N-methyl-D-aspartate (NMDA) receptors [153] contributes to the cognitive symptoms such as attentional, working memory, and dysexecutive impairments by reducing the depth of the basins of attraction of the prefrontal cortex networks involved in these functions, it has been proposed that the flattening of affect is produced by the same reduced NMDA receptor function, which decreases the neuronal firing rates, and in the orbitofrontal cortex and related areas would lead to decreased affect [1,154,155].

Conversely, it has been proposed that hyperfunctionality of the glutamate system in obsessive compulsive disorder [156,157] would contribute to overstability in prefrontal and related networks that would contribute to the perseverative/obsessional symptoms, and that the concomitant increased firing rates of neurons in the orbitofrontal cortex and related areas contributes to the increased emotionality that may be present in obsessive-compulsive disorder [158].

5.14   Beyond the representation of reward value to choice decision-making

In the neurophysiological studies described above, we have found that neuronal activity in the orbitofrontal cortex is related to the reward value of sensory stimuli, and how this changes when reward contingencies change, but is not related to the details of actions that are being performed, such as mouth or arm movements [1,17]. Wallis [159] and Padoa-Schioppa and Assad [160] have obtained evidence that supports this. An implication is that the orbitofrontal cortex represents the reward, affective (or, operationally, goal) value of a stimulus. Further, this value representation is on a continuous scale, as shown by the gradual decrease in orbitofrontal cortex neuronal responses to taste, olfactory, and visual rewarding stimuli during feeding to satiety [30,33,37,47]. Consistently, in humans the BOLD activations in different parts of the orbitofrontal cortex are continuously related to subjective pleasantness ratings of taste [39,86,161], olfactory [88], flavor [38,76,86,162], oral temperature [80], hand temperature [85], and face beauty [120] stimuli, and to monetary reward value [102,139], as shown by correlation analyses. An implication of these findings is that the orbitofrontal cortex may contribute to decision-making by representing on a continuous scale the value of each reward, with, as shown by the single neuron neurophysiology, different subsets of neurons for each different particular reward. It is, of course, essential to represent each reward separately, in order to make decisions about and between rewards, and separate representations (using distributed encoding [17]) of different rewards are present in the orbitofrontal cortex.

Approaches used in neuroeconomics help to define further the nature of the representation of reinforcers in the orbitofrontal cortex. When monkeys choose between different numbers of drops of two juices, one more preferred than the other, some neurons in the orbitofrontal cortex encode the offer value, some the choice value, and some the taste, but not the details of the motor response that is chosen [160]. Further, these neurons encode economic value, not relative preference, as shown by a study in which a particular reward was paired with other rewards. The fact that the neuronal responses are menu invariant suggests that transitivity, a fundamental trait of economic choice, may be rooted in the activity of individual neurons [163]. There is also evidence that relative reward value may be represented in the orbitofrontal cortex [164], and in what may provide a resolution of this, we are finding in a current study that some parts of the orbitofrontal cortex may represent the absolute pleasantness of stimuli and others the relative pleasantness of stimuli [165].

When a choice is made between stimuli with different reward probabilities, the choice made depends on the probability with which each reward will be obtained. In this probabilistic decision-making situation, we can define *expected value* as probability × reward magnitude) [166]. In an investigation of such a probabilistic choice decision task in which humans chose between two rewards, each available with different probabilities, it was found that the activation of the orbitofrontal cortex was related to expected value while the decision was being made, and also to the reward magnitude announced later on each trial [102]. Further evidence in a variety of tasks implicates a related and partly overlapping region of the ventromedial prefrontal cortex with expected value [105,167–169]. In contrast, the reward prediction errors or temporal difference errors as defined in reinforcement learning [104,170] are usually evident in the ventral striatum in imaging studies [102,105], though we should remember that negative reward prediction errors are represented by the error neurons in the primate orbitofrontal cortex [91] (see Section 5.9), and that the lateral orbitofrontal cortex is activated when a negative reward prediction error is generated in the reversal of a visual discrimination task [101].

Although it might be anticipated that the actual utility or "subjective utility" of an offer (a choice) to an individual approximately tracks the expected value, this is not exactly the case, with subjects typically undervaluing high rewards, and being over-sensitive to high punishments [171–177]. Subjects also typically have a subjective utility function that discounts rewards the further in the future they are delayed. Some parts of the ventromedial prefrontal cortex have activations that may follow the subjective utility of, for example, delayed rewards. In a study of this, it was found that activations in the ventromedial prefrontal cortex were correlated with the subjective utility of rewards delayed for different times, with the discount curve for each subject reconstructed from each subject's choices [178].

Clearly, a representation of reward magnitude, expected value, and even the subjective utility of a reward is an important input to a decision-making process, and the orbitofrontal cortex (with the ventromedial prefrontal area), appears to provide this information. When making a decision between two rewards, or whether to work for a reward that has an associated cost, it is important that the exact value of each reward is represented and enters the decision-making process. However, when a decision is reached, a system is needed that can make a binary choice, so that on one trial the decision might be reward 1, and on another trial reward 2, so that a particular action can be taken. For the evaluation, the neural activity needs to represent a stimulus in a way that continuously and faithfully represents the affective or reward value of the stimulus, and this could be present independently of whether a binary choice decision is being made or not. On the other hand, when a binary (choice) decision must be reached, a neural system is needed that does not continuously represent the reward value of the stimulus, but which instead falls into a binary state, in which for example the high firing of some neurons represents one decision (i.e., choice), and the high firing of other neurons represents a different choice. Processes such as this transition from spontaneous firing to a binary state of firing of neurons (fast versus slow) are known to occur in some premotor and related areas such as the macaque ventral premotor cortex when decisions are taken, in this case about which vibrotactile stimulus to choose [179–181].

It has been proposed that there may be a similar binary system, perhaps in another brain region, that becomes engaged when choice decisions are between rewards, or about rewards with which there is an associated cost [17]. To investigate whether representing the affective value of a reward on a continuous scale may occur before and separately from making a binary (for example, yes–no) decision about whether to choose the reward, Grabenhorst et al. [182] used fMRI to measure activations produced by pleasant warm, unpleasant cold, and affectively complex combinations of these stimuli applied to the hand. On some trials the affective value was rated on a continuous scale, and on different trials a yes–no (binary choice) decision was made about whether the stimulus should be repeated in future. Activations that were continuously related to the pleasantness ratings and that were not influenced when a binary (choice) decision was made were found in the orbitofrontal and pregenual cingulate cortex, implicating these regions in the continuous representation of affective value, consistent with the evidence described above. In this study, decision-making, contrasted with just rating the affective stimuli, revealed activations in the medial prefrontal cortex area 10, implicating this area in choice decision-making [182].

Support for a contribution of medial prefrontal cortex area 10 to taking binary (choice) decisions comes from a fMRI study in which two odors were separated by a delay, with instructions on different trials to decide which odor was more pleasant, or more intense, or to rate the pleasantness and intensity of the second odor on a continuous scale without making a binary (choice) decision. Activations in the medial prefrontal cortex area 10, and in regions to which it projects, including the anterior cingulate cortex and insula, were higher when binary choice decisions were being made compared to making ratings on a continuous scale, further implicating these regions in choice decision-making [183].

Different brain systems were implicated in different types of choice decision-making [183]. Decision-making about the affective value of odors produced larger effects in the dorsal part of medial prefrontal cortex area 10 and the agranular insula, whereas decisions about intensity produced larger effects in the dorsolateral prefrontal cortex, ventral premotor cortex, and anterior insula.

Consistent with these findings, patients with medial prefrontal cortex lesions are impaired in a decision-making shopping task, as reflected for example by visits to previously visited locations [184–186]. In another imaging study, area 10 activation has been related to moral decision-making [187].

In the study with warm and cold stimuli, and mixtures of the two, when a (choice) decision was yes versus no, effects were found in the dorsal anterior cingulate cortex [182], an area implicated by many other studies in decision-making [188,189]. The anterior cingulate cortex has been implicated in action-outcome learning [190,191], and the study with warm and cold stimuli shows that the contribution of the anterior cingulate cortex is in the choice decision-making itself, and that its activation does not occur just in relation to the pleasantness or intensity of the stimuli [182].

The implications are that the orbitofrontal cortex, and the pregenual cingulate cortex to which it projects, are involved in making decisions primarily by representing reward value on a continuous scale. Although the orbitofrontal cortex can have activations in decision-making tasks [192–194], it is important to separate processes involved in representing reward value from those involved in reaching a choice decision, which are separate computational processes [17]. The evidence we describe indicates that another tier of processing beyond the affective value stages becomes engaged in relation to taking binary (choice) decisions, and these areas include the medial prefrontal cortex area 10. Having separable systems for these types of processing appears to be computationally appropriate, for at the same time that one brain system is entering a binary decision state, that on this trial the choice is probabilistically one or another, in a way that could be implemented by the settling of an attractor network into one of its two or more high firing rate attractor states, each representing a choice [17,195,196], another brain system (involving the orbitofrontal and pregenual cingulate cortex) can still be representing faithfully the reward or affective value of the stimuli on a continuous scale [25].

We may ask why, if the activations in the orbitofrontal cortex and the pregenual cingulate cortex are somewhat similar in their continuous representations of reward or affective value, are there these two different areas? A suggestion is that the orbitofrontal cortex is the region that computes the rewards, expected rewards, and so on, and updates these rapidly when the reinforcement contingencies change, based on its inputs about primary reinforcers from the primary taste cortex [44], the primary olfactory cortex [197], the somatosensory cortex [198], etc. The orbitofrontal cortex makes explicit in its representations the reward value, based on these inputs, and in a situation where reward value is not represented at the previous tier, but instead where the representation is about the physical properties of the stimuli, their intensity, and so on [39,82,85,86,88,199] (see Fig. 5.1). The orbitofrontal cortex computes the expected value of previously neutral stimuli, and updates these representations rapidly when the reinforcement contingencies change, as described in this review. Thus, the orbitofrontal cortex is the computer of reward magnitude and expected reward value. It can thus represent outcomes, and expected outcomes, but it does not represent actions such as motor responses or movements. It is suggested that the representations of outcomes, and expected outcomes, are projected from the orbitofrontal cortex to the pregenual cingulate cortex, as the cingulate cortex has longitudinal connections, which allows this outcome information to be linked to the information about actions that is represented in the midcingulate cortex, and that the outcome information derived from the orbitofrontal cortex can contribute to action-outcome learning implemented in the cingulate cortex [17,25,190,191]. Although the anterior cingulate cortex is activated in relation to autonomic function [200], its functions clearly extend much beyond this, as shown also, for example, by the emotional changes that follow damage to the anterior cingulate cortex and related areas in humans [122].

Why, then, are there also outputs from the orbitofrontal cortex to medial area 10 (directly [201] and via pregenual cingulate cortex [13,201])? We suggest, based on the choice decision-making studies described here [25,182,183], that when a binary decision must be made between two (or more) rewards, then area 10 becomes involved. If it is simply a case of linking an action to a reward (and thus deciding which response to perform), the mid-cingulate cortex may be engaged. But if a prior decision must be made, not about which action to take to obtain an outcome, but instead between different rewards or expected rewards, or whether or not to choose a reward, then the medial prefrontal cortex area 10 may be involved [182,183]. The implication here is that there are many decision systems in the brain, and that we must specify exactly what type of decision is being made when relating a brain area to decision-making [17,181]. Consistent with this, in the odor decision-making study, when the decision between the first and second odor was not about which was more pleasant, but instead about which was more intense, the dorsolateral prefrontal cortex became engaged, rather than medial prefrontal cortex, area 10 [183].

5.15   Cortical networks that make choices between rewards: is there a common currency?

Attractor networks implemented by the recurrent collateral connections between cortical pyramidal cells provide a way to understand choice decision-making in the brain and its probabilistic nature [17,181,195,196]. Each set of neurons in the network that, if in the high firing rate state, represents one of the attractors corresponds to one of the decisions, and is biased on by the evidence for that decision, which might be the reward outcome expected if that decision is taken (i.e., the expected value). Because of the inhibitory interneurons, only one high firing rate attractor state can be active at any one time, so a choice is made on each trial. The state reached on a trial, that is, the decision taken, depends on the relative strength of the different expected rewards and on the noise within the network caused by the spiking of the neurons in the network. The network is essentially a short-term memory network, accumulating the evidence over short time periods (of, for example, 1 s) before finally falling into an attractor state in which one population of neurons only has won the competition on that trial, and is left with a high firing rate that represents the choice made.

In the application of this type of decision-making to rewards, the different inputs are the different rewards. One input might be an expected taste reward, another an expected monetary reward, another a social reward. Some authors have talked about a common currency for rewards [202–204]. What might this mean with this type of neuronal processing? In the neuronal decision mechanism described, the decision state is high firing activity of the representation of the particular reward that has won. This is excellent, because then action systems are provided with the information about the particular reward that is the goal of the action, and, of course, the actions selected will have to depend on the goal that has been selected. The fact that it is an attractor network that represents the reward selected is also very useful, for the short-term memory properties of the attractor network will keep the goal representation active while an action is being selected and performed. We can note that it would not be at all helpful to change the rewards into a common currency (such as points or dollars) as part of the selection process, as this would leave the selected goal just a number of points, or a number of dollars, which would not be useful to guide particular actions.

What is needed is that the different expected rewards that are the inputs to the decision networks must be on approximately the same scale. If food reward were to always be much stronger than other rewards, then the animal's genes would not survive, for it would never drink water, reproduce, etc. It has therefore been suggested that genes that specify rewards must be selected to ensure that the rewards they specify are approximately of the same maximum value, so that they will all be selected at some time [1]. There are, of course, factors that modulate the current value of each reward, such as hunger for food reward, thirst for water reward, etc. Also important in the modulation of the value of each reward is sensory-specific satiety, an adaptive property it is suggested all reward types to help selection of different rewards. The opposite is also a useful principle, namely incentive motivation, the shorter term increase in the reward value of a particular reward after a particular reward has been obtained (the salted nut phenomenon [205]), which has the adaptive utility of helping behavior to lock on to a goal for a useful and efficient amount of time, rather than continually switching between rewards [1]. Thus, we might speak of a common currency for different rewards in that each reward type must have a maximal value similar to other rewards as inputs that can drive the attractor decision-making network, so that each reward is selected at least sometimes. But there is no need to talk of a situation in which all specific rewards are converted into a common currency such as points. We can note that although the rewards that are specified as primary reinforcers by the genes should be specified to be approximately equipotent, learning mechanisms can adjust the reward value of what starts as a primary reinforcer, as when a taste is associated with sickness in taste aversion learning. As we shall see next, the costs associated with each reward can also be a factor.

Now in fMRI studies, it is frequently found that many different reward types (including taste, olfactory, flavor, texture, somatosensory, monetary, face expression, and social reputation rewards) activate rather similar brain areas, which often include the medial orbitofrontal cortex and pregenual cingulate cortex [1,25,59,204]. Does this provide evidence for a common reward representation of, for example, points? The evidence is that is does not, for all the single-neuron recording studies described above and elsewhere show that specific rewards are represented by each neuron, which often responds to a particular combination of sensory inputs. So why may all these different specific rewards be represented close together in, for example, the medial orbitofrontal cortex?

The answer, I suggest, is that the implementation of decision-making between rewards by an attractor network means that all the different reinforcers have to be brought spatially close together to compete with each other in a single network. The spatial constraint is that cortical networks operate over a short range of a few mm (for very good computational reasons, described by Rolls [17]), and this is why in this case the different rewards, to compete within the same network using the short-range inhibitory interneurons, and to support each other using the short range cortical excitatory recurrent collaterals, need to be represented close together in the cerebral cortex [17].

I note that the decision-making need not be between two rewards, and in principle an attractor-based decision network can make a single choice between multiple inputs [17,181,196].

How are costs taken into account in this decision-making process between different rewards? I suggest that the costs incurred in obtaining each goal need to be subtracted from the reward value of each goal, before they enter the decision-making network. The reason for this is that the costs are different for each type of reward, and so it would not make sense to choose the best reward independently of the cost of obtaining that reward. And to choose the best reward independent of cost, and then to go through a process of evaluating the cost for the highest reward, then if that does not exceed some criterion moving to the second highest reward, would also be computationally very time consuming as well as difficult to implement. For these reasons, the cost specific to each reward should be subtracted from the expected value of that reward to produce a net value for that reward-cost pair before the decision-making network that makes the choice selection. It will be very interesting to discover whether there are such representations of net reward-cost value in the brain, and if they are the inputs to the choice decision-making networks.

What factors influence whether a network is likely to be involved in choice decision-making versus representing expected reward value (or expected net reward value) on a continuous scale? I propose that if there is a strong forward input to the pyramidal cells that drives them hard, the firing rates will tend to reflect on a continuous scale the magnitude of the forward input. If the recurrent collaterals are particularly efficacious in any area, this will tend to make the cortical area more likely to produce "choices," that is, to end up with high firing rates for a winning population, with other cells inhibited. This may be a feature that, in terms of functional cortical architecture, may make some cortical areas more likely to represent inputs on a continuous scale, behaving perhaps linearly, whereas other areas may operate more nonlinearly, falling into an attractor state. Which is more likely may also be set dynamically, perhaps by acetylcholine and other modulators that may alter the relative efficacy of the recurrent collateral connections [25,206].

5.16 A computational basis for stimulus–reinforcer association learning and reversal in the orbitofrontal cortex involving conditional reward neurons and negative reward prediction error neurons

The neurophysiological, imaging, and lesion evidence described above suggests that one function implemented by the orbitofrontal cortex is rapid stimulus–reinforcement association learning and the correction of these associations when reinforcement contingencies in the environment change. How might this rapid stimulus–reinforcer association learning and reversal be implemented at the neuronal and neuronal network level? One

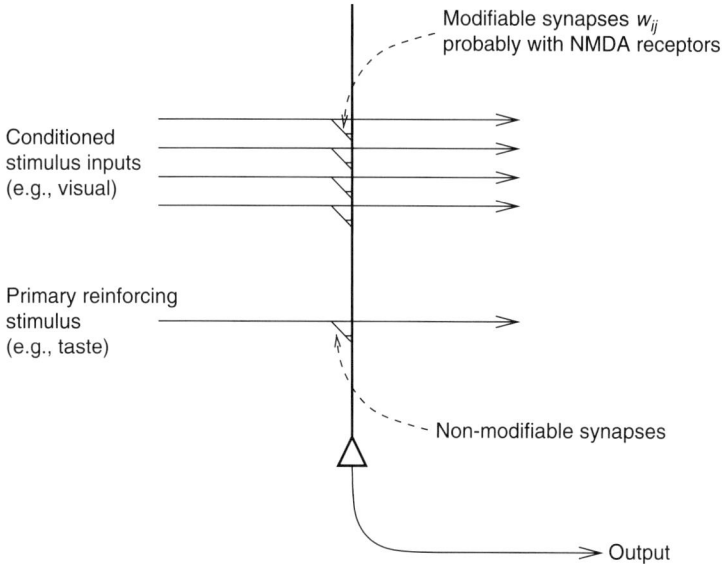

Figure 5.6 Pattern association between a primary reinforcer, such as the taste of food, which activates neurons through non-modifiable synapses, and a potential secondary reinforcer, such as the sight of food, which has modifiable synapses onto the same neurons. The associative rule for the synaptic modification is that if there is both presynaptic and post-synaptic firing, then that synapse should increase in strength. Such a mechanism appears to be implemented in the amygdala and orbitofrontal cortex. (Homosynaptic) long-term depression (produced by presynaptic firing in the absence of strong postsynaptic firing) in the pattern associator could account for the response to the no-longer reinforced stimulus becoming weaker. For further details, see [1].

mechanism could be implemented by Hebbian modification of synapses conveying visual input onto taste-responsive neurons, implementing a pattern association network [1,7,17,18,94,207]. Long-term potentiation would strengthen synapses from active conditioned stimulus neurons onto neurons responding to a primary reinforcer, such as a sweet taste, and homosynaptic long-term depression would weaken synapses from the same active visual inputs if the neuron was not responding because an aversive primary reinforcer (e.g., a taste of saline) was being presented (Fig. 5.6).

As described above, the conditional reward neurons in the orbitofrontal cortex convey information about the current reinforcement status of particular stimuli. In a new theory of how the orbitofrontal cortex implements rapid, one-trial, reversal, these neurons play a key part, for particular conditional reward neurons (responding to, e.g., "green is now rewarding"; see example in Fig. 5.4C) are biased on by a rule set of neurons if the association is being run direct, and are biased off if the association is being run reversed ("green is now not rewarding") [95]. One set of rule neurons in the short-term memory attractor network is active when the rule is direct, and a different set of neurons when the association is reversed. The state of the rule network is reversed when the error neurons fire in reversal, because the firing of the error neurons quenches the attractor by activating inhibitory neurons, and the opposite set of rule neurons emerge to activity after the quenching because of some adaptation in the synapses or neurons in the rule attractor that have just been active. The error-detection neurons themselves may be triggered by a mismatch between what was expected when the visual stimulus was shown and the primary reinforcer that was obtained, both of which are represented in the primate orbitofrontal cortex [91]. The whole system maps stimuli (such as green and blue) through a biased competition layer of conditional reward neurons in which the mapping is controlled by the biasing input from the rule neurons, to output neurons that fire if a stimulus is being shown that is currently associated with reward [95].

The model gives an account of the presence of conditional reward and error neurons in the orbitofrontal cortex, as well as neurons that respond to whichever visual stimulus is currently associated with reward, and neurons that signal whether a (e.g., taste) reward or punishment has just been obtained. The model also suggests that the orbitofrontal cortex may be especially appropriate for this rapid reversal mechanism, because, in contrast to the amygdala, the orbitofrontal cortex as a cortical structure has a well-developed system of recurrent collateral synapses between the pyramidal cells, providing an appropriate basis for implementing a working memory to hold the current rule. The model also shows how when on a reversal trial a reward is not obtained to a previously rewarded stimulus, on the very next trial when the recently punished stimulus is shown, it is treated as a reward, and it is chosen. This type of behavior at the behavioral level is in fact illustrated in Fig. 5.5 (e.g., trials 4 and 14), and cannot be accounted for by a new association of the now to be rewarded stimulus with reward, for in its recent past it has been associated with saline. Thus, this type of one-trial rapid reversal cannot be accounted for by direct stimulus–reward association learning, and a rule-based system, such as the type implemented in the model, is needed. The model has been worked out in detail at the level of integrate-and-fire spiking neurons, and makes predictions about further types of neuron expected to be present in the orbitofrontal cortex [1,95].

In conclusion, some foundations for understanding reward processing and decision-making have been described. A fuller approach to understanding reward processing and emotion is provided by Rolls [1], a rigorous computational approach is provided by Rolls [17], and future directions are suggested by Rolls and Grabenhorst [25].

Summary

I consider where sensory representations are transformed into reward based representations in the brain; how associations are learned and reversed between stimuli (that thereby become secondary reinforcers) and primary reinforcers such as taste and touch; how these processes lead to representations of reward magnitude, expected reward value, and reward prediction error; how cognition and attention specifically modulate these processes; and then how decisions which involve a choice are made between different rewards.

Acknowledgements

The author has worked on some of the experiments described here with I. Araujo, G.C. Baylis, L.L. Baylis, A. Bilderbeck, R. Bowtell, A.D. Browning, H.D. Critchley, S. Francis, F. Grabenhorst, M.E. Hasselmo, J. Hornak, M. Kadohisa, M. Kringelbach, C.M. Leonard, C. Margot, C. McCabe, F. McGlone, F. Mora, J. O'Doherty, B.A. Parris, D.I. Perrett, T.R. Scott, S.J. Thorpe, M.I. Velazco, J.V. Verhagen, E.A. Wakeman and F.A.W. Wilson, and their collaboration is sincerely acknowledged. Some of the research described was supported by the Medical Research Council, PG8513790 and PG9826105.

References

[1] E.T. Rolls, Emotion Explained, Oxford University Press, Oxford, 2005.

[2] J.A. Gray, Elements of a Two-Process Theory of Learning, Academic Press, London, 1975.

[3] A. Dickinson, Contemporary Animal Learning Theory, Cambridge University Press, Cambridge, 1980.

[4] N.J. Mackintosh, Conditioning and Associative Learning, Oxford University Press, Oxford, 1983.

[5] J.E. Mazur, Learning and Behavior, fourth ed., Prentice Hall, Upper Saddle River, NJ, 1998.

[6] D.A. Lieberman, Learning, Wadsworth, Belmont, CA, 2000.

[7] E.T. Rolls, The Brain and Emotion, Oxford University Press, Oxford, 1999.

[8] L. Weiskrantz, Emotion, in: L. Weiskrantz (Ed.), Analysis of Behavioural Change, Harper and Row, New York and London, 1968, pp. 50–90.

[9] S.T. Carmichael, J.L. Price, Architectonic subdivision of the orbital and medial prefrontal cortex in the macaque monkey, J. Comp. Neurol. 346 (1994) 366–402.

[10] M. Petrides, D.N. Pandya, Comparative architectonic analysis of the human and macaque frontal cortex, in: F. Boller, J. Grafman (Eds.), Handbook of Neuropsychology, Elsevier Science, Amsterdam, 1995, pp. 17–58.

[11] D. Öngür, J.L. Price, The organisation of networks within the orbital and medial prefrontal cortex of rats, monkeys and humans, Cereb. Cortex 10 (2000) 206–219.

[12] M.L. Kringelbach, E.T. Rolls, The functional neuroanatomy of the human orbitofrontal cortex: evidence from neuroimaging and neuropsychology, Prog. Neurobiol. 72 (2004) 341–372.

[13] J.L. Price, Connections of orbital cortex, in: D.H. Zald, S.L. Rauch (Eds.), The Orbitofrontal Cortex, Oxford University Press, Oxford, 2006, pp. 39–55.

[14] J.L. Price, Definition of the orbital cortex in relation to specific connections with limbic and visceral structures and other cortical regions, Ann. NY Acad. Sci. 1121 (2007) 54–71.

[15] E.T. Rolls, Functions of the primate temporal lobe cortical visual areas in invariant visual object and face recognition, Neuron 27 (2000) 205–218.

[16] E.T. Rolls, The representation of information about faces in the temporal and frontal lobes, Neuropsychologia 45 (2007) 125–143.

[17] E.T. Rolls, Memory, Attention, and Decision-making: A Unifying Computational Neuroscience Approach, Oxford University Press, Oxford, 2008.

[18] E.T. Rolls, G. Deco, Computational Neuroscience of Vision, Oxford University Press, Oxford, 2002.

[19] E.T. Rolls, S.M. Stringer, Invariant visual object recognition: a model, with lighting invariance, J. Physiol. Paris 100 (2006) 43–62.

[20] R. Norgren, Central neural mechanisms of taste, in: I. Darien-Smith (Ed.), Handbook of Physiology – The Nervous System III, Sensory Processes 1, American Physiological Society, Washington, DC, 1984, pp. 1087–1128.

[21] E.T. Rolls, T.R. Scott, Central taste anatomy and neurophysiology, in: R.L. Doty (Ed.), Handbook of Olfaction and Gustation, second ed., Dekker, New York, 2003, pp. 679–705.

[22] S.T. Carmichael, J.L. Price, Sensory and premotor connections of the orbital and medial prefrontal cortex of macaque monkeys, J. Comp. Neurol. 363 (1995) 642–664.

[23] H. Barbas, Anatomic basis of cognitive-emotional interactions in the primate prefrontal cortex, Neurosci. Biobehav. Rev. 19 (1995) 499–510.

[24] D.N. Pandya, E.H. Yeterian, Comparison of prefrontal architecture and connections, Philos. Trans. R. Soc. Lond. B Biol. Sci. 351 (1996) 1423–1431.

[25] E.T. Rolls, F. Grabenhorst, The orbitofrontal cortex and beyond: from affect to decision-making, Prog. Neurobiol. 86 (2008) 216–244.

[26] E.T. Rolls, The functions of the orbitofrontal cortex, Brain Cogn. 55 (2004) 11–29.

[27] E.T. Rolls, S. Yaxley, Z.J. Sienkiewicz, Gustatory responses of single neurons in the caudolateral orbitofrontal cortex of the macaque monkey, J. Neurophysiol. 64 (1990) 1055–1066.

[28] L.L. Baylis, E.T. Rolls, Responses of neurons in the primate taste cortex to glutamate, Physiol. Behav. 49 (1991) 973–979.

[29] E.T. Rolls, The representation of umami taste in the taste cortex, J. Nutr. 130 (2000) S960–S965.

[30] E.T. Rolls, H. Critchley, E.A. Wakeman, R. Mason, Responses of neurons in the primate taste cortex to the glutamate ion and to inosine 5'-monophosphate, Physiol. Behav. 59 (1996) 991–1000.

[31] E.T. Rolls, H.D. Critchley, A. Browning, I. Hernadi, The neurophysiology of taste and olfaction in primates, and umami flavor, Ann. NY Acad. Sci. 855 (1998) 426–437.

[32] E.T. Rolls, J.V. Verhagen, M. Kadohisa, Representations of the texture of food in the primate orbitofrontal cortex: neurons responding to viscosity, grittiness and capsaicin, J. Neurophysiol. 90 (2003) 3711–3724.

[33] E.T. Rolls, H.D. Critchley, A.S. Browning, A. Hernadi, L. Lenard, Responses to the sensory properties of fat of neurons in the primate orbitofrontal cortex, J. Neurosci. 19 (1999) 1532–1540.

[34] J.V. Verhagen, E.T. Rolls, M. Kadohisa, Neurons in the primate orbitofrontal cortex respond to fat texture independently of viscosity, J. Neurophysiol. 90 (2003) 1514–1525.

[35] H.D. Critchley, E.T. Rolls, Responses of primate taste cortex neurons to the astringent tastant tannic acid, Chem. Senses 21 (1996) 135–145.

[36] S.A. Simon, I.E. de Araujo, R. Gutierrez, M.A. Nicolelis, The neural mechanisms of gustation: a distributed processing code, Nat. Rev. Neurosci. 7 (2006) 890–901.

[37] E.T. Rolls, Z.J. Sienkiewicz, S. Yaxley, Hunger modulates the responses to gustatory stimuli of single neurons in the caudolateral orbitofrontal cortex of the macaque monkey, Eur. J. Neurosci. 1 (1989) 53–60.

[38] M.L. Kringelbach, J. O'Doherty, E.T. Rolls, C. Andrews, Activation of the human orbitofrontal cortex to a liquid food stimulus is correlated with its subjective pleasantness, Cereb. Cortex 13 (2003) 1064–1071.

[39] F. Grabenhorst, E.T. Rolls, Selective attention to affective value alters how the brain processes taste stimuli, Eur. J. Neurosci. 27 (2008) 723–729.

[40] F. Mora, D.B. Avrith, A.G. Phillips, E.T. Rolls, Effects of satiety on self-stimulation of the orbitofrontal cortex in the monkey, Neurosci. Lett. 13 (1979) 141–145.

[41] F. Mora, D.B. Avrith, E.T. Rolls, An electrophysiological and behavioural study of self-stimulation in the orbitofrontal cortex of the rhesus monkey, Brain Res. Bull. 5 (1980) 111–115.

[42] E.T. Rolls, M.J. Burton, F. Mora, Neurophysiological analysis of brain-stimulation reward in the monkey, Brain Res. 194 (1980) 339–357.

[43] E.T. Rolls, Understanding the mechanisms of food intake and obesity, Obes. Rev. 8 (2007) 67–72.

[44] L.L. Baylis, E.T. Rolls, G.C. Baylis, Afferent connections of the orbitofrontal cortex taste area of the primate, Neuroscience 64 (1995) 801–812.

[45] E.T. Rolls, H.D. Critchley, R. Mason, E.A. Wakeman, Orbitofrontal cortex neurons: role in olfactory and visual association learning, J. Neurophysiol. 75 (1996) 1970–1981.

[46] E.T. Rolls, L.L. Baylis, Gustatory, olfactory, and visual convergence within the primate orbitofrontal cortex, J. Neurosci. 14 (1994) 5437–5452.

[47] H.D. Critchley, E.T. Rolls, Hunger and satiety modify the responses of olfactory and visual neurons in the primate orbitofrontal cortex, J. Neurophysiol. 75 (1996) 1673–1686.

[48] T.C. Pritchard, E.M. Edwards, C.A. Smith, K.G. Hilgert, A.M. Gavlick, T.D. Maryniak, G.J. Schwartz, T.R. Scott, Gustatory neural responses in the medial orbitofrontal cortex of the old world monkey, J. Neurosci. 25 (2005) 6047–6056.

[49] T.C. Pritchard, G.J. Schwartz, T.R. Scott, Taste in the medial orbitofrontal cortex of the macaque, Ann. NY Acad. Sci. 1121 (2007) 121–135.

[50] E.T. Rolls, Functions of the orbitofrontal and pregenual cingulate cortex in taste, olfaction, appetite and emotion, Acta Physiol. Hung. 95 (2008) 131–164.

[51] T.C. Pritchard, E.N. Nedderman, E.M. Edwards, A.C. Petticoffer, G.J. Schwartz, T.R. Scott, Satiety-responsive neurons in the medial orbitofrontal cortex of the macaque, Behav. Neurosci. 122 (2008) 174–182.

[52] M.K. Sanghera, E.T. Rolls, A. Roper-Hall, Visual responses of neurons in the dorsolateral amygdala of the alert monkey, Exp. Neurol. 63 (1979) 610–626.

[53] T.R. Scott, Z. Karadi, Y. Oomura, H. Nishino, C.R. Plata-Salaman, L. Lenard, B.K. Giza, S. Ao, Gustatory neural coding in the amygdala of the alert monkey, J. Neurophysiol. 69 (1993) 1810–1820.

[54] M. Kadohisa, E.T. Rolls, J.V. Verhagen, Neuronal representations of stimuli in the mouth: the primate insular taste cortex, orbitofrontal cortex, and amygdala, Chem. Senses 30 (2005) 401–419.

[55] M. Kadohisa, E.T. Rolls, J.V. Verhagen, The primate amygdala: neuronal representations of the viscosity, fat texture, temperature, grittiness and taste of foods, Neuroscience 132 (2005) 33–48.

[56] J. Yan, T.R. Scott, The effect of satiety on responses of gustatory neurons in the amygdala of alert cynomolgus macaques, Brain Res. 740 (1996) 193–200.

[57] M.J. Burton, E.T. Rolls, F. Mora, Effects of hunger on the responses of neurones in the lateral hypothalamus to the sight and taste of food, Exp. Neurol. 51 (1976) 668–677.

[58] J. O'Doherty, E.T. Rolls, S. Francis, R. Bowtell, F. McGlone, The representation of pleasant and aversive taste in the human brain, J. Neurophysiol. 85 (2001) 1315–1321.

[59] E.T. Rolls, The anterior and midcingulate cortices and reward, in: B.A. Vogt (Ed.), Cingulate Neurobiology & Disease, Oxford University Press, Oxford, 2008.

[60] M. Jones-Gotman, R.J. Zatorre, Olfactory identification in patients with focal cerebral excision, Neuropsychologia 26 (1988) 387–400.

[61] R.J. Zatorre, M. Jones-Gotman, A.C. Evans, E. Meyer, Functional localization of human olfactory cortex, Nature 360 (1992) 339–340.

[62] S.F. Takagi, Olfactory frontal cortex and multiple olfactory processing in primates, in: A. Peters, E.G. Jones (Eds.), Cerebral Cortex, Plenum Press, New York, 1991, pp. 133–152.

[63] H.D. Critchley, E.T. Rolls, Olfactory neuronal responses in the primate orbitofrontal cortex: analysis in an olfactory discrimination task, J. Neurophysiol. 75 (1996) 1659–1672.

[64] G. Schoenbaum, M.P. Saddoris, T.A. Stalnaker, Reconciling the roles of orbitofrontal cortex in reversal learning and the encoding of outcome expectancies, Ann. NY Acad. Sci. 1121 (2007) 320–335.

[65] G. Schoenbaum, H. Eichenbaum, Information encoding in the rodent prefrontal cortex .1. Single-neuron activity in orbitofrontal cortex compared with that in pyriform cortex, J. Neurophysiol. 74 (1995) 733–750.

[66] E.T. Rolls, M.L. Kringelbach, I.E.T. de Araujo, Different representations of pleasant and unpleasant odors in the human brain, Eur. J. Neurosci. 18 (2003) 695–703.

[67] S. Francis, E.T. Rolls, R. Bowtell, F. McGlone, J. O'Doherty, A. Browning, S. Clare, E. Smith, The representation of pleasant touch in the brain and its relationship with taste and olfactory areas, Neuroreport 10 (1999) 453–459.

[68] J. O'Doherty, E.T. Rolls, S. Francis, R. Bowtell, F. McGlone, G. Kobal, B. Renner, G. Ahne, Sensory-specific satiety related olfactory activation of the human orbitofrontal cortex, Neuroreport 11 (2000) 893–897.

[69] J.S. Morris, R.J. Dolan, Involvement of human amygdala and orbitofrontal cortex in hunger-enhanced memory for food stimuli, J. Neurosci. 21 (2001) 5304–5310.

[70] I.E.T. de Araujo, E.T. Rolls, M.L. Kringelbach, F. McGlone, N. Phillips, Taste-olfactory convergence, and the representation of the pleasantness of flavour, in the human brain, Eur. J. Neurosci. 18 (2003) 2374–2390.

[71] J.V. Verhagen, M. Kadohisa, E.T. Rolls, The primate insular/opercular taste cortex: neuronal representations of the viscosity, fat texture, grittiness, temperature and taste of foods, J. Neurophysiol. 92 (2004) 1685–1699.

[72] N. Chaudhari, A.M. Landin, S.D. Roper, A metabotropic glutamate receptor variant functions as a taste receptor, Nat. Neurosci. 3 (2000) 113–119.

[73] G.Q. Zhao, Y. Zhang, M.A. Hoon, J. Chandrashekar, I. Erlenbach, N.J. Ryba, C.S. Zuker, The receptors for mammalian sweet and umami taste, Cell 115 (2003) 255–266.

[74] Y. Maruyama, E. Pereira, R.F. Margolskee, N. Chaudhari, S.D. Roper, Umami responses in mouse taste cells indicate more than one receptor, J. Neurosci. 26 (2006) 2227–2234.

[75] I.E.T. de Araujo, M.L. Kringelbach, E.T. Rolls, P. Hobden, The representation of umami taste in the human brain, J. Neurophysiol. 90 (2003) 313–319.

[76] C. McCabe, E.T. Rolls, Umami: a delicious flavor formed by convergence of taste and olfactory pathways in the human brain, Eur. J. Neurosci. 25 (2007) 1855–1864.

[77] E.T. Rolls, Taste, olfactory, visual and somatosensory representations of the sensory properties of foods in the brain, and their relation to the control of food intake, in: H-R. Berthoud, R.J. Seeley (Eds.), Neural and Metabolic Control of Macronutrient Intake, CRC Press, Boca-Raton, FL, 2000, pp. 247–262.

[78] M. Kadohisa, E.T. Rolls, J.V. Verhagen, Orbitofrontal cortex neuronal representation of temperature and capsaicin in the mouth, Neuroscience 127 (2004) 207–221.

[79] I.E.T. de Araujo, E.T. Rolls, The representation in the human brain of food texture and oral fat, J. Neurosci. 24 (2004) 3086–3093.

[80] S. Guest, F. Grabenhorst, G. Essick, Y. Chen, M. Young, F. McGlone, I. de Araujo, E.T. Rolls, Human cortical representation of oral temperature, Physiol. Behav. 92 (2007) 975–984.

[81] B.J. Rolls, R.J. Wood, E.T. Rolls, Thirst: the initiation, maintenance, and termination of drinking, Prog. Psychobiol. Physiol. Psychol. 9 (1980) 263–321.

[82] E.T. Rolls, J. O'Doherty, M.L. Kringelbach, S. Francis, R. Bowtell, F. McGlone, Representations of pleasant and painful touch in the human orbitofrontal and cingulate cortices, Cereb. Cortex 13 (2003) 308–317.

[83] H. Olausson, Y. Lamarre, H. Backlund, C. Morin, B.G. Wallin, G. Starck, S. Ekholm, I. Strigo, K. Worsley, A.B. Vallbo, M.C. Bushnell, Unmyelinated tactile afferents signal touch and project to insular cortex, Nat. Neurosci. 5 (2002) 900–904.

[84] C. McCabe, E.T. Rolls, A. Bilderbeck, F. McGlone, Cognitive influences on the affective representation of touch and the sight of touch in the human brain, Soc. Cogn. Affect. Neurosci. 3 (2008) 97–108.

[85] E.T. Rolls, F. Grabenhorst, B.A. Parris, Warm pleasant feelings in the brain, Neuroimage 41 (2008) 1504–1513.

[86] F. Grabenhorst, E.T. Rolls, A. Bilderbeck, How cognition modulates affective responses to taste and flavor: top down influences on the orbitofrontal and pregenual cingulate cortices, Cereb. Cortex 18 (2008) 1549–1559.

[87] A.K. Anderson, K. Christoff, I. Stappen, D. Panitz, D.G. Ghahremani, G. Glover, J.D. Gabrieli, N. Sobel, Dissociated neural representations of intensity and valence in human olfaction, Nat. Neurosci. 6 (2003) 196–202.

[88] F. Grabenhorst, E.T. Rolls, C. Margot, M.A. da Silva, M.I.A.P. Velazco, How pleasant and unpleasant stimuli combine in different brain regions: odor mixtures, J. Neurosci. 27 (2007) 13532–13540.

[89] E.T. Rolls, The affective and cognitive processing of touch, oral texture, and temperature in the brain, Neurosci. Biobehav. Rev. (2008), April 3, Epub ahead of print.

[90] E.T. Rolls, Face processing in different brain areas, and critical band masking, J. Neuropsychol. 2 (2008) 325–360.

[91] S.J. Thorpe, E.T. Rolls, S. Maddison, Neuronal activity in the orbitofrontal cortex of the behaving monkey, Exp. Brain Res. 49 (1983) 93–115.

[92] J.P. O'Doherty, R. Deichmann, H.D. Critchley, R.J. Dolan, Neural responses during anticipation of a primary taste reward, Neuron 33 (2002) 815–826.

[93] E.T. Rolls, S.J. Judge, M. Sanghera, Activity of neurones in the inferotemporal cortex of the alert monkey, Brain Res. 130 (1977) 229–238.

[94] E.T. Rolls, A. Treves, Neural Networks and Brain Function, Oxford University Press, Oxford, 1998.

[95] G. Deco, E.T. Rolls, Synaptic and spiking dynamics underlying reward reversal in orbitofrontal cortex, Cereb. Cortex 15 (2005) 15–30.

[96] M. Roesch, G. Schoenbaum, From associations to expectancies: orbitofrontal cortex as gateway between the limbic system and representational memory, in: D.H. Zald, S.L. Rauch (Eds.), The Orbitofrontal Cortex, Oxford University Press, Oxford, 2006, pp. 199–236.

[97] E.T. Rolls, J. Hornak, D. Wade, J. McGrath, Emotion-related learning in patients with social and emotional changes associated with frontal lobe damage, J. Neurol. Neurosurg. Psychiatry 57 (1994) 1518–1524.

[98] L.K. Fellows, M.J. Farah, Ventromedial frontal cortex mediates affective shifting in humans: evidence from a reversal learning paradigm, Brain 126 (2003) 1830–1837.

[99] J. Hornak, J. O'Doherty, J. Bramham, E.T. Rolls, R.G. Morris, P.R. Bullock, C.E. Polkey, Reward-related reversal learning after surgical excisions in orbitofrontal and dorsolateral prefrontal cortex in humans, J. Cogn. Neurosci. 16 (2004) 463–478.

[100] J.J. Paton, M.A. Belova, S.E. Morrison, C.D. Salzman, The primate amygdala represents the positive and negative value of visual stimuli during learning, Nature 439 (2006) 865–870.

[101] M.L. Kringelbach, E.T. Rolls, Neural correlates of rapid reversal learning in a simple model of human social interaction, Neuroimage 20 (2003) 1371–1383.

[102] E.T. Rolls, C. McCabe, J. Redoute, Expected value, reward outcome, and temporal difference error representations in a probabilistic decision task, Cereb. Cortex 18 (2008) 652–663.

[103] W. Schultz, Neural coding of basic reward terms of animal learning theory, game theory, microeconomics and behavioural ecology, Curr. Opin. Neurobiol. 14 (2004) 139–147.

[104] W. Schultz, Behavioral theories and the neurophysiology of reward, Annu. Rev. Psychol. 57 (2006) 87–115.

[105] T.A. Hare, J. O'Doherty, C.F. Camerer, W. Schultz, A. Rangel, Dissociating the role of the orbitofrontal cortex and the striatum in the computation of goal values and prediction errors, J. Neurosci. 28 (2008) 5623–5630.

[106] W. Schultz, L. Tremblay, J.R. Hollerman, Reward processing in primate orbitofrontal cortex and basal ganglia, Cereb. Cortex 10 (2000) 272–284.

[107] H. Niki, M. Watanabe, Prefrontal and cingulate unit activity during timing behavior in the monkey, Brain Res. 171 (1979) 213–224.

[108] K. Shima, J. Tanji, Role for cingulate motor area cells in voluntary movement selection based on reward, Science 282 (1998) 1335–1338.

[109] G. Bush, B.A. Vogt, J. Holmes, A.M. Dale, D. Greve, M.A. Jenike, B.R. Rosen, Dorsal anterior cingulate cortex: a role in reward-based decision making, Proc. Natl. Acad. Sci. USA 99 (2002) 523–528.

[110] M.F. Rushworth, M.E. Walton, S.W. Kennerley, D.M. Bannerman, Action sets and decisions in the medial frontal cortex, Trends Cogn. Sci. 8 (2004) 410–417.

[111] M. Matsumoto, K. Matsumoto, H. Abe, K. Tanaka, Medial prefrontal selectivity signalling prediction errors of action values, Nat. Neurosci. 10 (2007) 647–656.

[112] M.F. Rushworth, T.E. Behrens, Choice, uncertainty and value in prefrontal and cingulate cortex, Nat. Neurosci. 11 (2008) 389–397.

[113] B.A. Vogt (Ed.), Cingulate Neurobiology & Disease, Oxford University Press, Oxford, 2008.

[114] E.T. Rolls, Neurons in the cortex of the temporal lobe and in the amygdala of the monkey with responses selective for faces, Hum. Neurobiol. 3 (1984) 209–222.

[115] E.T. Rolls, Neurophysiological mechanisms underlying face processing within and beyond the temporal cortical visual areas, Philos. Trans. R. Soc. Lond. B Biol. Sci. 335 (1992) 11–21.

[116] E.T. Rolls, The orbitofrontal cortex, Philos. Trans. R. Soc. Lond. B Biol. Sci. 351 (1996) 1433–1444.

[117] E.T. Rolls, H.D. Critchley, A.S. Browning, K. Inoue, Face-selective and auditory neurons in the primate orbitofrontal cortex, Exp. Brain Res. 170 (2006) 74–87.

[118] E.T. Rolls, G.C. Baylis, Size and contrast have only small effects on the responses to faces of neurons in the cortex of the superior temporal sulcus of the monkey, Exp. Brain Res. 65 (1986) 38–48.

[119] M.E. Hasselmo, E.T. Rolls, G.C. Baylis, The role of expression and identity in the face-selective responses of neurons in the temporal visual cortex of the monkey, Behav. Brain Res. 32 (1989) 203–218.

[120] J. O'Doherty, J. Winston, H. Critchley, D. Perrett, D.M. Burt, R.J. Dolan, Beauty in a smile: the role of medial orbitofrontal cortex in facial attractiveness, Neuropsychologia 41 (2003) 147–155.

[121] J. Hornak, E.T. Rolls, D. Wade, Face and voice expression identification in patients with emotional and behavioural changes following ventral frontal lobe damage, Neuropsychologia 34 (1996) 247–261.

[122] J. Hornak, J. Bramham, E.T. Rolls, R.G. Morris, J. O'Doherty, P.R. Bullock, C.E. Polkey, Changes in emotion after circumscribed surgical lesions of the orbitofrontal and cingulate cortices, Brain 126 (2003) 1691–1712.

[123] I.E.T. de Araujo, E.T. Rolls, M.I. Velazco, C. Margot, I. Cayeux, Cognitive modulation of olfactory processing, Neuron 46 (2005) 671–679.

[124] E.T. Rolls, Sensory processing in the brain related to the control of food intake, Proc. Nutr. Soc. 66 (2007) 96–112.

[125] E.T. Rolls, F. Grabenhorst, C. Margot, M.A.A.P. da Silva, M.I. Velazco, Selective attention to affective value alters how the brain processes olfactory stimuli, J. Cogn. Neurosci. 20 (2008) 1815–1826.

[126] G. Deco, E.T. Rolls, Attention, short-term memory, and action selection: a unifying theory, Prog. Neurobiol. 76 (2005) 236–256.

[127] R. Desimone, J. Duncan, Neural mechanisms of selective visual attention, Annu. Rev. Neurosci. 18 (1995) 193–222.

[128] G. Deco, E.T. Rolls, Neurodynamics of biased competition and co-operation for attention: a model with spiking neurons, J. Neurophysiol. 94 (2005) 295–313.

[129] E.T. Rolls, Top-down control of visual perception: attention in natural vision, Perception 37 (2008) 333–354.

[130] J.R. Millenson, Principles of Behavioral Analysis, MacMillan, New York, 1967.

[131] E.T. Rolls, A theory of emotion, and its application to understanding the neural basis of emotion, in: Y. Oomura (Ed.), Emotions. Neural and Chemical Control, Karger, Basel, 1986, pp. 325–344.

[132] E.T. Rolls, Neural systems involved in emotion in primates, in: R. Plutchik, H. Kellerman (Eds.), Emotion: theory, research, and experience, Vol. 3. Biological foundations of emotion, Academic Press, New York, 1986, pp. 125–143.

[133] E.T. Rolls, A theory of emotion, and its application to understanding the neural basis of emotion, Cogn. Emotion 4 (1990) 161–190.

[134] E.T. Rolls, The functions of the orbitofrontal cortex, Neurocase 5 (1999) 301–312.

[135] E.T. Rolls, Précis of The brain and emotion, Behav. Brain Sci. 23 (2000) 177–233.

[136] L.K. Fellows, M.J. Farah, Different underlying impairments in decision-making following ventromedial and dorsolateral frontal lobe damage in humans, Cereb. Cortex 15 (2005) 58–63.

[137] H. Berlin, E.T. Rolls, U. Kischka, Impulsivity, time perception, emotion, and reinforcement sensitivity in patients with orbitofrontal cortex lesions, Brain 127 (2004) 1108–1126.

[138] L.K. Fellows, The role of orbitofrontal cortex in decision making: a component process account, Ann. NY Acad. Sci. 1121 (2007) 421–430.

[139] J. O'Doherty, M.L. Kringelbach, E.T. Rolls, J. Hornak, C. Andrews, Abstract reward and punishment representations in the human orbitofrontal cortex, Nat. Neurosci. 4 (2001) 95–102.

[140] R. Adolphs, F. Gosselin, T.W. Buchanan, D. Tranel, P. Schyns, A.R. Damasio, A mechanism for impaired fear recognition after amygdala damage, Nature 433 (2005) 68–72.

[141] M.L. Spezio, P.Y. Huang, F. Castelli, R. Adolphs, Amygdala damage impairs eye contact during conversations with real people, J. Neurosci. 27 (2007) 3994–3997.

[142] A. Bechara, H. Damasio, A.R. Damasio, G.P. Lee, Different contributions of the human amygdala and ventromedial prefrontal cortex to decision-making, J. Neurosci. 19 (1999) 5473–5481.

[143] M. Brand, F. Grabenhorst, K. Starcke, M.M. Vandekerckhove, H.J. Markowitsch, Role of the amygdala in decisions under ambiguity and decisions under risk: evidence from patients with Urbach-Wiethe disease, Neuropsychologia 45 (2007) 1305–1317.

[144] E.A. Phelps, J.E. LeDoux, Contributions of the amygdala to emotion processing: from animal models to human behavior, Neuron 48 (2005) 175–187.

[145] B. Seymour, R. Dolan, Emotion, decision making, and the amygdala, Neuron 58 (2008) 662–671.

[146] E.T. Rolls, Emotion, higher order syntactic thoughts, and consciousness, in: L. Weiskrantz, M.K. Davies (Eds.), Frontiers of Consciousness, Oxford University Press, Oxford, 2008, pp. 131–167.

[147] E.T. Rolls, C. McCabe, Enhanced affective brain representations of chocolate in cravers vs non-cravers, Eur. J. Neurosci. 26 (2007) 1067–1076.

[148] J.D. Beaver, A.D. Lawrence, Jv. Ditzhuijzen, M.H. Davis, A. Woods, A.J. Calder, Individual differences in reward drive predict neural responses to images of food, J. Neurosci. 26 (2006) 5160–5166.

[149] H. Berlin, E.T. Rolls, Time perception, impulsivity, emotionality, and personality in self-harming borderline personality disorder patients, J. Pers. Disord. 18 (2004) 358–378.

[150] H. Berlin, E.T. Rolls, S.D. Iversen, Borderline personality disorder, impulsivity and the orbitofrontal cortex, Am. J. Psychiatry 162 (2005) 2360–2373.

[151] S. Rahman, B.J. Sahakian, J.R. Hodges, R.D. Rogers, T.W. Robbins, Specific cognitive deficits in mild frontal variant frontotemporal dementia, Brain 122 (1999) 1469–1493.

[152] I.V. Viskontas, K.L. Possin, B.L. Miller, Symptoms of frontotemporal dementia provide insights into orbitofrontal cortex function and social behavior, Ann. NY Acad. Sci. 1121 (2007) 528–545.

[153] J.T. Coyle, G. Tsai, D. Goff, Converging evidence of NMDA receptor hypofunction in the pathophysiology of schizophrenia, Ann. NY Acad. Sci. 1003 (2003) 318–327.

[154] M. Loh, E.T. Rolls, G. Deco, A dynamical systems hypothesis of schizophrenia, PLoS Comput. Biol. 3 (2007) e228. doi:210.1371/journal.pcbi.0030228.

[155] E.T. Rolls, M. Loh, G. Deco, G. Winterer, Computational models of schizophrenia and dopamine modulation in the prefrontal cortex, Nat. Rev. Neurosci. 9 (2008) 696–709.

[156] K. Chakrabarty, S. Bhattacharyya, R. Christopher, S. Khanna, Glutamatergic dysfunction in OCD, Neuropsychopharmacology 30 (2005) 1735–1740.

[157] C. Pittenger, J.H. Krystal, V. Coric, Glutamate-modulating drugs as novel pharmacotherapeutic agents in the treatment of obsessive-compulsive disorder, NeuroRx 3 (2006) 69–81.

[158] E.T. Rolls, M. Loh, G. Deco, An attractor hypothesis of obsessive-compulsive disorder, Eur. J. Neurosci. 28 (2008) 782–793.

[159] J.D. Wallis, Neuronal mechanisms in prefrontal cortex underlying adaptive choice behavior, Ann. NY Acad. Sci. 1121 (2007) 447–460.

[160] C. Padoa-Schioppa, J.A. Assad, Neurons in the orbitofrontal cortex encode economic value, Nature 441 (2006) 223–226.

[161] I.E.T. de Araujo, M.L. Kringelbach, E.T. Rolls, F. McGlone, Human cortical responses to water in the mouth, and the effects of thirst, J. Neurophysiol. 90 (2003) 1865–1876.

[162] H. Plassmann, J. O'Doherty, B. Shiv, A. Rangel, Marketing actions can modulate neural representations of experienced pleasantness, Proc. Natl. Acad. Sci. USA 105 (2008) 1050–1054.

[163] C. Padoa-Schioppa, J.A. Assad, The representation of economic value in the orbitofrontal cortex is invariant for changes of menu, Nat. Neurosci. 11 (2008) 95–102.

[164] L. Tremblay, W. Schultz, Relative reward preference in primate orbitofrontal cortex, Nature 398 (1999) 704–708.

[165] F. Grabenhorst, E.T. Rolls, Different representations of relative and absolute value in the human brain, (2009) (in press).

[166] P. Glimcher, Decisions, Uncertainty, and the Brain, MIT Press, Cambridge, MA, 2004.

[167] S.C. Tanaka, K. Doya, G. Okada, K. Ueda, Y. Okamoto, S. Yamawaki, Prediction of immediate and future rewards differentially recruits cortico-basal ganglia loops, Nat. Neurosci. 7 (2004) 887–893.

[168] N.D. Daw, J.P. O'Doherty, P. Dayan, B. Seymour, R.J. Dolan, Cortical substrates for exploratory decisions in humans, Nature 441 (2006) 876–879.

[169] H. Kim, S. Shimojo, J.P. O'Doherty, Is avoiding an aversive outcome rewarding? Neural substrates of avoidance learning in the human brain, PLoS Biol. 4 (2006) e233.

[170] R.S. Sutton, A.G. Barto, Reinforcement Learning, MIT Press, Cambridge, MA, 1998.

[171] J. Bernoulli, Exposition of a new theory on the measurement of risk, Econometrica 22 (1738/1954) 23–36.

[172] J. von Neumann, O. Morgenstern, The Theory of Games and Economic Behavior, Princeton University Press, Princeton, NJ, 1944.

[173] D. Kahneman, A. Tversky, Prospect theory: an analysis of decision under risk, Econometrica 47 (1979) 263–292.

[174] D. Kahneman, A. Tversky, Choices, values, and frames, Am. Psychol. 4 (1984) 341–350.

[175] A. Tversky, D. Kahneman, Rational choice and the framing of decisions, J. Bus. 59 (1986) 251–278.

[176] H. Gintis, Game Theory Evolving, Princeton University Press, Princeton, NJ, 2000.

[177] A. Rangel, C. Camerer, P.R. Montague, A framework for studying the neurobiology of value-based decision making, Nat. Rev. Neurosci. 9 (2008) 545–556.

[178] J.W. Kable, P.W. Glimcher, The neural correlates of subjective value during intertemporal choice, Nat. Neurosci. 10 (2007) 1625–1633.

[179] R. Romo, A. Hernandez, A. Zainos, Neuronal correlates of a perceptual decision in ventral premotor cortex, Neuron 41 (2004) 165–173.

[180] V. de Lafuente, R. Romo, Neural correlate of subjective sensory experience gradually builds up across cortical areas, Proc. Natl. Acad. Sci. USA 103 (2006) 14266–14271.

[181] G. Deco, E.T. Rolls, R. Romo, Stochastic dynamics as a principle of brain function, (2009) Prog. Neurobiol. doi: 10.1016./j.pneurobio.2009.01.006.

[182] F. Grabenhorst, E.T. Rolls, B.A. Parris, From affective value to decision-making in the prefrontal cortex, Eur. J. Neurosci. 28 (2008) 1930–1939.

[183] E.T. Rolls, F. Grabenhorst, B.A. Parris, Neural systems underlying decisions about affective odors, (2009), J. Cogn. Neurosci. Epub 25 March 2009.

[184] T. Shallice, P.W. Burgess, Deficits in strategy application following frontal lobe damage in man, Brain 114 (Pt 2) (1991) 727–741.

[185] P.W. Burgess, Strategy application disorder: the role of the frontal lobes in human multitasking, Psychol. Res. 63 (2000) 279–288.

[186] P.W. Burgess, I. Dumontheil, S.J. Gilbert, The gateway hypothesis of rostral prefrontal cortex (area 10) function, Trends Cogn. Sci. 11 (2007) 290–298.

[187] H.R. Heekeren, I. Wartenburger, H. Schmidt, K. Prehn, H.P. Schwintowski, A. Villringer, Influence of bodily harm on neural correlates of semantic and moral decision-making, Neuroimage 24 (2005) 887–897.

[188] T.E. Behrens, M.W. Woolrich, M.E. Walton, M.F. Rushworth, Learning the value of information in an uncertain world, Nat. Neurosci. 10 (2007) 1214–1221.

[189] A.A. Marsh, K.S. Blair, M. Vythilingam, S. Busis, R.J. Blair, Response options and expectations of reward in decision-making: the differential roles of dorsal and rostral anterior cingulate cortex, Neuroimage 35 (2007) 979–988.

[190] M.F. Rushworth, T.E. Behrens, P.H. Rudebeck, M.E. Walton, Contrasting roles for cingulate and orbitofrontal cortex in decisions and social behaviour, Trends Cogn. Sci. 11 (2007) 168–176.

[191] M.F. Rushworth, M.J. Buckley, T.E. Behrens, M.E. Walton, D.M. Bannerman, Functional organization of the medial frontal cortex, Curr. Opin. Neurobiol. 17 (2007) 220–227.

[192] F.S. Arana, J.A. Parkinson, E. Hinton, A.J. Holland, A.M. Owen, A.C. Roberts, Dissociable contributions of the human amygdala and orbitofrontal cortex to incentive motivation and goal selection, J. Neurosci. 23 (2003) 9632–9638.

[193] J. Moll, F. Krueger, R. Zahn, M. Pardini, R. de Oliveira-Souza, J. Grafman, Human fronto-mesolimbic networks guide decisions about charitable donation, Proc. Natl. Acad. Sci. USA 103 (2006) 15623–15628.

[194] H. Kim, R. Adolphs, J.P. O'Doherty, S. Shimojo, Temporal isolation of neural processes underlying face preference decisions, Proc. Natl. Acad. Sci. USA 104 (2007) 18253–18258.

[195] X.J. Wang, Probabilistic decision making by slow reverberation in cortical circuits, Neuron 36 (2002) 955–968.

[196] G. Deco, E.T. Rolls, Decision-making and Weber's Law: a neurophysiological model, Eur. J. Neurosci. 24 (2006) 901–916.

[197] S.T. Carmichael, M-C. Clugnet, J.L. Price, Central olfactory connections in the macaque monkey, J. Comp. Neurol. 346 (1994) 403–434.

[198] R.J. Morecraft, C. Geula, M-M. Mesulam, Cytoarchitecture and neural afferents of orbitofrontal cortex in the brain of the monkey, J. Comp. Neurol. 232 (1992) 341–358.

[199] D.M. Small, M.D. Gregory, Y.E. Mak, D. Gitelman, M.M. Mesulam, T. Parrish, Dissociation of neural representation of intensity and affective valuation in human gustation, Neuron 39 (2003) 701–711.

[200] H.D. Critchley, S. Wiens, P. Rotshtein, A. Ohman, R.J. Dolan, Neural systems supporting interoceptive awareness, Nat. Neurosci. 7 (2004) 189–195.

[201] S.T. Carmichael, J.L. Price, Connectional networks within the orbital and medial prefrontal cortex of macaque monkeys, J. Comp. Neurol. 371 (1996) 179–207.

[202] D.J. McFarland, Problems of Animal Behaviour, Longman, Harlow, 1989.

[203] P.R. Montague, G.S. Berns, Neural economics and the biological substrates of valuation, Neuron 36 (2002) 265–284.

[204] K. Izuma, D.N. Saito, N. Sadato, Processing of social and monetary rewards in the human striatum, Neuron 58 (2008) 284–294.

[205] D.O. Hebb, The Organization of Behavior: A Neuropsychological Theory, Wiley, New York, 1949.

[206] L.M. Giocomo, M.E. Hasselmo, Neuromodulation by glutamate and acetylcholine can change circuit dynamics by regulating the relative influence of afferent input and excitatory feedback, Mol. Neurobiol. 36 (2007) 184–200.

[207] E.T. Rolls, Memory systems in the brain, Annu. Rev. Psychol. 51 (2000) 599–630.

[208] S. Rodriguez, C.S. Warren, S. Moreno, A. Cepeda-Benito, D.H. Gleaves, M. Del Carmen Fernandez, J. Vila, Adaptation of the food-craving questionnaire trait for the assessment of chocolate cravings: Validation across British and Spanish Women, Appetite 49 (2007) 245–250.

Part Two

fMRI Studies on Reward and Decision Making

6 Decomposing brain signals involved in value-based decision making

Jean-Claude Dreher

Reward and decision making group, Cognitive Neuroscience Center, CNRS UMR5229, Lyon 1 University 67, Bd Pinel 69675 Bron, France

Abstract

Deciding between options leading to rewards of different nature depends both upon our internal needs and upon the subjective value of available options. Because there is no single sense organ transducing all types of rewards, our brain may compare different goods using a "common reward currency," allowing us to choose the option with the highest subjective value. Here, we analyze the neural substrates of different value-related signals involved when processing and deciding between rewards of different nature, such as prediction error, uncertainty, subjective value of each option, goal, and decision value. Some of these value signals are computed even without choice, and all of them eventually influence the decision-making process. We review recent neuroimaging work investigating the neural substrates of these different value signals and present recent results showing how genetically-influenced variations in dopamine transmission also influence the response of the reward system in humans.

Key points

1. Electrophysiological and neuroimaging data show that prediction error is modulated by several factors (probability, magnitude, delay) and is computed regardless of reward type.
2. Reward uncertainty and prediction error are computed in distinct brain networks, and several uncertainty signals co-exist in the brain.
3. Distinct value-based signals (distance between subjective value of different options, goal-value and decision-value) are computed in partially overlapping brain regions.
4. Primary and secondary rewards both activate a common brain network ("common neural currency") and reveal a new functional organization of the orbitofrontal cortex according to reward type (anterior obitofrontal cortex for secondary rewards and posterior orbitofrontal cortex for primary rewards).
5. Genetic variations in dopamine-related genes influence the response of the reward system and may contribute to individual differences in reward-seeking behavior and in predisposition to neuropsychiatric disorders.

6.1 Basic computations involved in decision making

When presented with several options, we need to assign subjective values to each of them to make a choice. Based on existing theoretical models of decision making, recent reviews

Choice   Value-based decision making

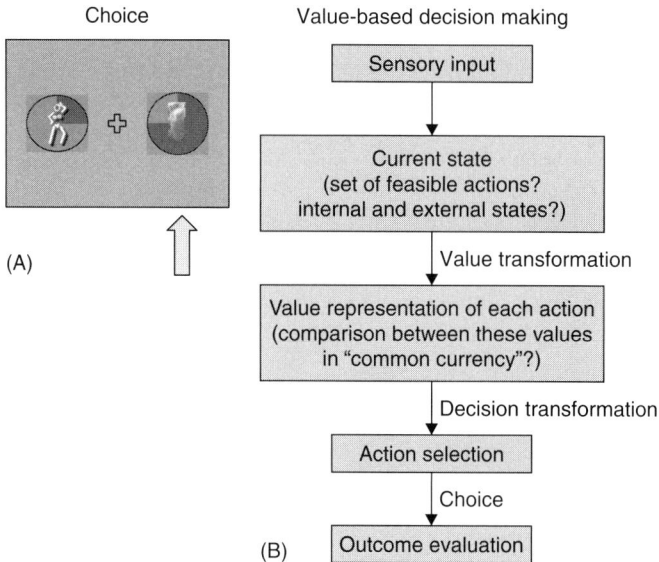

(A)

(B)

Figure 6.1 (A) Choosing between options leading to rewards of different nature. Example of a simple choice in which the brain needs to weigh the probability of each option and the nature of potential rewards (here, erotic stimuli or fruit juice) according to internal needs (see paragraph 6.7 for description of fMRI experiment). (B) Basic computations involved in value-based decision making. Based on existing theoretical models of decision making, value-based decision making can be decomposed into basic processes. First, one recognizes the current situation (or state), including internal (e.g., hunger) and external states (e.g., cold), and potential courses of actions (e.g., purchase food). Second, a valuation system needs to weigh available options in terms of cost and benefit (reward/punishment). Third, action selection is implemented based on this valuation. Finally, the chosen action may be re-evaluated based on the actual outcome, leading to updating of the other processes through learning to improve subsequent decisions.

proposed a framework that decomposes value-based decision making into basic processes [1–3] (Fig. 6.1).

The first stage includes a representation of the current situation (or state), including the identification of internal state (e.g., hunger), external state (e.g., cold), and potential courses of actions (e.g., purchase food). Second, a valuation system needs to weigh available options in terms of reward and punishment, as well as cost and benefit. Third, the agent selects an action on the basis of this valuation. Finally, the chosen action may be re-evaluated based on the actual outcome, eventually leading to update the other processes through learning to improve subsequent decisions. Although these processes may occur in parallel, this simplified framework is nonetheless useful to decompose basic computations performed by the brain.

It is still unclear whether there are separate valuation systems in the brain, but a number of studies distinguish between at least two systems: Pavlovian and instrumental conditioning. In Pavlovian (or classical) conditioning, subjects learn to predict outcomes without having the opportunity to act. In instrumental conditioning, animals learn to choose actions to obtain rewards and avoid punishments. Various strategies are possible, such as optimizing the average rate of acquisition of rewards minus punishments or optimizing the expected sum of future rewards, where outcomes received in the far future are discounted compared with outcomes received more immediately.

The focus of this chapter is to define different value signals that are used by the brain to make a decision and to review our current understanding of their possible neuronal implementation. The brain must perform multiple value computations to make decisions. Even without having to decide between options leading to different rewards, the brain computes a prediction of the value of potential outcomes and compares this prediction with the actual outcome (prediction error signal). This expected value and the reward prediction error signal are modulated by a number of factors, such as the magnitude and probability of reward, the timing uncertainty of the reward delivery, and the delay period between the cue associated with the reward and the outcome delivery. Each of these factors also influence the computation of signals necessary to make a decision, such as goal values, decision values, subjective distance between available options, subjective value of the chosen option, and choice uncertainty.

Below, we review the recent literature on the neural substrates of these different value signals and discuss our own results, showing their contributions to decision making between rewards of different nature or between costly options.

6.2   Computing reward prediction error

6.2.1   Animal electrophysiology on prediction error

Prediction errors measure deviations from previous reward expectations. Thus, prediction error can be either positive (when the reward delivered is better than expected) or negative (less or no reward delivered at the expected time) [96, 97]. Prediction errors are used to learn the value of states of the world and are critical for learning how to make better choices in the future. Electrophysiological studies in monkeys indicate that dopaminergic neurons code such a prediction error signal in a transient fashion. This signal may be sent to the striatum and prefrontal cortex to influence reward-dependent learning [4–6].

In classical conditioning experiments, where an association has to be learnt between a visual predictor (conditioned stimulus) and a rewarding outcome (unconditioned stimulus), each of the factors mentioned before (magnitude, probability, timing uncertainty, and delay) influences the phasic prediction signal occurring at the time of the conditioned stimuli. That is, the phasic response of dopamine neurons to the conditioned stimuli monotonically increases with probability and magnitude [7] and decreases with the reward delay in temporal discounting paradigms, both in Pavlovian conditioning [8] (see Chapter 2) and in intertemporal choice [9]. Moreover, at the time of the outcome, the response of dopamine neurons increases with reward delay and magnitude and decreases with increasing reward probability [8,10]. However, the magnitude of activation or suppression of dopaminergic neurons response appears to be identical for different magnitudes that are delivered with maximal uncertainty ($P = 0.5$), despite the fact that the absolute difference between actual and expected volume magnitude varied over a large range [7]. Thus, the responses of dopamine neurons do not appear to scale according to the absolute difference between actual and expected reward. Rather, the sensitivity of the neural responses appears to adapt according to the discrepancy in magnitude between two potential outcomes. Taken together, these results suggest that the dopamine response reflects the subjective value of the reward and may be sent to a number of neural structures involved in computing value-based signals involved in decision making.

In rodents, recent results also indicate that midbrain dopamine neurons encode decisions for future action [11], as well as the most valuable option in choice situations (reward of shorter delay or larger magnitude), consistently with their proposed role in coding the value of the chosen option post-choice [9]. In this experiment, rats could choose to respond for either a high-value or a low-value reward, and dopamine neurons response reflected the value of the best possible option, independent of which was ultimately selected.

Of particular importance for understanding the functional properties of dopaminergic neurons are two recent findings concerning the roles of the lateral habenula and the globus pallidus (internal segment) in the reward circuitry. The lateral habenula, which provides a key source of input to dopaminergic neurons [12] may suppress the activity of dopamine neurons, inducing pauses in the burst firing of dopamine cells that might be responsible for their negative prediction errors. Lateral habenula neurons respond to conditioned stimuli associated with the absence of reward or the presence of punishment and to punishment itself. They are also inhibited by rewarding outcomes, especially when these are less predictable [13]. Thus, the lateral habenula may control both reward-seeking (associated with the dopaminergic system) and punishment-avoidance behavior (associated with the serotoninergic system), through its projections to these two systems. Moreover, globus pallidus cells may drive the reward-negative responses of lateral habenula neurons [14]. These results help to understand the functional neuroanatomy underlying the response of dopaminergic neurons.

6.2.2   Human neuroimaging studies on prediction error

Recent human neuroimaging studies have investigated the neural correlates of the prediction error signal. A number of these studies suggest that activity in the ventral striatum and the prefrontal cortex correlates with prediction errors related to stimulus–response associations or rewards of different types, such as faces, money, or juice [15–21]. When examining the influence of reward magnitude during reward anticipation and at the time of rewarded outcome, increased activity has been observed in several brain regions, particularly in the ventral striatum. For example, increased ventral striatal activation was found with increasing magnitude of anticipated gains but not losses [22,23]. Several studies also investigated the influence of reward probability on brain activation. Some gambling studies found that ventral striatal activity increased with reward probability [19,24,25] while a cued reaction time study failed to find ventral striatal activation as a function of increasing probability [23]. In some of these studies, a region of the medial prefrontal cortex also showed increasing activation during anticipation of rewards with increasing probability [23,25].

In a recent monetary fMRI study using slot machines varying known reward probability and magnitude, we could distinguish between transient and sustained signals using a fixed long anticipatory period [20]. We found that the midbrain was activated both transiently with the prediction error signal and in a sustained fashion with reward uncertainty (see section 6.3). Moreover, distinct activity dynamics were observed in post-synaptic midbrain projection sites: the prefrontal cortex responded to the transient prediction error signal while the ventral striatum covaried with the sustained reward uncertainty signal (Fig. 6.2).

S1   Delay   S2

Win $20
(P = 0.5 $20) > (P = 0.25 $20)   (P = 0.25 $20) > (P = 0.5 $20)

y=−23   y=−23   y=−19

Midbrain   Midbrain   Midbrain

(A)

y=23   z=−11

Lateral prefrontal   Bilateral ventral   Lateral prefrontal
and cingulate cortex   striatum   and cingulate cortex

(B)

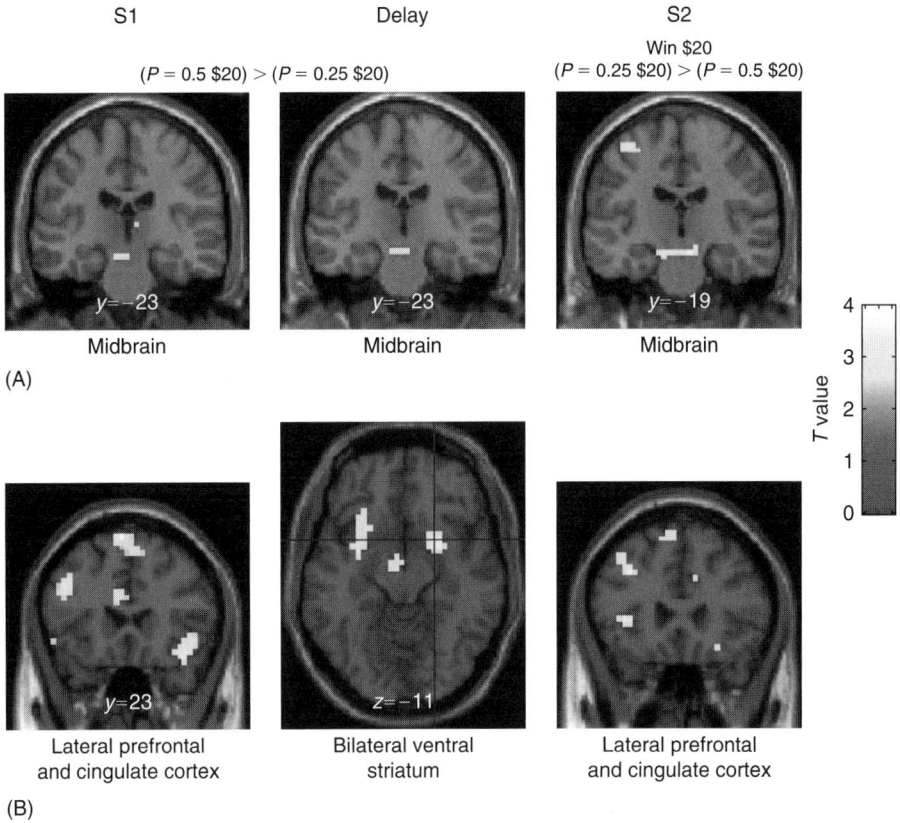

Figure 6.2 (A) Transient and sustained midbrain activities. Location of transient midbrain responses covarying with the error prediction signal at the cue S1 (*Left*) and at the rewarded outcome S2 (*Right*). Consistent with electrophysiological recordings [10], the human midbrain region was transiently activated with higher reward probability at the cue S1 and with lower reward probability at the rewarded outcome S2. Moreover, the midbrain region showed higher sustained activity with reward uncertainty during the delay [20]. (B) Location of transient midbrain and prefrontal responses covarying with the error prediction signal at the cue S1 (*Left*) and at the rewarded outcome S2 (*Right*). Middle: location of sustained bilateral ventral striatum activites covarying with the reward uncertainty signal during the delay period.

The frontal network we observed both at the time of the cue and at the time of the outcome was specifically involved with the reward prediction error signal because it was not significantly activated by reward uncertainty during the delay, and was significantly more activated in association with these phasically-modeled responses than in association with a sustained-modeled response related to reward uncertainty during the delay period. Our results extend previous fMRI reports that the dorsolateral prefrontal cortex, inferior frontal gyrus, and orbitofrontal cortex activity correlates with a prediction error signal related to abstract stimulus–response associations or taste reward, although some of these studies focused more on ventral striatal activity [15–21]. The lateral prefrontal cortex may generate the reward prediction because neurons from this brain region represent predictions about expected rewards according to the context [26,27].

In two recent fMRI studies, we then investigated how prediction error is modulated not only by reward probability and magnitude but also by reward type (money, fruit juice, and erotic stimuli) and by reinforcement nature (reward *versus* punishment). In a first study, we explicitly informed subjects on subsequent reward type (erotic stimuli or monetary reward), probability, and intensity. We found that activity in the ventral striatum not only correlated with reward magnitude for both monetary and erotic rewards, but also with reward prediction error regardless of reward nature (primary or secondary reinforcers) [28] (see Fig. 6.6).

In another fMRI study, we used temporal difference modeling during a classical conditioning learning paradigm. This study investigated prediction error related to different types of reinforcement nature and also compared prediction error for rewards and punishments [29]. Previous fMRI studies using models of reinforcement learning have shown that distinct components of the reward system have a response profile consistent with the temporal difference prediction error signal. However, it was still unclear whether: (1) the reward system discriminates between prediction errors related to reward and punishment or (2) common and distinct brain regions code prediction errors related to different types of outcome. To address these questions, we used a 2×2 fMRI factorial design crossing the valence (reward and punishment) and the type (taste and vision) of outcomes. Subjects were engaged in a Pavlovian conditioning procedure with four conditions (apple juice, salty water, money, and aversive picture), each with a 50% reinforcement schedule. Trials consisted in two phases: an anticipatory period followed by presentation of the outcome. The results showed that the putamen, the insula, and the anterior cingulate cortex (ACC) code the taste prediction error regardless of valence, that is, respond for both the appetitive and the aversive liquids (juice and salty water). A different pattern of activation was observed in the amygdala, which coded a prediction error only for the primary/immediate reinforcers (apple juice, salty water, and aversive pictures). Finally, the lateral and medial orbitofrontal cortex differentially coded the prediction error for different types of primary reinforcers (liquid versus aversive picture). Indeed, the Blood-oxygen-level (BOLD) activity in the orbitofrontal cortex correlated positively with the prediction error signal for the aversive picture condition and correlated negatively with the prediction error signal for the apple juice and salty water conditions. Taken together, these results demonstrate the different contributions made by distinct brain regions in computing prediction error depending upon the type and valence of the reinforcement (Fig. 6.3).

Finally, a recent approach proposed that temporal-difference signals are not the only learning signals encoded in the brain, in particular when needing to compute the difference between experienced outcomes and outcomes that could have been experienced if decisions had been different (that is a learning signal associated with the actions not taken, i.e., a fictive learning signal) [30]. The authors used a sequential investment task in which after each decision, information was revealed to the subject, regarding whether higher or lower investments would have been a better choice. The natural learning signal for criticizing each choice was the difference between the best return that could have been obtained and the actual gain or loss—that is, the fictive error. Behaviorally, the fictive error was found to be an important determinant for the next investment. The fictive error signal was associated with increasing BOLD response in the ventral caudate nucleus that was not explained by the temporal difference error signal. This fictive error signals may help us to understand the specific roles played by a number of brain regions when making decisions that are subsequently compared to an alternative outcome or decision (counterfactual effect) (see also Chapter 20).

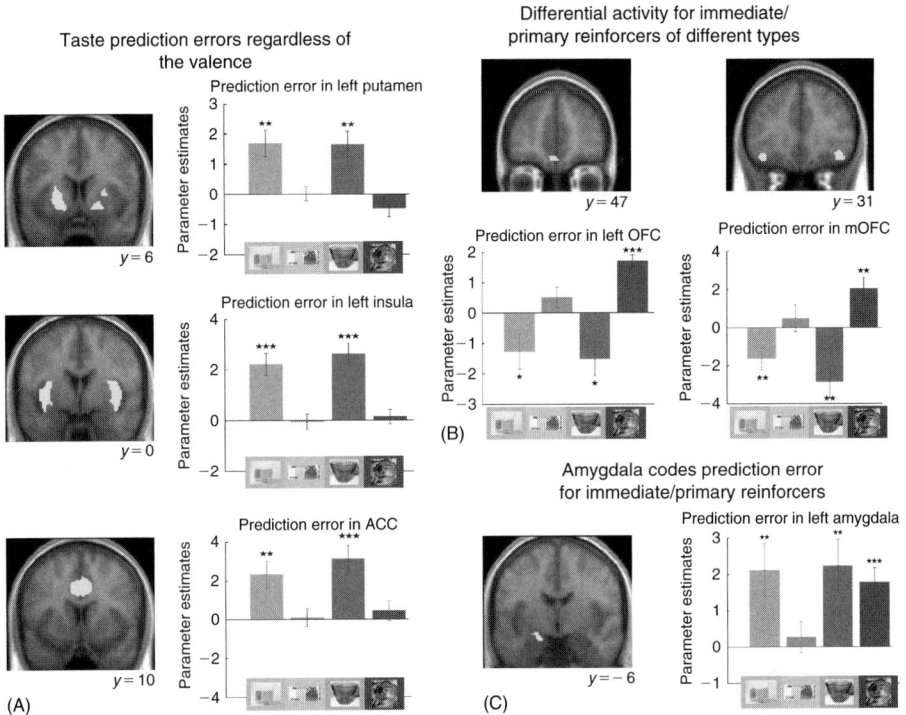

Figure 6.3 (A) The putamen, the insula, and the ACC code taste prediction error regardless of valence, that is, for both the appetitive and the aversive liquids (juice and salty water). (B) The lateral and medial orbitofrontal cortices differentially code the prediction error for different types of primary reinforcers (liquid versus aversive picture). BOLD activity in the orbitofrontal cortex correlated positively with the prediction error signal for the aversive picture condition and correlated negatively with the prediction error signal for the apple juice and salty water conditions. (C) The amygdala coded a prediction error only for primary/immediate reinforcers (apple juice, salty water, and aversive pictures). Thus, distinct brain regions compute prediction errors depending upon the type and valence of the reinforcement [29].

6.3 Computing various uncertainty signals in the brain

We have seen that the prediction error and expected value are crucial signals coded in a number of brain regions, including midbrain dopaminergic neurons and their projection sites. However, recent electrophysiological studies in monkeys indicate that dopaminergic neurons not only code a transient reward prediction error signal but also a sustained signal covarying with reward uncertainty (i.e., reward probability = 0.5) that may be functionally important for risk-seeking behavior and/or exploratory behavior [10]. Until recently, it was unknown whether these two modes of activity could also be observed in humans and whether they could be distinguished by post-synaptic dopaminergic projection sites. Using functional neuroimaging, we have successfully distinguished transient and sustained dynamics of the dopaminergic system in healthy young humans using a new reward task based on the monkey electrophysiology study, which systematically varied monetary reward probability and magnitude in the absence of choice [20]. The results showed that the human dopaminergic midbrain exhibits similar activity dynamics than midbrain from non-human primates. Moreover, specific dopaminergic projection sites were activated: (a) the ventral striatum, during anticipation of rewards with maximal uncertainty (reward probability = 0.5), (b) the prefrontal cortex and ACCs at the time of the outcome, correlating with a transient prediction error signal coding the difference between expected and obtained rewards (Fig. 6.2). These results indicate that specific functional brain networks subserve the coding of sustained and transient aspects of reward information in humans. These results are important because they support a unified cross-species view in which dopaminergic neurons obey common basic principles of neural computation and provide important new insights into human reward information processing.

It has been proposed that gambling, with its intrinsic reward uncertainty characteristics, has reinforcing properties that may share common mechanisms with addictive drugs [10]. Our results also offers an account for previous reports of human ventral striatum activation during anticipation of monetary and taste rewards for coding, at least in part, the expectation of reward information [22,31,32]. This signal could gain access to striatal neurons through ascending dopamine fibers as well as structures implicated in the evaluation of the motivational significance of stimuli, especially the amygdala and the orbitofrontal cortex.

Our finding of two networks covarying with different reward information signals may indicate that dopaminergic projection sites can distinguish between the two signals. It is also possible that these targets show independent transient (prefrontal cortex) and sustained (ventral striatum) activities related to the two signals and/or that they help to shape dopaminergic neuronal activity by differentially modulating their phasic and sustained modes of firing, which occur independently in individuals neurons [10]. This latter hypothesis is supported by anatomical observations that different populations of dopaminergic neurons are innervated predominantly by the target areas to which they project, or by the regions that, in functional terms, are the most closely linked to the target areas [33]. For example, in rodents, dopaminergic neurons projecting to the prefrontal cortex receive direct reciprocal inputs from this brain region, but not from the striatum, while dopaminergic neurons projecting to the striatum receive afferents from that brain region, but not from the prefrontal cortex, thereby forming two projection systems [33]. This suggests a general principle for midbrain dopaminergic neuronal afferents regulation, the prefrontal cortex and the striatum being responsible for regulating and controlling different modes of dopaminergic neuronal firing.

Another study involving choice behavior investigated the neural correlates of risk, modeled as outcome variance (risk being maximal at 50% probability) found increased activation in the insula, lateral orbitofrontal cortex, and midbrain [24] (see also Chapter 22). Insula activity also correlated with uncertainty in other paradigms involving money and non-monetary stimuli [34,35].

The discrepancy between the different findings of the ventral striatum coding either prediction error or reward uncertainty may be due to several factors. First, most fMRI studies investigating prediction signal used temporal-difference modeling in the context of learning paradigms. In contrast, in our early monetary reward fMRI paradigm [20], there was no learning of cue–outcome associations. So, the putamen activation we observed during anticipation with maximal uncertainty cannot be attributed to a learning effect. Second, one limitation of most fMRI studies varying reward probability is that they could not clearly separate the transient and sustained signals because the delay duration between the conditioned stimulus and the outcome was either too short or randomly jittered (which is a problem since transient dopaminergic responses are known to depend upon timing uncertainty) [19,24]. To address this problem, we have recently used intracranial recordings in humans to investigate the neural coding of prediction error and uncertainty with a more precise temporal definition (see Fig. 6.4) [36,37].

Although hippocampal–midbrain functional interactions are well documented and the hippocampus receives reward-related information not only from midbrain dopaminergic neurons but also from other components of the reward system, such as the amygdala and orbitofrontal cortex [38], it was still unknown whether it codes statistical properties of reward information, such as prediction error or reward uncertainty. To answer this question, we recorded hippocampal activity in epileptic patients implanted with depth electrodes while they learned to associate cues of slot machines with various monetary reward probabilities (*P*) (unlike our early fMRI monetary reward paradigm in which probability were explicitly given to the subjects) [37] (Fig. 6.4).

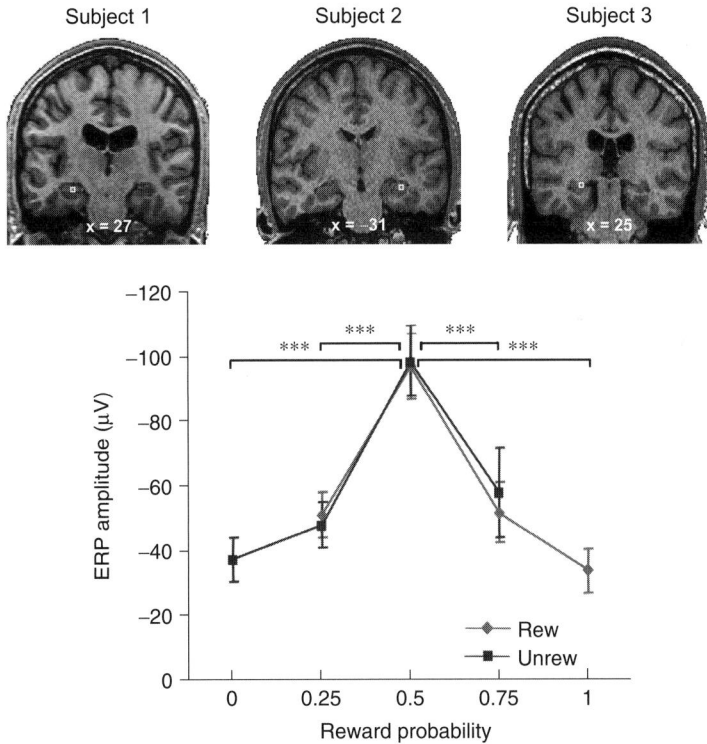

Figure 6.4 (Top) Location of intracranial electrode contacts. Coronal MRI slices from the three subjects showing the location of the intracranial electrode contacts in the hippocampus. The contacts in the hippocampus yielding the largest potentials are shown in bold square. (Bottom) Uncertainty coding in the human hippocampus. Hippocampal ERP amplitudes code uncertainty at the outcome, regardless of winning or not. Mean peak ERP amplitudes averaged across subjects at the outcome, as a function of reward probability, both for rewarded and for unrewarded trials [37].

Subjects estimated the reward probability of five types of slot machines that varied with respect to monetary reward probabilities P (0 to 1) and that could be discriminated by specific fractal images on top of them. Trials were self-paced and were composed of four distinct phases: (1) Slot machine presentation (S1): subjects pressed one of two response keys to estimate whether the slot machine frequently delivered 20€ or not, based on the outcomes of all the past trials; (2) Delay period (1.5 s): subject's key press triggered three spinners to roll around and to successively stop every 0.5 s during 0.5 s; (3) Outcome S2 (lasting 0.5€): the third spinner stopped and revealed the trial outcome (i.e., fully informing the subject on subsequent reward or no-reward delivery). Only two configurations were possible at the time the third spinner stopped: "bar, bar, seven" (no reward) or "bar, bar, bar" (rewarded trial); (4) Reward/No-reward delivery (1 s): picture of 20€ bill or rectangle with 0€ written inside.

The results showed that the amplitudes of hippocampal negative event related potentials (ERP), co-varied with uncertainty at the outcome, being maximal for $P = 0.5$ and minimal for $P = 0$ and $P = 1$, regardless of winning or not (Figure 6.4). This inverted U-shape relationship is typical of uncertainty coding and is incompatible with prediction error, novelty, or surprise coding, which would have predicted a negative monotonic correlation between ERP amplitudes and increasing reward probability [10,20]. This uncertainty coding of cue–outcome associations by the hippocampus may constitute a fundamental mechanism underlying the role of this brain region in a number of functions, including attention-based learning, associative learning, probabilistic classification, and binding of stimulus elements, that until now, have received no unified explanation concerning the underlying information processing performed by the hippocampus to achieve them. We propose that the uncertainty coding of cue-outcome associations may constitute the general computational mechanism used by the hippocampus to achieve these different functions. The transient uncertainty signal emitted by the hippocampus at the outcome may play a complementary role to the sustained uncertainty signal emitted by midbrain dopaminergic neurons during the delay period between the cue and the outcome. This finding constitutes a major advance in the knowledge of the functional properties of the human hippocampus and has crucial implications for understanding the basic neural mechanisms used by the brain to extract structural relationships from the environment. It is clear that an ubiquitous coding of uncertainty exists in the human brain, particularly in the midbrain, ventral striatum, insula, ACC, and orbitofrontal cortex [20,24,39–41] and the present study revealed that the hippocampus also participates to uncertainty processing. Future studies are needed to pinpoint the specific roles and time course of each structure in computing uncertainty in different contexts.

6.4 Discounting the value of costly options in delay and effort discounting studies

When deciding to engage in a given action, our choice is guided both by the prospect of reward and by the costs that this action entails. Psychological and economic studies have shown that outcome values are discounted with longer delays, an effect known as temporal discounting. A recent electrophysiological study demonstrated that when monkeys choose between sooner smaller available rewards and later larger rewards, the longer the delay of the later larger reward, the less firing of dopaminergic neurons at the time of the conditioned stimuli [8] (see also Chapter 2). Moreover, this reduction in firing rate followed a hyperbolic decay function similar to that observed in choice behavior. In addition, dopamine responses increased with longer delays at the time of the delayed larger reward delivery, interpreted as reflecting temporal uncertainty and partial learning. These fundamental results establish that dopamine responses reflect the subjective reward value discounted by delay and may provide useful inputs to neural structures involved in intertemporal choices.

Recent fMRI findings on delay-discounting support two opposite theories. According to the first set of experiments, there may be two separate systems in the brain: a limbic system computing the value of rewards delivered immediately or in the near future based on a small discount factor, and a cortical system computing the value of distant rewards based on a high discount factor [17,42–45]. Discounting would result from the interaction of these two systems associated with different value-signals. According to the second theory, based on a recent fMRI study, there would be a single valuation system simply discounting future rewards [46]. One way to conciliate these apparent opposite views is that the striato-prefrontal network might integrate information that is encoded elsewhere in the brain into a single value signal, but that immediate and delayed outcomes activate different types of information that are used to compute the reward value [3]. One further recent finding is that the orbitofrontal cortex may separate the representation of the temporal discount factor applied to distant rewards from the representation of the magnitude of the reward, suggesting that these quantities may be integrated elsewhere in the brain.

Although a few neuroimaging studies start to shed some light on the neural substrates involved in processing subjective value during delay discounting, virtually nothing is known about how effort is discounted in humans. Animal studies demonstrated that the ACC, the ventral striatum, and the orbitofrontal cortex make specific contributions to decision when costly options involve an effort or a delay [47,48]. However, in humans, it is unclear whether there are dissociable pathways underlying different types of costs such as effort and delay to reward. In order to answer this question, we designed a delay/effort discounting task involving primary rewards (visual erotic stimuli) [49]. Heterosexual men were scanned in an event-related fMRI paradigm while performing the task. On every trial, an incentive cue (fuzzy pictures of naked women) briefly appeared on a screen and was followed by the instruction (delay or effort), together with a thermometer indicating the level of delay or effort. Depending on the incentive cue and the proposed cost level, subjects decided whether to invest in the proposed effort (respectively to tolerate the proposed delay) to view the erotic image in clear for 3 s or to perform a minimal effort (respectively to wait for only 1.5 s) to view it for 1 s only. Then, subjects either waited passively in the delay condition (range: 1.5–9 s) or squeezed a hand-grip in the effort condition. We found that choices of the costly option depended upon the subjective value of incentive cues, as indexed by post-scan ratings of these cues, and upon the required level of delay and effort. Thus, decision makers combined two types of information about the benefit (incentive) and cost (level of delay or effort) associated with each option. When investigating the brain regions involved when choosing the costly option regardless of the nature of the cost (delay and effort), we observed stronger activity in the medial anterior prefrontal cortex and in the ventral striatum. These results indicate that choosing the costly option for both types of cost activates common brain regions associated with subjective value coding.

6.5   The concept of common neural currency

As noted previously, our behavior is motivated by rewards of different nature among which we frequently need to choose. Because there is no single-sense organ transducing rewards of different types, our brain must integrate and compare them to choose the options with the highest subjective value. It has been proposed that the brain may use a "common reward currency" that can be used as a common scale to value diverse behavioral acts and sensory stimuli [1]. The need for this common currency arises from the variety of choice we face in our daily life.

Recent behavioral studies in monkeys showed that monkeys differentially value the opportunity to acquire visual information about particular classes of social images. Male rhesus macaques sacrificed fluid for the opportunity to view female perinea and faces of high-status monkeys, but required fluid overpayment to view the faces of low-status monkeys. This work uses a behavioral method to quantify how non-human primates are likely to weigh one type of reward against another [50]. In humans, looking at other people can also be described as rewarding, and that the opportunity to view pictures of the opposite sex is discounted by delay to viewing, substitutes for money, and reinforces work [51]. Attributing value to available options is impaired by orbitofrontal cortex lesion; recent electrophysiological results indicate that some neurons in the orbitofrontal cortex encode the values of offered and chosen goods [52]. Moreover, when a monkey is offered one raisin versus one piece of apple, neurons in the orbitofrontal cortex encode the value of the two goods independently of visuospatial factors and motor responses (contrary to other brain areas in which value modulates activity related to sensory or motor processes). These results make an essential distinction between choosing between goods and choosing between actions. In addition, a classical and general question is how the neuronal representation of value depends upon behavioral context. Although some authors have proposed that the encoded value in the orbitofrontal cortex is relative [53], recent work suggests that neuronal responses in the orbitofrontal cortex are typically invariant for changes of menu—that is, orbitofrontal neuronal response to one particular good usually does not depend on which other goods are available at the same time [54]. These authors proposed that orbitofrontal neuronal activity encodes economic value rather than relative preference.

Because of the properties mentioned previously, the orbitofrontal cortex is likely to be an important brain structure involved in the comparison between different types of goods. However, all the electrophysiological and brain imaging studies published so far compared choices between goods of identical nature (e.g., only food items). Yet, based on the "common currency" concept, there should be a common brain network coding for different types of goods. Many fMRI studies are consistent with this idea, because common brain structures are involved in reward processing, regardless of reward nature. For example, increased midbrain, ventral striatum, and orbitofrontal activities have been observed with different types of rewards, such as monetary gains [19,20,55], pleasant taste [17,18,56], visual erotic stimuli [57,58], beautiful faces [21,59], drugs such as cocaine [60,61] as well as pain relief [62–64]. However, all these neuroimaging studies only investigated one reinforcer at a time and did not compare any two of these reinforcers directly. This was precisely the goal of a recent fMRI study that we performed to compare the common and distinct brain networks involved in processing primary and secondary rewards [28] (see section 6.6).

6.6 Common and distinct brain regions involved in processing primary and secondary rewards

Humans are motivated by a wide range of vegetative rewards (such as food and sex) and nonvegetative rewards (such as money, power, fame, and so on). However, it is unclear whether different types of reinforcers recruit distinct or common neural circuits. In a recent study [28], we compared brain activations to monetary gains and erotic pictures in an incentive delay task. Despite their critical sociobiological importance, visual sexual stimuli have never been studied as reinforcers, but rather as arousing stimuli in passive viewing paradigms focusing on sexual function. They can be considered as "primary rewards," in the sense that they have an innate value and satisfy biological needs. Conversely, money is defined as a "secondary reward," because its value is more abstract and needs to be learned by association with primary rewards.

We hypothesized that monetary and erotic outcomes would activate both shared and distinct cerebral networks. Based on recent fMRI studies, we hypothesized that core components of the reward system, such as the midbrain, ventral striatum, and ACC, would form the core of the shared network ("common currency" network). We also hypothesized a functional dissociation within the orbitofrontal cortex based on a meta-analysis of neuroimaging studies involving different types of rewards. This meta-analysis proposed a postero-anterior dissociation in the orbitofrontal cortex, with more complex or abstract reinforcers being represented more anteriorly than less complex reinforcers [65]. That is, we expected erotic rewards to activate more robustly the posterior part of the orbitofrontal cortex, while the more anterior part of this brain region would be more engaged by secondary rewards. In addition, a crucial question was to know whether the neural correlates of prediction error and expected value could be identified for visual erotic stimuli, which cannot be ascribed an objective value (unlike the amount of monetary reward).

To test our hypotheses, we designed an fMRI experiment comparing brain responses to monetary and visually erotic rewards. Young heterosexual males performed a new event-related fMRI paradigm varying reward nature (money versus erotic stimuli), reward probability, and reward intensity. The structure of each trial was as follows. During anticipation, a cue carried information about the type (monetary or erotic), the probability (0.25, 0.50, or 0.75) and the intensity (high or low) of the upcoming reward. Subjects then had to perform a simple discrimination task by pressing a specified response button for a visual target. At the time of the outcome, they were presented either with "scrambled" pictures (no reward), erotic images, or a picture of a safe indicating an amount of money. At that time, they also had to rate the reward value (of money or erotic stimuli) on a continuous scale.

At the time of outcome, robust BOLD signal was observed for both rewards in a brain circuit including the striatum, the ACC, the midbrain, and the anterior insula. These regions showed a parametric response with the hedonic value, consistent with the idea of a "common neural currency." Moreover, as expected, an antero-posterior dissociation was observed in the lateral orbitofrontal cortex at the time of reward outcome, monetary gains being specifically represented in the anterior part of the orbitofrontal cortex while erotic pictures eliciting activation in its posterior part. This result is important because it identifies a new functional division within the orbitofrontal cortex, with more recent cortical circuits supporting symbolic representation of goods and evolutionary more ancient orbitofrontal region representing subjective value of primary reward (Fig. 6.5).

Another key finding of this study is that prediction error was computed in similar brain regions for monetary and for erotic rewards (Fig. 6.6). Prediction error was defined as the absolute difference between the outcome value and the prediction, where the outcome value was measured by the hedonic ratings and the prediction by the product of expected reward intensity by probability. Brain activity in the ventral striatum, anterior insula, and ACC was shown to positively correlate with prediction error, suggesting that

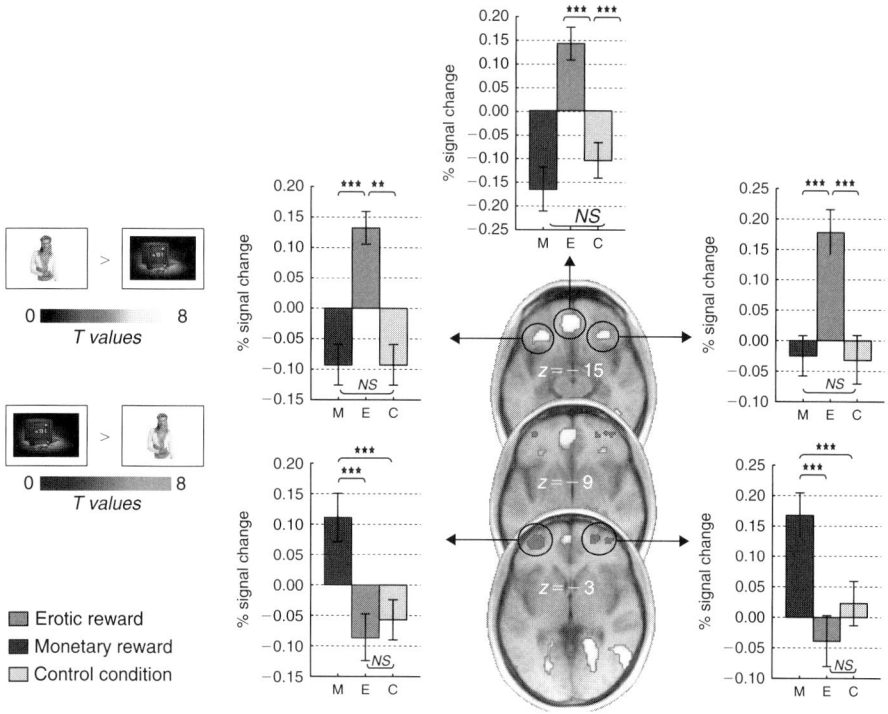

Figure 6.5 Antero-posterior dissociation within the orbitofrontal cortex according to reward nature. The anterior orbitofrontal cortex codes secondary reward (money) while the posterior and medial orbitofrontal cortex code primary reward (erotic stimuli). Brain regions specifically activated by monetary rewards outcomes are shown in blue-green, and those specifically activated by erotic rewards are shown in red-yellow. Mean percent signal change shows an interaction between reward type and orbitofrontal cortex (OFC) region in both the left and right sides of the brain. Functional maps are overlaid on axial slices of an average anatomical scan of all subjects and are significant at $P < 0.05$ family-wise error (FWE) corrected for multiple comparisons. Asterisks in the bar graphs denote significance of paired comparisons ($***P < 0.001$; $**P < 0.01$; NS, non-significant). Error bars indicate standard error to the mean (SEM) [28]. See Plate 4 of Color Plate section.

prediction error signals might be essentially computed in the brain regions commonly activated by both rewards. These results extend the concept of prediction error to erotic rewards and expand our understanding of reward functions by showing that a common brain network is activated by non-vegetative and vegetative rewards and that distinct orbitofrontal regions respond differentially to various kinds of rewards.

These results are interesting when considering a recent fMRI study suggesting that there may be a single valuation system that discounts future rewards [46]. Another fMRI study supports the idea of a "common neural currency" for two types of rewards [66]. This study showed that the acquisition of one's good reputation robustly activated reward-related brain areas, such as the striatum, and that these areas overlapped with those

Prediction error for primary and secondary rewards

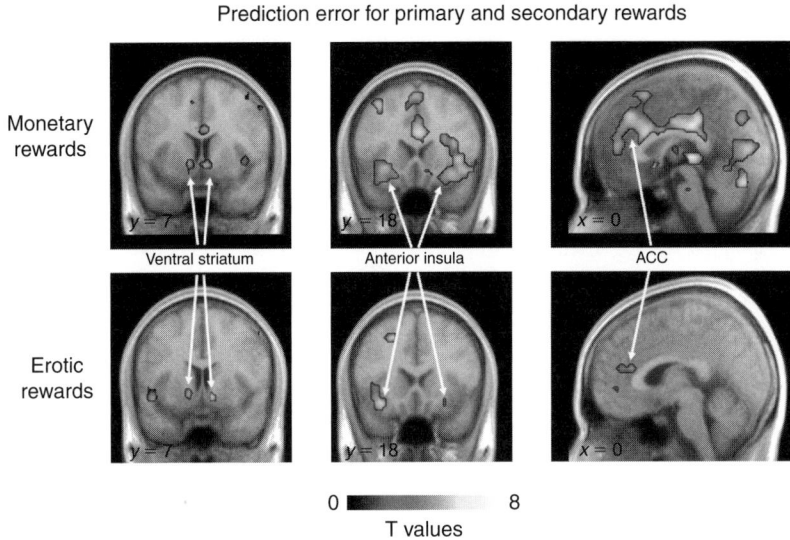

Figure 6.6 Brain regions responding parametrically with prediction error. Functional maps showing brain regions where BOLD response positively correlates with a measure of prediction error at the time of monetary reward (top) and erotic outcomes (bottom). Prediction error is computed as |Rating − (Probability × Expected intensity)|. Results are overlaid on an average anatomical scan of all subjects and survived a voxel-level threshold of $P < 0.001$ uncorrected for multiple comparisons [28].

activated by monetary rewards. In summary, recent advances in monkey electrophysiology (see Part One of this book) and in functional neuroimaging suggest that individuals use some of the same circuits to process money and other types of rewards, even in the absence of choice between them.

6.7 Distinguishing two brain systems involved in choosing between different types of rewards

Because the concept of "common currency" involves the notion of comparison between different types of goods, we have also recently characterized distinct value-based signals involved when choosing between different types of rewards [67]. One signal reflects the computation of the distance between the subjective values of each option. Another one codes the subjective value of the chosen option, while a third elementary signal involved in motivated choice codes choice uncertainty (maximal at the point of subjective equivalence between the two options).

Young heterosexual males, drink-deprived for 12 h, were scanned in a new fMRI paradigm while choosing between two gambles, one rewarded by a very small amount of fruit juice (0.5 ml) and the other by visual erotic stimuli (pictures of naked women) (Fig. 6.1A). Participants experienced both types of primary rewards directly inside the scanner. For each trial, two pie charts indicated the reward probabilities, varying independently (e.g., $P = 0.75$ juice versus $P = 0.5$ erotic stimulus) (Fig. 6.7.A). One important aspect of the task is that the magnitude of the reward was kept constant. Therefore, choices were made on the basis of preference for a type of reward and on the basis of reward probability.

We first estimated the preference of each participant for fruit juice over an erotic picture and expressed it as an equivalent offer by fitting, for each participant, a logistic model of the probability of choice that included the probability of being rewarded by the fruit juice, the erotic picture, and the trial number as explanatory variables. This last variable accounted for a possible drift of the preference during the experiment and was included in the model as a control. The preference was computed as the ratio of the parameter estimates for the picture and drink. Then, the subjective distance between options for each offer was computed as the difference between the subjective value of the juice option and the subjective value of the erotic picture option.

Behavioral results indicated that participants had heterogeneous preferences, some preferring juice over pictures, others pictures over juice. Response times increased linearly with choice uncertainty, indicating that the decision process slows down as the subjective distance between options decreases and as it becomes harder to discriminate which option is the best. Conversely, response times decreased as the subjective value of the chosen option increased, reflecting higher motivation for the favored choice. Moreover, the proportion of choice of a given option varied as a sigmoidal function of the distance between the subjective values of each option, showing that probability of choice is effectively modulated by the difference between subjective values of the available options (Fig. 6.7.B).

The brain imaging results revealed that, with increasing difference between subjective values, activity increased in the medial anterior and lateral parts of the orbitofrontal cortex and the midbrain, reflecting computation of the distance between options in a "common currency" space (Fig. 6.7.D). The same orbitofrontal regions coding the subjective distance between options at the time of decision also coded the subjective value of the chosen option. At the time of the rewarded outcome, the error prediction signal varied in the same direction as the subjective difference between options: it decreased when juice was delivered as compared to when it was not delivered, and it increased when a picture was delivered relative to when it was not (Fig. 6.7.E).

Moreover, brain regions coding choice uncertainty involved the ACC, the bilateral anterior insula and the inferior frontal gyri. This activity is likely to reflect the slowing down of the decision process observed behaviorally. Importantly, BOLD activity in the orbitofrontal cortex did not correlate with choice uncertainty, even when lowering the statistical threshold. Overall, these results indicate a functional dissociation between two brain networks: the orbitofrontal cortex, which codes the subjective values related to the goal of the decision, and the ACC/anterior insula network, which codes the uncertainty on these values.

Moreover, these results indicate that the same orbitofrontal cortex region codes different value-related signals and pinpoint a brain network composed of the ACC and the anterior insula that computes choice uncertainty.

6.8   Goal-value and decision-value signals

It is still unclear how many value-related signals are computed by the brain to make decisions. The computational complexity of these signals, as well as their possible reducibility to canonical signals remain also poorly characterized. Two value signals that may be computed during decision making are goal-value and decision-value signals, which may be used to choose the option with highest benefit. Goal values measure the predicted amount of reward associated with the outcome generated by each of the actions under consideration. Decision values measure the net value of taking the different actions, that

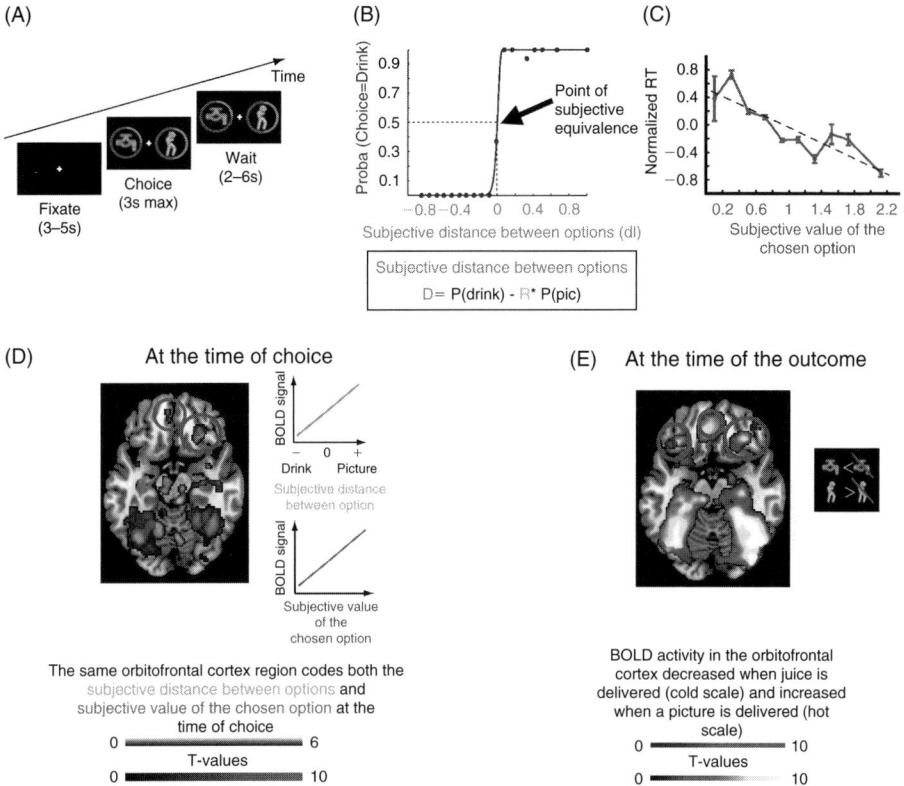

Figure 6.7 (A) Design of the experiment. Participants were asked to freely make motivated choices between two types of rewards with varying reward probability. For example, the offer consisted in a choice between an option rewarded 75% of the time by fruit juice and by an option rewarded 50% of the time by an erotic picture. The red part of the circle around each symbol indicates the reward probability. After a waiting period lasting 2-6 seconds, participants were probabilistically rewarded with juice or by viewing an erotic picture. (B) Estimation of the preference of each participant for drinking fruit juice over viewing erotic pictures was expressed as an equivalent offer by fitting a logistic model of the probability of choice that included the probability of being rewarded by a drink, by a picture and by the trial number. The preference was computed as the ratio of the betas for the picture and the drink. The subjective distance between options was computed for each offer as the difference between the subjective value of the drink option and the subjective value of the picture option. (C) Response times decreased as the subjective value of the chosen option increased. (D) At the time of choice, the same orbitofrontal regions coding the subjective distance (yellow scale) between options also coded the subjective value of the chosen option (red). (E) At the time of the outcome, the error prediction signal varied in the same direction as the subjective difference between options: it decreased at the time of reward when juice was delivered compared to when it was not delivered (cold scale), and it increased when a picture was delivered compared to when is was not viewed (hot scale). See plate 5 of color plate section.

is, the benefits *minus* the costs. In a recent fMRI study, goal value was computed by the willingness to pay for different food items, while decision values were computed by subtracting the price of the offered food items from the goal value [68]. These authors found that activity in the medial orbitofrontal cortex were correlated with goal values, that activity in the central orbitofrontal cortex correlated with decision values, and that activity in the ventral striatum correlated with prediction errors.

To conclude, the studies reviewed here indicate that the human orbitofrontal cortex is involved in processing a number of value signals, such as the subjective values of stimuli, but also contributes to processing signals related to the decision-making process itself, such as the distance between the subjective value of different options or the subjective distance of chosen option, thereby coding signals informing about what action to take next.

6.9   Variation in dopamine genes influence reward processing

Both reward processing and decision making engage brain structures that lie on the ascending dopaminergic pathways. An important axis of current research is to study the brain influence of genes that affect dopaminergic transmission in order to clarify the biological mechanisms underlying interindividual differences and vulnerability to pathology related to the dysfunction of the dopaminergic system. Although there are clear individual genetic differences regarding susceptibility to and manifestation of these neuropsychopathologies, the influence of genetic predispositions and variations on activation of the human reward system remains poorly understood. Recent neuroimaging and behavioral studies have focused on the genetic variations of dopamine receptors, especially DRD2 and DRD4, and other genes coding for enzymes and transporters involved in the dopaminergic transmission, such as the catechol-O-methyltransferase (COMT) and the dopamine transporter (DAT). For example, polymorphisms in dopamine receptor (DRD4) and monoamine oxidase A (MAOA) genes showed significant associations with efficiency of handling conflict as measured by reaction time differences in an attention task and modulate ACC activation [69]. Moreover, the role of the DRD2 polymorphism in monitoring negative action outcomes and feedback-based learning was tested during a probabilistic learning task [70]. A1-allele carriers, with reduced dopamine D2 receptor densities, showed lower posterior medial frontal cortex activity, involved in feedback monitoring, and learned to avoid actions with negative consequences less efficiently. The authors suggested that dopamine D2 receptor reduction seems to decrease sensitivity to negative action consequences, which may explain an increased risk of developing addictive behaviors in A1-allele carriers. Recent behavioral and computational modeling works also suggest independent gene effects (DARPP-32, DRD2, COMT) on reinforcement learning parameters that contribute to reward and avoidance learning in humans. These findings support a neurocomputational dissociation between striatal and prefrontal dopaminergic mechanisms in reinforcement learning [71] (see also Chapter 19).

Two important proteins contribute to terminating the action of intrasynaptic dopamine in the brain: COMT, which catabolizes released dopamine, and the DAT, which plays a crucial role in determining the duration and amplitude of dopamine action by rapidly recapturing extracellular dopamine into presynaptic terminals after release. In humans, the *COMT* gene contains a common and evolutionarily recent functional polymorphism that codes for the substitution of valine (val) by methionine (met) at codon 158, referred to as Val[158]Met polymorphism. The COMT enzyme is involved in the metabolic degradation of catecholamines, converting dopamine into 3-methoxytyramine and norepinephrine into normetanephrine. Because the COMT protein containing methionine is relatively thermolabile, its activity is lower at body temperatures than the COMT valine protein, which is fully active at body temperature. Hence, individuals with two copies of the met allele (met/met) have 25–75% reduction in COMT enzyme activity, and therefore presumptively more baseline synaptic dopamine, compared to individuals with two copies of the val allele (val/val) [72,73].

The *DAT*1 gene (SLC6A3) includes 15 exons, with a variable number of tandem repeat (VNTR) polymorphisms in the 15th exon, a region encoding the transcript's 3′ UTR [74]. The 40-bp VNTR element is repeated between 3 and 13 times but in most of the population occurs with greatest frequency in the 9- and 10-repeat forms. The expression of the *DAT*1 9-repeat allele is lower than the 10-repeat allele [75–77], although one study reported the opposite allelic associations [78]. Thus, the *DAT*1 10-repeat allele, associated with increased expression of the gene, presumably leads to relatively decreased extrasynaptic striatal dopamine levels. This is consistent with a human SPECT study reporting increased striatal DAT availability in 9-repeat carriers relative to 10-repeat carriers [79], although another study failed to support this [75]. Mice lacking the *DAT*1 gene show extensive adaptative changes in the dopaminergic system, the DAT controlling both the duration of extracellular dopamine signals and regulating presynaptic dopamine homeostasis [80].

Importantly, animal studies indicate differential functional localization of the COMT and DAT proteins. The COMT enzyme plays a particular role in modulating dopamine in the prefrontal cortex, where *DAT*1 expression is sparse [81,82]. *COMT* is expressed more abundantly in cortical neurons than in the striatum [83], but it is unclear to what extent *COMT* modulates catecholamine function outside the cortex. Recent studies in COMT knockout mice suggest that COMT has little if any role in striatal DA levels [84]. In contrast, animal research and human postmortem studies indicate that the *DAT*1 is expressed abundantly in midbrain, striatum, and hippocampus but sparsely in the prefrontal cortex (PFC) [85,86].

In parallel with the fundamental fMRI results concerning prediction error mentioned before, fMRI studies in healthy young subjects have documented that distinct reward anticipation- and outcome-processing phases are associated with differential patterns of specific midbrain dopaminergic postsynaptic targets [20,32,87]. Specifically, anticipation of reward robustly activates foci in the ventral striatum [32,87], particularly during anticipation of rewards with maximal uncertainty (i.e., reward probability = 0.5) [20] while rewarded outcomes activate the lateral and orbital parts of the PFC [20,87]. Despite the direct involvement of the COMT and DAT proteins in dopamine transmission, the influences of *COMT* and *DAT*1 functional polymorphisms on distinct components of the reward system have not been as systematically explored as have been the domains of working and episodic memory [86,88,89].

We recently used event-related fMRI and a recently developed reward paradigm to directly investigate the relationship between *COMT* and *DAT*1 functional polymorphisms and the response of the reward system during anticipation of uncertain rewards and at the time of reward delivery, bridging the gap between basic molecular genetics, fundamental electrophysiological findings, and functional neuroimaging in humans [90].

The results revealed a main effect of *COMT* genotype in the ventral striatum and lateral prefrontal cortex during reward anticipation and in the orbitofrontal cortex at the time of reward delivery, met/met individuals exhibiting the highest activation (Fig. 6.8).

The main effect of *DAT*1 genotype was seen in robust BOLD response differences in the caudate nucleus and ventral striatum during reward anticipation and in the lateral prefrontal cortex and midbrain at the time of reward delivery, with carriers of the *DAT*1 9-repeat allele showing the highest activity. Moreover, an interaction between the *COMT* and *DAT*1 genes was found in the ventral striatum and lateral prefrontal cortex during

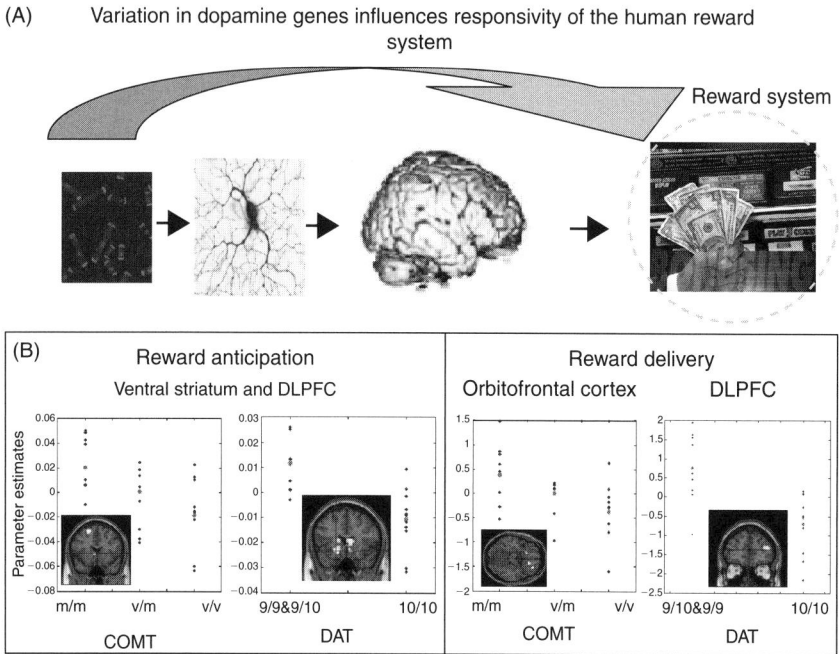

Figure 6.8 (A) Relationships between the effects of genetic variations and reward processing. Influence of the polymorphisms of the catecholamine-O-methyltransferase (COMT) (valine/valine; valine/methionine; methionine/methionine) and the dopamine transporter (DAT) (9/9&9/10; 10/10) on the reward system. (B) (Left) Main effect of *COMT* and *DAT* genotypes during anticipation of reward with maximal uncertainty. Negative relationship was observed between *COMT* val allele dosage (0_met/met, 1_val/met, or 2_val/val) and BOLD response in the ventral striatum, left superior PFC, and dorsolateral PFC during anticipation of reward with maximal uncertainty. More robust BOLD response was observed in 9-repeat carriers (including *DAT*1 9-repeat and 9/10) compared to 10-repeat individuals during reward anticipation in the bilateral ventral striatum. (Right) Main effect of *COMT* and *DAT* genotypes at the time of reward delivery. Negative relationship between *COMT* val allele dosage and orbitofrontal cortex activation at the time of reward delivery. Higher lateral prefrontal BOLD signal was observed in *DAT*1 9-repeat allele dosage compared to 10-repeat carriers at the time of reward delivery [90].

reward anticipation and in the lateral prefrontal and orbitofrontal cortices as well as in the midbrain at the time of reward delivery, with carriers of the *DAT*1 9-repeat allele and *COMT* met/met allele exhibiting the highest activation, presumably reflecting functional change consequent to higher synaptic dopamine availability.

One important insight provided by our data is a clear demonstration of interaction between the *DAT*1 and *COMT* genes that control a complex phenotype (activation of the reward system). This interaction likely reflects differences in dopaminergic level due to the combined effect of the *COMT* val/val and *DAT*1 10/10 alleles on elimination of DA in the fronto-striatal system. Interestingly, the effects on the BOLD signal of this presumed low DA level in val/val and 10-repeat alleles' carriers differ both according to brain regions and task phases.

These results indicate that genetically-influenced variations in dopamine transmission modulate the response of brain regions involved in anticipation and reception of rewards and suggest that these responses may contribute to individual differences in reward-seeking behavior and in predisposition to neuropsychiatric disorders.

A recent study used a guessing task to investigate how individual variation in *COMT* and *DAT*1 genes influences reward processing [91] (see also Chapters 16 and 17). In accordance with our results, this study reported that, during reward anticipation, the lateral PFC and the ventral striatum activities were *COMT* genotype-dependent: subjects homozygous for the met allele showed larger responses in these brain regions compared with volunteers homozygous for the val allele. This effect was observed when averaging all probabilities and magnitudes against baseline, but no main effect of *COMT* genotype was observed on ventral striatal sensitivity to reward uncertainty. Moreover, no main effect of *DAT*1 genotype was reported on striatal activity during reward anticipation, despite the well-established abundancy of DAT in the striatum. A gene–gene interaction between *COMT* and *DAT*1 was observed in the ventral striatum when sorting genotypes from met/met *DAT*1 10-repeat allele to val/val 9-repeat allele, interpreted as consistent with the notion that basal dopaminergic tone, regulated by *COMT*, interacts with phasic dopamine release, regulated by the *DAT*. It is difficult to directly compare our findings to these results because *COMT* and *DAT*1 genotypes may both directly influence distinct components of the human reward system (COMT modulating the dorsolateral prefrontal cortex (DLPFC) and DAT the striatum) and differentially affect their neurofunctional balance in a task-dependent manner. Finally, because this previous study did not report effects of genotype on fMRI results at the time of reward delivery, it remains unclear whether distinct phases of this guessing task induce differential brain activity dependent upon *COMT* and *DAT*1 polymorphisms.

It should be noted that our fMRI results on COMT/DAT genotypes cannot establish the neurophysiological mechanisms underlying the relationship between dopamine release and BOLD signal increase [92]. However, our study directly links genotype-dependent synaptic dopamine availability with BOLD signal change in humans and suggests that higher BOLD signal at prefronto-striatal sites is associated with greater dopamine synaptic availability (i.e., lower DA elimination), in agreement with recent studies observing: (a) that in young adults there is a tight coupling between increased midbrain dopamine synthesis and reward-related increase BOLD signal in the PFC both during reward anticipation and at the time of reward delivery [93]; and (b) that in animals, injection of dopamine-releasing agents increases BOLD signal in mesolimbic regions (frontal cortex, striatum, cingulate cortex) with a time course that parallels the changes observed by microdialysis measurements of striatal dopamine release [94].

6.10 Conclusions

Making choices requires processing of several value-related signals, such as prediction error, uncertainty, subjective value of different options and the distance between them, goal value, and decision value. In this review, we have described neuroimaging evidence showing the neural substrates of these different value signals. The integrity of the neural structures computing these value signals are crucial for efficient decision making and processing of reward information. Clinical areas of research in which the current knowledge on value-based decision making can be applied concern a variety of neuropathologies, such as schizophrenia, Parkinson's disease, pathological gambling, or drug addiction. A better knowledge of the neural basis of goal values, decision values, and prediction errors is likely to advance our understanding of the impact that different types of neuropathologies have on reward and decision making. For example, a recent neuroimaging study relates dysfunctions in motivational salience and prediction error signal to explain the abnormal mental experience of psychosis. Patients with psychosis exhibited abnormal physiological responses associated with reward prediction error in the dopaminergic midbrain, striatum, and limbic system, providing the first evidence linking abnormal mesolimbic activity, reward learning and psychosis [95] (see also Chapter 11). Future works should also investigate how genetically-influenced variations in different monoamine transmitters (dopamine, noradrenaline, serotonin), modulate the response of brain regions coding the various value signals involved in decision making outlined in this chapter.

Acknowledgments

I thank Philippe Domenech, Elise Météreau, Charlotte Prévost, Guillaume Sescousse and Dr Giovanna Vanni-Mercier for performing some of the experiments described here and for their helpful comments on early versions of this chapter. J-C Dreher is supported by the CNRS, the Fyssen foundation and by the "Fondation pour la Recherche Médicale".

References

[1] L.P. Sugrue, G.S. Corrado, W.T. Newsome, Choosing the greater of two goods: neural currencies for valuation and decision making, Nat. Rev. Neurosci. 6 (2005) 363–375.

[2] K. Doya, Modulators of decision making, Nat. Neurosci. 11 (2008) 410–416.

[3] A. Rangel, C. Camerer, P.R. Montague, A framework for studying the neurobiology of value-based decision making, Nat. Rev. Neurosci. 9 (2008) 545–556.

[4] W. Schultz, Multiple reward signals in the brain, Nat. Rev. Neurosci. 1 (2000) 199–207.

[5] W. Schultz, A. Dickinson, Neuronal coding of prediction errors, Annu. Rev. Neurosci. 23 (2000) 473–500.

[6] H.M. Bayer, B. Lau, P.W. Glimcher, Statistics of midbrain dopamine neuron spike trains in the awake primate, J. Neurophysiol. 98 (2007) 1428–1439.

[7] P.N. Tobler, C.D. Fiorillo, W. Schultz, Adaptive coding of reward value by dopamine neurons, Science 307 (2005) 1642–1645.

[8] S. Kobayashi, W. Schultz, Influence of reward delays on responses of dopamine neurons, J. Neurosci. 28 (2008) 7837–7846.

[9] M.R. Roesch, D.J. Calu, G. Schoenbaum, Dopamine neurons encode the better option in rats deciding between differently delayed or sized rewards, Nat. Neurosci. 10 (2007) 1615–1624.

[10] C.D. Fiorillo, P.N. Tobler, W. Schultz, Discrete coding of reward probability and uncertainty by dopamine neurons, Science 299 (2003) 1898–1902.

[11] G. Morris, A. Nevet, D. Arkadir, E. Vaadia, H. Bergman, Midbrain dopamine neurons encode decisions for future action, Nat. Neurosci. 9 (2006) 1057–1063.

[12] H. Ji, P.D. Shepard, Lateral habenula stimulation inhibits rat midbrain dopamine neurons through a GABA(A) receptor-mediated mechanism, J. Neurosci. 27 (2007) 6923–6930.

[13] M. Matsumoto, O. Hikosaka, Lateral habenula as a source of negative reward signals in dopamine neurons, Nature 447 (2007) 1111–1115.

[14] S. Hong, O. Hikosaka, The globus pallidus sends reward-related signals to the lateral habenula, Neuron 60 (2008) 720–729.

[15] G.S. Berns, S.M. McClure, G. Pagnoni, P.R. Montague, Predictability modulates human brain response to reward, J. Neurosci. 21 (2001) 2793–2798.

[16] P.C. Fletcher, J.M. Anderson, D.R. Shanks, R. Honey, T.A. Carpenter, T. Donovan, N. Papadakis, E.T. Bullmore, Responses of human frontal cortex to surprising events are predicted by formal associative learning theory, Nat. Neurosci. 4 (2001) 1043–1048.

[17] S.M. McClure, G.S. Berns, P.R. Montague, Temporal prediction errors in a passive learning task activate human striatum, Neuron 38 (2003) 339–346.

[18] J.P. O'Doherty, P. Dayan, K. Friston, H. Critchley, R.J. Dolan, Temporal difference models and reward-related learning in the human brain, Neuron 38 (2003) 329–337.

[19] B. Abler, H. Walter, S. Erk, H. Kammerer, M. Spitzer, Prediction error as a linear function of reward probability is coded in human nucleus accumbens, Neuroimage 31 (2006) 790–795.

[20] J.C. Dreher, P. Kohn, K.F. Berman, Neural coding of distinct statistical properties of reward information in humans, Cereb. Cortex 16 (2006) 561–573.

[21] S. Bray, J. O'Doherty, Neural coding of reward-prediction error signals during classical conditioning with attractive faces, J. Neurophysiol. 97 (2007) 3036–3045.

[22] B. Knutson, C.M. Adams, G.W. Fong, D. Hommer, Anticipation of increasing monetary reward selectively recruits nucleus accumbens, J. Neurosci. 21 (2001) RC159.

[23] B. Knutson, J. Taylor, M. Kaufman, R. Peterson, G. Glover, Distributed neural representation of expected value, J. Neurosci. 25 (2005) 4806–4812.

[24] K. Preuschoff, P. Bossaerts, S.R. Quartz, Neural differentiation of expected reward and risk in human subcortical structures, Neuron 51 (2006) 381–390.

[25] J. Yacubian, J. Glascher, K. Schroeder, T. Sommer, D.F. Braus, C. Buchel, Dissociable systems for gain- and loss-related value predictions and errors of prediction in the human brain, J. Neurosci. 26 (2006) 9530–9537.

[26] S. Kobayashi, J. Lauwereyns, M. Koizumi, M. Sakagami, O. Hikosaka, Influence of reward expectation on visuospatial processing in macaque lateral prefrontal cortex, J. Neurophysiol. 87 (2002) 1488–1498.

[27] M. Watanabe, K. Hikosaka, M. Sakagami, S. Shirakawa, Coding and monitoring of motivational context in the primate prefrontal cortex, J. Neurosci. 22 (2002) 2391–2400.

[28] G. Sescousse, J-C. Dreher, Coding of reward type along an antero-posterior gradient in the human orbitofrontal cortex, in: Exciting Biologies meeting, Chantilly, France, 2008. Biology of Cognition.

[29] E. Météreau, J-C. Dreher, Neural responses underlying predictive learning of different types of rewards and punishments, in: Society for Neuroscience, Washington DC, 2008.

[30] P.H. Chiu, T.M. Lohrenz, P.R. Montague, Smokers' brains compute, but ignore, a fictive error signal in a sequential investment task, Nat. Neurosci. 11 (2008) 514–520.

[31] H.C. Breiter, I. Aharon, D. Kahneman, A. Dale, P. Shizgal, Functional imaging of neural responses to expectancy and experience of monetary gains and losses, Neuron 30 (2001) 619–639.

[32] J.P. O'Doherty, R. Deichmann, H.D. Critchley, R.J. Dolan, Neural responses during anticipation of a primary taste reward, Neuron 33 (2002) 815–826.

[33] S.R. Sesack, D.B. Carr, N. Omelchenko, A. Pinto, Anatomical substrates for glutamate-dopamine interactions: evidence for specificity of connections and extrasynaptic actions, Ann. NY Acad. Sci. 1003 (2003) 36–52.

[34] S.A. Huettel, A.W. Song, G. McCarthy, Decisions under uncertainty: probabilistic context influences activation of prefrontal and parietal cortices, J. Neurosci. 25 (2005) 3304–3311.

[35] J. Grinband, J. Hirsch, V.P. Ferrera, A neural representation of categorization uncertainty in the human brain, Neuron 49 (2006) 757–763.

[36] J. Thomas, G. Vanni-Mercier, J-C. Dreher, Temporal dynamics of reward probability coding: a Magnetoencephalographic study in humans, in: Human Brain Mapping meeting, Melbourne, Australia, 2008.

[37] G. Vanni-Mercier, F. Mauguière, J. Isnard, J-C. Dreher, The hippocampus codes the uncertainty of cue-outcome associations: an intracranial electrophysiological study in humans. Journal of Neuroscience 29: 5287–5294.

[38] W.A. Suzuki, D.G. Amaral, Topographic organization of the reciprocal connections between the monkey entorhinal cortex and the perirhinal and parahippocampal cortices, J. Neurosci. 14 (1994) 1856–1877.

[39] M. Hsu, M. Bhatt, R. Adolphs, D. Tranel, C.F. Camerer, Neural systems responding to degrees of uncertainty in human decision-making, Science 310 (2005) 1680–1683.

[40] P.N. Tobler, J.P. O'Doherty, R.J. Dolan, W. Schultz, Reward value coding distinct from risk attitude-related uncertainty coding in human reward systems, J. Neurophysiol. 97 (2007) 1621–1632.

[41] K. Preuschoff, S.R. Quartz, P. Bossaerts, Human insula activation reflects risk prediction errors as well as risk, J. Neurosci. 28 (2008) 2745–2752.

[42] S.C. Tanaka, K. Doya, G. Okada, K. Ueda, Y. Okamoto, S. Yamawaki, Prediction of immediate and future rewards differentially recruits cortico-basal ganglia loops, Nat. Neurosci. 7 (2004) 887–893.

[43] S.M. McClure, K.M. Ericson, D.I. Laibson, G. Loewenstein, J.D. Cohen, Time discounting for primary rewards, J. Neurosci. 27 (2007) 5796–5804.

[44] N. Schweighofer, S.C. Tanaka, K. Doya, Serotonin and the evaluation of future rewards: theory, experiments, and possible neural mechanisms, Ann. NY Acad. Sci. 1104 (2007) 289–300.

[45] N. Schweighofer, M. Bertin, K. Shishida, Y. Okamoto, S.C. Tanaka, S. Yamawaki, K. Doya, Low-serotonin levels increase delayed reward discounting in humans, J. Neurosci. 28 (2008) 4528–4532.

[46] J.W. Kable, P.W. Glimcher, The neural correlates of subjective value during intertemporal choice, Nat. Neurosci. 10 (2007) 1625–1633.

[47] M.E. Walton, S.W. Kennerley, D.M. Bannerman, P.E. Phillips, M.F. Rushworth, Weighing up the benefits of work: behavioural and neural analyses of effort-related decision making, Neural Netw. 19 (2006) 1302–1314.

[48] M.F. Rushworth, T.E. Behrens, P.H. Rudebeck, M.E. Walton, Contrasting roles for cingulate and orbitofrontal cortex in decisions and social behaviour, Trends Cogn. Sci. 11 (2007) 168–176.

[49] C. Prévost, M. Pessiglione, M-C. Cléry-Melin, J-C. Dreher, Delay versus effort-discounting in the human brain, in: Society for Neuroscience, Washington DC, 2008.

[50] R.O. Deaner, A.V. Khera, M.L. Platt, Monkeys pay per view: adaptive valuation of social images by rhesus macaques, Curr. Biol. 15 (2005) 543–548.

[51] B.Y. Hayden, M.L. Platt, Temporal discounting predicts risk sensitivity in rhesus macaques, Curr. Biol. 17 (2007) 49–53.

[52] C. Padoa-Schioppa, J.A. Assad, Neurons in the orbitofrontal cortex encode economic value, Nature 441 (2006) 223–226.

[53] L. Tremblay, W. Schultz, Relative reward preference in primate orbitofrontal cortex, Nature 398 (1999) 704–708.

[54] C. Padoa-Schioppa, J.A. Assad, The representation of economic value in the orbitofrontal cortex is invariant for changes of menu, Nat. Neurosci. 11 (2008) 95–102.

[55] J.P. O'Doherty, Reward representations and reward-related learning in the human brain: insights from neuroimaging, Curr. Opin. Neurobiol. 14 (2004) 769–776.

[56] J. O'Doherty, Can't learn without you: predictive value coding in orbitofrontal cortex requires the basolateral amygdala, Neuron 39 (2003) 731–733.

[57] J. Redoute, S. Stoleru, M.C. Gregoire, N. Costes, L. Cinotti, F. Lavenne, D. Le Bars, M.G. Forest, J.F. Pujol, Brain processing of visual sexual stimuli in human males, Hum. Brain Mapp. 11 (2000) 162–177.

[58] S. Karama, A.R. Lecours, J.M. Leroux, P. Bourgouin, G. Beaudoin, S. Joubert, M. Beauregard, Areas of brain activation in males and females during viewing of erotic film excerpts, Hum. Brain Mapp. 16 (2002) 1–13.

[59] J.S. Winston, J. O'Doherty, J.M. Kilner, D.I. Perrett, R.J. Dolan, Brain systems for assessing facial attractiveness, Neuropsychologia 45 (2007) 195–206.

[60] R.C. Risinger, B.J. Salmeron, T.J. Ross, S.L. Amen, M. Sanfilipo, R.G. Hoffmann, A.S. Bloom, H. Garavan, E.A. Stein, Neural correlates of high and craving during cocaine self-administration using BOLD fMRI, Neuroimage 26 (2005) 1097–1108.

[61] P. Kufahl, Z. Li, R. Risinger, C. Rainey, L. Piacentine, G. Wu, A. Bloom, Z. Yang, S.J. Li, Expectation modulates human brain responses to acute cocaine: a functional magnetic resonance imaging study, Biol. Psychiatry 63 (2008) 222–230.

[62] B. Seymour, J.P. O'Doherty, P. Dayan, M. Koltzenburg, A.K. Jones, R.J. Dolan, K.J. Friston, R. S. Frackowiak, Temporal difference models describe higher-order learning in humans, Nature 429 (2004) 664–667.

[63] B. Seymour, J.P. O'Doherty, M. Koltzenburg, K. Wiech, R. Frackowiak, K. Friston, R. Dolan, Opponent appetitive-aversive neural processes underlie predictive learning of pain relief, Nat. Neurosci. 8 (2005) 1234–1240.

[64] B. Seymour, T. Singer, R. Dolan, The neurobiology of punishment, Nat. Rev. Neurosci. 8 (2007) 300–311.

[65] M.L. Kringelbach, The human orbitofrontal cortex: linking reward to hedonic experience, Nat. Rev. Neurosci. 6 (2005) 691–702.

[66] K. Izuma, D.N. Saito, N. Sadato, Processing of social and monetary rewards in the human striatum, Neuron 58 (2008) 284–294.

[67] P. Domenech, J-C. Dreher, Distinguishing two brain systems involved in choosing between different types of rewards, in: Society for Neuroscience, Washington DC, 2008.

[68] T.A. Hare, J. O'Doherty, C.F. Camerer, W. Schultz, A. Rangel, Dissociating the role of the orbitofrontal cortex and the striatum in the computation of goal values and prediction errors, J. Neurosci. 28 (2008) 5623–5630.

[69] J. Fan, J. Fossella, T. Sommer, Y. Wu, M.I. Posner, Mapping the genetic variation of executive attention onto brain activity, Proc. Natl. Acad. Sci. USA 100 (2003) 7406–7411.

[70] T.A. Klein, J. Neumann, M. Reuter, J. Hennig, D.Y. von Cramon, M. Ullsperger, Genetically determined differences in learning from errors, Science 318 (2007) 1642–1645.

[71] M.J. Frank, A.A. Moustafa, H.M. Haughey, T. Curran, K.E. Hutchison, Genetic triple dissociation reveals multiple roles for dopamine in reinforcement learning, Proc. Natl. Acad. Sci. USA 104 (2007) 16311–16316.

[72] H.M. Lachman, D.F. Papolos, T. Saito, Y.M. Yu, C.L. Szumlanski, R.M. Weinshilboum, Human catechol-O-methyltransferase pharmacogenetics: description of a functional polymorphism and its potential application to neuropsychiatric disorders, Pharmacogenetics 6 (1996) 243–250.

[73] J. Chen, B.K. Lipska, N. Halim, Q.D. Ma, M. Matsumoto, S. Melhem, B.S. Kolachana, T. M. Hyde, M.M. Herman, J. Apud, M.F. Egan, J.E. Kleinman, D.R. Weinberger, Functional analysis of genetic variation in catechol-O-methyltransferase (COMT): effects on mRNA, protein, and enzyme activity in postmortem human brain, Am. J. Hum. Genet. 75 (2004) 807–821.

[74] D.J. Vandenbergh, A.M. Persico, A.L. Hawkins, C.A. Griffin, X. Li, E.W. Jabs, G.R. Uhl, Human dopamine transporter gene (DAT1) maps to chromosome 5p15.3 and displays a VNTR, Genomics 14 (1992) 1104–1106.

[75] A. Heinz, D. Goldman, D.W. Jones, R. Palmour, D. Hommer, J.G. Gorey, K.S. Lee, M. Linnoila, D.R. Weinberger, Genotype influences in vivo dopamine transporter availability in human striatum, Neuropsychopharmacology 22 (2000) 133–139.

[76] J. Mill, P. Asherson, C. Browes, U. D'Souza, I. Craig, Expression of the dopamine transporter gene is regulated by the 3′ UTR VNTR: evidence from brain and lymphocytes using quantitative RT-PCR, Am. J. Med. Genet. 114 (2002) 975–979.

[77] S.H. VanNess, M.J. Owens, C.D. Kilts, The variable number of tandem repeats element in DAT1 regulates in vitro dopamine transporter density, BMC Genet. 6 (2005) 55.

[78] C.H. Van Dyck, R.T. Malison, L.K. Jacobsen, J.P. Seibyl, J.K. Staley, M. Laruelle, R.M. Baldwin, R.B. Innis, J. Gelernter, Increased dopamine transporter availability associated with the 9-repeat allele of the SLC6A3 gene, J. Nucl. Med. 46 (2005) 745–751.

[79] L.K. Jacobsen, J.K. Staley, S.S. Zoghbi, J.P. Seibyl, T.R. Kosten, R.B. Innis, J. Gelernter, Prediction of dopamine transporter binding availability by genotype: a preliminary report, Am. J. Psychiatry 157 (2000) 1700–1703.

[80] S.R. Jones, R.R. Gainetdinov, M. Jaber, B. Giros, R.M. Wightman, M.G. Caron, Profound neuronal plasticity in response to inactivation of the dopamine transporter, Proc. Natl. Acad. Sci. USA 95 (1998) 4029–4034.

[81] F. Karoum, S.J. Chrapusta, M.F. Egan, 3-Methoxytyramine is the major metabolite of released dopamine in the rat frontal cortex: reassessment of the effects of antipsychotics on the dynamics of dopamine release and metabolism in the frontal cortex, nucleus accumbens, and striatum by a simple two pool model, J. Neurochem. 63 (1994) 972–979.

[82] M. Matsumoto, C.S. Weickert, S. Beltaifa, B. Kolachana, J. Chen, T.M. Hyde, M.M. Herman, D.R. Weinberger, J.E. Kleinman, Catechol O-methyltransferase (COMT) mRNA expression in the dorsolateral prefrontal cortex of patients with schizophrenia, Neuropsychopharmacology 28 (2003) 1521–1530.

[83] M. Matsumoto, C.S. Weickert, M. Akil, B.K. Lipska, T.M. Hyde, M.M. Herman, J.E. Kleinman, D.R. Weinberger, Catechol O-methyltransferase mRNA expression in human and rat brain: evidence for a role in cortical neuronal function, Neuroscience 116 (2003) 127–137.

[84] L. Yavich, M.M. Forsberg, M. Karayiorgou, J.A. Gogos, P.T. Mannisto, Site-specific role of catechol-O-methyltransferase in dopamine overflow within prefrontal cortex and dorsal striatum, J. Neurosci. 27 (2007) 10196–10209.

[85] S.R. Sesack, V.A. Hawrylak, C. Matus, M.A. Guido, A.I. Levey, Dopamine axon varicosities in the prelimbic division of the rat prefrontal cortex exhibit sparse immunoreactivity for the dopamine transporter, J. Neurosci. 18 (1998) 2697–2708.

[86] B.H. Schott, C.I. Seidenbecher, D.B. Fenker, C.J. Lauer, N. Bunzeck, H.G. Bernstein, W. Tischmeyer, E.D. Gundelfinger, H.J. Heinze, E. Duzel, The dopaminergic midbrain participates in human episodic memory formation: evidence from genetic imaging, J. Neurosci. 26 (2006) 1407–1417.

[87] B. Knutson, G.W. Fong, S.M. Bennett, C.M. Adams, D. Hommer, A region of mesial prefrontal cortex tracks monetarily rewarding outcomes: characterization with rapid event-related fMRI, Neuroimage 18 (2003) 263–272.

[88] A. Bertolino, G. Blasi, V. Latorre, V. Rubino, A. Rampino, L. Sinibaldi, G. Caforio, V. Petruzzella, A. Pizzuti, T. Scarabino, M. Nardini, D.R. Weinberger, B. Dallapiccola, Additive effects of genetic variation in dopamine regulating genes on working memory cortical activity in human brain, J. Neurosci. 26 (2006) 3918–3922.

[89] X. Caldu, P. Vendrell, D. Bartres-Faz, I. Clemente, N. Bargallo, M.A. Jurado, J.M. Serra-Grabulosa, C. Junque, Impact of the COMT Val108/158 Met and DAT genotypes on prefrontal function in healthy subjects, Neuroimage 37 (2007) 1437–1444.

[90] J-C. Dreher, P. Kohn, B. Kolachana, D.R. Weinberger, K.F. Berman, Variation in dopamine genes influences responsivity of the human reward system, Proc. Natl. Acad. Sci. USA (2009) Sci USA 106:15106–15111.

[91] J. Yacubian, T. Sommer, K. Schroeder, J. Glascher, R. Kalisch, B. Leuenberger, D.F. Braus, C. Buchel, Gene-gene interaction associated with neural reward sensitivity, Proc. Natl. Acad. Sci. USA 104 (2007) 8125–8130.

[92] B. Knutson, S.E. Gibbs, Linking nucleus accumbens dopamine and blood oxygenation, Psychopharmacology (Berl) 191 (2007) 813–822.

[93] J-C. Dreher, A. Meyer-Lindenberg, P. Kohn, K.F. Berman, Age-related changes in midbrain dopaminergic regulation of the human reward system, Proc. Natl. Acad. Sci. USA 105 (2008) 15106–15111.

[94] Y.C. Chen, W.R. Galpern, A.L. Brownell, R.T. Matthews, M. Bogdanov, O. Isacson, J.R. Keltner, M.F. Beal, B.R. Rosen, B.G. Jenkins, Detection of dopaminergic neurotransmitter activity using pharmacologic MRI: correlation with PET, microdialysis, and behavioral data, Magn. Reson. Med. 38 (1997) 389–398.

[95] G.K. Murray, P.R. Corlett, L. Clark, M. Pessiglione, A.D. Blackwell, G. Honey, P.B. Jones, E. T. Bullmore, T.W. Robbins, P.C. Fletcher, Substantia nigra/ventral tegmental reward prediction error disruption in psychosis, Mol. Psychiatry 13 (239) (2008) 267–276.

[96] W. Schultz, P. Dayan, P.R. Montague, A neural substrate of prediction and reward, Science 275 (1997) 1593–1599.

[97] R.S. Sutton, A.G. Barto, Reinforcement learning: an introduction, IEEE Trans Neural Netw 9 (1998) 1054.

7 Reward processing in the human brain: insights from fMRI

Anthony J. Porcelli and Mauricio R. Delgado

Department of Psychology, Rutgers University, 101 Warren St., Newark, NJ 07102

Abstract

In recent years, an explosion of neuroimaging research has replicated and extended findings from a rich animal literature on basic brain reward systems to probe how such systems are modulated by more complex processes that typically influence goal-directed behaviors in human society (e.g., social and economic factors). These research questions have led to a blending of the disciplines of psychology, neuroscience and economics to investigate common questions pertaining to the neural basis of human reward processing and its relationship with decision-making. The goal of this chapter is to discuss and attempt to integrate neuroimaging studies of reward processing. Focus will be given to a cortical-striatal circuits involved in goal-directed behavior and the valuation of reward-related information. Additionally, we will highlight how cortical-striatal circuits and valuation signals can be modulated by the presence of more complex factors such as risk, time and social context. Finally, important directions for future research in the context of emerging disciplines of neuroeconomics and social neuroscience will be discussed.

Key points

1. Reward processing engages diverse brain regions, including multiple prefrontal regions and the basal ganglia (particularly the multifaceted striatum).
2. Corticostriatal circuits are involved in computation of subjective value for experienced rewards, leading to a valuation signal which can be used to guide future decisions via reinforcement-learning mechanisms.
3. Neuroimaging research has begun to highlight functional subdivisions within components of this corticostriatal circuitry.
4. Reward processing can be modulated by a number of additional factors, including magnitude of reward, risk, time, and social context.
5. Important directions for future research include the study of the complex modulation of reward processing by social factors, as well as processing of aversive information that can also modulate behavior.

7.1 Introduction

With the advent of neuroimaging technology, scientific understanding of human brain function has taken a great leap forward. One technique that has gained a prominent position among these new methodologies is functional magnetic resonance imaging (fMRI). Over the past two decades, a veritable explosion of fMRI research has deepened our understanding of the basic neural processes involved in learning, memory, and emotion. More recently, a blending of the disciplines of psychology, neuroscience, and economics has evoked a great deal of interest in the neural basis of reward processing in the context of economic decisions. The goal of this chapter is to examine and integrate recent fMRI findings on reward processing in order to augment current understanding of the topic and identify potentially productive future directions.

Reward-related information can be broadly classified into two categories that can have opposite effects on decision-making and goal-directed behavior. "Rewards" can be operationally defined as positively valenced stimuli that can evoke exploratory or approach behavior (e.g., searching for food). Punishments, on the other hand, are stimuli of a negative valence that may suppress behavior (e.g., not searching for foods that lead to sickness). Thus, an individual's ability to process rewards and punishments enables him or her to navigate through the environment in a goal-directed manner – resulting in observable behaviors that involve being drawn to rewards and repelled from punishments. As such, reward processing is intimately related to the ability to make decisions.

In order to use reward-related information to guide behavior, the brain must have some mechanism by which value can be computed. Complicating matters, however, is that "value" is a concept with multiple dimensions. For example, an important distinction can be drawn between the value of a reward that has been experienced (e.g., a sip of juice already consumed) and the value of a reward one expects to experience at some future point (e.g., a sip of juice not yet taken). In fact, an individual's subjective experience with the hedonic properties of a reward already received can lead to the development of an expectation of a similar reward in the future (i.e., via learning). Furthermore, the probability of such an expectation actually coming to pass contributes an element of risk to the entire computation. Researchers using fMRI have made much progress in gaining an understanding of the neural underpinnings of this highly complex process of valuation in the human brain.

Thus far the approach of investigators interested in examining the neural basis of reward processing in decision making has been to break the larger process into its constituent parts, allowing for targeted studies that aim to establish a network of regions mediating these valuation computations. While this has resulted in a multitude of interesting and well-designed studies on specific aspects of reward processing and decision making, it is useful to consider the common and distinct results across various studies and outline outstanding issues in the literature. In order to weave these diverse findings into a cohesive whole, this chapter will proceed in three stages. First, the general neuroanatomy of the human brain's reward circuitry as typically discussed in neuroimaging studies will be described. Having established this basic framework, fMRI research positing basic neural computations involved in reward processing will be presented. In the final part of the chapter, fMRI evidence for the modulation of reward processing in decision making by more complex factors (e.g., social and economic variables) will be discussed.

7.2 General neuroanatomy of reward processing

The fMRI research discussed in this chapter builds upon a rich animal literature that has identified a constellation of regions involved in the processing of rewards and reward-related learning (for review, see [1–7]). This "reward circuitry" consists of a diverse array of subcortical and cortical regions which most prominently features distributed prefrontal regions, the basal ganglia (particularly the multifaceted striatum), and the amygdala – all modulated by dopaminergic innervations from midbrain targets such as the substantia nigra and ventral tegmental area. When considering fMRI research involving these regions it is vital to note that each region is anatomically and functionally complex, and can be subdivided along subtle dimensions that are difficult to highlight given the restraints imposed by the technology. In light of that fact, however, attempts have been made using fMRI to devise clear criteria for differentiating between the two [8].

At the cortical level various loci within the prefrontal cortex (PFC) have been implicated as components of the brain's reward-processing circuitry. A number of these regions interact to form a large functional network in humans and non-human animals, referred to as the orbital and medial prefrontal cortex [9]. This swathe of cortex is functionally heterogeneous and exhibits connections to many brain regions. Within this larger network, the orbital prefrontal cortex (OFC) and medial prefrontal cortex (mPFC) have received a great deal of attention in the study of reward processing utilizing fMRI.

The anatomical boundaries between OFC and mPFC are somewhat blurred, in part because research indicates that they overlap [10]. Given the connectivity of these regions, and their integrative nature, a functional overlap is not necessarily surprising (for an extensive neuroanatomical review, refer back to [9]). These two regions, however, are not to be confused with the ventromedial prefrontal cortex [11]. Posited as playing a role in the use of emotional information in decision-making (i.e., somatic markers), this region overlaps both mPFC and OFC regions although it is centered more medially [12].

Located on the posterior, central, and lateral orbital surface of the frontal lobe of the brain, the human OFC is roughly composed of areas 11, 13, and 47/12 (Fig. 7.1; [9]). Involvement of this region in emotional processing and decision making is based in part on its diverse connectivity [5]. These include, but are not limited to, other PFC centers involved in cognitive control such as the dorsolateral prefrontal cortex [13,14], subcortical regions such as the amygdala [15] and striatum [16], and multimodal sensory input from primary cortical regions [13]. Thus, OFC is well-placed and connected to modulate behavior by integrating sensory, emotional, and cognitive information (for a review and meta-analysis, see [17]).

The neighboring mPFC has also been implicated in monitoring the outcome of rewards, especially with respect to processing of social information [18]. This may overlap some medial portions of cortex on the orbital wall, obscuring a clear-cut anatomical boundary between mPFC and OFC [10]. For example, mPFC has been defined as including parts of the areas just described with respect to OFC (medial 11, anterior 13, orbital 47/12). The medial network also includes areas 14, 24, 25, and 32 on the medial wall of the frontal lobe [9]. Regardless of the specific boundaries of this region, what is clear is that these mPFC areas innervate numerous visceromotor regions – perhaps in complement to the connections of the more sensory OFC, hearkening back to the aforementioned theory that these two regions form a single functional network.

Frontal pole

RS 10r

9

32h

24b 10m

Corpus
callosum 32m

24c

24a 25

CS

Temporal lobe

14r

14c

FMS

10o

OS

11m 11l 47/12r

46

13m 45

TOS 47/12l

13b 13l LOS HR

MOS 47/12m

13a 47/12s

AON Iam

lapm lai

lal

OC

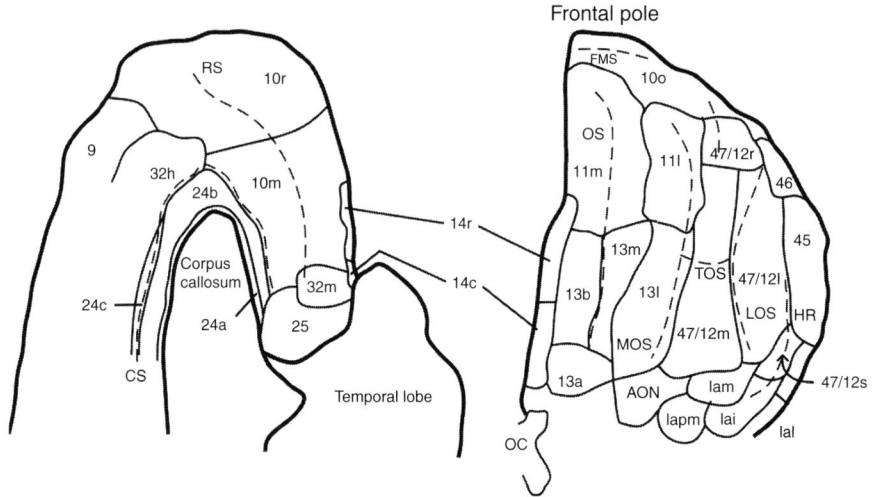

Figure 7.1 Map of human prefrontal cortex. *Source*: Adapted from Ongur & Price (2000) [9] with permission.

As previously mentioned, regions in the PFC are interconnected with subcortical structures involved in motor, cognitive, and motivational components of behavior – chiefly the basal ganglia. The connectivity between different loci within the striatum, the input unit of the basal ganglia, and various cortical sites gives rise to a vast array of corticostriatal loops integral in mediating the aforementioned aspects of goal-directed behavior [19–21]. The striatum is composed of three structures: the caudate nucleus, putamen, and nucleus accumbens. A dorsal/ventral distinction has been suggested for the striatum on functional grounds [2,13,22] with some support from anatomical studies. The dorsal striatum, consisting of the caudate and putamen, primarily connects with prefrontal regions involved in cognition and motor functions, while the ventral striatum, including the nucleus accumbens and more ventral portions of the putamen and caudate [23,24], is largely connected to ventral prefrontal and limbic regions thought to be involved in motivation and emotion, respectively [25]. Rather than a dorsal/ventral divide, however, an alternative proposal suggests that information flow within the striatum may follow a medial to lateral gradient that subserves the initial acquisition of reward-related associations to habit formation [26,27].

Corticostriatal loops are innervated by dopaminergic neurons from midbrain nuclei, with the ventral striatum receiving inputs mainly from the ventral tegmental area and dorsal striatum from the substantia nigra. Early work in non-human primates lead to the theory that the excitatory neurotransmitter dopamine plays an important role in reward processing (for a review, see [28]). Specifically, dopaminergic neurons respond to unexpected rewards and conditioned stimuli that signal a potential reward, but do not at the omission of an expected reward. These findings have led to the theory that dopamine neurons code prediction errors that aid goal-directed behaviors [29].

Finally, an additional subcortical region that has received much attention in fMRI studies of emotion is the amygdala. Consisting of a cluster of interconnected subnuclei in the anterior portion of the temporal lobe, the amygdala is a region previously implicated in processing emotional information, particularly fear [30–33]. It receives lower-level thalamic sensory input as well as interoceptive input from visceral sensory relays, the hypothalamus and higher-level sensory cortical regions such as OFC, while exteroceptive information reaches the amygdala via cortical association areas and the thalamus [34]. Research on the monkey brain also indicates the amygdala reciprocally connects with multiple neural regions that have also been identified as playing a role in processing of rewards and punishments and decision making, including OFC and ventral striatum [15].

7.3   The subjective value of rewards

In order to learn about, and adapt to, an ever-changing environment an individual must have a representation of current and future goals and an ability to evaluate the outcomes of past actions. Thus, evaluative and predictive computations of rewards and punishments are essential to guide future decisions and enable decision making to attain (and maintain) a goal-directed focus. It is through outcome evaluation (of an affective experience) that a value is attached to an experienced reward [35]. Such evaluations can lead to the establishment of predictive valuations that can be used to guide behavior. Although the subjective value of a reward is established when outcomes are evaluated, these evaluations are invoked prior to future choices. That information may then influence subsequent choices and become susceptible to updating, based on the accuracy of matches between predicted and experienced rewards (via learning mechanisms).

7.3.1   Orbital and medial prefrontal cortex

Numerous fMRI studies provide evidence that corticostriatal circuits (particularly between the OFC and the striatum) play a role in coding for the subjective value of a stimulus, across a wide range of modalities and types of reinforcers. In terms of outcome evaluation, for example, OFC activation has been observed during delivery of affectively pleasant compared to aversive gustatory stimuli (glucose versus salt, respectively) [36], with similar results observed in the olfactory domain [37]. Other such studies support the proposal that OFC is involved the representation of a stimulus' reward value in the domains of somatosensation [38] and more subjective modalities such as audition [39] and vision [40]. The results of sensory-specific satiation studies, where hungry participants are presented with food-related stimuli and then fed one type until satisfied, provide additional evidence in this direction. When individuals in that context are exposed to a conditioned stimulus predicting a satiated food, OFC exhibits decreases in blood-oxygen-level-dependent (BOLD) signal associated with the devaluation of that food post-feeding [41,42].

Interestingly, a few dissociations within the OFC have been proposed. A medial/lateral distinction has been suggested with respect to valence [17]. Specifically, medial OFC has been suggested to code for primary [37] and secondary [36] appetitive stimuli, while lateral OFC has been suggested to code for aversive stimuli. Another potential dissociation that has been proposed highlights an anterior/posterior gradient, with studies utilizing more abstract rewards (e.g., money) tending to report more anterior OFC activation while those involving more concrete primary rewards (e.g., taste or odor) report activity located in more posterior parts of OFC [17]. However, these dissociations are topics of future research as other studies find OFC activity primarily linked with valence or goal values irrespective of localization or type of stimuli [43,44].

A neighboring prefrontal region, mPFC, may also be involved in coding for the value of rewards. One study observed BOLD activation increases in mPFC when participants received an anticipated reward [45]. It has also been proposed that mPFC is involved in the computation of appetitive "goal values" (the predicted subjective value of a reward contingent on some action) [46]. While medial portions of OFC have also been implicated in processing of goal values [35], the aforementioned difficulty in distinguishing a clear functional and anatomical boundary between OFC and mPFC leaves such assertions open to interpretation. Research in non-human primates does indicate, however, that a distinction of this type is appropriate in that corticostriatal projections to these two regions may be functionally organized along the lines of a dissociation established within the subcortical striatum [22,47].

7.3.2   Dorsal and ventral striatum

The striatum is another brain region implicated in subjective value coding (see [48] for a review). In terms of outcome evaluation, early studies suggested involvement of both dorsal and ventral striatum irrespective of type of reinforcer. For example, Delgado et al. [49] observed differential responses in both dorsal and ventral striatum in response to feedback granting monetary rewards, compared to monetary punishments or losses (Fig. 7.2A). Similar patterns in striatum BOLD signals have been observed with primary reinforcers ranging from beautiful faces [50] to more gustatory rewards and punishments [42,51].

The role of the striatum in coding subjective value is also displayed in paradigms where a conditioned cue signals a potential reward. In such studies, the representation of the subjective value of a potential reward is predicted by a conditioned stimulus, at times influencing future decision making. Increases in BOLD signal in the striatum are often reported in such paradigms using various types of reinforcers [52]. For instance, dorsal and ventral striatum activation correlates with cues that predict monetary rewards contingent on a rapid response [53–55] and with cues that predict juice rewards [56].

One important functional distinction between dorsal and ventral striatum that has been proposed in such conditioning paradigms and others suggests that subjective value representations may be coded with respect to task requirements. Specifically, the dorsal striatum has been linked primarily with appetitive conditioning paradigms that require an action component (response–reward associations), a function it is well-suited for due to its connections with motor and dorsal prefrontal cortices [19], while the ventral striatum appears to be critical to creating stimulus–reward contingencies (see [2,57] for review of relevant animal data; [58]).

In support of this distinction, a contingency between motivation and action has been found to correlate with BOLD signals in the human dorsal striatum. Tricomi and colleagues [59] used an oddball-like paradigm to attempt to explain previous results linking striatum and reward processes [49]. It was suggested that differential responses between reward and punishment outcomes previously observed in the dorsal striatum could be explained by the perception of control inherent in the experimental design. Participants receiving non-contingent delivery of rewards and punishments (masked as oddballs) did not recruit dorsal striatum activation. Instead, the dorsal striatum response to rewarding outcomes was only observed when a contingency existed between behavior and reward (via a response that was perceived to lead to the desirable outcome). This study and others [22,60,61] indicated that the dorsal striatum was involved in the processing of the reinforcement of an action, rather than the reward *per se*.

In another study, O'Doherty and colleagues [22] further suggested that the human dorsal striatum plays the role of an "actor," maintaining information about response–reward

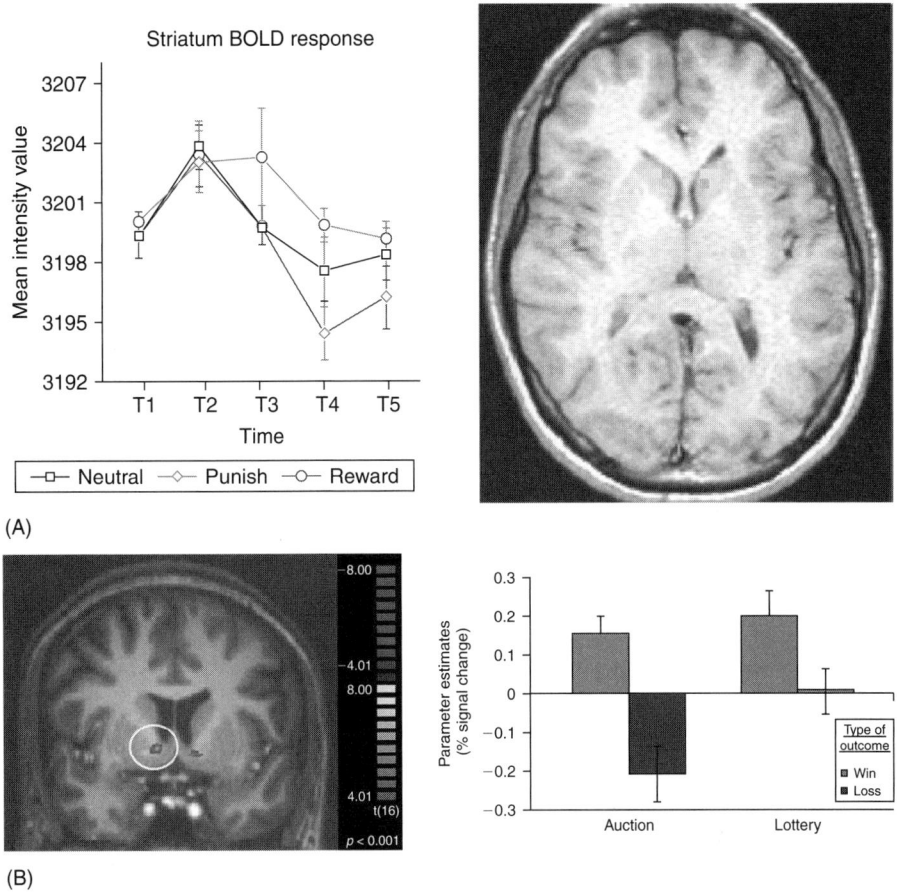

(A)

(B)

Figure 7.2 (A) Differential responses to reward and punishment in the striatum. Figure depicts activation in dorsal striatum and hemodynamic response graph with reward, neutral, and punish responses. A typical trial was 15 s and each time point (e.g., T1) represents 3-s bins. Differential responses are observed at T3 and T4 6–9 s after delivery of outcome. (B) BOLD signals in the ventral caudate nucleus during the outcome phase of an auction or lottery game. No differences between auction and lottery games were observed when the outcome was positive ("wins"). Instead, a negative outcome ("losses") during the competitive environment of an auction lead to a greater decrease in signals in the striatum compared to lottery games, which correlated with overbidding behavior. *Source*: For A, adapted from Delgado et al. (2000) [49] with permission; for B, adapted from Delgado et al. (2008) [115] with permission. See Plate 6 of Color Plate section.

associations to enable better choices in the future, while the ventral striatum serves as the "critic" and predicts future rewards. This study employed two yoked conditioning tasks in which participants made choices between stimuli predicting delivery of a juice reward or neutral solution at high and low probabilities (instrumental conditioning), or simply indicated which stimulus the computer had selected for them (classical conditioning). In accord with ideas put forth by actor–critic models [62,63] it was observed that BOLD activity in a dorsal striatal "actor" correlated with prediction error signals particularly during the instrumental task. The ventral striatal "critic," on the other hand, demonstrated this relationship during both tasks. These results provide support for the proposition that dorsal and ventral striatum interact to guide behavior, by establishing a link between dorsal striatum and instrumental conditioning (the role of the actor) and ventral striatum and both instrumental and classical conditioning (critic).

Having established a stable representation of the expected reward value of the reward contingent upon a decision, it is critical that the brain's reward circuitry be able to code for deviations from such predictions when that reward is actually received. Deviations of this type are termed "prediction errors." By carrying out such a computation, the brain can update expectations based on prior experience to reflect a changing environment. Based on reinforcement learning models from the field of computer science [63] the theory of prediction error, previously alluded to, elegantly explains how the brain's reward circuitry fosters learning. For example, if an individual expects a cup of coffee to have a high subjective value but it turns out to be terrible upon evaluation, the expected reward value of the coffee is adjusted during subsequent (predictive) valuations. This could bias subsequent decision making away from options leading to that outcome in the future. Thus it may be that the ability to generate prediction errors is essential for an individual to learn from, and modulate future behaviors based on, the outcome of past decisions.

As previously described, work by Schultz and colleagues provide a neural basis for understanding how prediction errors are computed in the brain, chiefly through dopaminergic neurons [29]. In humans, prediction errors are observed in dopaminergic projection sites such as the striatum using fMRI [46,64–66]. Coding of prediction errors in the striatum is consistent with previous studies suggesting that striatum signals processing of reinforcement information, rather than the pure value of a reward, in a dynamic fashion [59,67–69].

While early studies mimicked the aforementioned animal paradigms [64,65], more recent studies have highlighted the role of computational-modeling to generate estimates of the temporal profile of the creation of stimulus–response–reward associations, and subsequent prediction error signals, from participant's behavioral data – acquired during fMRI scanning. In one such study, it was observed that stimulus–response–reward associations correlated with activation increases in the putamen of the dorsal striatum, while activity in the ventral striatum correlated with calculations of prediction error [70]. These results support the proposed roles of the dorsal and ventral striatum, as they have been discussed thus far.

7.3.3 Dissociating OFC and striatum contributions to subjective value calculations

More recently, researchers have attempted to decompose decision making into its basic computations to dissociate the roles of the OFC and striatum in that process [46]. In order to obtain a measure of the expected value of various foods (designated the goal value), hungry participants took part in an auction procedure prior to fMRI scanning that established their willingness to pay for each item. During the scan, participants were offered those same food items at various prices paired with a random monetary gain or loss – with the understanding that they would be able to consume only the item they purchased at the end of the experiment. Based on their novel experimental design, Hare and colleagues were able to calculate separable estimates of subjects' goal values (i.e., willingness to pay), decision values (i.e., the net value of a decision or the goal value minus the cost of the item), and prediction errors for each decision. It was observed that calculations of goal and decision values correlated with medial and central OFC BOLD activity respectively, while prediction errors correlated with ventral striatal activation.

Thus, it appears that the ventral striatum is essential for the computation of prediction errors that enable an individual to update expectations regarding the outcome of their actions to learn about, and adapt to, their current environment. Cortical prefrontal regions such as OFC are involved in the encoding of the subjective values of experienced stimuli, information which can then be used in the representation and valuation of future decision options in the form of expected reward values associated with a given stimulus and/or action. Furthermore, OFC subregions involved in the calculation of such values may conform to a medial/lateral functional dissociation by the valence of a reward or punishment. Although valence of a stimulus has largely been the focus of this chapter up to this point, there are other dimensions along which the processing of rewards can be modulated.

7.3.4 The amygdala and aversive processing

The amygdala's role in coding subjective value is prominent mostly in the domain of aversive processing. Specifically, the amygdala has been implicated as an "emotion" structure given its involvement in fear conditioning paradigms (see [32] for a review). Amygdala-related findings from a rich animal literature extend to humans, as amygdala activation has been found to correlate with conditioned stimuli that predict aversive outcomes [71–73] and patients with amygdala lesions are unable to acquire fearful responses (as measured by skin conductance responses) [74]. Thus, it may be that the amygdala adaptively codes for subjective value of potential threat to build affective evaluations of environment, others, and context [75].

While studies across species support a role for the amygdala in learning about negative stimuli, both positron emission tomography [76,77] and fMRI [78] studies link the amygdala with positively valenced stimuli involved in appetitive or reward learning. Based on results of this type, it has been argued that the amygdala actually codes for intensity, rather than valence of an affective stimulus, and negative stimuli used in conditioning studies (e.g., shock) are typically more intense than positive ones (e.g., a pellet of food). For example, one study [43] capitalized on the nature of olfactory stimuli to dissociate the contributions of valence and intensity (of a stimulus) to the subjective value of rewards. It was observed that while BOLD activity in OFC was associated with valence of an olfactory stimulus, the amygdala exhibited a pattern of activation associated with intensity alone. Additional evidence indicates that the human striatum is also involved in the processing of aversive stimuli, rather than just appetitive or reward processing (for a review, see [79]). Therefore, the neural basis of aversive processing is a topic still of great debate – and the role of the amygdala in this process may be unrelated to valence.

7.4 Decision-making computations that contribute to valuation

Other than the ability of the brain's reward circuitry to assign value to rewards or expected rewards in terms of subjective value, additional computations may exist that utilize reward-related information in the decision-making process. Rangel and colleagues

[35] theorize that, in addition to outcome evaluation and valuation, the brain performs "representation" and "action selection" computations. According to this framework representational computations (not to be confused with representation of rewards themselves) generate sets of feasible decision options for subsequent valuation, in addition to incorporating interoceptive and exteroceptive information in those valuations. After representation and valuation, at the time of choice, a specific decision option is selected and enacted via the process of action selection. A greater understanding of the neural correlates of these computations and their possible independence from subjective value would clarify what may be important steps in the decision-making process.

7.4.1 Representation of decision options

Although an individual may often need to generate sets of decision options in the context of day-to-day decision making, in the laboratory setting research participants tend to be explicitly given a set of options from which to choose [80]. That being said, some behavioral research has been conducted in an attempt to circumvent this problem [81]. In one such study, participants verbalized their thought processes as they occurred in an attempt to quantify their generation of decision options, and it was observed that those with higher levels of knowledge generated more high-quality decision options [82]. Another study involving the presentation of large amounts of decision-relevant information indicated that participants utilized a "stopping heuristic" based on how many attributes considered of core importance to the decision had been met [83]. Unfortunately, though both studies provide interesting directions for future research the former paradigm is not easily adaptable to fMRI while the latter has not yet been conducted in that context.

One might make the argument that the generation of a set of decision options and internal/external state information is inextricably linked with, perhaps even defined by, the valuations with which they are associated. In fact, it may even be that such valuations dictate those representations that will be generated. Conversely, another interpretation might posit that during representation only the motor (i.e., the actions inherent in a given decision) and visceral (i.e., peripheral sensory information) components of those behaviors are established – and that values are attached at a later point. This question is one that requires further clarification and research.

7.4.2 Action selection

The manner in which a specific action is selected and initiated is a topic that researchers are just beginning to address. One proposal states that action selection can best be explained via a dual process framework [84]. Based on this framework, a network of corticostriatal circuits composed of the caudate, dorsolateral striatum, and various association cortices (i.e., premotor, anterior cingulate, medial, and orbitomedial) may support the deliberative and flexible types of decision-making processes [70,85]. Conversely, more habitual and automatic types of decision-making processes may be subserved by a different corticostriatal circuit reciprocally connecting the putamen, dorsolateral striatum, and sensorimotor cortices [86,87]. An alternative, yet compatible, proposal based on work using computational modeling techniques states that the basal ganglia may interact with cortical areas by providing information on alternative action choices – serving as a central switch in the gating of different behavioral options [88]. While these theories provide an excellent platform for future research and hypothesis generation, the process of action selection has not yet been well studied using fMRI.

7.5 Modulation of reward processing and decision making

Up to this point reward processing has largely been discussed in terms of coding for subjective value via valuation and outcome evaluation. Additional factors exist, however, that can modulate calculation of subjective value, enhancing, depressing, or even suppressing this signal entirely at the neural level. Such factors could bias the representation and/or action selection process away from specific decision options independent of subjective value calculations. Thus, while it is possible to characterize reward processing simply in terms of classically or instrumentally conditioned responses to specific stimuli leading to the reinforcement of future actions it may be that a more complex operational definition is needed to probe the process' neural underpinnings. More complex decisions, therefore, are those where the calculation of subjective value is influenced by additional factors such as magnitude, risk, time, and social interactions.

7.5.1 Magnitude

Magnitude may be defined as the quantity of a given reward or punishment. In one study, magnitude was operationalized as parametrically increasing monetary rewards and punishments (i.e., ranging between −$5.00 and +$5.00; [55]). When participants were asked to respond to stimuli associated with specific members of this range of dollar amounts during fMRI scanning, it was observed that BOLD activation in the dorsal striatum (caudate) scaled to anticipation of increasing magnitude for both positively and negatively valenced potential outcomes. Another study extended this interesting result beyond an anticipatory period by examining the response profile of the caudate post-reward delivery [89]. In this experiment, analysis of the time course of left caudate BOLD activation during feedback on a prior choice indicated that responses were strongest for high-magnitude rewards and weakest for high-magnitude punishments. Subsequent research, however, indicates that reward-related caudate activity is context-dependent rather than absolute magnitude [90].

An alternative, but compatible, interpretation of magnitude is that it may be subjectively appraised by an individual as the "intensity" of a stimulus in some situations. In fMRI studies in which stimuli (gustatory and olfactory) are matched for magnitude but vary in valence, or are matched for valence but vary in magnitude, a dissociation was observed such that OFC activated in the former case while amygdala activated in the latter [43,51]. Therefore, it may be that in simple decision making the amygdala codes for magnitude solely on the basis of the hedonic intensity of a stimulus. On the other hand, in complex decision-making rational appraisals of the quantity of a reward may also become an important motivating factor, modulating decision making in a top-down manner. These situations are analogous to those discussed earlier in the context of magnitude and monetary rewards or punishments. In addition, this leads one to the interesting conclusion that the subjective value of a stimulus may, in fact, be a composed of neural responses to both valence and magnitude of reward.

7.5.2 Risk: uncertainty and ambiguity

It was established earlier that predictive subjective valuations (expected reward values) based on learned stimulus–response–reward associations contribute to decision making. Because such associations are probabilistic in nature and not perfectly accurate, it is sensible that decisions based on them would be imperfect, resulting in prediction errors that can be used to guide future decisions. One way to conceptualize risk is as an individual's assessment of his or her likelihood to make a prediction error in an upcoming choice [91]. Another compatible description from the field of economics states that risk is analogous to the variance exhibited by the outcomes of past decisions (i.e., the spread of subjective values from past rewards around the expected or mean reward value) [92]. If expected reward value is analogous to the mean of past rewards received, and risk the variance surrounding that mean, it is plausible that the subjective value of expected rewards may be comprised of an amalgam of computations coding for reward valence, magnitude, and risk.

In addition, there are two different categories of risky decisions – those made under uncertainty (or pure risk) versus ambiguity [91]. A decision made under uncertainty is one where the probabilities are explicitly known, either because they were given to the decision maker or perhaps learned due to previous experience with (or training on) that type of decision. Ambiguous decisions, on the other hand, are those made when an individual does not have any decision-related knowledge [91]. Also of interest is that there appear to be large differences between individuals' attitudes with respect to risk [93]. While some individuals exhibit risk-averse tendencies, others may be risk seeking.

In one study examining financial risk taking, participants underwent fMRI scanning while making a choice between one of three options (risk-neutral, -averse, or -seeking) [94]. By calculating probabilistic estimates of the optimal choice for each trial, the researchers were able to identify when participants made risk-seeking or risk-averse mistakes. Interestingly, increased BOLD activity was observed in the ventral striatum (nucleus accumbens) preceding risky choices and risk-seeking mistakes. On the other hand, a region not yet discussed exhibited increased activation prior to risk less choices and risk-averse mistakes – the anterior insula. These results indicate that separable neural circuits may underlie risk-seeking versus risk-averse behavior – perhaps implying that calculations of subjective value for the expected reward value of uncertain decisions would be enhanced in the former but depressed in the latter.

Multiple fMRI studies implicate the insula in assessment of risk and risk-taking behavior [95,96]. This region is bilaterally located deep within the lateral (or sylvian) fissure, enclosed by a major infolding of the temporal and inferior parietal lobes. One interesting proposal states that the insula calculates what have been termed "risk prediction errors" – the difference between expected prediction errors and experienced prediction errors [97]. Therefore, as the brain uses prediction errors to learn about expected reward values (or the mean value of past rewards) it may also use risk prediction errors to learn about risk (or the variance of past rewards). It must be noted, however, that some research disputes such a role for the insula. For example, in one study BOLD activation increases were observed in the ventral striatum prior to a risky decision whereas choices not made under risk were preceded by activation of the anterior insula [94]. Another experiment observed BOLD activation increases associated with risk-averse choices in lateral OFC, while risk-seeking choices correlated with more medial OFC activation [98]. Additional research is necessary to clarify the complex interaction of risk with reward processing and decision making.

While it appears that decisions made under uncertainty involve separable computations for expected reward value and risk, originating in different neural regions and then integrated at a later point, less is known about the neural underpinnings of ambiguous decisions. One feasible proposal states that the same areas involved in decision making under uncertainty are involved when an individual makes an ambiguous decision – save that the actual patterns or intensity of activation within these regions may differ [91]. In one fMRI study on this topic, BOLD activity in OFC and the amygdala positively correlated with levels of ambiguity, whereas striatal activity and ambiguity were negatively correlated [99]. Although this particular question is just beginning to be examined using fMRI, a number of sophisticated models from the field of economics may provide excellent platforms for hypothesis generation and experimentation. One model useful in this regard is the α-maxmin utility model [100], which states that decisions made under ambiguity are anchored by either a best-case or worst-case scenario interpretation of the possible outcome of a decision. Under this theory, individual differences between decision makers can explain their reactions to ambiguous decisions (i.e., ambiguity loving, averse, or neutral), a metric that can be helpful in interpretation of both behavior and patterns of BOLD activation in future fMRI research.

7.5.3 Time and intertemporal decisions

Time is an additional factor that can exert an influence over the processing of rewards, and thus decision making. Much evidence indicates that rewards are devalued by the brain's reward circuitry as function of the delay between the time a decision is made to pursue a reward and reward delivery, a phenomenon known as time (or delay) discounting [101–103]. Effectively, this means that the value of immediate rewards is enhanced at a neural level, and that delays in the receipt of a reward exert a potent modulatory effect over decision making. Thus, an intertemporal decision is one whose outcome extends beyond the selection of a specific decision and performance of its associated action(s).

Research on this topic has yielded an interesting and fruitful debate regarding the nature of the neural systems involved in immediate versus delayed rewards. One camp posits a dual-process interpretation based on the relevant fMRI research, stating that prefrontal and posterior parietal regions are involved in subjective value coding for delayed rewards whereas subcortical structures perform such computations for immediate rewards [104–107]. Under this interpretation, the former system discounts (devalues) rewards at a high rate while the latter discounts rewards at a low rate, thus explaining the phenomenon of time discounting. Furthermore, this theory is consistent with concepts previously discussed in terms of simple (immediate) as compared to complex (long-term) decision making.

In contrast, another theory states that a unitary corticostriatal network codes for the subjective value of both immediate and delayed rewards, with discounting occurring at an exponential or hyperbolic rate as a function of time [108]. In an attempt to integrate these very different standpoints, Rangel and colleagues [35] have proposed that corticostriatal circuitry integrates information from disperse brain regions into a single value signal, and as the type of information inherent to immediate versus delayed rewards differs so do the extended regions involved in such computations. Although additional research is necessary to clearly define the nature of time discounting in reward processing and decision making, the research just described has laid the groundwork for a sophisticated understanding of this phenomenon.

7.5.4 Social interactions

The social environment surrounding a decision maker is another factor that has been observed to influence reward processing. Most interestingly, research indicates that social interactions can modulate not only behavior but neural activity as well. While the fields of neuroeconomics and social neuroscience are still in their infancies, they have yielded fascinating insights into the social nature of decision making. At a simple level this may be related to hedonically positive or negative values of such experiences, but it is apparent that social interactions can also be highly nuanced and less hedonically based, possibly resulting in a more complex interaction with decision making. One possibility that merits exploration is that some social interactions are based on reinforcement-learning mechanisms, but can be encoded in a more declarative manner based on prior trial-and-error experiences, after which they are resistant to the activity of said mechanisms.

For example, research in the field of economics indicates that trust (even of an unknown counterpart) is vital to reciprocity between two individuals in financial decision making, which allows for a maximization of financial gains [109]. Building on this research, it has been observed that BOLD activation in the dorsal striatum mirrors this interaction, which can be conceptually defined as the building of a reputation between two partners engaged in a financial exchange [110]. Other research supports these findings. In one study, participants were provided with vignettes characterizing their (fictional) trading partners as "good", "bad", or "neutral", and were then asked to make risky decisions to share or keep money, in the knowledge that their partner could either keep those funds or return them in kind for a maximization of reward [67]. It was observed that BOLD activity in the caudate nucleus differentiated between feedback indicating whether the partner had returned or kept the money, but for the "neutral" partner only. This result is notable in that it suggests that reputation can not only influence reward processing at the neural level, but can diminish reliance on experience-based reinforcement-learning mechanisms. Although it may be the case that social interactions originate in hedonically oriented reinforcement learning, this research indicates that it is possible for such factors to supersede those mechanisms.

7.6 Future directions and open questions

With the development of neuroimaging technology, sophisticated models of economic decision-making and an exponentially increasing knowledge of the brains of humans and other species, much progress has been made towards a clear understanding the neural basis of decision-making. What is also apparent, however, is that there is much more to learn. Reviewing some of the questions posed over the course of this chapter alone yields enough material to require years of research. For instance, can subtle anatomical boundaries between OFC and mPFC (as well as subdivisions of the complex striatum) be distinguished using fMRI in terms of function? Are the processes of representation and action selection independent from valuation – or are they part of the brain's valuation circuitry? These regions do not work alone; what are the connectivity patterns that allow reward-related processing and goal-directed behavior to occur? And how is this circuitry modulated by more basic factors that influence valuation, such as magnitude, delay, and risk, as well as more complex factors such as social and economic variables.

While this chapter has focused on the processing of rewards, aversive processing is a topic that merits an equal amount of attention. Valuation systems must account for punishments just as much as rewards when calculating decisions; yet fMRI research on the neural basis of human decision making has mostly focused on reward processes. Economic theorists have developed sophisticated models accounting for the processing of aversive information, which indicate that such information exerts a stronger influence over behavior than rewards (i.e., loss aversion) [111]. Moving towards an integration of economic and neuroscientific theories one novel fMRI study examined loss aversion, testing the hypothesis that the phenomenon results from emotional processes evoked by losses [112]. This study yielded results of interest to both communities, indicating that loss aversion was neurally represented – but in brain regions related to valuation and not emotion, *per se*. Other integrative research supports the idea that a neural basis can be elucidated for economic theories (e.g., the role of the amygdala in framing effects) [113]. Yet, this interaction is not a one-way street – neuroscience can inform economic theory as well [114]. For example, in one recent study, knowledge of the brain's reward circuitry was employed to examine a question of great interest to economists: why people often "overbid" in an auction. The neuroimaging study suggested that overbidding is associated with enhanced striatal activity in response to the competitive social context of an auction [115], yielding a hypotheses that was confirmed in a behavioral economic design where participants in a loss frame overbid at greater frequency than other groups (Fig. 7.2B). Thus, a potential future direction of research is to further investigate the impact of aversive processing on valuation and decision making.

Perhaps some of the most interesting questions relate to the topic of the social brain, which recent research indicates may share a common currency with decision making via the brain's reward circuitry [116]. Empirical study of this aspect of brain function is especially important for a number of reasons. For example, the neural correlates of various psychopathologies (e.g., anxiety disorders) may be found in the very same brain regions highlighted in this chapter (OFC, mPFC, and amygdala) [117]. In addition, a greater understanding of the neural circuitry underlying social aspects of the human condition could even lead to advances in social policy and ethics [118]. As new questions are asked and new scientific discoveries made, the impact of this knowledge on society will be both pervasive and highly constructive.

References

[1] S.N. Haber, K. Kunishio, M. Mizobuchi, E. Lynd-Balta, The orbital and medial prefrontal circuit through the primate basal ganglia, J. Neurosci. 15 (1995) 4851–4867.

[2] T.W. Robbins, B.J. Everitt, Neurobehavioural mechanisms of reward and motivation, Curr. Opin. Neurobiol. 6 (1996) 228–236.

[3] W. Schultz, Multiple reward signals in the brain, Nat. Rev. Neurosci. 1 (2000) 199–207.

[4] R.A. Wise, D.C. Hoffman, Localization of drug reward mechanisms by intracranial injections, Synapse 10 (1992) 247–263.

[5] E.T. Rolls, The Brain and Emotion, Oxford University Press, Oxford, 1999.

[6] A. Dickinson, B. Balleine, Motivational control of goal-directed action, Anim. Learn. Behav. 22 (1994) 1–18.

[7] K.C. Berridge, T.E. Robinson, Parsing reward, Trends Neurosci. 26 (2003) 507–513.

[8] H.C. Breiter, R.L. Gollub, R.M. Weisskoff, D.N. Kennedy, N. Makris, J.D. Berke, J.M. Goodman, H.L. Kantor, D.R. Gastfriend, J.P. Riorden, R.T. Mathew, B.R. Rosen, S.E. Hyman, Acute effects of cocaine on human brain activity and emotion, Neuron 19 (1997) 591–611.

[9] D. Ongur, J.L. Price, The organization of networks within the orbital and medial prefrontal cortex of rats, monkeys and humans, Cereb. Cortex 10 (2000) 206–219.

[10] M.L. Kringelbach, The human orbitofrontal cortex: linking reward to hedonic experience, Nat. Rev. Neurosci. 6 (2005) 691–702.

[11] A. Bechara, A.R. Damasio, H. Damasio, S.W. Anderson, Insensitivity to future consequences following damage to human prefrontal cortex, Cognition 50 (1994) 7–15.

[12] L. Clark, A. Bechara, H. Damasio, M.R. Aitken, B.J. Sahakian, T.W. Robbins, Differential effects of insular and ventromedial prefrontal cortex lesions on risky decision-making, Brain 131 (2008) 1311–1322.

[13] S.T. Carmichael, J.L. Price, Sensory and premotor connections of the orbital and medial prefrontal cortex of macaque monkeys, J. Comp. Neurol. 363 (1995) 642–664.

[14] E.K. Miller, J.D. Cohen, An integrative theory of prefrontal cortex function, Annu. Rev. Neurosci. 24 (2001) 167–202.

[15] D.G. Amaral, J.L. Price, Amygdalo-cortical projections in the monkey (*Macaca fascicularis*), J. Comp. Neurol. 230 (1984) 465–496.

[16] F. Eblen, A.M. Graybiel, Highly restricted origin of prefrontal cortical inputs to striosomes in the macaque monkey, J. Neurosci. 15 (1995) 5999–6013.

[17] M.L. Kringelbach, E.T. Rolls, The functional neuroanatomy of the human orbitofrontal cortex: evidence from neuroimaging and neuropsychology, Prog. Neurobiol. 72 (2004) 341–372.

[18] D.M. Amodio, C.D. Frith, Meeting of minds: the medial frontal cortex and social cognition, Nat. Rev. Neurosci. 7 (2006) 268–277.

[19] G.E. Alexander, M.D. Crutcher, Functional architecture of basal ganglia circuits: neural substrates of parallel processing, Trends Neurosci. 13 (1990) 266–271.

[20] B.W. Balleine, M.R. Delgado, O. Hikosaka, The role of the dorsal striatum in reward and decision-making, J. Neurosci. 27 (2007) 8161–8165.

[21] F.A. Middleton, P.L. Strick, Basal ganglia output and cognition: evidence from anatomical, behavioral, and clinical studies, Brain Cogn. 42 (2000) 183–200.

[22] J. O'Doherty, P. Dayan, J. Schultz, R. Deichmann, K. Friston, R.J. Dolan, Dissociable roles of ventral and dorsal striatum in instrumental conditioning, Science 304 (2004) 452–454.

[23] J.L. Fudge, S.N. Haber, Defining the caudal ventral striatum in primates: cellular and histochemical features, J. Neurosci. 22 (2002) 10078–10082.

[24] S.N. Haber, K.S. Kim, P. Mailly, R. Calzavara, Reward-related cortical inputs define a large striatal region in primates that interface with associative cortical connections, providing a substrate for incentive-based learning, J. Neurosci. 26 (2006) 8368–8376.

[25] H.J. Groenewegen, H.B. Uylings, The prefrontal cortex and the integration of sensory, limbic and autonomic information, Prog. Brain Res. 126 (2000) 3–28.

[26] S.N. Haber, J.L. Fudge, N.R. McFarland, Striatonigrostriatal pathways in primates form an ascending spiral from the shell to the dorsolateral striatum, J. Neurosci. 20 (2000) 2369–2382.

[27] P. Voorn, L.J. Vanderschuren, H.J. Groenewegen, T.W. Robbins, C.M. Pennartz, Putting a spin on the dorsal-ventral divide of the striatum, Trends Neurosci. 27 (2004) 468–474.

[28] W. Schultz, Behavioral dopamine signals, Trends Neurosci. 30 (2007) 203–210.

[29] W. Schultz, P. Dayan, P.R. Montague, A neural substrate of prediction and reward, Science 275 (1997) 1593–1599.

[30] M. Davis, The role of the amygdala in fear and anxiety, Annu. Rev. Neurosci. 15 (1992) 353–375.

[31] M.R. Delgado, A. Olsson, E.A. Phelps, Extending animal models of fear conditioning to humans, Biol. Psychol. 73 (2006) 39–48.

[32] J.E. LeDoux, Emotion circuits in the brain, Annu. Rev. Neurosci. 23 (2000) 155–184.

[33] J.S. Morris, K.J. Friston, C. Buchel, C.D. Frith, A.W. Young, A.J. Calder, R.J. Dolan, A neuromodulatory role for the human amygdala in processing emotional facial expressions, Brain 121 (Pt 1) (1998) 47–57.

[34] D. Derryberry, D.M. Tucker, Neural mechanisms of emotion, J. Consult. Clin. Psychol. 60 (1992) 329–338.

[35] A. Rangel, C. Camerer, P.R. Montague, A framework for studying the neurobiology of value-based decision making, Nat. Rev. Neurosci. 9 (2008) 545–556.

[36] J. O'Doherty, E.T. Rolls, S. Francis, R. Bowtell, F. McGlone, Representation of pleasant and aversive taste in the human brain, J. Neurophysiol. 85 (2001) 1315–1321.

[37] E.T. Rolls, M.L. Kringelbach, I.E.T. de Araujo, Different representations of pleasant and unpleasant odours in the human brain, Eur. J. Neurosci. 18 (2003) 695–703.

[38] E.T. Rolls, J. O'Doherty, M.L. Kringelbach, S. Francis, R. Bowtell, F. McGlone, Representations of pleasant and painful touch in the human orbitofrontal and cingulate cortices, Cereb. Cortex 13 (2003) 308–317.

[39] A.J. Blood, R.J. Zatorre, P. Bermudez, A.C. Evans, Emotional responses to pleasant and unpleasant music correlate with activity in paralimbic brain regions, Nat. Neurosci. 2 (1999) 382–387.

[40] J. O'Doherty, J. Winston, H. Critchley, D. Perrett, D.M. Burt, R.J. Dolan, Beauty in a smile: the role of medial orbitofrontal cortex in facial attractiveness, Neuropsychologia 41 (2003) 147–155.

[41] M.L. Kringelbach, J. O'Doherty, E.T. Rolls, C. Andrews, Activation of the Human Orbitofrontal Cortex to a Liquid Food Stimulus is Correlated with its Subjective Pleasantness, Cereb. Cortex 13 (2003) 1064–1071.

[42] J. O'Doherty, E.T. Rolls, S. Francis, R. Bowtell, F. McGlone, G. Kobal, B. Renner, G. Ahne, Sensory-specific satiety-related olfactory activation of the human orbitofrontal cortex, Neuroreport 11 (2000) 399–403.

[43] A.K. Anderson, K. Christoff, I. Stappen, D. Panitz, D.G. Ghahremani, G. Glover, J.D. Gabrieli, N. Sobel, Dissociated neural representations of intensity and valence in human olfaction, Nat. Neurosci. 6 (2003) 196–202.

[44] H. Plassmann, J. O'Doherty, A. Rangel, Orbitofrontal cortex encodes willingness to pay in everyday economic transactions, J. Neurosci. 27 (2007) 9984–9988.

[45] B. Knutson, G.W. Fong, S.M. Bennett, C.M. Adams, D. Hommer, A region of mesial prefrontal cortex tracks monetarily rewarding outcomes: characterization with rapid event-related fMRI, Neuroimage 18 (2003) 263–272.

[46] T.A. Hare, J. O'Doherty, C.F. Camerer, W. Schultz, A. Rangel, Dissociating the role of the orbitofrontal cortex and the striatum in the computation of goal values and prediction errors, J. Neurosci. 28 (2008) 5623–5630.

[47] A.T. Ferry, D. Öngür, A. Xinhai, J.L. Price, Prefrontal cortical projections to the striatum in macaque monkeys: evidence for an organization related to prefrontal networks, J. Comp. Neurol. 425 (2000) 447–470.

[48] B. Knutson, M.R. Delgado, P.E.M. Phillips, Representation of subjective value in the striatum, in: P.W. Glimcher, C. Camerer, E. Fehr, R.A. Poldrack (Eds.), Neuroeconomics: Decision Making and the Brain, Academic Press, New York, 2008, pp. 389–403.

[49] M.R. Delgado, L.E. Nystrom, C. Fissell, D.C. Noll, J.A. Fiez, Tracking the hemodynamic responses to reward and punishment in the striatum, J. Neurophysiol. 84 (2000) 3072–3077.

[50] I. Aharon, N. Etcoff, D. Ariely, C.F. Chabris, E. O'Connor, H.C. Breiter, Beautiful faces have variable reward value: fMRI and behavioral evidence, Neuron 32 (2001) 537–551.

[51] D.M. Small, M.D. Gregory, Y.E. Mak, D. Gitelman, M.M. Mesulam, T. Parrish, Dissociation of neural representation of intensity and affective valuation in human gustation, Neuron 39 (2003) 701–711.

[52] J.P. O'Doherty, Reward representations and reward-related learning in the human brain: insights from neuroimaging, Curr. Opin. Neurobiol. 14 (2004) 769–776.

[53] M.R. Delgado, V.A. Stenger, J.A. Fiez, Motivation-dependent responses in the human caudate nucleus, Cereb. Cortex 14 (2004) 1022–1030.

[54] P. Kirsch, A. Schienle, R. Stark, G. Sammer, C. Blecker, B. Walter, U. Ott, J. Burkart, D. Vaitl, Anticipation of reward in a nonaversive differential conditioning paradigm and the brain reward system: an event-related fMRI study, Neuroimage 20 (2003) 1086–1095.

[55] B. Knutson, C.M. Adams, G.W. Fong, D. Hommer, Anticipation of increasing monetary reward selectively recruits nucleus accumbens, J. Neurosci. 21 (2001) RC159.

[56] J.P. O'Doherty, R. Deichmann, H.D. Critchley, R.J. Dolan, Neural responses during anticipation of a primary taste reward, Neuron 33 (2002) 815–826.

[57] B.W. Balleine, A. Dickinson, Goal-directed instrumental action: contingency and incentive learning and their cortical substrates, Neuropharmacology 37 (1998) 407–419.

[58] M.G. Packard, B.J. Knowlton, Learning and memory functions of the Basal Ganglia, Annu. Rev. Neurosci. 25 (2002) 563–593.

[59] E.M. Tricomi, M.R. Delgado, J.A. Fiez, Modulation of caudate activity by action contingency, Neuron 41 (2004) 281–292.

[60] R. Elliott, J.L. Newman, O.A. Longe, J.F. William Deakin, Instrumental responding for rewards is associated with enhanced neuronal response in subcortical reward systems, Neuroimage 21 (2004) 984–990.

[61] C.F. Zink, G. Pagnoni, M.E. Martin-Skurski, J.C. Chappelow, G.S. Berns, Human striatal responses to monetary reward depend on saliency, Neuron 42 (2004) 509–517.

[62] A.G. Barto, Adaptive critics and the basal ganglia, in: J. Houk, L. Davis, B.G. Beiser (Eds.), Models of Information Processing in the Basal Ganglia, MIT Press, Cambridge, MA, 1996, pp. 215–232.

[63] R.S. Sutton, A.G. Barto, Reinforcement Learning, MIT Press, Cambridge, MA, 1998.

[64] S.M. McClure, G.S. Berns, P.R. Montague, Temporal prediction errors in a passive learning task activate human striatum, Neuron 38 (2003) 339–346.

[65] J.P. O'Doherty, P. Dayan, K. Friston, H. Critchley, R.J. Dolan, Temporal difference models and reward-related learning in the human brain, Neuron 38 (2003) 329–337.

[66] G. Pagnoni, C.F. Zink, P.R. Montague, G.S. Berns, Activity in human ventral striatum locked to errors of reward prediction, Nat. Neurosci. 5 (2002) 97–98.

[67] M.R. Delgado, M.M. Miller, S. Inati, E.A. Phelps, An fMRI study of reward-related probability learning, Neuroimage 24 (2005) 862–873.

[68] M. Haruno, T. Kuroda, K. Doya, K. Toyama, M. Kimura, K. Samejima, H. Imamizu, M. Kawato, A neural correlate of reward-based behavioral learning in caudate nucleus: a functional magnetic resonance imaging study of a stochastic decision task, J. Neurosci. 24 (2004) 1660–1665.

[69] K. Koch, C. Schachtzabel, G. Wagner, J.R. Reichenbach, H. Sauer, R. Schlosser, The neural correlates of reward-related trial-and-error learning: an fMRI study with a probabilistic learning task, Learn. Mem. 15 (2008) 728–732.

[70] M. Haruno, M. Kawato, Different neural correlates of reward expectation and reward expectation error in the putamen and caudate nucleus during stimulus-action-reward association learning, J. Neurophysiol. 95 (2006) 948–959.

[71] K.S. LaBar, J.C. Gatenby, J.C. Gore, J.E. LeDoux, E.A. Phelps, Human amygdala activation during conditioned fear acquisition and extinction: a mixed-trial fMRI study, Neuron 20 (1998) 937–945.

[72] J.S. Morris, A. Ohman, R.J. Dolan, A subcortical pathway to the right amygdala mediating "unseen" fear, Proc. Natl. Acad. Sci. USA 96 (1999) 1680–1685.

[73] E.A. Phelps, K.J. O'Connor, J.C. Gatenby, J.C. Gore, C. Grillon, M. Davis, Activation of the left amygdala to a cognitive representation of fear, Nat. Neurosci. 4 (2001) 437–441.

[74] K.S. LaBar, J.E. LeDoux, D.D. Spencer, E.A. Phelps, Impaired fear conditioning following unilateral temporal lobectomy in humans, J. Neurosci. 15 (1995) 6846–6855.

[75] P. Petrovic, R. Kalisch, M. Pessiglione, T. Singer, R.J. Dolan, Learning affective values for faces is expressed in amygdala and fusiform gyrus, Soc. Cogn. Affect. Neurosci. 3 (2008) 109–118.

[76] S.B. Hamann, T.D. Ely, S.T. Grafton, C.D. Kilts, Amygdala activity related to enhanced memory for pleasant and aversive stimuli, Nat. Neurosci. 2 (1999) 289–293.

[77] J.P. Royet, D. Zald, R. Versace, N. Costes, F. Lavenne, O. Koenig, R. Gervais, Emotional responses to pleasant and unpleasant olfactory, visual, and auditory stimuli: a positron emission tomography study, J. Neurosci. 20 (2000) 7752–7759.

[78] F. Dolcos, K.S. LaBar, R. Cabeza, Interaction between the amygdala and the medial temporal lobe memory system predicts better memory for emotional events, Neuron 42 (2004) 855–863.

[79] M.R. Delgado, J. Li, D. Schiller, E.A. Phelps, The role of the striatum in aversive learning and aversive prediction errors, Philos. Trans. R. Soc. Lond. B Biol. Sci. 363 (2008) 3787–3800.

[80] L.K. Fellows, The cognitive neuroscience of human decision making: a review and conceptual framework, Behav. Cogn. Neurosci. Rev. 3 (2004) 159–172.

[81] J.G. Johnson, M. Raab, Take the first: option-generation and resulting choices, Organ. Behav. Hum. Decis. Process. 91 (2003) 215–229.

[82] A.B. Butler, L.L. Scherer, The effects of elicitation aids, knowledge, and problem content on option quantity and quality, Organ. Behav. Hum. Decis. Process. 72 (1997) 184–202.

[83] G. Saad, J. Russo, Stopping criteria in sequential choice, Organ. Behav. Hum. Decis. Process. 67 (1996) 258–270.

[84] K.R. Ridderinkhof, M. Ullsperger, E.A. Crone, S. Nieuwenhuis, The role of the medial frontal cortex in cognitive control, Science 306 (2004) 443–447.

[85] R. Levy, B. Dubois, Apathy and the functional anatomy of the prefrontal cortex-basal ganglia circuits, Cereb. Cortex 16 (2006) 916–928.

[86] M.S. Jog, Y. Kubota, C.I. Connolly, V. Hillegaart, A.M. Graybiel, Building neural representations of habits, Science 286 (1999) 1745–1749.

[87] R.A. Poldrack, J. Clark, E.J. Pare-Blagoev, D. Shohamy, J.C. Moyano, C. Myers, M.A. Gluck, Interactive memory systems in the human brain, Nature 414 (2001) 546–550.

[88] R. Bogacz, K. Gurney, The basal ganglia and cortex implement optimal decision making between alternative actions, Neural Comput. 19 (2007) 442–477.

[89] M.R. Delgado, H.M. Locke, V.A. Stenger, J.A. Fiez, Dorsal striatum responses to reward and punishment: effects of valence and magnitude manipulations, Cogn. Affect. Behav. Neurosci. 3 (2003) 27–38.

[90] S. Nieuwenhuis, H.A. Slagter, N.J. von Geusau, D.J. Heslenfeld, C.B. Holroyd, Knowing good from bad: differential activation of human cortical areas by positive and negative outcomes, Eur. J. Neurosci. 21 (2005) 3161–3168.

[91] P. Bossaerts, K. Preuschoff, M. Hsu, The neurobiological foundations of valuation in human decision making under uncertainty, in: P.W. Glimcher, C. Camerer, E. Fehr, R.A. Poldrack (Eds.), Neuroeconomics: Decision Making and the Brain, Academic Press, New York, 2008, pp. 353–366.

[92] D.M. Kreps, A Course in Microeconomic Theory, Princeton University Press, New York, 1990.

[93] E.U. Weber, A. Blais, N.E. Betz, Measuring risk perceptions and risk behaviors, J. Behav. Decis. Making 15 (2002) 263–290.

[94] C.M. Kuhnen, B. Knutson, The neural basis of financial risk taking, Neuron 47 (2005) 763–770.

[95] S.A. Huettel, A.W. Song, G. McCarthy, Decisions under uncertainty: probabilistic context influences activation of prefrontal and parietal cortices, J. Neurosci. 25 (2005) 3304–3311.

[96] M.P. Paulus, C. Rogalsky, A. Simmons, J.S. Feinstein, M.B. Stein, Increased activation in the right insula during risk-taking decision making is related to harm avoidance and neuroticism, Neuroimage 19 (2003) 1439–1448.

[97] K. Preuschoff, S.R. Quartz, P. Bossaerts, Human insula activation reflects risk prediction errors as well as risk, J. Neurosci. 28 (2008) 2745–2752.

[98] P.N. Tobler, J.P. O'Doherty, R.J. Dolan, W. Schultz, Reward value coding distinct from risk attitude-related uncertainty coding in human reward systems, J. Neurophysiol. 97 (2007) 1621–1632.

[99] M. Hsu, M. Bhatt, R. Adolphs, D. Tranel, C.F. Camerer, Neural systems responding to degrees of uncertainty in human decision-making, Science 310 (2005) 1680–1683.

[100] P. Ghirardato, F. Maccheroni, M. Marinacci, Differentiating ambiguity and ambiguity attitude, J. Econ. Theor. 118 (2004) 133–173.

[101] S. Frederick, G. Loewenstein, T. O'Donoghue, Time discounting and time preference: a critical review, J. Econ. Lit. 40 (2002) 351–401.

[102] L. Green, J. Myerson, A discounting framework for choice with delayed and probabilistic rewards, Psychol. Bull. 130 (2004) 769–792.

[103] D. Laibson, Golden eggs and hyperbolic discounting, Q. J. Econ. 112 (1997) 443–477.

[104] G.S. Berns, D. Laibson, G. Loewenstein, Intertemporal choice – toward an integrative framework, Trends Cogn. Sci. 11 (2007) 482–488.

[105] J. Li, S.M. McClure, B. King-Casas, P.R. Montague, Policy adjustment in a dynamic economic game, PLoS ONE 1 (2006) e103.

[106] S.M. McClure, K.M. Ericson, D.I. Laibson, G. Loewenstein, J.D. Cohen, Time discounting for primary rewards, J. Neurosci. 27 (2007) 5796–5804.

[107] S.M. McClure, M.K. York, P.R. Montague, The neural substrates of reward processing in humans: the modern role of FMRI, Neuroscientist 10 (2004) 260–268.

[108] J.W. Kable, P.W. Glimcher, The neural correlates of subjective value during intertemporal choice, Nat. Neurosci. 10 (2007) 1625–1633.

[109] J. Berg, J. Dickhaut, K. McCabe, Trust, reciprocity, and social History, Game. Econ. Behav. 10 (1995) 122–142.

[110] B. King-Casas, D. Tomlin, C. Anen, C.F. Camerer, S.R. Quartz, P.R. Montague, Getting to know you: reputation and trust in a two-person economic exchange, Science 308 (2005) 78–83.

[111] D. Kahneman, A. Tversky, Prospect theory: an analysis of decision under risk, Econometrica 47 (1979) 263–291.

[112] S.M. Tom, C.R. Fox, C. Trepel, R.A. Poldrack, The neural basis of loss aversion in decision-making under risk, Science 315 (2007) 515–518.

[113] B. De Martino, D. Kumaran, B. Seymour, R.J. Dolan, Frames, biases, and rational decision-making in the human brain, Science 313 (2006) 684–687.

[114] C. Camerer, G. Loewenstein, D. Prelec, Neuroeconomics: how neuroscience can inform economics, J. Econ. Lit. 43 (2005) 9–64.

[115] M.R. Delgado, A. Schotter, E.Y. Ozbay, E.A. Phelps, Understanding overbidding: using the neural circuitry of reward to design economic auctions, Science 321 (2008) 1849–1852.

[116] K. Izuma, D.N. Saito, N. Sadato, Processing of social and monetary rewards in the human striatum, Neuron 58 (2008) 284–294.

[117] M.R. Milad, S.L. Rauch, The role of the orbitofrontal cortex in anxiety disorders, Ann. NY Acad. Sci. 1121 (2007) 546–561.

[118] J. Illes, M.P. Kirschen, J.D. Gabrieli, From neuroimaging to neuroethics, Nat. Neurosci. 6 (2003) 205.

8 Spatiotemporal characteristics of perceptual decision making in the human brain

Marios G. Philiastides and Hauke R. Heekeren

Neurocognition of Decision Making Group, Max Planck Institute for Human Development, Lentzeallee 94, 14195 Berlin, Germany

Abstract

Perceptual decision making is the process by which information gathered from sensory systems is combined and used to influence our behavior. In recent years, the fields of systems and cognitive neuroscience have aggressively sought to examine the neural correlates of this process. As a result, significant contributions in the area of perceptual decision making have emerged. In this chapter we briefly review the major contributions made to this area by monkey neurophysiology and discuss how these animal experiments have inspired scientists to study the neural correlates of perceptual decision making in humans using non-invasive methods such as fMRI, EEG, and MEG. We present findings primarily from the visual and somatosensory domains, which we use as supporting evidence in proposing a new theoretical model of perceptual decision making. The latter part of the chapter focuses on how to best integrate EEG with fMRI to achieve both high spatial and high temporal resolution to help inform theories of the neurobiology of perceptual decision making. We conclude by providing a motivation on how this framework for perceptual decision making in combination with the techniques presented here can be extended to study the interaction of sensory and reward systems as well as to study value-based decision making in humans.

Key points

1. Perceptual decision making is the process by which information gathered from sensory systems is combined and used to influence our behavior.
2. Findings from monkey physiology experiments parallel those from human neuroimaging experiments.
3. Sensory evidence is represented in sensory processing areas.
4. Accumulation of sensory evidence occurs in decision-making areas that are downstream of the sensory processing areas; these decision-making areas form a decision by comparing outputs from sensory neurons.
5. The functional architecture for human perceptual decision making consists of separate processes that interact in a heterarchical manner in which at least some of the processes happen in parallel.
6. Simultaneous EEG/fMRI measurements and EEG-informed fMRI analysis techniques allow us to characterize the spatiotemporal characteristics of the network processes underlying perceptual decision making in humans.

8.1   Introduction

Perceptual decision making is the process by which incoming sensory information is combined and used to influence how we behave in the world. The neural correlates of perceptual decision making in the human brain are currently under intense investigation by systems and cognitive neuroscience. Fortunately, animal neurophysiology has already laid the foundation upon which critical new hypotheses about human decision making can be based. Specifically, results of single and multi-unit recordings in primates have already proposed that decision making involves three main processing stages: representation of sensory evidence, integration of the available sensory information across time, and a comparison of the accumulated evidence to a decision threshold [1]. Furthermore, some psychological theories suggest that these stages of decision formation are likely to occur in a serial fashion [2,3].

Though the overall simplicity of this hierarchical model is admittedly appealing, perceptual decision making in the human brain is likely to involve a more complex, non-serial cascade of events that includes sensory processing, attention, prior information, reward, evidence accumulation, and motor response networks [4]. An alternative model, as outlined in Fig. 8.1A, involves at least four complementary and partially overlapping systems which interact in a heterarchical manner, with some of the processes occurring in parallel.

In addition to the main processing modules of the simple hierarchical architecture, this four-compartment model includes a system that detects perceptual uncertainty or task difficulty as well as a performance monitoring system. In this chapter we will discuss recent findings from human neuroimaging studies, which use new data analysis techniques to identify the spatiotemporal characteristics of these different systems, to provide support for the extended model proposed here.

The majority of human studies that have addressed this problem use functional magnetic resonance imaging (fMRI) to identify the cortical regions that are participating in decision making [5–8]. The low temporal resolution of fMRI however, imposes limitations on inferring causation as little can be said about the sequence of neural activation in these regions, which is also needed to ultimately infer the true underlying neural network. A different approach to deciphering the temporal characteristics of perceptual decision making is provided by non-invasive measurements of the human electro- and magneto-encephalograms (EEG/MEG). Though the spatial resolution of these imaging modalities is rather low, they possess temporal resolution on the order of milliseconds and in conjunction with advanced single-trial analysis techniques can be used to map out temporally distinct components related to different events during decision formation [9–11].

Though significant progress has already been made using each of these modalities in isolation, the localization restrictions of EEG and MEG and the temporal precision constraints of fMRI, suggest that only a combination of these approaches can ultimately enable the recovery of the spatiotemporal characteristics of the network processes underlying perceptual decision making in humans. This can potentially be achieved by simultaneous EEG/fMRI measurements or by EEG-informed fMRI analysis techniques where EEG-derived regressors are used to model the fMRI data [12–14]. As the across-trial and across-condition variability seen in the identified EEG components may carry important information regarding the underlying neural processes, correlating EEG component activity with the blood-oxygenation-level-dependent (BOLD) fMRI signal could provide images of the source of this variability with high spatial resolution. Figure 8.1B illustrates

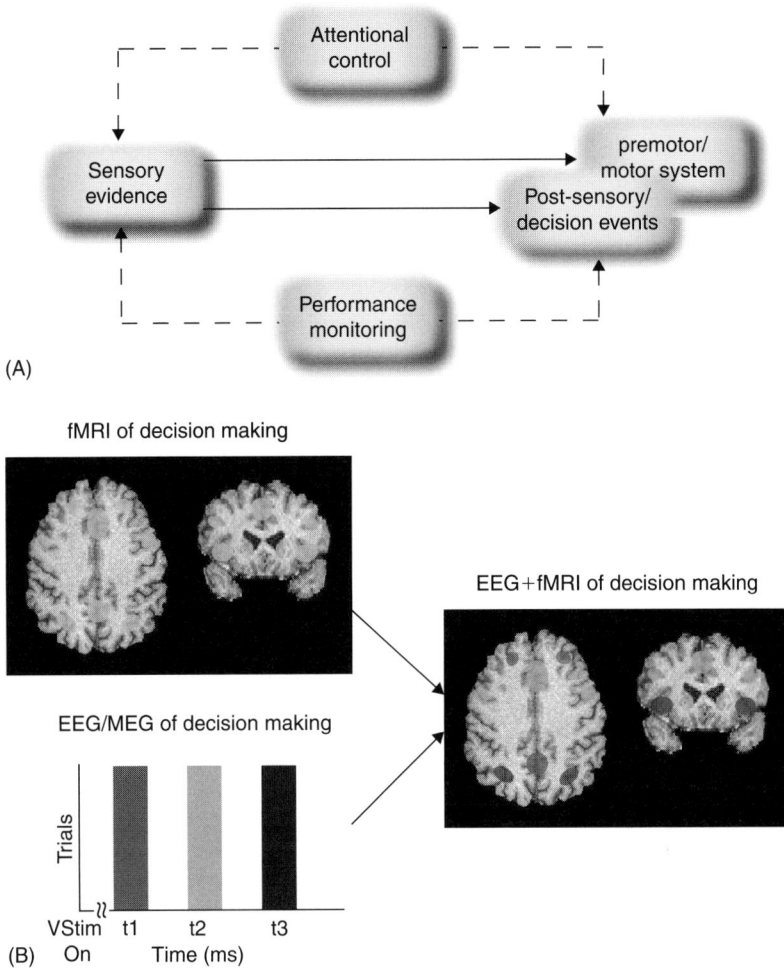

(A)

fMRI of decision making

EEG+fMRI of decision making

EEG/MEG of decision making

Trials

VStim   t1   t2   t3
(B)   On   Time (ms)

Figure 8.1 A theoretical model for human perceptual decision making. Integrating EEG with fMRI can help reveal the spatiotemporal characteristics of this model. (A) A four-compartment model of perceptual decision making in the human brain. In contrast to traditional hierarchical models of decision making [2,3] the main processes of some of these compartments can happen in parallel. The model includes a system for representing the early sensory evidence, and a system for post-sensory, decision-related processing including comparison and accumulation of sensory evidence and computation of decision variables. As in many tasks, decisions are usually expressed through action; this system includes motor and premotor structures. In addition, it incorporates a system for detecting perceptual uncertainty or difficulty to signal for recruitment of more attentional resources when task demands are increased, and a system for performance monitoring to detect when errors occur and when decision strategies need to be adjusted to improve performance. (B) Identifying the spatiotemporal characteristics of the model presented in (A) requires imaging the brain at both high spatial and high temporal resolution. fMRI can provide the desired spatial resolution while single-trial EEG can identify temporally well-localized features of this model. Developing new techniques to integrate EEG with fMRI can ultimately enable the recovery of the spatiotemporal characteristics of the network processes underlying human perceptual decision making.

the benefits of combining EEG and fMRI in inferring the spatiotemporal characteristics of human decision making.

This chapter is organized as follows. We start out by briefly reviewing the major contributions of monkey neurophysiology to our current knowledge of perceptual decision making. We then discuss how the concepts derived from this animal work also apply to human decision making by providing evidence from a number of recent fMRI, EEG and MEG studies. Where appropriate we use these findings to make references in support of the model outlined in Fig. 8.1A.The latter part of the chapter focuses on how to best integrate EEG and fMRI and provides an example of how the EEG-derived fMRI analysis approach can be a valuable tool in achieving high spatiotemporal characterization of the neural correlates of perceptual decision making in humans. We conclude by providing a motivation on how this framework for perceptual decision making in combination with the techniques presented here can be extended to study reward- and value-based decision making in humans.

8.2   Perceptual decision making in monkeys

8.2.1   *Sensory evidence representation*

A number of single-unit experiments in primates have already established a clear relationship between neuronal activity in sensory regions and psychophysical judgments. In a discrimination task in which monkeys had to decide the direction of motion from random dot kinetograms consisting of varying amounts of coherent motion, Newsome and colleagues showed that the activity of direction-selective neurons in middle temporal area (MT/V5) can provide a satisfactory account of behavioral performance [15–17]. In addition, trial-to-trial variability in these neuronal signals was correlated with the monkeys' actual choices [18]. That is, when a neuron in area MT fired more vigorously, the monkeys were more likely to make a decision in favor of that neuron's preferred direction of motion. In line with this idea, electrical microstimulation of MT neurons biased the monkeys to commit more and faster choices towards the neurons' preferred direction [19–21]. Taken together, these findings lend support to the notion that neuronal signals in area MT provide the sensory evidence upon which monkeys base their decision regarding the direction of stimulus motion.

Interestingly, this pattern of neural responses appears to extend to even highly complex visual stimuli such as faces. A study, using a rapid serial visual presentation (RSVP) task, identified activity of individual neurons in macaque temporal cortex which predicted whether the monkey responded that it saw a face in the stimulus or not [22]. More recently, and for a similar face versus no-face categorization task, microstimulation of face-selective neurons in inferotemporal (IT) cortex biased the monkeys' choices towards the face category [23]. The magnitude of the effect depended on the degree of face selectivity and the size of the stimulated cluster of face-selective neurons. Moreover, the early time, relative to stimulus onset, at which microstimulation had an effect suggested that neurons in IT can provide the sensory evidence needed for object-based decision making.

In the somatosensory domain, Romo and colleagues used a task in which monkeys had to discriminate the vibration frequency of two sequentially presented tactile stimuli and report which one was the highest. As with the MT experiments, here too, the sensitivity of the average responses in primary somatosensory cortex (S1) was similar to the behavioral sensitivity of the monkeys and the trial-to-trial fluctuations in the neural responses

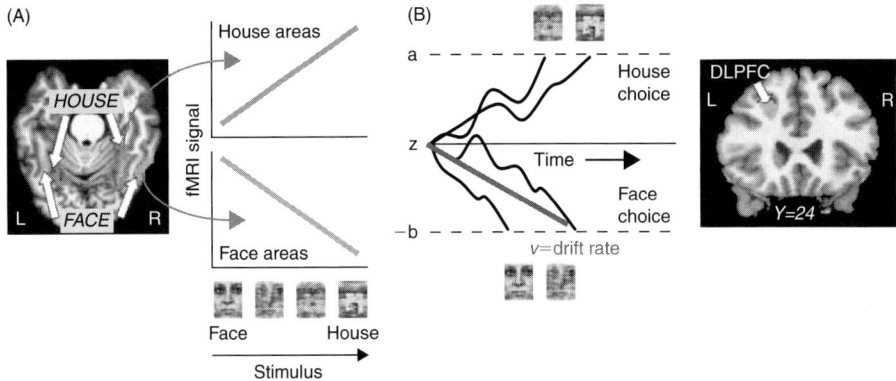

Figure 8.2 Representation and integration of sensory evidence during perceptual decision making in humans. (A) Using fMRI, Heekeren et al. [5] identified face- and house-selective regions (orange and green clusters, respectively) that are thought to represent the sensory evidence required to make a face-house discrimination. Specifically, they found a greater response in face-selective areas to clear images of faces than to noisy images of faces. Conversely, house-selective areas showed a greater response to clear images of houses than to noisy images of house. The orange and green lines illustrate this point in a cartoon-like fashion. (B) Decision making in higher-level brain regions is thought to involve an integration of sensory evidence over time. The diffusion model for simple decision making [27,28] assumes that decisions are made by continuously accumulating sensory information until one of two response criteria (a or b) is reached as illustrated graphically in this panel. Moment-to-moment fluctuations in the sample path reflect noise in the decision process. The accumulation rate, termed drift rate (v) in the model, reflects the quality of the available sensory evidence. For example, clear images of faces/houses contain more sensory evidence than noisy images, and therefore have a higher drift rate. Heekeren et al. [5] showed that such computations are carried out in the DLPFC. See Plate 7 of Color Plate section.

predicted the animals' choices to a small but significant degree [24]. Furthermore, micro-stimulation of S1 neurons, in the absence of physical stimulation, was sufficient to reproduce the behavioral patterns seen under normal conditions [25,26]. These results demonstrate that signals in S1 represent the evidence used by the monkeys to form the decision.

8.2.2   Accumulation of sensory evidence and decision formation

How can the sensory evidence provided by sensory regions, such as MT and S1, be used to drive the later stages of decision formation? Computational models of decision making, including diffusion and race models, have already proposed that decisions regarding ambiguous sensory evidence can benefit from an accumulation of information over time [27–31] (see Chapter 18). The diffusion model, for two-choice decisions, in particular assumes that in the decision process, evidence is integrated over time to one of two decision thresholds corresponding to the two choices (see Fig. 8.2B for an illustration). The rate of accumulation is called drift rate, and it is determined by the quality of the sensory information. The better the information quality, the larger the drift rate toward the appropriate decision boundary and the faster and more accurate the response. Moreover, trial-to-trial variability in the accumulation of information could result in processes with the same mean drift rate but terminate at different times (producing different response times) and sometimes at different boundaries (producing errors).

As it turns out there are indeed brain regions in which the neural activity matches predictions made by the model. One such region, which appears to be critically involved in the direction discrimination task, is localized in the lateral wall of the intraparietal sulcus (IPS) and is commonly referred to as lateral intraparietal (LIP) area. LIP was originally shown to be involved in linking sensory and motor processing stages. Furthermore its activity is predictive of the time and direction of a monkey's saccadic eye movements [32–34]. As monkeys are typically trained to indicate their choice by making an eye movement (saccade) towards a target on the side of the perceived direction of motion, this area was studied further for its potential role in decision making.

Single-unit recordings in LIP [34–37] have shown that, for saccades made towards the response field of the neuron under consideration, neural activity increased in a ramp-like fashion, consistent with an accumulator process. The rate at which responses increased was proportional to the amount of coherent motion in the stimulus. This build-up of activity may represent the accumulated difference in firing rates of two opposed pools of direction selective MT neurons. This difference is thought to approximate the logarithm of the likelihood ratio (logLR) in favor of one alternative over another [1,38,39]. More important, by the time the monkey was committed to a particular eye movement response, neural responses in LIP achieved a common value regardless of motion strength, consistent with the idea of a decision boundary that is common to both easy and difficult choices. More recently, these results were extended from a two- to a four-choice direction discrimination task [40]. This pattern of activity was also reported in the frontal eye fields (FEF) and the dorsolateral prefrontal cortex (DLPFC) [41] and is regarded as evidence that all of these areas are involved in the conversion of an analog motion representation into a binary decision variable.

Correspondingly, for the vibrotactile frequency discrimination experiments, regions in the secondary somatosensory (S2), medial premotor cortex (MPC), ventral premotor cortex (VPC), and in the DLPFC were reported as being involved in decision formation [42–45]. As with the motion experiments, responses in these regions are likely to reflect a comparison between the two frequencies under consideration. Similarly to the LIP, responses the MPC and VPC were also shown to form a decision by computing the difference between the activities of neurons in S2 that code for each of the frequencies used for stimulation [44,45]. In addition, neurons in S2 itself responded as a function of both the first (remembered) and second (current) stimulus and their activity was correlated with the monkeys' decisions shortly after both frequencies were presented. This suggested that at least some S2 neurons may combine past and present sensory information to form a decision [43]. Finally, time-dependent persistent activity in the DLPFC during the delay period between the two stimuli, correlated with the monkeys' behavior, suggesting an active role of short-term memory representation in decision making [42,46].

8.3 Perceptual decision making in humans

In this section we review human neuroimaging evidence showing that the principles that have emerged from the neurophysiology work in monkeys also hold for the human brain.

8.3.1   fMRI studies on perceptual decision making

Representation of visual evidence

Heekeren and colleagues used fMRI and a face-house categorization task to investigate perceptual decision making in the visual domain [5]. Previous neuroimaging studies had identified regions in the human ventral temporal cortex that are activated more by faces than by houses, and vice versa: the fusiform face area (FFA) and the parahippocampal place area (PPA), respectively [47–51]. The face-house task can thus be used to identify two brain regions, and to test whether they represent the sensory evidence relevant for the task. There was a greater response in face-selective regions to clearer images of faces ("easy" trials) than to degraded images of faces ("difficult" trials), whereas degraded houses showed a greater response than clearer houses in these face-selective areas. The opposite pattern was found in house-selective regions, namely, a greater response to clearer images of houses ("easy" trials) than to degraded images of houses ("difficult" trials), but a greater response to degraded than to clearer images of faces (Fig. 8.2A).

These results support the concept that face- and house-selective regions represent the sensory evidence for the two respective categories, consistent with the initial processing module of the model in Fig. 8.1A.

Representation of somatosensory evidence

Inspired by the work of Romo and colleagues, recent fMRI studies have used vibrotactile frequency tasks to study somatosensory decision making in the human brain. In this task, individuals had to decide which of two successive vibratory stimuli had a higher frequency. Consistent with neurophysiological data in monkeys, the primary somatosensory cortex exhibited increased activity during the encoding phase (processing of the first stimulus) in tactile decision making [52]. Similarly, using a somatosensory discrimination task, in which participants had to compare the frequency of two successive electrical tactile stimuli, Pleger and associates found that tactile stimuli *per se* evoked activity in, among other regions, somatosensory cortex [7].

The most direct evidence in support of the concept of representation of sensory evidence in the somatosensory domain comes from a transcranial magnetic stimulation (TMS) study which showed that stimulation of primary somatosensory cortex lowered two-point discrimination thresholds of the right index finger and enlarged its neural representation as assessed with fMRI [53]. Notably, this enlargement correlated with the individual TMS-induced perceptual improvement. Taken together, the results of the studies described above provide support for the idea that, similar to the findings in monkeys, primary somatosensory cortex represents the sensory evidence during tactile decision making. Next, we review recent human neuroimaging studies that provide evidence for a comparison of accumulated sensory evidence as a mechanism for perceptual decision making.

Integration of sensory evidence and formation of the decision variable

The single-unit recording studies in monkeys have shown that neuronal activity in areas involved in decision making gradually increases and then remains elevated until a response is made. Importantly, the rate of increase in neural activity is slower during more difficult trials than during easier trials. Furthermore, these studies have shown that downstream cortical regions (i.e., further along the processing chain), such as LIP and the DLPFC, could form a decision by comparing the output of pools of selectively tuned sensory neurons.

A recent fMRI study showed how the BOLD signal can be used to examine the process of accumulation of sensory evidence [8]. Pictures were revealed gradually over the course of 12–20 s and participants signaled the time of recognition with a button press. In several occipital regions, the fMRI signal increased primarily as stimulus information increased, suggesting a role in lower-level sensory processing. There was a gradual build-up in fMRI signal peaking in correspondence with the time of recognition in inferior temporal, frontal, and parietal regions, suggesting that these regions accumulate sensory evidence.

Heekeren and colleagues directly tested whether a comparison operation is also at work in the human brain using the face-house discrimination task described previously [5]. Specifically, based on the neurophysiological data in monkeys, Heekeren proposed that higher-level decision areas should fulfill two criteria. First, they should show the greatest BOLD activity on trials in which the weight of evidence for a given perceptual category is greatest, namely, a higher fMRI signal during decisions about clear images of faces and houses ("easy trials") than during decisions about degraded images of these stimuli ("hard trials"). Second, their BOLD signals should correlate with the difference between the signals in brain areas selectively tuned to the different categories involved; that is, those in face- and house-responsive regions.

Only one brain region fulfilled both criteria [5]: the posterior portion of the left DLPFC uniquely responded more to clear relative to degraded stimuli, and the activity of this region correlated with the difference between the output signals of face- and house-responsive regions (Fig. 8.2B).

Thus, when people make categorical decisions about face and house stimuli, this brain region appears to integrate the outputs from lower-level sensory regions and use a subtraction operation to compute perceptual decisions. Notably, activity in the left DLPFC also predicted behavioral performance in the categorization task [5]. Hence, even for complex object categories, the comparison of the outputs of different pools of selectively tuned neurons appears to be a general mechanism by which the human brain computes perceptual decisions.

Uncertainty, attention, and task difficulty

The human neuroimaging studies reviewed so far have used single-unit recording findings as a constraint to predict decision-related changes in fMRI signals [35]. Specifically, neuronal activity in areas involved in decision making gradually increases with increasing sensory evidence and then remains elevated until a response is made, with a greater rate of increase during easier trials than during more difficult trials. This leads to the prediction of an enhanced fMRI response during easy relative to hard trials in decision-making areas.

Other investigators took a different approach to the identification of regions involved in perceptual decision making: they characterized decision-making regions on the basis of correlations of the BOLD signal with accuracy or response time (RT) [54]. This approach is based on Donders' theory that the time an individual needs to deliberate before responding to a stimulus increases with task difficulty, and thus can be used to differentiate sensory and decision processes. Therefore, in contrast to the neurophysiological work and neuroimaging studies reviewed previously, these investigators have reasoned that BOLD activity in decision-related regions should be correlated with RT; namely, they should show a greater response during difficult trials than during easy trials.

Binder and associates manipulated difficulty so as to affect both accuracy and RT in a phonetic discrimination task [54]. As task difficulty decreased, accuracy increased sigmoidally from chance performance to nearly perfect with easy trials. In contrast, RT was biphasic, with shorter RTs for very easy items and very hard items, and longer RTs for items of intermediate difficulty. These authors found that BOLD activity in regions just adjacent to primary auditory cortex correlated with accuracy, whereas BOLD activity in the anterior insula and the inferior frontal gyrus positively correlated with RT. These data were interpreted to support a sensory processing role (auditory identification) for the areas where BOLD signal correlated with accuracy and a decision-related role for areas where BOLD signal correlated with RT.

A related goal of some investigators has been to eliminate differences between trials in terms of stimulus evidence and thereby reduce the overall influence of either attention or task difficulty on the fluctuations in BOLD signal, which characterize decision-making regions. For instance, Thielscher and Pessoa [55] asked study participants to decide whether a given face expressed fear or disgust. They focused their analysis on trials where there was no facial expression visible in the stimuli (i.e., neutral faces) and therefore no trial-to-trial difference in the amount of sensory evidence [55]. Similar to Binder and colleagues [54], they postulated that decision-related regions should show a positive correlation between RT and fMRI signal amplitude. They too found that BOLD activity was positively correlated with RT in the inferior frontal gyrus/anterior insula, as well as in the anterior cingulate cortex (ACC).

A related strategy was adopted by Grinband and associates [56] who manipulated perceptual uncertainty independently of stimulus evidence. They asked individuals to classify a line segment as being either long or short, based on a learned, abstract categorical boundary. They reported regions in a fronto-striatal-thalamic network, including a large region of the medial frontal gyrus, whose activity increased with perceptual uncertainty independent of stimulus evidence, and suggested that these regions may be involved in comparing a stimulus to a categorical boundary.

All of the studies cited here [54–56] as well as [8] have associated the medial frontal gyrus and the inferior frontal gyrus/anterior insula with perceptual decision-making, based on the finding of a greater response during difficult than easy trials. Heekeren et al. have found a similar response pattern in these regions [5,6]. However, they have suggested that their role in perceptual decision making is to bring to bear additional attentional resources to maintain accuracy in decision making when the task becomes more difficult. Their interpretation is congruent with the attentional control module illustrated in Fig. 8.1A. Recent studies by Philiastides and colleagues [10,14] may provide a resolution for these different conceptualizations (see following).

The role of the motor system

Neurophysiological studies in monkeys as well as modeling studies suggest that the brain regions involved in selecting and planning a certain action play an important role in forming decisions that lead to that action. To test whether this result also holds for the human brain, Heekeren et al. [57] asked human observers to make direction-of-motion judgments about dynamic random-dot motion stimuli and to indicate their judgment with an eye movement to one of two visual targets. In each individual, the authors localized regions that are part of the oculomotor network, namely, the FEF and an eye-movement related region in the IPS, presumably corresponding to area LIP of monkeys [58]. Importantly, during the period of decision formation, between the onset of visual motion and the cue to respond, the percent BOLD change in both the FEF and IPS was highly correlated with the strength of the motion signal in the stimuli [57]. These data are thus consistent with the single-unit studies in monkeys reporting that FEF and LIP participate in the process of forming a perceptual decision.

The results are also similar to a study of oculomotor decision making by Heinen and colleagues [59] who had participants play "ocular baseball" while undergoing fMRI. In this game, the subjects had to indicate whether they thought a dot moving across a computer screen would cross into a visible strike zone or not. Subjects scored a point when they correctly predicted a "strike," so that their eye movements pursued a dot that eventually crossed into the strike zone. Subjects also scored a point on trials when they correctly predicted a "ball" and withheld an eye movement (e.g., remained fixated) when the dot missed the strike zone. When the results of a task with identical motor behavior were compared to the "baseball" trials, decision-related signals were found in the superior parietal lobule, FEF, and ventrolateral prefrontal cortex. In line with the monkey data, these results suggest that, when a decision is associated with a specific movement, formation of the decision and preparation of the behavioral response share a common neural substrate. Put more generally, the findings support the view that the human motor system also plays an important role in perceptual decision making (cf. Green and Heekeren, forthcoming).

More recently, Heekeren et al. have investigated whether decisions may be transformed into motor actions in the human brain independent of motor planning and execution – that is, at an abstract level [6]. Individuals performed the direction-of-motion discrimination task and responded either with button presses or saccadic eye movements. Areas that represent decision variables at a more abstract level should show a greater response to high coherence (easy) relative to low coherence (difficult) trials, independent of the motor system that is used to express the decision. Heekeren and associates found four such areas: left posterior DLPFC, left posterior cingulate cortex, left IPS, and left fusiform/parahippocampal gyrus. Most important, the increase in BOLD activity in these regions was independent of the motor system the participants used to express their decision. The results from this fMRI study are in line with the finding by Kim and Shadlen in monkeys that neural activity increases proportionally to the strength of the motion signal in the stimulus [41]. However, the findings in humans suggest that the posterior DLPFC is an important component of a network that not only accumulates sensory evidence to compute a decision but also translates this evidence into an action independent of response modality.

Notably to date, neurophysiological studies in monkeys have not found neurons whose activity reflects decisions independently of response modality. In fact, one could conclude from the neurophysiological studies in monkeys that "to see and decide is, in effect, to plan a motor-response" [60]. In contrast, in humans, Heekeren et al. found regions of the cortex that responded independently of the motor effectors used [6]. Based on these findings, one could speculate that humans may have evolved a more abstract decision-making network, thereby allowing a more flexible link between decision and action.

Performance and error monitoring

Neuroimaging studies have corroborated neurophysiological findings in monkeys in showing that the posterior medial prefrontal cortex (also referred to as ACC), plays an important role in performance monitoring, error monitoring, and signaling the need for adjustments of behavior [12,61] (see also [62]). An intriguing possibility is that these monitoring systems may selectively adjust the sensitivity in sensory brain regions rather than changing decision criteria. Evidence for this comes from a recent fMRI study, which showed that monitoring mechanisms enhance performance by transiently amplifying cortical responses to task-relevant information. In that study, Egner and Hirsch monitored fMRI activity in the FFA while participants performed a task in which face information was sometimes relevant and sometimes irrelevant [63]. Brain activity during trials that followed incongruent trials (where the face information was a possible confound with the non-face information) was compared with activity during trials that followed congruent trials. Egner and Hirsch found that the BOLD-response in the FFA was significantly increased by task relevance. This study also showed that amplification of FFA activity was mediated by the DLPFC, as the level of interaction between DLPFC and FFA was greater during the high FFA activity trials immediately following incongruent trials. Thus, this study shows how the performance-monitoring system and the system that represents sensory evidence interact during perceptual decision making as highlighted in Fig. 8.1A.

8.3.2   EEG/MEG studies on perceptual decision making

Even though fMRI provides millimeter spatial resolution, due to slow scanning rates and the low-pass nature of the BOLD response, its temporal resolution is rather limited. To overcome this limitation advanced methods that use EEG and MEG measurements have been developed to study the temporal characteristics of perceptual decision making in humans.

Single-trial EEG reveals temporal characteristics of decision making

Traditionally, the analysis of EEG has relied on averaging event-locked data across hundreds of trials as well as across subjects, to uncover the neural signatures of the neurocognitive process under investigation. The underlying assumption of this approach is that trial averaging increases signal-to-noise ratio (SNR) by minimizing the background EEG activity relative to the neural activity correlated with experimental events. While this assumption is generally valid, it also carries a major detriment; it conceals inter-trial and inter-subject response variability which may carry important information regarding the underlying neural processes. In contrast, single-trial methods usually exploit the large number of sensor arrays by spatially integrating information across the scalp to identify EEG components that optimally discriminate between experimental conditions. Spatial integration enhances the signal quality without loss of temporal precision common to trial averaging. The resulting discriminating components describe the spatial extent but, more important, the temporal evolution of the underlying cortical activity.

Methods that have been used for such analysis include independent component analysis (ICA) [64–66], common spatial patterns (CSP) [67,68], support vector machines (SVM) [69,70], and linear discrimination (LD) based on logistic regression [71,72]. LD in particular can be used to compute a set of spatial weights, which maximally discriminate between experimental conditions over several different temporal windows, thus allowing the monitoring of the temporal evolution of discriminating activity. Unlike CSP, which tries to identify orientations in sensor space that maximize power, LD tries to maximize discrimination between two classes. Also unlike ICA, which is designed to minimize the correlation between spatial components (i.e., make spatial components as independent as possible [73]), LD is used to identify components that maximize the correlation with relevant experimental events. All of these techniques linearly transform the original EEG signal via the following transformation:

$$\mathbf{Y} = \mathbf{WX}, \tag{8.1}$$

where $\mathbf{X}$ is the original data matrix, $\mathbf{W}$ is the transformation matrix (or vector) calculated using the different techniques, and $\mathbf{Y}$ is the resulting source matrix (or vector). Figure 8.3 illustrates how the technique can be used for a binary discrimination.

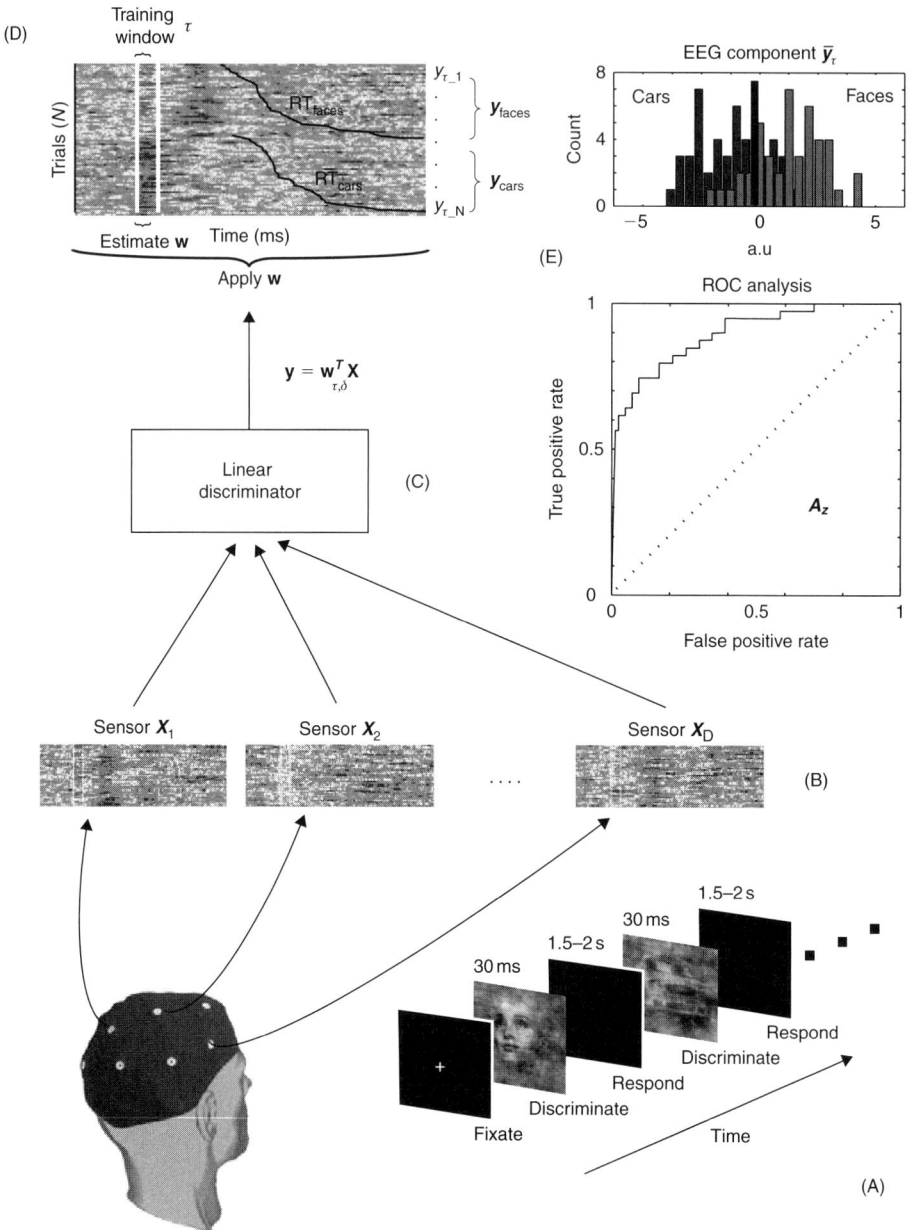

Figure 8.3 Summary of the single-trial EEG linear discrimination approach. (A) Subjects are discriminating between two classes of images while EEG is simultaneously recorded from D sensors. (B) EEG trials are locked to stimulus onset and a time window is defined with a latency, τ, relative to the stimulus and a width, δ (typically 50 ms wide). (C) EEG data from each sensor ($X_1 \to {}_D$) and each window are used to train a linear classifier (i.e., estimate spatial filters $\mathbf{w}_{\tau,\delta}$), to discriminate labeled trials (here, faces versus cars). (D) The linear classifier, through application of $\mathbf{w}_{\tau,\delta}$ on the

One of the first studies to use single-trial analysis of the EEG to explore the temporal characteristics of perceptual decision making in humans and to precisely quantify the relationship between neural activity and behavioral output was that of Philiastides et al. [9]. Motivated from the early work of Newsome and colleagues in primates [15,18], these authors reported the first non-invasive neural measurements of perceptual decision making in humans, which lead to neurometric functions predictive of psychophysical performance on a face versus car categorization task (Fig. 8.3A).

Similar to Heekeren and colleagues [5], Philiastides et al. manipulated the difficulty of the task by changing the spatial phase coherence of the stimuli in a range that spanned psychophysical threshold. Carrying out the LD approach (as outlined in Fig. 8.3) at different time windows and coherence levels revealed two EEG components that discriminated maximally between faces and cars as seen in Fig. 8.4A for one subject.

The early component was consistent with the well-known face-selective N170 [74–78] and its temporal onset appeared to be unaffected by task difficulty. The late component, appeared on average around 300 ms post-stimulus at the easiest condition, and it systematically shifted later in time and became more persistent as a function of task difficulty. Both of these components were sensitive to decision accuracy in that a high positive and a high negative discriminator output value ($\bar{y}_{\tau\_i}$, see Fig. 8.3B–D for details) indicated an easy face and car trial, respectively, whereas values near zero indicated more difficult decisions.

To directly compare the neuronal performance at these two times to the psychophysical sensitivity as captured by each subject's psychometric function, the authors constructed neurometric functions for each of the two components. Analogous to Britten et al. [15], receiver operating characteristic (ROC) analysis was used to quantify the discriminator's performance at each coherence level. The neurometric functions were then obtained by plotting the area under each of the ROC curves (i.e. A_z values, see Fig. 8.3E) against the corresponding coherence level. Neurometric functions from the late component were a better match to the psychophysical data than those from the early component (Fig. 8.4B). A third neurometric function, which was obtained by training a linear discriminator while integrating data across both time windows, was found to be an excellent predictor of overall behavioral performance. Finally, choice probability analysis [18] revealed that the late component also predicted the subjects' actual choices more reliably than the early one, indicating that this component reflects the content of the final decision.

Figure 8.3 (*Continued*)

D sensors, collapses the *D*–dimensional EEG space into a 1–dimensional discriminating component space **y**. Compared to individual sensors this 1–dimensional projection is considered a better estimator of the underlying neural activity, as it usually carries a higher SNR and reduces interference from other sources. To visualize the profile of the discriminating component across trials (indexed by $i = 1 \rightarrow N$), the classifier, trained only on EEG within each of the selected windows, is applied across all time points to construct the component map seen here. Trials of class 1 (i.e., faces) are mapped to positive **y**–values (red), whereas those of class 2 (i.e., cars) to negative ones (blue). In this example the sigmoidal curves represent the subject's reaction time profile for each of the two image classes. (E) The discriminating components are validated using a ROC analysis based on a leave-one-out procedure. Specifically, left-out single-trial discriminating components, averaged within the training window (i.e., $\bar{y}_{\tau\_i}$), are used to generate discriminator output distributions for each of the two classes. The area under the ROC curve, also known as an A_z value, is used to quantify the degree of separation between the two distributions and can be used to establish a relationship between behavioral and neuronal responses as in [15,144]. See Plate 8 of Color Plate section.

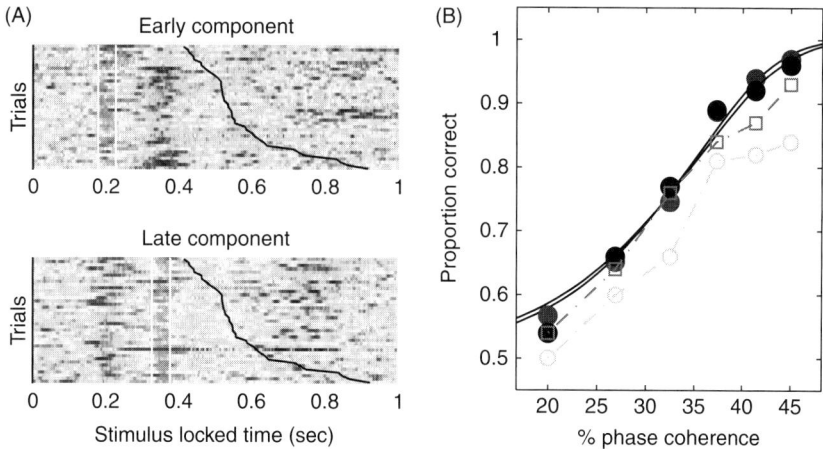

Figure 8.4 Single-trial EEG components correlate with decision accuracy on a face versus car discrimination task. (A) Discriminant component maps for the early ($\approx$170 ms) and late ($\approx$300 ms) decision accuracy components identified by [9]. All trials are aligned to the onset of visual stimulation (time 0 ms) and sorted by RT (black sigmoidal curves). Unlike the discriminant component maps in Fig. 8.3 only half the trials are represented here. Specifically, each row of these maps represents the output of the linear discriminator for a single face trial with the mean of all car trials subtracted (i.e., $\mathbf{y}_{face\_i} - \overline{\mathbf{y}}_{cars}$). (B) Comparison of one subject's psychometric function (gray solid line) with neurometric functions obtained from the early component (light-gray dotted line), the late component (dark-gray dotted line), and a combination of the two (black solid line). Note that integrating data across both time windows helped produce a neurometric function that was statistically indistinguishable from its corresponding psychometric curve. In addition, the neurometric function from the late component alone was a better match to the psychophysical data than that of the early one. See Plate 9 of Color Plate section.

Situated somewhere between the early and late components, around 220 ms post-stimulus, there was yet a third component the strength of which systematically increased with increasing task demands. This decision difficulty component was a good predictor of the onset time of the late decision accuracy component. Philiastides and colleagues speculated that this component reflects a top-down influence of attention on decision making rather than a mere bottom-up processing of the stimulus evidence. To substantiate this claim they used a variant of the original behavioral paradigm where the same stimuli were colored red or green, and the subjects were either cued to perform a color discrimination or the original face categorization task [10]. While leaving the stimulus evidence unchanged, they compared the amplitude of the difficulty component during a challenging face discrimination with that of a trivial color discrimination. They found that the difficulty component was significantly reduced when the subjects were merely discriminating the color of the stimulus. As the images were identical in the two tasks, these results ruled out the possibility that this component simply reflects the early processing of the stimulus.

Additionally, this new version of the experiment has produced further evidence on the role of the early and late components. The authors found that the early component remained unaffected by task demands, in that for the color discrimination the response of this component to face versus car stimuli was unchanged. In contrast, the response of the late component was largely eliminated when subjects were making a color decision. Finally, the response of the late component was correlated with mean drift rate in a diffusion model simulation [10, 144]. This was the first study to link human brain signals with parameters of the diffusion model, suggesting that the late EEG component reflects the post-sensory evidence that is fed into the diffusion process, which ultimately determines the decision.

These results taken together suggest that the different EEG components can be thought of as representing distinct cognitive events during perceptual decision making. Specifically, the early component appears to reflect the stimulus quality independent of the task (face/car or color discrimination) and is likely to provide the early sensory evidence, consistent with the first processing stage in the four-compartment model of perceptual decision making presented in Fig. 8.1.A. In contrast, the late component better represents information in the actual face/car decision process as it was shown to be a good predictor of overall behavioral performance during face categorization (Fig. 8.4B) while its responses to the color discrimination were virtually diminished. Consistent with a top-down attentional control system (Fig. 8.1.A, the difficulty component appears to be implicated in the recruitment of the relevant attentional and other neuronal resources required to make a difficult decision. It further predicts the onset time of the late component, which is consistent with the idea that as the brain is engaging additional resources a delay in the next processing module (e.g., late component) is observed.

The role of synchronized activity in perceptual decision making

EEG and MEG signals are thought to arise primarily from oscillatory components in the brain [79]. This oscillatory activity often exhibits power changes in response to different experimental events. Moreover, these changes are not necessarily phase-locked to the events that caused them and they would therefore tend to cancel out in the average evoked potentials [80]. Time-frequency decomposition of EEG/MEG data has recently gained much popularity as it can ultimately capture these changes when applied on single-trial data prior to averaging.

A time-frequency representation (TFR) describes the variation of the spectral energy of the signal over time and is a valuable tool for interpreting non-stationary signals. There are many approaches to obtain a TFR, however for the analysis of neural data the two most commonly used methods are wavelets [81] and multitapers [82,83]. Wavelet decomposition involves convolving the data with a basis function (usually a Morlet wavelet). Wavelets have a length that scales inversely with frequency such that the time-frequency product remains unchanged. This means that for higher frequencies the temporal resolution increases in the expense of frequency resolution (i.e., time-frequency resolution trade-off). In contrast, multitapers are based on a windowed Fourier transform where a set of Slepian windows or discrete prolate spheroidal sequences (DPSS) are chosen so that power bleeding into neighboring frequencies is minimized. Unlike wavelets the temporal and frequency specificity of multitapers does not scale with frequency. Wavelets can be quite sensitive to low-amplitude signals, whereas multitapers have a high degree of frequency specificity and are better suited for detecting high-amplitude transients [84].

A recent MEG study using time-frequency analysis techniques based on multitapers [85] has shown that during the same motion discrimination task used in monkey experiments neural activity in the high gamma range, namely 60–100 Hz, was monotonically increasing with respect to the strength (i.e., coherence) of the visual motion. The analysis was restricted to the early stages of visual presentation to ensure that only those regions involved in encoding the intensity of the physical stimulus were represented. Using "beam forming" source reconstruction techniques [86,87], the authors were able to attribute the strongest gamma-band modulation to several motion-responsive regions in occipitoparietal and occipitotemporal cortex. Of particular interest was the prevalence of such modulation in area V5/MT + , which is thought to represent the human-homologue of monkey MT. These findings are seminal in that they begin to bridge the gap between monkey electrophysiology and human neuroimaging. They also provide support that motion-selective regions, such as MT + , represent the sensory evidence (Fig. 8.1A) upon which human observers base their decisions regarding direction discrimination.

In a separate study, Donner et al. [11] have also used multitaper-based TFR of MEG data to explore the neural correlates of perceptual decision making in humans. They used a visual motion detection task where subjects reported whether a small amount of coherent motion was present or not (yes/no paradigm) in a conventional random-dot kinetogram. The TFR approach revealed an induced steady-state response, reflective of non-phase locked fluctuations of ongoing oscillatory activity, in response to the stimulus. This activity was sustained for the entire period that the dynamic random dot patterns remained on the screen.

The authors then tested whether this activity covaried with behavioral performance. They found MEG activity in the beta band (12–24 Hz) to be larger before correct than error trials. Similar to [9,18] they used signal detection theory, namely ROC analysis (on correct versus error choices), to quantify the association between neural data and behavioral choices. They showed that data from the 12–24 Hz range could predict behavioral choices on a single-trial basis. A closer look at the time course of this beta band activity revealed a gradual build-up in the difference signal between correct and error choices consistent with accumulator models [29,38]. Finally, activity in this frequency band was also shown to reflect the accuracy of the decision, rather than the content (i.e., yes or no), by virtue of the fact that it was higher before "correct rejects" than before "false alarms" in the physical absence of the motion target. Taken together, these results clearly implicate the source of this oscillatory activity in the actual decision-making process (Fig. 1A). A source reconstruction based on "beam formers" [86,87] identified the posterior IPS (pIPS) and DLPFC as potential sources.

The findings from the fMRI, EEG, and MEG studies presented in this section provide converging insights into the neural basis of perceptual decision making in humans as outlined in the model of Fig. 8.1A. At the same time they emphasize the importance of combining these imaging modalities to infer the spatiotemporal profile of the interactions between the different processing modules of this model. In the next section we present a new approach on how to best integrate single-trial EEG with fMRI to decipher the spatiotemporal characteristics of perceptual decision making.

8.4   Spatiotemporal characterization of decision making by integrating EEG with fMRI

Simultaneous EEG/fMRI measurements can potentially enable the fusion of EEG and fMRI in a manner that circumvents the disparate space and time scales on which the two datasets are acquired. Animal experiments have already demonstrated that hemodynamic signals are more closely coupled to synaptic than spiking activity and that changes in the fMRI BOLD signal can correlate tightly with synchronized oscillatory activity recorded from local field potentials (LFPs) [88–91]. Under these premises, it is reasonable to

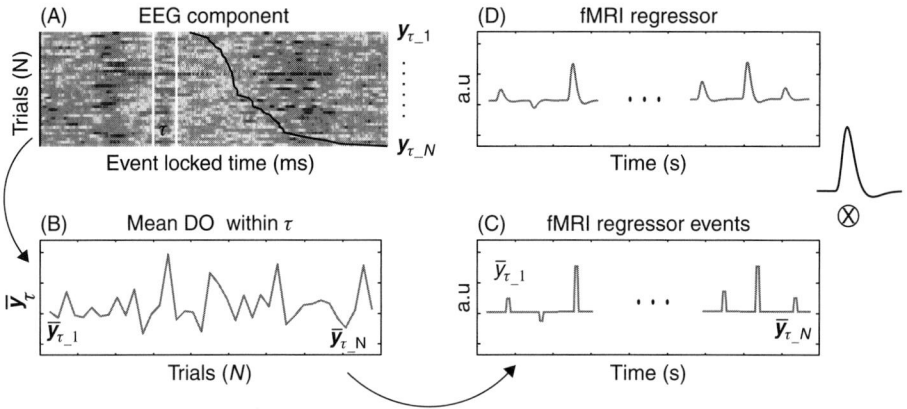

Figure 8.5 Graphical representation of how single-trial EEG can be used to construct fMRI regressors. The discriminator output (DO) can be used to derive as many fMRI regressors as there are temporally distinct EEG components. The onset time and duration of each of the regressor events are determined by the onset time (τ) and duration (δ) of the EEG components as identified by the single-trial EEG analysis (as in Fig. 8.3). More important, the amplitude of each regressor event will be based on the output of the linear discriminator $\mathbf{y}_\tau$ as defined in Eq. 8.2. See Plate 10 of Color Plate section.

assume that neural activity reflected in the EEG could also correlate well with the underlying BOLD hemodynamic response. In that case, constructing EEG-derived fMRI regressors based on pre-defined, highly discriminating EEG components could yield the desired high spatiotemporal information needed to describe the neural correlates of perceptual decision making, as well as other neurocognitive processes, non-invasively in humans.

One way to construct EEG-derived fMRI activation maps that will depend on task and subject specific electrophysiological source variability is to take advantage of the single-trial discrimination approach described earlier. Specifically, the discriminator output for each trial can be used as the basis for parametrically modulating the amplitude of the different fMRI regressor events. Figure 8.5 outlines the main steps involved in this process.

Single-trial discrimination of the EEG is initially performed to identify components of interest (Fig. 8.5A). Assuming the discriminator is trained with T samples within each window (τ) of interest, the output $\mathbf{y}_\tau$ has dimensions $T \times N$, where N is the total number of trials. To achieve more robust single-trial estimates for $\mathbf{y}_\tau$, averaging across all training samples is performed:

$$\bar{\mathbf{y}}_{\tau\_i} = \frac{1}{T}\sum_{j=1}^{T}\mathbf{y}_{\tau\_ij},$$

(8.2)

where i is used to index trials and j training samples. This is shown graphically in Fig. 8.5B. $\bar{\mathbf{y}}_\tau$ is then used to modulate the amplitude of the different fMRI regressor events (Fig. 8.5C). Finally, the parametric regressor is convolved with a prototypical hemodynamic response function (Fig. 8.5D), which is used to model the fMRI data in the context of a general linear model (GLM). This process can be repeated for multiple windows/components (τ's), each resulting in a separate regressor. Identifying the brain regions that correlate with each of these regressors will enable a comprehensive characterization of the cortical network involved in the neurocognitive process under investigation.

In the absence of simultaneous EEG/fMRI measurements, however, one could still combine knowledge acquired from the single-trial EEG analysis with fMRI to achieve both high temporal and high spatial resolution information on decision making. Assuming multiple EEG components are identified *a priori* as part of a continuum of cognitive stages involved in decision making, an EEG-informed fMRI study can potentially reveal the cortical regions involved in each stage. In this case, an important requirement is that the different EEG components respond uniquely to different experimental manipulations/ conditions so that the EEG-derived regressors are independent. After all this is a requirement that every sensible fMRI experimental design should satisfy. Then averaging the discriminator output associated with each component and each experimental condition across trials can be used to modulate the amplitude of the different regressor events:

$$\bar{y}_\tau^c = \frac{1}{N}\frac{1}{T}\sum_{i=1}^{N}\sum_{j=1}^{T}\mathbf{y}_{\tau\_ij}^c, \tag{8.3}$$

where c is used to index the different experimental conditions. Also note that $\bar{y}_\tau^c$ is now a scalar – that is, all similar trials are modeled in the same way. Though the inter-trial variability will ultimately be concealed in this formulation, important information regarding the localization of each of the EEG components that would otherwise be unattainable using EEG or fMRI alone can now be achieved.

The experimental observations from the cued version of the behavioral task used in [10] were well suited for this approach. The strength of the early component was proportional to stimulus evidence and it remained unchanged between the face/car and color discriminations. The late component also responded as a function of stimulus evidence during face categorization but it was stronger across all difficulty levels relative to the early one. It was, however, virtually eliminated during the color discrimination. Unlike the early and late components, the strength of the difficulty component was proportional to the difficulty of the task. The authors repeated the same paradigm during fMRI and used their earlier EEG results to inform the analysis of the functional data. Specifically, they introduced three parametric regressors (one for each of their early, difficulty, and late components) and they used Eq. 8.3 to estimate the relative strengths of each of their components with respect to the difficulty (i.e., low [L] versus high [H] coherence) and the type of task (i.e., face versus car [FC] or red versus green [RG]) to modulate the heights of the corresponding regressor events (i.e., $\bar{y}_\tau^{FC,L}, \bar{y}_\tau^{FC,H}, \bar{y}_\tau^{RG,L}, \bar{y}_\tau^{RG,H}, \tau = \{early, difficulty, late\}$).

For the early component, they reported significant activations in areas implicated in early visual processing of objects/faces. In particular, they found bilateral activations in an area around the fusiform gyrus (FG), activations in superior temporal gyrus/sulcus (STG/STS) as well as significant activations in the cuneus (CU). In addition, an independent localizer scan was used to identify the FFA. A region of interest (ROI) analysis revealed that the signal change in this area was predominantly explained by the early component. Both the FFA and STS have previously been implicated in early visual processing of faces using neuroimaging [48,92–94] and field potentials recorded directly from the cortical surface [95–97]. The CU was also shown to be critical in early visual processing [98,99], including evidence from studies on visual extinction and spatial neglect of faces [100]. These results verify the hypothesized role of the early component in processing the incoming sensory evidence, consistent with the initial processing module of the four-compartment model introduced in this chapter.

For the difficulty component, a number of brain regions that are typically associated with the human attentional network were activated, providing support for the attentional control system shown in Fig. 8.1A. These included the supplementary and frontal eye fields (SEF/FEF), the ACC, the DLPFC, as well as the anterior insula (INS). Attention-related fluctuations were previously found in oculomotor structures such as the SEF and FEF [101–103] while microstimulation experiments in primates have revealed causal links between these areas and regions involved in early visual processing [104,105]. Though these findings have yet to be demonstrated in humans, they suggest that there might exist reciprocal interactions between the attention-related system and the early sensory evidence module, as shown in Fig. 8.1A.

The ACC has previously been shown to participate in conflict monitoring and error detection and to signal the need for greater cognitive adjustments [106–109], suggesting an active role of a performance monitoring system in decision making as highlighted in Fig. 8.1A. The DLPFC was also shown to exert attentional control by representing and maintaining the attentional demands of a task [107,110]. DLPFC was also implicated in directing efficient [111,112] and successful [113,114] working memory encoding and maintenance. The anterior INS on the other hand, is likely to participate in the integration of multimodal information as evident by its widespread projections to and from both the frontal and parietal cortices [115–117]. Taken together, these observations substantiate the authors' earlier claim regarding the presence of an attentional control system that exerts top-down influence on decision making.

Finally, activations correlating with the late component were found in the lateral occipital complex (LOC) and in the right ventrolateral prefrontal cortex (rVLPFC). Aside from its involvement in object categorization [118–122], the LOC has been implicated in "perceptual persistence" [123,124], a process in which a percept assembled by lower visual areas is allowed to remain in the visual system as a form of iconic memory [125,126]. A possible mechanism of this "persistence" involves feedback pathways in the ventral stream, which allow a visual representation to reverberate via "local" loops [125–127]. The brief stimulus durations used in these experiments suggest that perceptual persistence is a likely mechanism by which rapid object decision making is instigated. That is, for brief presentations the accumulation of evidence is not based on the decaying stimulus traces themselves but rather on a durable representation of the stimulus retained in short-term memory. This interpretation explains why the late component was a better predictor of overall behavioral performance than the early one, why it correlated with mean drift rate in a diffusion model simulation, and why it disappeared when a demanding face versus car discrimination was no longer required (e.g., during color discrimination).

The other activation that correlated with the late component was in the rVLPFC. Current evidence implicates VLPFC in decision-making tasks that involve uncertainty or risk [128]. Moreover, activity in VLPFC appears to subserve the active maintenance and retrieval of information held in short-term memory to facilitate executive processes such as active selection, comparison, and judgment of stimuli [129–131]. Hence, the pattern of activity in VLPFC appears to be in line with the perceptual persistence interpretation, also seen in LOC, as a means of driving the final decision-making stages. Figure 8.6 summarizes these findings in a form of a spatiotemporal diagram.

Note the striking similarities between this diagram and the theoretical model for perceptual decision making introduced in Fig. 8.1A, which suggest that the EEG-informed

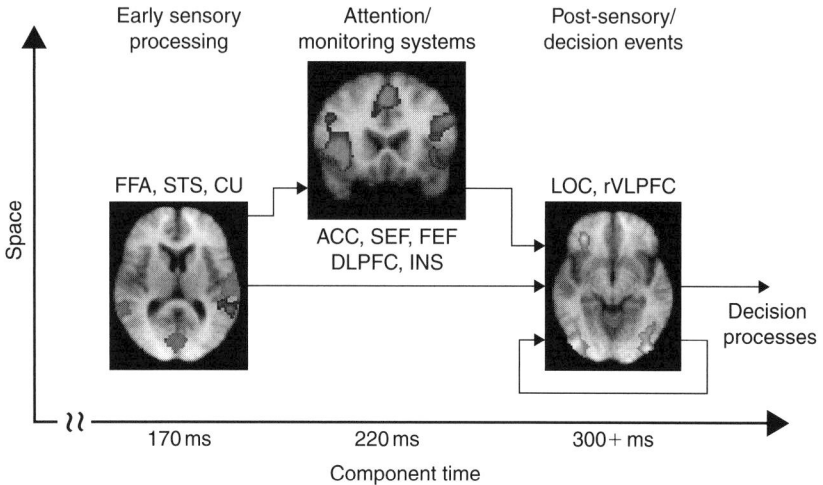

Figure 8.6 Spatiotemporal diagram of perceptual decision making during a face versus car discrimination task [14]. Using an EEG-informed fMRI analysis, Philiastides and associates identified the cortical regions correlating with each of their EEG temporally specific components, and in doing so, they demonstrated that a cascade of events associated with perceptual decision making, which included early sensory processing (early component), task difficulty and attention (difficulty component), and post-sensory/decision-related events (late component), takes place in a highly distributed neural network. The interactions between the different compartments are in part based on their experimental observations and in part based on anatomical and functional connectivity evidence from the literature. The similarities between this spatiotemporal diagram and the model introduced in Fig. 8.1.A suggest that the EEG-informed fMRI approach can enable the recovery of the spatiotemporal characteristics of different neurocognitive processes in the human brain.

fMRI approach is a promising new tool in mapping out the spatiotemporal characteristics of different neurocognitive processes in the human brain.

8.5   From perceptual to reward-based decision making

In this chapter we presented recent findings from fMRI, EEG, and MEG studies on perceptual decision making in humans. We also presented a method for integrating EEG with fMRI and we demonstrated its efficacy in achieving high spatiotemporal characterization of perceptual decision making. We now briefly present new research directions that look at other factors thought to influence perceptual decision making, such as neuromodulation, reward, and prior probability that can benefit from this new technique.

8.5.1   Neuromodulation of perceptual decision making

Although diffusion models of perceptual decision making postulate noise as a fundamental aspect of signal processing the neurobiological sources of noise and their contribution to cortical dynamics remain elusive. Patient studies, neurocognitive aging research, and genomic imaging studies indicate that the neurotransmitter dopamine (DA) modulates noise in information processing [132–136]. It will thus be important to investigate how dopaminergic neuromodulation affects perceptual decision making. The *COMT* gene for example regulates DA levels in the prefrontal cortex by affecting DA catabolism, which in turn might have an effect on the neuronal SNR in the different decision-making processing modules. Investigating how individual differences in DA-related genes modulate neural information processing will further our understanding of the neural correlates of perceptual decision making in humans.

8.5.2   Modulation of perceptual decision making by reward information

Reward-based decision making in humans, especially in the context of reinforcement learning and reward-related activity in dopaminergic systems [62,137–140], has already been studied, mostly using fMRI. Surprisingly, however, little research has been done to explore the potential effects of reward on perceptual decision making, whether on sensory function or motor planning and action selection. One hypothesis is that in situations where rewarding outcomes depend on decisions associated with different perceptual tasks, reward signals are propagated back to sensory systems, in the form of a "teaching signal," where they can shape early sensory representations to optimize reward outcome.

To date the only study that addressed this issue is by Pleger et al. [141]. They used a tactile discrimination task, in which subjects had to discriminate the relative frequency of two successive somatosensory stimuli applied to the same finger, while manipulating the reward rate received at the end of each trial. Not only did higher rewards improve behavioral performance but they also led to increased BOLD responses in the ventral striatum, a key component of the human reward system. More important, however, these authors demonstrated that during reward delivery and in the absence of somatosensory stimulation, the S1 controlateral to the judged finger was re-activated and this re-activation was proportional to the amount of reward. Finally, they showed that reward magnitude on a particular trial influenced responses on the subsequent trial, with better behavioral performance and greater controlateral S1 BOLD responses for higher rewards.

These results clearly demonstrate that the systems involved in valuation interact with early sensory systems; however, it still remains elusive how these interactions are mediated. It also remains unclear whether reward signals also interact with other modules of the four compartment model presented in Fig. 8.1A. Designing new paradigms that can benefit from the EEG-informed fMRI approach presented in this review can help provide answers to these questions.

8.5.3   Valuation-based/reward-based decision making

Often when we make decisions, the benefit of an option needs to be weighed against accompanying costs. So far, little is known about how the brain does this [142]. Notably, the only available theoretical models to date come from the literature on perceptual decision making, which has modeled binary perceptual choices as a race-to-barrier diffusion process (as reviewed in this chapter). It is, however, unclear whether this class of model also applies to value-based decision making.

References

[1] J. Gold, M. Shadlen, The neural basis of decision making, Annu. Rev. Neurosci. 30 (2007) 535–574.

[2] A. Tversky, D. Kahneman, The framing of decisions and the psychology of choice, Science 211 (1981) 453–458.

[3] I. Opris, C. Bruce, Neural circuitry of judgment and decision mechanisms, Brain Res. Rev. 48 (2005) 509–526.

[4] H. Heekeren, S. Marrett, L. Ungerleider, The neural systems that mediate human perceptual decision making, Nat. Rev. Neurosci. 9 (2008) 467–479.

[5] H. Heekeren, S. Marrett, P. Bandettini, L. Ungerleider, A general mechanism for perceptual decision-making in the human brain, Nature 431 (2004) 859–862.

[6] H. Heekeren, S. Marrett, D. Ruff, P. Bandettini, L. Ungerleider, Involvement of human left dorsolateral prefrontal cortex in perceptual decision making is independent of response modality, Proc. Natl. Acad. Sci. USA 103 (2006) 10023–10028.

[7] B. Pleger, C. Ruff, F. Blankenburg, S. Bestmann, K. Wiech, K. Stephan, A. Capilla, K. Friston, R. Dolan, Neural coding of tactile decisions in the human prefrontal cortex, J. Neurosci. 26 (2006) 12596–12601.

[8] E. Ploran, S. Nelson, K. Velanova, D. Donaldson, S. Petersen, M. Wheeler, Evidence accumulation and the moment of recognition: dissociating perceptual recognition processes using fMRI, J. Neurosci. 27 (2007) 11912–11924.

[9] M. Philiastides, P. Sajda, Temporal characterization of the neural correlates of perceptual decision making in the human brain, Cereb. Cortex 16 (2006) 509–518.

[10] M. Philiastides, R. Ratcliff, P. Sajda, Neural representation of task difficulty and decision-making during perceptual categorization: a timing diagram, J. Neurosci. 26 (2006) 8965–8975.

[11] T. Donner, M. Siegel, R. Oostenveld, P. Fries, M. Bauer, A. Engel, Population activity in the human dorsal pathway predicts the accuracy of visual motion detection, J. Neurophysiol. 98 (2007) 345–359.

[12] S. Debener, M. Ullsperger, M. Siegel, K. Fiehler, D. von Cramon, A. Engel, Trial-by-trial coupling of concurrent electroencephalogram and functional magnetic resonance imaging identifies the dynamics of performance monitoring, J. Neurosci. 25 (2005) 11730–11737.

[13] S. Debener, M. Ullsperger, M. Siegel, A. Engel, Single-trial EEG-fMRI reveals the dynamics of cognitive function, Trends Cogn. Sci. 10 (2006) 558–563.

[14] M. Philiastides, P. Sajda, EEG-informed fMRI reveals spatiotemporal characteristics of perceptual decision making, J. Neurosci. 27 (2007) 13082–13091.

[15] K. Britten, M. Shadlen, W. Newsome, J. Movshon, The analysis of visual motion: a comparison of neuronal and psychophysical performance, J. Neurosci. 12 (1992) 4745–4765.

[16] K. Britten, M. Shadlen, W. Newsome, J. Movshon, Responses of neurons in macaque MT to stochastic motion signals, Vis. Neurosci. 10 (1993) 4745–4765.

[17] M. Shadlen, W. Newsome, Motion perception: seeing and deciding, Proc. Natl. Acad. Sci. USA 93 (1996) 628–633.

[18] K. Britten, W. Newsome, M. Shadlen, S. Celebrini, J. Movshon, A relationship between behavioral choice and visual responses of neurons in macaque MT, Vis. Neurosci. 14 (1996) 87–100.

[19] C. Salzman, K. Britten, W. Newsome, Cortical microstimulation influences perceptual judgements of motion direction, Nature 346 (1990) 174–177.

[20] C. Salzman, C. Murasugi, K. Britten, W. Newsome, Microstimulation in visual area mt: effects on direction discrimination performance, J. Neurosci. 12 (1992) 2331–2355.

[21] J. Ditterich, M. Mazurek, M. Shadlen, Microstimulation of visual cortex affects the speed of perceptual decisions, Nat. Neurosci. 6 (2003) 891–898.

[22] C. Keysers, D.-K. Xiao, P. Foldiak, D. Perrett, The speed of sight, J. Cogn. Neurosci. 13 (2001) 90–101.

[23] S. Afraz, R. Kiani, H. Esteky, Microstimulation of inferotemporal cortex influences face categorization, Nature 442 (2006) 692–695.

[24] E. Salinas, A. Hernandez, A. Zainos, R. Romo, Periodicity and firing rate as candidate neural codes for the frequency of vibrotactile stimuli., J. Neurosci. 20 (2000) 5503–5515.

[25] R. Romo, A. Hernandez, A. Zainos, E. Salinas, Somatosensory discrimination based on cortical microstimulation, Nature 392 (1998) 387–390.

[26] R. Romo, A. Hernandez, A. Zainos, C. Brody, L. Lemus, Sensing without touching: psychophysical perfrormance based on cortical microstimulation, Neuron 26 (2000) 273–278.

[27] R. Ratcliff, A theory of memory retrieval, Psychol. Rev. 85 (1978) 59–108.

[28] R. Ratcliff, F. Tuerlinckx, Estimating parameters of the diffusion model: approaches to dealing with contaminant reaction times and parameters variability, Psychon. Bull. Rev. 9 (2002) 438–481.

[29] M. Mazurek, J. Roitman, J. Ditterich, M. Shadlen, A role for neural integrators in perceptual decision making, Cereb. Cortex 13 (2003) 1257–1269.

[30] R. Bogacz, Optimal decision making theories: linking neurobiology with behaviour, Trends Cogn. Sci. 11 (2007) 118–125.

[31] S. Grossberg, P. Pilly, Temporal dynamics of decision-making during motion perception in the visual cortex, Vision Res. 48 (2008) 1345–1373.

[32] J. Schall, Neural basis of saccade target selection, Rev. Neurosci. 6 (1995) 63–85.

[33] C. Colby, J. Duhamel, M. Goldberg, Visual, presaccadic, and cognitive activation of single neurons in monkey lateral intraparietal area, J. Neurophysiol. 76 (1996) 2841–2852.

[34] M. Shadlen, W. Newsome, Neural basis of perceptual decision making in the parietal cortex (area LIP) of the rhesus monkey, J. Neurophysiol. 86 (2001) 1916–1936.

[35] J. Roitman, M. Shadlen, Response of neurons in the lateral intraparietal area during a combined visual discrimination reaction time task, J. Neurosci. 22 (2002) 9475–9489.

[36] A. Huk, M. Shadlen, Neural activity in the macaque parietal cortex reflects temporal integration of visual motion signals during perceptual decision making, J. Neurosci. 25 (2005) 10420–10436.

[37] T. Hanks, J. Ditterich, M. Shadlen, Microstimulation of macaque area lip affects decision-making in a motion discrimination task, Nat. Neurosci. 9 (2006) 682–689.

[38] J. Gold, M. Shadlen, Neural computations that underlie decisions about sensory stimuli, Trends Cogn. Sci. 5 (2001) 10–16.

[39] T. Yang, M. Shadlen, Probabilistic reasoning by neurons, Nature 447 (2007) 1075–1080.

[40] A. Churchland, R. Kiani, M. Shadlen, Decision-making with multiple alternatives, Nat. Neurosci. 11 (2008) 693–702.

[41] J. Kim, M. Shadlen, Neural correlates of decision making in the dorsolateral prefrontal cortex of the macaque, Nat. Neurosci. 2 (1999) 176–185.

[42] R. Romo, C. Brody, A. Hernandez, L. Lemus, Neuronal correlates of parametric working memory in prefrontal cortex, Nature 399 (1999) 470–473.

[43] R. Romo, A. Hernandez, A. Zainos, L. Lemus, C. Brody, Neuronal correlates of decision-making in secondary somatosensory cortex, Nat. Neurosci. 5 (2002) 1217–1224.

[44] R. Romo, A. Hernandez, A. Zainos, Neuronal correlates of decisionmaking in ventral premotor cortex, Neuron 41 (2004) 165–173.

[45] A. Hernandez, A. Zainos, R. Romo, Temporal evolution of a decision-making process in medial premotor cortex, Neuron 33 (2002) 959–972.

[46] C. Brody, A. Hernandez, A. Zainos, R. Romo, Timing and neural encoding of somatosensory parametric working memory in macaque prefrontal cortex, Cereb. Cortex 13 (2003) 1196–1207.

[47] J. Haxby, The functional organization of human extrastriate cortex: a PET-rCBF study of selective attention to faces and locations, J. Neurosci. 14 (1994) 6336–6353.

[48] N. Kanwisher, J. McDermott, M. Chun, The fusiform face area: a module in human extrastriate cortex specialized for face perception, J. Neurosci. 17 (1997) 4302–4311.

[49] G. McCarthy, A. Puce, J. Gore, T. Allison, Face-specific processing in the human fusiform gyrus, J. Cogn. Neurosci. 9 (1997) 605–611.

[50] R. Epstein, N. Kanwisher, A cortical representation of the local visual environment, Nature 392 (1998) 598–601.

[51] A. Ishai, L. Ungerleider, A. Martin, J. Schouten, J. Haxby, Distributed representation of objects in the human ventral visual pathway, Proc. Natl. Acad. Sci. USA 96 (1999) 9379–9384.

[52] C. Preuschhof, H. Heekeren, B. Taskin, T. Schubert, A. Villringer, Neural correlates of vibro-tactile working memory in the human brain, J. Neurosci. 26 (2006) 13231–13239.

[53] M. Tegenthoff, P. Ragert, B. Pleger, P. Schwenkreis, A. Forster, V. Nicolas, H. Dinse, Improvement of tactile discrimination performance and enlargement of cortical somatosensory maps after 5 Hz rTMS, PLoS Biol. 3 (2005) 2031–2040.

[54] J. Binder, E. Liebenthal, E. Possing, D. Medler, B. Ward, Neural correlates of sensory and decision processes in auditory object identification, Nat. Neurosci. 7 (2004) 295–301.

[55] A. Thielscher, L. Pessoa, Neural correlates of perceptual choice and decision making during fear-disgust discrimination, J. Neurosci. 27 (2007) 2908–2917.

[56] J. Grinband, J. Hirsch, V.P. Ferrera, A neural representation of categorization uncertainty in the human brain, Neuron 49 (2006) 757–763.

[57] H. Heekeren, S. Marrett, P. Bandettini, L. Ungerleider, Human fMRI evidence for representation of a perceptual decision in oculomotor areas, in: Society for Neuroscience, 35th Annual Meeting Abst. 228.8, 2005.

[58] M. Sereno, S. Pitzalis, A. Martinez, Mapping of controlateral space in retinotopic coordinates by a parietal cortical area in humans, Science 294 (2001) 1350–1354.

[59] S. Heinen, J. Rowland, B. Lee, A. Wade, An oculomotor decision process revealed by functional magnetic resonance imaging, J. Neurosci. 26 (2006) 13515–13522.

[60] A. Rorie, W. Newsome, A general mechanism for perceptual decision-making in the human brain?, Trends Cogn. Sci. 9 (2005) 41–43.

[61] K. Ridderinkhof, M. Ullsperger, E. Crone, S. Nieuwenhuis, The role of the medial frontal cortex in cognitive control, Science 306 (2004) 443–447.

[62] M. Rushworth, T. Behrens, Choice, uncertainty and value in prefrontal and cingulate cortex, Nat. Neurosci. 11 (2008) 389–397.

[63] T. Egner, J. Hirsch, Cognitive control mechanisms resolve conflict through cortical amplification of task-relevant information, Nat. Neurosci. 8 (2005) 1784–1790.

[64] S. Makeig, M. Westrfield, T. Jung, S. Enghoff, J. Townsend, E. Courchesne, T. Sejnowski, Dynamic brain sources of visual evoked responses, Science 295 (2002) 690–694.

[65] T. Jung, S. Makeig, M. McKeown, A. Bell, T. Lee, T. Sejnowski, Imaging brain dynamics using independent component analysis, Proc. IEEE. 89 (2001) 1107–1122.

[66] J. Onton, M. Westerfield, J. Townsend, S. Makeig, Imaging human EEG dynamics using independent component analysis, Neurosci. Biobehav. Rev. 30 (2006) 802–822.

[67] C. Guger, H. Ramoser, G. Pfurtscheller, Real-time EEG analysis with subject-specific spatial patterns for a brain computer interface BCI, IEEE. Trans. Rehabil. Eng. 8 (2000) 441–446.

[68] H. Ramoser, J.M.-G.G. Pfurtscheller, Optimal spatial filtering of single trial EEG during imagined hand movement, IEEE. Trans. Rehabil. Eng. 8 (2000) 441–446.

[69] T. Lal, M. Schroder, T. Hinterberger, J. Weston, M. Bogdan, N. Birbaumer, B. Scholkopf, Support vector channel selection in BCI, IEEE. Trans. Biomed. Eng. 51 (2004) 1003–1010.

[70] M. Thulasidas, C. Guan, J. Wu, Robust classification of EEG signals for brain-computer interface, IEEE. Trans. Neural Syst. Rehabil. Eng. 14 (2006) 24–29.

[71] L. Parra, C. Alvino, A. Tang, B. Pearlmutter, N. Young, A. Osman, P. Sajda, Linear spatial integration for single-trial detection in encephalography, Neuroimage 17 (2002) 223–230.

[72] L. Parra, C. Spence, A. Gerson, P. Sajda, Recipes for the linear analysis of EEG, Neuroimage 28 (2005) 326–341.

[73] A. Hyvarinen, J. Karhunen, E. Oja, Independent Component Analysis, John Wiley and Sons, New York, 2001.

[74] D. Jeffreys, Evoked studies of face and object processing, Vis. Cogn. 3 (1996) 1–38.

[75] S. Bentin, T. Allison, A. Puce, A. Perez, G. McCarthy, Electrophysiological studies of face perception in humans, J. Cogn. Neurosci. 8 (1996) 551–565.

[76] E. Halgren, T. Raij, K. Marinkovic, V. Jousmaki, R. Hari, Cognitive response profile of the human fusiform face area as determined by MEG, Cereb. Cortex 10 (2000) 69–81.

[77] J. Liu, M. Higuchi, A. Marantz, N. Kanwisher, The selectivity of the occipitotemporal M170 for faces, Neuroreport 11 (2000) 337–341.

[78] B. Rossion, C. Joyce, G. Cottrell, M. Tarr, Early laterization and orientation tuning for face, word, and object processing in the visual cortex, Neuroimage 20 (2003) 1609–1624.

[79] P. Nunez, R. Srinivasan, Electric Fields of the Brain: The Neurophysics of EEG, Oxford University Press, New York, 2005.

[80] C. Tallon-Baudry, O. Bertrand, Oscillatory gamma activity in humans and its role in object representation, Trends Cogn. Sci. 3 (1999) 151–162.

[81] S. Schiff, A. Aldroubi, M. Unser, S. Sato, Fast wavelet transformation of eeg, Electroencephalogr. Clin. Neurophysiol. 91 (1994) 442–455.

[82] D. Thomson, Spectrum estimation and harmonic analysis, Proc. IEEE. 70 (1982) 1055–1096.

[83] P. Mitra, B. Pesaran, Analysis of dynamic brain imaging data, Biophys. J. 76 (1999) 691–708.

[84] M. van Vugt, P. Sederberg, M. Kahana, Comparison of spectral analysis methods for characterizing brain oscillations, J. Neurosci. Methods 162 (2007) 49–63.

[85] M. Siegel, T. Donner, R. Oostenveld, P. Fries, A. Engel, High-frequency activity in human visual cortex is modulated by visual motion strength, Cereb. Cortex 17 (2007) 732–741.

[86] B. Van Veen, W. van Drongelen, M. Yuchtman, A. Suzuki, Localization of brain electrical activity via linearly constrained minimum variance spatial filtering, IEEE. Trans. Biomed. Eng. 44 (1997) 867–880.

[87] J. Gross, J. Kujala, M. Hamalainen, L. Timmermann, A. Schnitzler, R. Salmelin, Dynamic imaging of coherent sources: studying neural interactions in the human brain, Proc. Natl. Acad. Sci. USA 98 (2001) 694–699.

[88] N. Logothetis, J. Pauls, M.A. Augath, T. Trinath and A. Oeltermann, Neurophysiological investigation of the basis of the fMRI signal, Nature 412 (2001) 150–157.

[89] N. Logothetis, What we can do and what we cannot do with fMRI, Nature 453 (2008) 869–878.

[90] J. Niessing, B. Ebisch, K. Schmidt, M. Niessing, W. Singer, R. Galuske, Hemodynamic signals correlate tightly with synchronized gamma oscillations, Science 309 (2005) 948–951.

[91] A. Viswanathan, R. Freeman, Neurometabolic coupling in cerebral cortex reflects synaptic more than spiking activity. neurometabolic coupling in cerebral cortex reflects synaptic more than spiking activity, Nat. Neurosci. 10 (2007) 1308–1312.

[92] A. Puce, T. Allison, S. Bentin, J. Gore, G. McCarthy, Temporal cortex activation in humans viewing eye and mouth movements, J. Neurosci. 18 (1998) 2188–2199.

[93] J. Haxby, E. Hoffman, M. Gobbini, The distributed human neural system for face perception, Trends Cogn. Sci. 4 (2000) 223–233.

[94] E. Hoffman, J. Haxby, Distinct representation of eye gaze and identity in the distributed human neural system for face perception, Nat. Neurosci. 3 (2000) 80–84.

[95] T. Allison, A. Puce, D. Spencer, G. McCarthy, Electrophysiological studies of human face perception: potentials generated in occipitotemporal cortex by face and nonface stimuli, Cereb. Cortex 9 (1999) 415–430.

[96] A. Puce, T. Allison, G. McCarthy, Electrophysiological studies of human face perception. III. effects of top-down processing on face-specific potentials, Cereb. Cortex 9 (1999) 445–458.

[97] A. Puce, T. Allison, G. McCarthy, Electrophysiological studies of human face perception. II. response properties of face specific potentials generated in occipitotemporal cortex, Cereb. Cortex 9 (1999) 431–444.

[98] J. Cohen, W. Peristein, T. Braver, L. Nystrom, D. Noll, J. Jonides, E. Smith, Temporal dynamics of brain activation during working memory task, Nature 386 (1997) 604–608.

[99] G. Ganis, W. Thompson, S. Kosslyn, Brain areas underlying visual mental imagery and visual perception: an fMRI study, Brain Res. Cogn. Brain Res. 20 (2004) 226–241.

[100] P. Vuilleumier, N. Sagiv, E. Hazeltine, R. Poldrack, D. Swick, R.D. Rafal, J. Gabrieli, Neural fate of seen and unseen faces in visuospatial neglect: a combined event-related functional MRI and event-related potential study, Proc. Natl. Acad. Sci. USA 98 (2001) 3495–3500.

[101] M. Corbetta, E. Akbudak, T. Conturo, A. Snyder, J. Ollinger, H. Drury, M. Linenweber, S. Petersen, M. Raichle, S. Petersen, M. Raichle, D. Essen, G. Shulman, A common network of functional areas for attention and eye movements, Neuron 21 (1998) 761–773.

[102] J. Schall, V. Stuphorn, J. Brown, Monitoring and control of action by the frontal lobes, Neuron 36 (2002) 309–322.

[103] T. Kelley, J. Serences, B. Giesbrecht, S. Yantis, Cortical mechanisms for shifting and holding visuospatial attention, Cereb. Cortex 18 (2008) 114–125.

[104] T. Moore, K. Armstrong, M. Fallah, Visuomotor origins of covert spatial attention, Neuron 40 (2003) 671–683.

[105] T. Moore, K. Armstrong, Selective gating of visual signals by microstimulation of frontal cortex, Nature 421 (2003) 370–373.

[106] C. Carter, T. Braver, D. Barch, M. Botvinick, D. Noll, J. Cohen, Anterior cingulate cortex, error detection, and the online monitoring of performance, Science 280 (1998) 747–749.

[107] A. MacDonald III, J. Cohen, V. Stenger, C. Carter, Dissociating the role of the dorsolateral prefrontal and anterior cingulate cortex in cognitive control, Science 288 (2000) 1835–1838.

[108] J. Kerns, J. Cohen, A. MacDonald, R. Cho, V. Stenger, C. Carter, Anterior cingulate conflict monitoring and adjustments in control, Science 303 (2004) 1023–1026.

[109] J. Brown, T. Braver, Learned predictions of error likelihood in the anterior cingulate cortex, Science 307 (2005) 1118–1121.

[110] M. Milham, M. Banich, A. Webb, V. Barad, N. Cohen, T. Wszalek, A. Kramer, The relative involvement of anterior cingulate and prefrontal cortex in attentional control depends on nature conflict, Cogn. Brain Res. 12 (2001) 467–473.

[111] D. Bor, J. Duncan, R. Wiseman, A. Owen, Encoding strategies dissociate prefrontal activity from working memory demand, Neuron 37 (2003) 361–367.

[112] P. Olesen, H. Westerberg, T. Klingberg, Increased prefrontal and parietal activity after training of working memory, Nat. Neurosci. 7 (2004) 75–79.

[113] L. Pessoa, E. Gutierrez, P. Bandettini, L. Ungerleider, Neural correlates of visual working memory: fMRI amplitude predicts task performance, Neuron 35 (2002) 975–987.

[114] K. Sakai, J. Rowe, R. Passingham, Active maintenance in prefrontal area 46 creates distractor-resistant memory, Nat. Neurosci. 5 (2002) 479–484.

[115] M. Mesulam, E. Mufson, Insula of the old world monkey. II: afferent cortical output and comments on function, J. Comp. Neurol. 212 (1982) 23–37.

[116] M. Mesulam, E. Mufson, Insula of the old world monkey. II: efferent cortical output and comments on function, J. Comp. Neurol. 212 (1982) 38–52.

[117] L. Selemon, P. Goldman-Rakic, Common cortical and subcortical targets of the dorsolateral prefrontal and posterior parietal cortices in the rhesus monkey: evidence for a distributed neural network subserving spatially guided behavior, J. Neurosci. 8 (1988) 4049–4068.

[118] T. James, G. Humphrey, J. Gati, R. Menon, M. Goodale, The effects of visual object priming on brain activation before and after recognition, Curr. Biol. 10 (2000) 1017–1024.

[119] T. James, G. Humphrey, J. Gati, R. Menon, M. Goodale, Differential effects of viewpoint on object-driven activation in dorsal and ventral streams, Neuron 35 (2002) 793–801.

[120] K. Grill-Spector, T. Kushnir, T. Hendler, R. Malach, The dynamics of object-selective activation correlate with recognition performance in humans, Nat. Neurosci. 3 (2000) 837–843.

[121] K. Grill-Spector, Z. Kourtzi, N. Kanwisher, The lateral occipital complex and its role in object recognition, Vision Res. 41 (2001) 1409–1422.

[122] K. Grill-Spector, N. Knouf, N. Kanwisher, The fusiform face area subserves face perception, not generic within-category identification, Nat. Neurosci. 7 (2004) 555–562.

[123] S. Ferber, G. Humphrey, T. Vilis, The lateral occipital complex subserves the perceptual persistence of motion-defined groupings, Cereb. Cortex 35 (2002) 793–801.

[124] M. Large, A. Aldcroft, T. Vilis, Perceptual continuity and the emergence of perceptual persistence in the ventral visual pathway, J. Neurophysiol. 93 (2005) 3453–3462.

[125] V.D. Lollo, Temporal characteristics of iconic memory, Nature 267 (1977) 241–243.

[126] M. Coltheart, The persistences of vision, Philos. Trans. R. Soc. Lond. B Biol. Sci. 290 (1980) 57–69.

[127] R. VanRullen, C. Koch, Visual selective behavior can be triggered by a feed-forward process, J. Cogn. Neurosci. 15 (2003) 209–217.

[128] S. McClure, D. Laibson, G. Loewenstein, J. Cohen, Separate neural systems value immediate and delayed monetary rewards, Science 306 (2004) 503–507.

[129] M. Petrides, The mid-ventrolateral prefrontal cortex and active mnemonic retrieval, Neurobiol. Learn. Mem. 78 (2002) 528–538.

[130] S. Prince, S. Daselaar, R. Cabeza, Neural correlates of relational memory: successful encoding and retrieval of semantic and perceptual associations, J. Neurosci. 25 (2005) 1203–1210.

[131] T. Hanakawa, M. Honda, G. Zito, M. Dimyan, M. Hallett, Brain activity during visuomotor behavior triggered by arbitrary and spatial constrained cues: an fMRI study in humans, Exp. Brain Res. 172 (2006) 275–282.

[132] G. Winterer, D. Weinberger, Genes, dopamine and cortical signal-to-noise ratio in schizophrenia, Trend Neurosci. 27 (2004) 683–690.

[133] G. Winterer, F. Musso, G. Vucurevic, P. Stoeter, A. Konrad, B. Seker, J. Gallinat, Dahmen, D. Weinberger, COMT genotype predicts BOLD signal and noise characteristics in prefrontal circuits, Neuroimage 32 (2006) 1722–1732.

[134] A. Meyer-Lindenberg, D. Weinberger, Intermediate phenotypes and genetic mechanisms of psychiatric disorders, Nat. Rev. Neurosci. 7 (2006) 818–827.

[135] T. Lotta, J. Vidgren, C. Tilgmann, I. Ulmanen, K. Melen, I. Julkunen, J. Taskinen, Kinetics of human soluble and membrane-bound catechol omethyltransferase: a revised mechanism and description of the thermolabile variant of the enzyme, Biochemistry 34 (1995) 4202–4210.

[136] S. MacDonald, L. Nyberg, L. Backman, Intra-individual variability in behavior: links to brain structure, neurotransmission and neuronal activity, Trend Neurosci. 29 (2006) 474–480.

[137] J. O'Doherty, Reward representations and reward-related learning in the human brain: insights from human neuroimaging, Curr. Opin. Neurobiol. 14 (2004) 769–776.

[138] J. O'Doherty, A. Hampton, H. Kim, Model-based fMRI and its application to reward learning and decision making, Ann. NY Acad. Sci. 1104 (2007) 35–53.

[139] N. Daw, J. O'Doherty, P. Dayan, B. Seymour, R. Dolan, Cortical substrates for exploratory decisions in humans, Nature 441 (2006) 876–879.

[140] P. Montague, B. King-Casas, J. Cohen, Imaging valuation models in human choice, Annu. Rev. Neurosci. 29 (2006) 417–448.

[141] B. Pleger, F. Blankenburg, C. Ruff, J. Driver, R. Dolan, Reward facilitates tactile judgments and modulates hemodynamic responses in human primary somatosensory cortex, J. Neurosci. 28 (2008) 8161–8168.

[142] A. Rangel, C. Camerer, P. Montague, A framework for studying the neurobiology of value-based decision making, Nat. Rev. Neurosci. (2008) 545–556.

[143] D. Green, J. Swets, Signal Detection Theory and Psychophysics, John Wiley & Sons, New York, 1966.

[144] R. Ratcliff, M.G. Philiastides and P. Sajda, Quality of evidence for perceptual decision making is indexed by trial-to-trial variability of the EEG, Proceedings of National Academy of Science (PNAS), 2009, doi:10.1073/pnas.0812580106.

9 Feedback valuation processing within the prefrontal cortex

Céline Amiez and Michael Petrides

Montreal Neurological Institute, McGill University, 3801 University Street, Montreal, Quebec H3A 2B4, Canada

Abstract

In an uncertain environment, numerous factors must be evaluated to allow the selection of the best possible response: the valence, the size, the probability, and the salience of the expected or obtained outcomes. In the present article, we review functional neuroimaging and single-neuron recording data on the role of three regions of the frontal cortex in reward-based decision processes: the anterior cingulate cortex, the orbitofrontal cortex, and the mid-dorsolateral prefrontal cortex. These data suggest that the anterior cingulate cortex has a role in the decision making process *per se*, and not simply an evaluative role, as previously thought. The orbitofrontal cortex may be necessary to monitor stimulus–feedback associations, and the mid-dorsolateral prefrontal cortex, which is critical for the monitoring of information in working memory in general, tracks the reward history in working memory of a series of actions.

Key points

1. Appropriate decision-making requires the evaluation of critical parameters (i.e. the expected value of each choice, the risk associated with each choice, the prediction error).
2. Neuroimaging studies in human and electrophysiological studies in monkey have shown the involvement of the anterior cingulate cortex, the orbitofrontal cortex, and the dorsolateral prefrontal cortex in reward-based decision-making.

9.1 Introduction

When decisions have to be made in the face of multiple complex choices, the evaluation of the potential outcome of each available option is required. Numerous parameters have to be evaluated to allow the selection of the best possible option, such as the valence, size, probability, and salience of the expected outcomes. In addition, efficient analysis of the outcomes obtained (i.e., the rewards and errors), the history of the outcomes, and evaluation of the difference between the expected and the obtained outcomes (i.e., the prediction error) are central to appropriate adjustment of subsequent behavior.

There is a long history of outstanding research in the field of experimental psychology dealing with the effect of reinforcement on behavior [1]. Learning theory aims to predict decisions on the basis of the outcome history of behavioral responses in uncertain environments [1,2]. In addition to the estimation of the immediate goal of an action, the estimation of the overall goal that must be reached at the end of a course of actions is necessary if an appropriate decision is to be made. In any learning situation, the subject initially engages in exploratory behavior in order to discover the options offered as well as their respective value. Three variables are of importance in reinforcement learning theory: the expected value of each option (i.e., the value of the outcome X the probability of obtaining it), the volatility/uncertainty associated with each choice (i.e., how risky the decision might be), and the prediction error (i.e., the discrepancy between the expected and the obtained outcome). In a probabilistic environment, the prediction error on one trial will modify the expected value on subsequent trials, which will consequently be modified also. Such a dynamic system allows the optimization of decision-making processes.

There is evidence that the prediction error is encoded by dopaminergic neurons in the ventral tegmental area (VTA) and the substantia nigra pars compacta (SNc) [3–5]. Several prefrontal cortical areas receive dopaminergic innervations [6], indicating that the prefrontal cortex receives information related to reinforcement. In addition, different dopaminergic populations project to the various prefrontal areas, suggesting distinct neural reward related inputs to the various prefrontal areas (e.g., [7,8]). Several studies have implicated the orbitofrontal cortex (OFC), the anterior cingulate cortex (ACC), and the lateral prefrontal cortex in both the monkey and the human brains in reward-based decision-making processes [9–13]. Despite the fact that progress has been made, the exact roles of these regions in decision-making remain unclear. In the present article, we review some aspects of the possible role of each one of these three frontal cortical regions, focusing on studies of single-neuron recording in monkeys and functional neuroimaging in human subjects that examined activity during the outcome expectation period and the outcome occurrence period, namely the periods during which the expected value and riskiness of the choice (outcome expectation period) and the prediction error (outcome occurrence period) are being assessed.

9.2   Anterior cingulate cortex

Many studies have implicated the ACC in decision-making and its possible role in cognitive processing in general [10,11,14]. The "anterior cingulate cortex" is used rather loosely in the research field to refer to the cortex that lies above and around the anterior part of the corpus callosum. This large region includes the agranular cingulate cortex proper (area 24), the dysgranular transitional paracingulate cortex that surrounds it (area 32) and in many studies also the subcallosal cortex (area 25) (Fig. 9.1). With regard to decision-making, single-neuron recording studies in the monkey have suggested that the ACC is involved during the exploratory period in a learning situation when the subject is discovering the environment, but not when the environment is well known [15]. The involvement of the ACC in exploratory behavior has also been shown in fMRI studies with human subjects [16].

9.2.1   Activity related to the anticipation of the outcome

The demonstration of the involvement of the ACC in the anticipation of the outcome of a decision comes from electrophysiological studies in monkeys. Matsumoto et al. [18] have

Human   Monkey

(A)

(B)

(C)

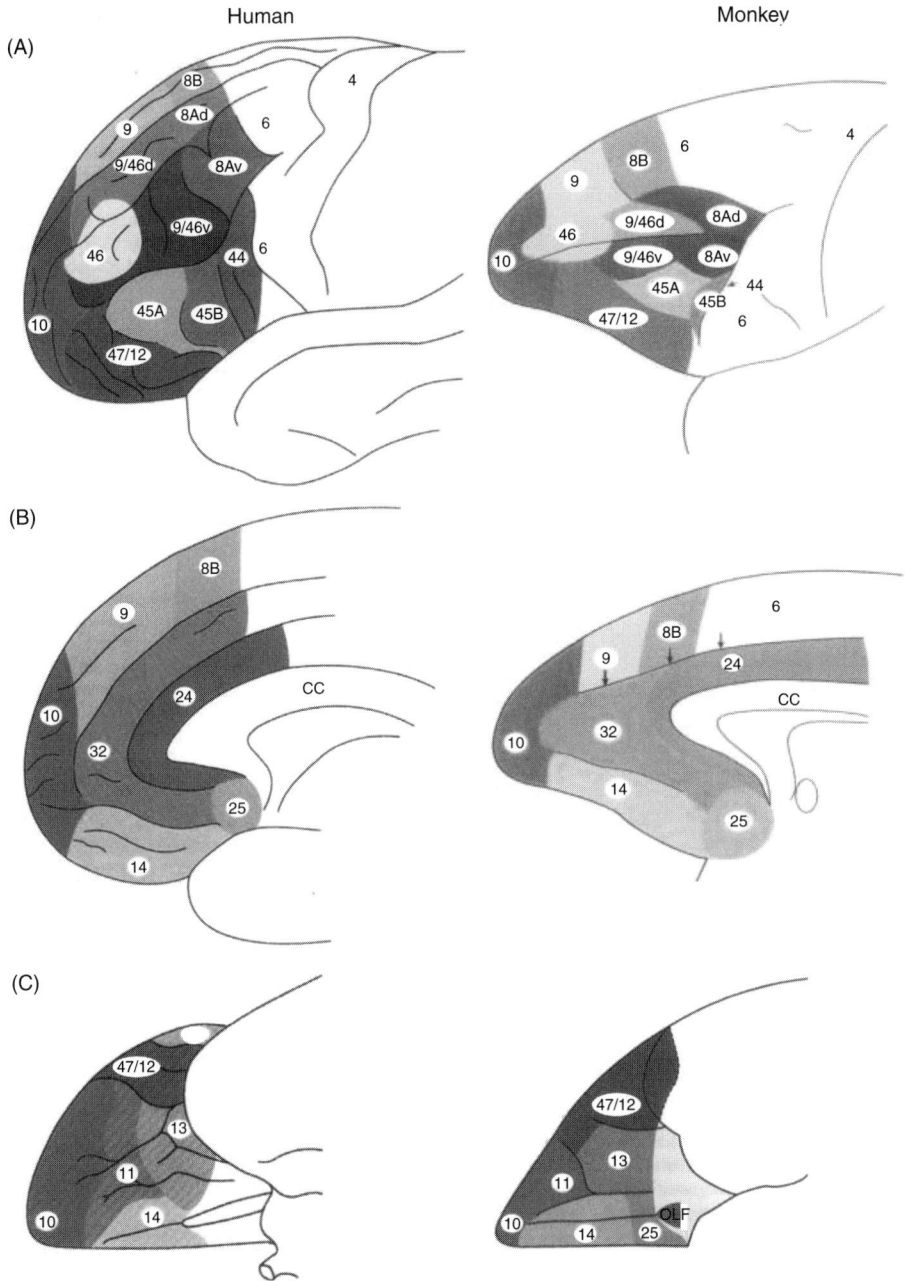

Figure 9.1 Comparative cytoarchitectonic map of the lateral (A), medial (B), and orbital (C) surfaces of the human and macaque monkey frontal cortex by Petrides and Pandya [17]. See Plate 11 of Color Plate section.

shown that the activity of ACC neurons reflected the expected reward in a GO/NO-GO task in which the monkeys could choose their responses on the basis of cues which predicted the reward. Furthermore, Matsumoto et al. [18] demonstrated that ACC neurons reflected the type of the performed action (GO or NO-GO), as well as the interaction between the action type and the expected reward. Deviations from expectation also appeared to be coded by ACC neurons, such as when the monkey is instructed that the response is going to be more or less rewarded than what is expected [19]. These results suggest that the ACC encodes the linkage between action and expected reward. In addition, Amiez et al. [20] have shown, in an electrophysiological study, that outcome anticipatory ACC activity reflects the average value of rewards associated with the monkey's choice. In the task used, the monkey had to discover which one of two presented stimuli was the most rewarded in the long run. This detection was rendered difficult because of the probabilities of the rewards associated with each stimulus: One stimulus (A) yielded 1.2 ml of fruit juice (reward) in 70% of trials and 0.4 ml in 30% of trials; the other stimulus (B) yielded 1.2 ml in 30% of trials and 0.4 ml in 70% of trials. Monkeys were able to detect the best stimulus in such a situation, and the ACC activity reflected the average value of the best choice. Together, the above results suggest that the ACC encodes the immediate and the overall goal that must be reached and that the ACC has access to the representation of the reward history. Thus, the ACC has the representations required to guide modifications in behavior on subsequent trials in the exploratory phase of a series of actions. The few fMRI studies in human subjects that have examined the involvement of the ACC during the anticipatory period have shown that it appears to encode the uncertainty of the outcome [21], the expected outcome value [22], and the subjective value of potential rewards [23].

9.2.2   Activity related to the occurrence of the outcome

Several neuroimaging and electroencephalographic studies on human subjects suggest that the ACC is involved in the detection of errors, regardless of whether the subjects are aware of these errors, as well as the detection of the errors of others [24–37]. The ACC error-related activity appears to depend on dopaminergic signals coming from the VTA and the SNc [30], where the prediction error is thought to be encoded [3–5]. Importantly, several neuroimaging studies in humans have suggested that the role of the ACC was restricted not only to error detection but also to detection of the positive or negative outcome of a response and adjusting an action [4,10,13,16,22,38,39].

   Similarly, studies in the monkey have confirmed that neuronal activity in the ACC is related not only to error detection but also to the evaluation of the current feedback to adjust behavior accordingly on subsequent trials. It has been demonstrated that ACC neurons discharge in response to both the commission of errors and the occurrence of rewards [40,41]. In addition, the magnitude of the error-related activity is known to correlate with the expected reward that the monkey would have received if the trial were correct [42]. Finally, the feedback-related activity is modulated by the difference between the expected feedback and the correctness of the response [43]. All these findings indicate that the ACC is involved in the processing of the prediction error signal.

9.3   Orbitofrontal cortex

It is widely believed that the OFC plays an important role in reward-based decision-making; this belief is based largely on results obtained from studies of human patients who suffered damage that included the OFC [44–48], as well as from studies of lesions of the OFC in monkeys [49]. For instance, subjects with lesions that include the OFC make perseverative choices of actions that are no longer rewarded or lead systematically to losses. The OFC is a large and anatomically and functionally heterogeneous region of the frontal lobe. It can be subdivided in areas 11, 12, 13, and 14 in both the monkey and the human brains (see Fig. 9.1). The caudal part of the OFC, which includes area 13, has the strongest connections with the limbic system and may be expected to play a critical role in the evaluation of the value of stimuli. In the human brain, positron emission tomography (PET) studies have indicated that the caudal OFC is involved when the stimuli presented were modified so that they differed from what the subject expected [50]. In addition, it has been shown that the OFC is involved in situations requiring readjustment of stimulus–feedback associations in visual attention tasks [51]. Such data suggest that the OFC is involved in the evaluation of novel sensory information and in assigning value to this information (for review, [52]).

9.3.1   Activity related to the anticipation of the outcome

Functional neuroimaging studies in human subjects during the performance of gambling tasks in which the outcomes were monetary gains and losses and in which the uncertainty was high have shown increased activity in the OFC in relation to the expected monetary reward value and the uncertainty of the outcome [21,39,53–57]. Comparable observations have been made in functional neuroimaging studies when the expected rewards were pleasant taste [58], food [59,60], or touch [61]. Finally, Ursu and Carter [62] have shown that the OFC is involved in the comparison between the available choices and the emotional weight associated with each choice in guiding a decision. Comparable electrophysiological studies in the monkey using tasks in which stimuli predict the upcoming reward showed that OFC neuronal activity during the presentation of the stimuli varies depending on the value of the expected reward, namely, its magnitude and the extent to which the monkey prefers the particular reward [63–73].

9.3.2   Activity related to the occurrence of the outcome

The OFC is also involved during the presentation of feedback, as demonstrated in functional neuroimaging studies in which the magnitude of its activity was modulated by the amount of the monetary reward received [21,53–56]. Similar observations have been made when the received rewards were pleasant taste [58], food [59,60], or touch [61]. In addition, Walton et al. [16] have shown in an fMRI study using a response switching task that the OFC is involved in readjusting stimulus–reward associations. These conclusions receive support from single-neuron recording studies in the monkey showing that OFC neurons discharge during the presentation of the feedback and appear to code the magnitude, the nature, and the preference for the reward [63,66–73]. Note that there is no evidence for involvement of the OFC in the coding of the feedback history, suggesting that it may not have access to a representation of the overall goal to be reached, as the ACC appears to have (see above). Finally, there is only weak evidence of coding of the prediction error in the OFC. One electrophysiological study in the monkey reported the presence of error cells in the medial part of the OFC [74], and one lesion study has shown an alteration in an error-related potential and some impairment in the ability to correct errors in a patient with a ventromedial frontal lesion [75].

9.4   Lateral prefrontal cortex

Although the dorsolateral prefrontal has not traditionally been thought to play a direct role in reward processing and has been discussed more in terms of working memory processing, several single-neuron recording studies in macaque monkeys have shown that it does have access to reward-related information and that motivational information can affect the firing of lateral frontal neurons coding various aspects of delay-related activity and response selection. For instance, it has been demonstrated that delay-related neuronal activity can be modulated by the monkey's reward expectancy [76], the magnitude of the expected rewards [77–80], and the uncertainty of the reward [81,82]. It should be noted here that observations of the modulation of cognitive-related neuronal activity in the lateral prefrontal cortex by motivational manipulations do not prove that lateral prefrontal neurons code reward *per se*. Manipulating reward expectation inevitably changes the subject's level of interest in the current trial and thus the level of attention, and it is likely that these changes in attention modulate the activity of lateral prefrontal neurons. For instance, feedback suggesting to the monkey that the reward will increase on the upcoming trial will inevitably increase the animal's level of interest and attention on that trial, and these changes in attention are reflected in the neuronal activity recorded from the dorsolateral prefrontal cortex. Several electrophysiological studies have shown that lateral prefrontal neurons discharge in relation to the delivery of the feedback [83,84] and that this feedback-related activity can be modulated by the animal's previous choices [85] and the reward history [86,87], providing some evidence that the dorsolateral frontal cortex may be involved in the monitoring the value of the choice-outcome associations.

Inspired by the animal studies, a few functional neuroimaging studies on human subjects have attempted to provide evidence of modulations of cognitive activity in the lateral frontal cortex by reward-related manipulations. A PET study examined activity in normal human subjects performing a delayed go-no go task under two different reinforcement conditions: Correct responses were rewarded with money or a simple "ok" [56]. Comparison of the monetary reward condition with the simple "ok" condition resulted in greater activity in the left hemisphere in the frontal pole (area 10), area 44 (Broca's area), and the left lateral OFC. As the investigators pointed out, these results may reflect the reward manipulation or greater arousal (attention) in the monetary reward condition. We should also point out that the activity in area 44 (Broca's area) may reflect subvocal processing of the number displayed on the screen indicating the value of the monetary reward.

Ramnani and Miall [89] showed that manual performance is enhanced when monetary rewards were provided; they used fMRI to examine activity related to action preparation and selection that was influenced by the reward. There was a significant interaction between reward and preparation in the premotor cortex, the prestriate cortex, and the frontal polar region. Pochon et al. [88] used a working memory task in an fMRI study to show that lateral frontal areas with increased activation in working memory tasks had their activity modulated by reward manipulations.

Sailer et al. [90] have shown in an fMRI study with normal human subjects that neural activation was more pronounced during feedback processing in the exploratory phase of a decision-making task (DM task) in several brain regions, including lateral prefrontal and parietal cortex and the striatum. Furthermore, the activation in these regions changed more following gains rather than losses. Similarly, Landmann et al. [91], using a motor task in which subjects had to discover by trial and error the correct sequence in which four buttons had to be pressed, showed that activity in several brain regions, including lateral prefrontal, parietal, cingulated, and striatum, were modulated, bilaterally, by reward prediction error signals.

The above studies in both the monkey and human subjects suggest that activity in the lateral frontal cortex is modulated by the expected reward value, the level of uncertainty of the reward, prediction error signals, and the subject's choice history. However, neither the monkey studies nor the studies with human subjects have as yet permitted a more precise specification of the role of any one of the many lateral frontal cortical areas in the interaction between cognitive processing and reward processing.

9.5   Dissociation of the role of OFC, ACC, and dorsolateral prefrontal cortex (DLPFC) in reward-based decision-making

Functional neuroimaging studies comparing the outcome anticipation period with the period of outcome occurrence are rare. In addition, most neuroimaging studies in human subjects assessing brain activity related to reward-based decision-making used tasks in which the decision was made on information available on the current trial only. Such protocols do not provide insight into brain activity related to the accumulation of evidence in order to make the best decision. We carried out an experiment that attempted to respond to the issues mentioned above and also to highlight differences between the mid-dorsolateral prefrontal cortex (area 46 and 9/46) and the ACC in a reward-based DM task (Amiez and Petrides, unpublished experiment). The behavioral task used in this fMRI study was adapted from a task developed by Amiez and colleagues for the monkey [20,42,92]. On each trial of this adapted reward-based DM task, the subjects were faced with two unknown stimuli and had to discover which stimulus was associated with the best financial reward in the long run. The detection of the optimal stimulus was not easy because the magnitudes of the rewards provided by both stimuli were probabilistic. In order to remove the uncertainty parameter, the amounts of the rewards and the probabilities of obtaining them were explained in detail to the subject. Normal right-handed volunteers were trained in the task during a 1-h session before the fMRI scanning.

Each trial started with the appearance of two visual abstract stimuli that were not known to the subject (question period). One of these stimuli appeared on the left side of the screen and the other on the right side, and each stimulus occupied randomly the left or right position 50% of the time. The subjects had 2 s to select one of these stimuli and indicate their selection by pressing the left or right button of a computer mouse, corresponding to the left and right positions of the stimuli. After a delay varying from 4 to 6 s, the amount of money associated with the previous choice was presented for 1 s (feedback period). An intertrial interval varying from 7 to 9 s followed. Selecting stimulus A yielded $1 with probability 0.7, and 10 cents with probability 0.3. The reinforcement ratio for stimulus B was the opposite (Fig. 9.2). The distribution of the probabilities was such that the choice of stimulus A (the most-rewarded stimulus overall) on successive trials would be the best strategy to adopt. The same two stimuli were presented during 12 successive trials. Thus, the subjects had 12 trials during which to discover the best stimulus. In this task, there was a search period during which the subjects searched for the best stimulus, and a repetition period during which they had discovered the best stimulus and generally chose it on successive trials. The subjects were asked to press a specific key of the computer mouse during the intertrial interval following the trial during which they discovered

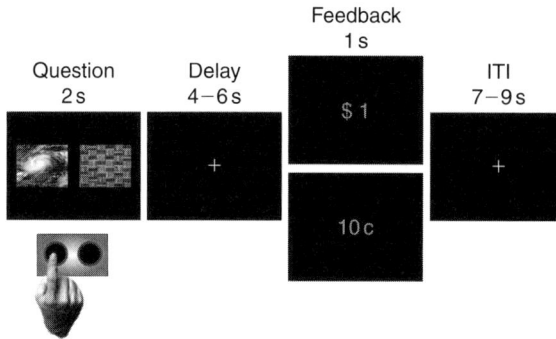

Figure 9.2 Decision-making task. Two stimuli (A and B) unknown to the subjects were presented for 2 s on each trial. The left/right position of these two stimuli was randomly determined. During this time, the subjects had to indicate their selection of one of the two stimuli by pressing on the left or the right button of a computer mouse, depending on whether the selected stimuli occupied the left or right position. After a delay varying from 4 to 6 s, the amount of money associated with the previous choice (i.e., feedback) was presented for 1 s. Selecting stimulus A (the stimulus presented on the left in the specific trial displayed) yielded $1 with probability 0.7, and 10 cents with probability 0.3. The reinforcement ratio for stimulus B was the opposite. The same two stimuli were presented across 12 successive trials with their left/right position varying randomly. The subjects had to discover which of the two stimuli was the most rewarded in the long run. In the particular example, they had to discover that stimulus A leads to the larger reward overall. An intertrial interval (ITI) varying from 7 to 9 s followed each trial.

which one was the best stimulus, and this key press marked the beginning of the repetition period. The beginning of a new search was instructed by the appearance of a phrase written on the screen for 2 s (e.g., "First search," "Second search," etc.). The mean number of searches in the DM task during which the best stimulus was discovered was 89.6%. A search period lasted on average 7.4 ($\pm$1.1, standard deviation (STD)) trials.

During the search trials, the subject is trying to discover which one of the two stimuli is most rewarded. Thus, the subject must carefully monitor (i.e., track) in working memory both the occurrence of stimuli A and B across a series of trials and the reward that was associated with each of them. For instance, the subject must monitor the fact that, in the last X number of trials, stimulus A occurred several times with $1 reward (e.g., on three of the four trials), whereas stimulus B occurred three times and was linked with 10 cents on two of the three trials. Monitoring demands within working memory are minimal in the repetition trials, that is, once the subject has discovered which one is the best-rewarded stimulus (e.g., stimulus A). Following the discovery of the most-rewarded stimulus, the subject must simply keep selecting that stimulus (e.g., stimulus A) on all successive repetition trials without the need to monitor in working memory the preceding trials. Thus, the comparison of activity in the search trials with activity in the repetition trials should yield greater activity in the mid-dorsolateral prefrontal cortex (areas 46 and 9/46). This prediction is based on earlier lesion work in the monkey showing that the critical role of the mid-dorsolateral prefrontal cortex lies in the monitoring of information in working memory and functional neuroimaging research showing that this region of the human frontal lobe shows greater activity when the monitoring demands in working memory tasks increase [93,94] (see Fig. 9.1). In order to determine the cerebral structures

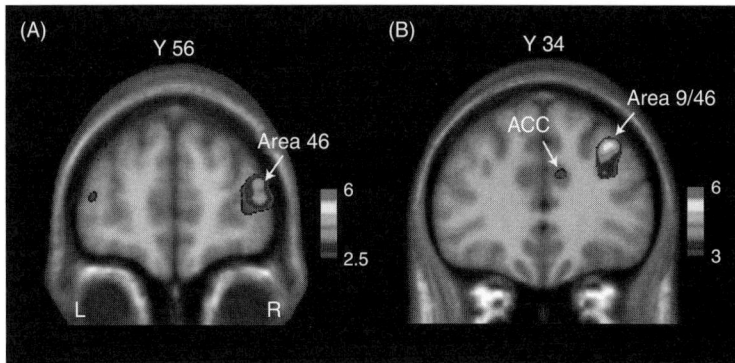

Figure 9.3 Results from the search minus repetition period comparison during the period of presentation of the stimuli (A) and the period of presentation of the feedback (B). The increased activity in the mid-dorsolateral prefrontal cortex and the anterior cingulate cortex (ACC) are represented on coronal sections. The Y value refers to the anteroposterior level in the Montreal Neurological Institute standard stereotaxic space. The color scale indicates the range for the *t*-statistic. L and R, left and right hemisphere. See Plate 12 of Color Plate section.

involved in making the decision in the DM task, the two periods (i.e., the question and the feedback periods) were analyzed separately.

First, the comparison between the blood oxygenation level dependent (BOLD) signal obtained during the question period in the search trials with that obtained during the repetition trials revealed specific increases in activity in the mid-dorsolateral prefrontal area 46 (Fig. 9.3A) and area 9/46 in the right hemisphere, and in area 11 in the OFC bilaterally. Importantly, the ACC did not exhibit greater activity when the BOLD signal obtained during the question period in the search trials was compared with that obtained during the repetition trials. The latter finding is consistent with results from a previous electrophysiological study in the monkey using a similar task [20]. In that study, we showed that ACC activity preceding the reward delivery encoded the average reward value associated with the best choice (i.e., the overall goal that the animal had to reach) and that this coding occurred during both the search and the repetition trials. It was therefore expected that no activity would be observed in the ACC from the comparison of the search and repetition trials during the question period in the functional neuroimaging study with human subjects. As pointed out above, we also observed activity in the OFC in the search trials during the question period. Importantly, electrophysiological studies in the monkey have shown that the OFC does not have neurons discharging in relation to the performance of motor acts. Since in the present study the stimulus presentation cannot be dissociated from the motor act, it is reasonable to suggest that the activity observed here is not linked to the motor act, but rather to the stimulus presentation. Thus, our data confirm the involvement of the OFC in associating stimuli with feedback during exploratory situations, as previously shown in neuroimaging studies in human subjects [21,22,39,53–56,95] and in electrophysiological studies on monkeys [63,65–73,96].

When we compared the BOLD signal obtained during the feedback period in the search trials with the signal obtained during the repetition trials, there were specific increases in activity in the mid-dorsolateral prefrontal area 46 bilaterally, in the mid-dorsolateral prefrontal area 9/46 in the right hemisphere, and in the ACC in the right hemisphere (see Fig. 9.3B). The involvement of the mid-dorsolateral prefrontal cortex during the feedback period in the search trials is again consistent with the prediction that it will be involved in the monitoring within working memory of the reward values associated with the two stimuli during the search trials. Indeed, the subject monitors the fact that, on trials X, $X - 1$, and $X - 4$, \$1 was received for stimulus A, but on trial $X - 5$ stimulus A received 10 cents, whereas stimulus B occurred on two preceding trials and received only 10 cents reward. Once the subject has decided that stimulus A is the best-rewarded stimulus, no intense monitoring of recent occurrences of stimuli A and B is necessary because the subject already knows that stimulus A is the best rewarded and will keep choosing this stimulus across the remaining trials (i.e., repetition trials).

The fact that there was greater activity in the mid-dorsolateral prefrontal cortex in both the search minus repetition trials during the question period and also in the search minus repetition trials during the feedback period is consistent with the known role of this part of the frontal cortex in the monitoring of information that is in working memory [94]. What is particularly interesting in the results of the present study is the difference in activity in the ACC in these two comparisons. There was no difference in activity in the ACC in the comparison between the search and the repetition trials during the question period as expected from electrophysiological results obtained in monkeys [20] (see above); but, in sharp contrast, the search minus repetition trials comparison during the feedback period showed increased activity in the ACC. This latter result is consistent with the suggestion that it is involved in analyzing the value of the feedback and the readjustment of the value of the action-outcome associations [12]. Note that, in a DM task in which the decision can be made only after several trials, we can hypothesize that the ACC may be involved in the readjustment of the value of the action-outcome associations across trials. Finally, the absence of increased activity in the OFC in the comparison search minus repetition trials during the feedback period suggests that the OFC

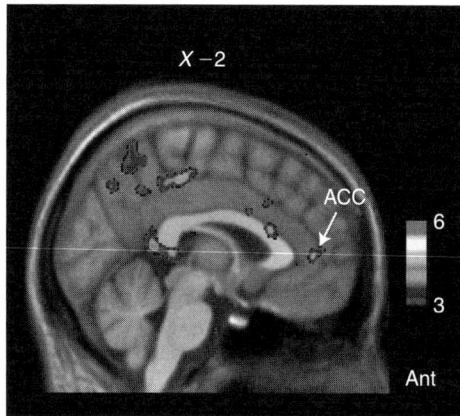

Figure 9.4 Results from the comparison of the decision intertrial interval minus the search period intertrial interval. Increased activity peak in the ACC is represented on a sagittal section. The X value corresponds to the mediolateral level in the Montreal Neurological Institute standard stereotaxic space. The color scale indicates the range for the t-statistic. Ant, anterior; ACC, anterior cingulate cortex. See Plate 13 of Color Plate section.

may not encode prediction error values or the reward history. Thus, it appears that the OFC may not have a representation of the overall goal to be reached in decision-making problems.

In order to assess the prefrontal regions involved in the decision process *per se*, we then compared the BOLD signal obtained during the intertrial interval, when the decision of which stimulus was the best had already been made, with the signal obtained during the intertrial interval in the search trials, when the decision had not yet been made. This contrast revealed specific increases in activity in the ACC bilaterally, in a region located just in front of the genu of the corpus callosum (Fig. 9.4). Note that no increased activity was observed from this comparison anywhere in the lateral or orbital prefrontal cortex. These data indicate that the ACC plays a crucial role in making a decision and adapt subsequent behavior, in contrast to the lateral prefrontal cortex, which plays a role in monitoring the reward history in working memory. This result is consistent with the hypothesis by Holroyd and Cole [4] that the ACC is responsible for selecting the best choice among competing choices based on the reward prediction error signals that it receives from the midbrain dopaminergic system [5]. As such, the ACC does not have only an evaluative role but also a critical role in the decision process *per se*.

9.6 Conclusions

In reward-based DM tasks, the ACC and the mid-DLPFC work in tandem to monitor action-feedback associations by encoding the local and overall goals to attain, the outcome uncertainty/volatility of a decision, and the prediction error values allowing adjustments to behavior on subsequent trials. By contrast, the OFC may monitor primarily stimulus–feedback associations by encoding the local goal to be reached and the uncertainty of the outcome. Finally, our results suggest that the ACC does not have only an evaluative role but has also a specific role in the decision-making process *per se*. The lack of studies dissociating the outcome expectation period from the outcome occurrence period raised major issues in our understanding of the role of the prefrontal cortex in reward-based decision-making processes. As such, future neuroimaging studies should focus on assessing this dissociation as well as on varying only one reinforcement learning parameter at a time to disentangle the role of various prefrontal cortical areas.

Acknowledgements

This research was supported from CIHR grant FRN 37753 to Michael Petrides. Céline Amiez was supported by a Fyssen Foundation fellowship. We would like to thank J. Sallet for helpful comment on the manuscript.

References

[1] N.J. Mackintosh, The Psychology of Animal Learning, Academic Press, London, 1974.
[2] R.S. Sutton, A.G. Barto, Reinforcement Learning: An Introduction, MIT Press, Cambridge, MA, 1998.
[3] C.D. Fiorillo, P.N. Tobler, W. Schultz, Discrete coding of reward probability and uncertainty by dopamine neurons, Science 299 (2003) 1898–1902.

[4] C.B. Holroyd, M.G. Coles, The neural basis of human error processing: reinforcement learning, dopamine, and the error-related negativity, Psychol. Rev. 109 (2002) 679–709.

[5] W. Schultz, A. Dickinson, Neuronal coding of prediction errors, Annu. Rev. Neurosci. 23 (2000) 473–500.

[6] S.M. Williams, P.S. Goldman-Rakic, Widespread origin of the primate mesofrontal dopamine system, Cereb. Cortex 8 (1998) 321–345.

[7] T.W. Robbins, A.C. Roberts, Differential regulation of fronto-executive function by the monoamines and acetylcholine, Cereb. Cortex 17 (Suppl 1) (2007) i151–i160.

[8] S.C. Walker, T.W. Robbins, A.C. Roberts, Differential contributions of dopamine and serotonin to orbitofrontal cortex function in the marmoset, Cereb. Cortex (2008).

[9] D.C. Krawczyk, Contributions of the prefrontal cortex to the neural basis of human decision making, Neurosci. Biobehav. Rev. 26 (2002) 631–664.

[10] M.F. Rushworth, T.E. Behrens, Choice, uncertainty and value in prefrontal and cingulate cortex, Nat. Neurosci. 11 (2008) 389–397.

[11] M.F. Rushworth, T.E. Behrens, P.H. Rudebeck, M.E. Walton, Contrasting roles for cingulate and orbitofrontal cortex in decisions and social behaviour, Trends Cogn. Sci. 11 (2007) 168–176.

[12] M.F. Rushworth, M.J. Buckley, T.E. Behrens, M.E. Walton, D.M. Bannerman, Functional organization of the medial frontal cortex, Curr. Opin. Neurobiol. 17 (2007) 220–227.

[13] M.F. Rushworth, M.E. Walton, S.W. Kennerley, D.M. Bannerman, Action sets and decisions in the medial frontal cortex, Trends Cogn. Sci. 8 (2004) 410–417.

[14] T. Paus, Primate anterior cingulate cortex: where motor control, drive and cognition interface, Nat. Rev. Neurosci. 2 (2001) 417–424.

[15] E. Procyk, P. Ford Dominey, C. Amiez, J.P. Joseph, The effects of sequence structure and reward schedule on serial reaction time learning in the monkey, Brain Res. Cogn. Brain Res. 9 (2000) 239–248.

[16] M.E. Walton, J.T. Devlin, M.F. Rushworth, Interactions between decision making and performance monitoring within prefrontal cortex, Nat. Neurosci. 7 (2004) 1259–1265.

[17] M. Petrides, D.N. Pandya, Comparative architectonic analysis of the human and the macaque frontal cortex, Handbook Neuropsychol. 9 (1994) 17–58.

[18] K. Matsumoto, W. Suzuki, K. Tanaka, Neuronal correlates of goal-based motor selection in the prefrontal cortex, Science 301 (2003) 229–232.

[19] J. Sallet, R. Quilodran, M. Rothe, J. Vezoli, J.P. Joseph, E. Procyk, Expectations, gains, and losses in the anterior cingulate cortex, Cogn. Affect. Behav. Neurosci. 7 (2007) 327–336.

[20] C. Amiez, J.P. Joseph, E. Procyk, Reward encoding in the monkey anterior cingulate cortex, Cereb. Cortex 16 (2006) 1040–1055.

[21] H.D. Critchley, C.J. Mathias, R.J. Dolan, Neural activity in the human brain relating to uncertainty and arousal during anticipation, Neuron 29 (2001) 537–545.

[22] R.D. Rogers, N. Ramnani, C. Mackay, J.L. Wilson, P. Jezzard, C.S. Carter, S.M. Smith, Distinct portions of anterior cingulate cortex and medial prefrontal cortex are activated by reward processing in separable phases of decision-making cognition, Biol. Psychiatry 55 (2004) 594–602.

[23] J.W. Kable, P.W. Glimcher, The neural correlates of subjective value during intertemporal choice, Nat. Neurosci. 10 (2007) 1625–1633.

[24] J.C. Dreher, P. Kohn, K.F. Berman, Neural coding of distinct statistical properties of reward information in humans, Cereb. Cortex 16 (2006) 561–573.

[25] M. Falkenstein, J. Hohnsbein, J. Hoormann, L. Blanke, Effects of crossmodal divided attention on late ERP components. II. Error processing in choice reaction tasks, Electroencephalogr. Clin. Neurophysiol. 78 (1991) 447–455.

[26] K. Fiehler, M. Ullsperger, D.Y. von Cramon, Neural correlates of error detection and error correction: is there a common neuroanatomical substrate?, Eur. J. Neurosci. 19 (2004) 3081–3087.

[27] H. Garavan, T.J. Ross, J. Kaufman, E.A. Stein, A midline dissociation between error-processing and response-conflict monitoring, Neuroimage 20 (2003) 1132–1139.

[28] W.J. Gehring, B. Goss, M.G.H. Coles, D.E. Meyer, E. Donchin, A neural system for error-detection and compensation, Psychol. Sci. 4 (1993) 385–390.

[29] R. Hester, J.J. Foxe, S. Molholm, M. Shpaner, H. Garavan, Neural mechanisms involved in error processing: a comparison of errors made with and without awareness, Neuroimage 27 (2005) 602–608.

[30] C.B. Holroyd, S. Nieuwenhuis, N. Yeung, L. Nystrom, R.B. Mars, M.G. Coles, J.D. Cohen, Dorsal anterior cingulate cortex shows fMRI response to internal and external error signals, Nat. Neurosci. 7 (2004) 497–498.

[31] T.A. Klein, T. Endrass, N. Kathmann, J. Neumann, D.Y. von Cramon, M. Ullsperger, Neural correlates of error awareness, Neuroimage 34 (2007) 1774–1781.

[32] E. Magno, J.J. Foxe, S. Molholm, I.H. Robertson, H. Garavan, The anterior cingulate and error avoidance, J. Neurosci. 26 (2006) 4769–4773.

[33] O. Monchi, M. Petrides, V. Petre, K. Worsley, A. Dagher, Wisconsin Card Sorting revisited: distinct neural circuits participating in different stages of the task identified by event-related functional magnetic resonance imaging, J. Neurosci. 21 (2001) 7733–7741.

[34] S.F. Taylor, B. Martis, K.D. Fitzgerald, R.C. Welsh, J.L. Abelson, I. Liberzon, J.A. Himle, W.J. Gehring, Medial frontal cortex activity and loss-related responses to errors, J. Neurosci. 26 (2006) 4063–4070.

[35] M. Ullsperger, H. Nittono, D.Y. von Cramon, When goals are missed: dealing with self-generated and externally induced failure, Neuroimage 35 (2007) 1356–1364.

[36] M. Ullsperger, D.Y. von Cramon, Error monitoring using external feedback: specific roles of the habenular complex, the reward system, and the cingulate motor area revealed by functional magnetic resonance imaging, J. Neurosci. 23 (2003) 4308–4314.

[37] M. Ullsperger, D.Y. von Cramon, Subprocesses of performance monitoring: a dissociation of error processing and response competition revealed by event-related fMRI and ERPs, Neuroimage 14 (2001) 1387–1401.

[38] T.E. Behrens, M.W. Woolrich, M.E. Walton, M.F. Rushworth, Learning the value of information in an uncertain world, Nat. Neurosci. 10 (2007) 1214–1221.

[39] M.X. Cohen, Individual differences and the neural representations of reward expectation and reward prediction error, Soc. Cogn. Affect. Neurosci. 2 (2007) 20–30.

[40] S. Ito, V. Stuphorn, J.W. Brown, J.D. Schall, Performance monitoring by the anterior cingulate cortex during saccade countermanding, Science 302 (2003) 120–122.

[41] R. Quilodran, M. Rothe, E. Procyk, Behavioral shifts and action valuation in the anterior cingulate cortex, Neuron 57 (2008) 314–325.

[42] C. Amiez, J.P. Joseph, E. Procyk, Anterior cingulate error-related activity is modulated by predicted reward, Eur. J. Neurosci. 21 (2005) 3447–3452.

[43] M. Matsumoto, K. Matsumoto, H. Abe, K. Tanaka, Medial prefrontal cell activity signaling prediction errors of action values, Nat. Neurosci. 10 (2007) 647–656.

[44] A. Bechara, A.R. Damasio, H. Damasio, S.W. Anderson, Insensitivity to future consequences following damage to human prefrontal cortex, Cognition 50 (1994) 7–15.

[45] A. Bechara, H. Damasio, D. Tranel, A.R. Damasio, Deciding advantageously before knowing the advantageous strategy, Science 275 (1997) 1293–1295.

[46] A. Bechara, D. Tranel, H. Damasio, Characterization of the decision-making deficit of patients with ventromedial prefrontal cortex lesions, Brain 123 (Pt 11) (2000) 2189–2202.

[47] J. Hornak, J. O'Doherty, J. Bramham, E.T. Rolls, R.G. Morris, P.R. Bullock, C.E. Polkey, Reward-related reversal learning after surgical excisions in orbito-frontal or dorsolateral pre-frontal cortex in humans, J. Cogn. Neurosci. 16 (2004) 463–478.

[48] E.T. Rolls, J. Hornak, D. Wade, J. McGrath, Emotion-related learning in patients with social and emotional changes associated with frontal lobe damage, J. Neurol. Neurosurg. Psychiatry 57 (1994) 1518–1524.

[49] A. Izquierdo, R.K. Suda, E.A. Murray, Bilateral orbital prefrontal cortex lesions in rhesus mon-keys disrupt choices guided by both reward value and reward contingency, J. Neurosci. 24 (2004) 7540–7548.

[50] M. Petrides, B. Alivisatos, S. Frey, Differential activation of the human orbital, mid-ventrolateral, and mid-dorsolateral prefrontal cortex during the processing of visual stimuli, Proc. Natl. Acad. Sci. USA 99 (2002) 5649–5654.

[51] A.C. Nobre, J.T. Coull, C.D. Frith, M.M. Mesulam, Orbitofrontal cortex is activated during breaches of expectation in tasks of visual attention, Nat. Neurosci. 2 (1999) 11–12.

[52] M. Petrides, The orbitofrontal cortex: novelty, deviation from expectation, and memory, Ann. NY Acad. Sci. 1121 (2007) 33–53.

[53] H.C. Breiter, I. Aharon, D. Kahneman, A. Dale, P. Shizgal, Functional imaging of neural responses to expectancy and experience of monetary gains and losses, Neuron 30 (2001) 619–639.

[54] J. O'Doherty, H. Critchley, R. Deichmann, R.J. Dolan, Dissociating valence of outcome from behavioral control in human orbital and ventral prefrontal cortices, J. Neurosci. 23 (2003) 7931–7939.

[55] J. O'Doherty, M.L. Kringelbach, E.T. Rolls, J. Hornak, C. Andrews, Abstract reward and pun-ishment representations in the human orbitofrontal cortex, Nat. Neurosci. 4 (2001) 95–102.

[56] G. Thut, W. Schultz, U. Roelcke, M. Nienhusmeier, J. Missimer, R.P. Maguire, K.L. Leenders, Activation of the human brain by monetary reward, Neuroreport 8 (1997) 1225–1228.

[57] P.N. Tobler, J.P. O'Doherty, R.J. Dolan, W. Schultz, Reward value coding distinct from risk attitude-related uncertainty coding in human reward systems, J. Neurophysiol. 97 (2007) 1621–1632.

[58] J.P. O'Doherty, R. Deichmann, H.D. Critchley, R.J. Dolan, Neural responses during anticipa-tion of a primary taste reward, Neuron 33 (2002) 815–826.

[59] I.E. De Araujo, E.T. Rolls, Representation in the human brain of food texture and oral fat, J. Neurosci. 24 (2004) 3086–3093.

[60] D.M. Small, R.J. Zatorre, A. Dagher, A.C. Evans, M. Jones-Gotman, Changes in brain activity related to eating chocolate: from pleasure to aversion, Brain 124 (2001) 1720–1733.

[61] E.T. Rolls, J. O'Doherty, M.L. Kringelbach, S. Francis, R. Bowtell, F. McGlone, Representations of pleasant and painful touch in the human orbitofrontal and cingulate cortices, Cereb. Cortex 13 (2003) 308–317.

[62] S. Ursu, C.S. Carter, Outcome representations, counterfactual comparisons and the human orbitofrontal cortex: implications for neuroimaging studies of decision-making, Brain Res. Cogn. Brain Res. 23 (2005) 51–60.

[63] K. Hikosaka, M. Watanabe, Delay activity of orbital and lateral prefrontal neurons of the monkey varying with different rewards, Cereb. Cortex 10 (2000) 263–271.

[64] C. Padoa-Schioppa, J.A. Assad, Neurons in the orbitofrontal cortex encode economic value, Nature 441 (2006) 223–226.

[65] E. Procyk, C. Amiez, R. Quilodran, J.P. Joseph, Modulations of prefrontal activity related to cognitive control and performance monitoring, in: Y. Rossetti, P. Haggard, M. Kawato (Eds.), Attention and Performance XXII: Sensorimotor Foundations of Higher Cognition, Oxford University Press, Oxford, 2007, pp. 235–250.

[66] M.R. Roesch, C.R. Olson, Neuronal activity related to reward value and motivation in primate frontal cortex, Science 304 (2004) 307–310.

[67] E.T. Rolls, The orbitofrontal cortex, Philos. Trans. R. Soc. Lond. B Biol. Sci. 351 (1996) 1433–1443 discussion 1443–1434.

[68] E.T. Rolls, S. Yaxley, Z.J. Sienkiewicz, Gustatory responses of single neurons in the caudolateral orbitofrontal cortex of the macaque monkey, J. Neurophysiol. 64 (1990) 1055–1066.

[69] W. Schultz, L. Tremblay, J.R. Hollerman, Reward processing in primate orbitofrontal cortex and basal ganglia, Cereb. Cortex 10 (2000) 272–284.

[70] S.J. Thorpe, E.T. Rolls, S. Maddison, The orbitofrontal cortex: neuronal activity in the behaving monkey, Exp. Brain Res. 49 (1983) 93–115.

[71] L. Tremblay, W. Schultz, Modifications of reward expectation-related neuronal activity during learning in primate orbitofrontal cortex, J. Neurophysiol. 83 (2000) 1877–1885.

[72] L. Tremblay, W. Schultz, Relative reward preference in primate orbitofrontal cortex, Nature 398 (1999) 704–708.

[73] L. Tremblay, W. Schultz, Reward-related neuronal activity during go-nogo task performance in primate orbitofrontal cortex, J. Neurophysiol. 83 (2000) 1864–1876.

[74] H. Niki, M. Sakai, K. Kubota, Delayed alternation performance and unit activity of the caudate head and medial orbitofrontal gyrus in the monkey, Brain Res. 38 (1972) 343–353.

[75] A.U. Turken, D. Swick, The effect of orbitofrontal lesions on the error-related negativity, Neurosci. Lett. 441 (2008) 7–10.

[76] M. Watanabe, Reward expectancy in primate prefrontal neurons, Nature 382 (1996) 629–632.

[77] K. Amemori, T. Sawaguchi, Contrasting effects of reward expectation on sensory and motor memories in primate prefrontal neurons, Cereb. Cortex 16 (2006) 1002–1015.

[78] S. Kobayashi, J. Lauwereyns, M. Koizumi, M. Sakagami, O. Hikosaka, Influence of reward expectation on visuospatial processing in macaque lateral prefrontal cortex, J. Neurophysiol. 87 (2002) 1488–1498.

[79] M.I. Leon, M.N. Shadlen, Effect of expected reward magnitude on the response of neurons in the dorsolateral prefrontal cortex of the macaque, Neuron 24 (1999) 415–425.

[80] M. Watanabe, M. Sakagami, Integration of cognitive and motivational context information in the primate prefrontal cortex, Cereb. Cortex 17 (Suppl 1) (2007) i101–i109.

[81] D. Lee, M.F. Rushworth, M.E. Walton, M. Watanabe, M. Sakagami, Functional specialization of the primate frontal cortex during decision making, J. Neurosci. 27 (2007) 8170–8173.

[82] E. Procyk, P.S. Goldman-Rakic, Modulation of dorsolateral prefrontal delay activity during self-organized behavior, J. Neurosci. 26 (2006) 11313–11323.

[83] H. Niki, M. Watanabe, Prefrontal unit activity and delayed response: relation to cue location versus direction of response, Brain Res. 105 (1976) 79–88.

[84] M. Watanabe, Prefrontal unit activity during associative learning in the monkey, Exp. Brain Res. 80 (1990) 296–309.

[85] S. Tsujimoto, T. Sawaguchi, Neuronal representation of response-outcome in the primate prefrontal cortex, Cereb. Cortex 14 (2004) 47–55.

[86] D.J. Barraclough, M.L. Conroy, D. Lee, Prefrontal cortex and decision making in a mixed-strategy game, Nat. Neurosci. 7 (2004) 404–410.

[87] H. Seo, D.J. Barraclough, D. Lee, Dynamic signals related to choices and outcomes in the dorsolateral prefrontal cortex, Cereb. Cortex 17 (Suppl 1) (2007) i110–i117.

[88] J.B. Pochon, R. Levy, P. Fossati, S. Lehericy, J.B. Poline, B. Pillon, D. Le Bihan, B. Dubois, The neural system that bridges reward and cognition in humans: an fMRI study, Proc. Natl. Acad. Sci. USA, 99 (8) (2002) 5669–5674.

[89] N. Ramnani, R.C. Miall, Instructed delay activity in the human prefrontal cortex is modulated by monetary reward expectation, Cereb. Cortex 13 (3) (2003) 318–327.

[90] U. Sailer, S. Robinson, F.P. Fischmeister, E. Moser, I. Kryspin-Exner, H. Bauer, Imaging the changing role of feedback during learning in decision-making, Neuroimage 37 (4) (2007) 1474–1486.

[91] C. Landmann, S. Dehaene, S. Pappata, A. Jobert, M. Bottlaender, D. Roumenov, D. Le Bihan, Dynamics of prefrontal and cingulate activity during a reward-based logical deduction task, Cereb. Cortex 17 (2007) 749–759.

[92] C. Amiez, E. Procyk, J. Honore, H. Sequeira, J.P. Joseph, Reward anticipation, cognition, and electrodermal activity in the conditioned monkey, Exp. Brain Res. 149 (2003) 267–275.

[93] M. Petrides, Frontal lobes and working memory: evidence from investigations of the effects of cortical excisions in non-human primates, in: F. Boller, J. Grafman (Eds.), Handbook of Neuropsychology, Elsevier, Amsterdam, 1994, pp. 59–82.

[94] M. Petrides, Lateral prefrontal cortex: architectonic and functional organization, Philos. Trans. R. Soc. Lond. B Biol. Sci. 360 (2005) 781–795.

[95] P.N. Tobler, C.D. Fiorillo, W. Schultz, Adaptive coding of reward value by dopamine neurons, Science 307 (2005) 1642–1645.

[96] C. Padoa-Schioppa, Orbitofrontal cortex and the computation of economic value, Ann. NY Acad. Sci. 1121 (2007) 232–253.

10 Computational neuroimaging: monitoring reward learning with blood flow

Samuel M. McClure[1] and Kimberlee D'Ardenne[2]

[1]Department of Psychology, Stanford University, Stanford, CA 94305
[2]Department of Neuroscience, Baylor College of Medicine, Houston, TX 77030

Abstract

The reward prediction error theory of dopamine function is one of the great recent advances in neuroscience. It has spurred research on reinforcement learning at all levels of investigation that has now localized many components of the associated computational algorithms to specific neural processes. With these advances, interest has expanded to include the neural basis of human reward learning and decision-making. Functional MRI (fMRI) has become the method of choice for these experiments since it offers the desired combination of spatial and temporal resolution. We discuss the strengths and limitations of fMRI in the study of reward processing and review recent advances in using fMRI to map, and in some instances extend, reinforcement learning models of human brain function.

Key points

1. Overview of reinforcement learning algorithms.
2. Relationship of reinforcement learning algorithms to dopamine neuron activity.
3. Challenges in relating neuronal recordings to fMRI experiments.
4. Recent advances in tracking reinforcement learning using fMRI.

10.1 Introduction

Of several responses made to the same situation, those which are accompanied or closely followed by satisfaction to the animal will, other things being equal, be more firmly connected with the situation, so that, when it recurs, they will be more likely to recur; those which are accompanied or closely followed by discomfort to the animal will, other things being equal, have their connections with that situation weakened, so that, when it recurs, they will be less likely to occur. The greater the satisfaction or discomfort, the greater the strengthening or weakening of the bond.

E.L. Thorndike [1]

Reinforcement learning refers to the general problem of how to learn from intermittent positive and negative events in order to improve behavior though time and experience. It is an old problem in psychology; Thorndike's law of effect, quoted above, encompasses the main principles underlying modern reinforcement learning algorithms[1] see Chapter 2. Our terminology has now changed: Satisfiers are referred to as rewards and annoyers as punishments (although Thorndike uses these terms as well). Nonetheless, the principle that the magnitude and valence of outcomes tend to strengthen or weaken their associated basic mode of updating that underlies all reinforcement learning algorithms.

Formal models of reinforcement learning function around reward predictions and reward prediction errors. In the learning model developed by Rescorla and Wagner [2], estimates of expected reward are maintained in a variable which we call V. Reward estimates are compared on every trial of learning with the reward that is actually obtained, which we call r. Since any number of stimuli could function as predictors of reward, independent estimates are maintained by having V be a function of the state of the world, s: [$V(s)$]. For any trial, the prediction error is the difference between obtained and expected reward. We refer to error with the Greek letter δ, so that the reward prediction error is given by

$$\delta(t) = r(t) - V(s_t). \tag{10.1}$$

The variable t is time, or trial number, and s_t is the stimulus (or, more precisely, the conditioned stimulus, CS) that occurred on the trial.

The reward prediction error is used primarily for learning. If reward predictions are updated in proportion to the prediction error, so that

$$V(s_t) \leftarrow V(s_t) + \alpha\,\delta(t) \tag{10.2}$$

(where "$\leftarrow$" indicates the change that occurs before the next trial), then the reward predictions V will converge to the expected reward averaged over all occurrences. The learning rate, α, is a number between 0 and 1 that determines how fast learning occurs. If α is small, then learning progresses more slowly but V also fluctuates less for variable rewards.

Since learning in this model depends strictly on the occurrence of an unconditioned stimulus, then some forms of animal learning cannot be readily accounted for. The classic example is secondary conditioning [3]. In secondary conditioning, learning first occurs to associate a conditioned stimulus with a reward (CS1-US). Once learning has occurred, a second CS is associated with the first CS (CS2-CS1). With this procedure, animals learn to predict a reward after the occurrence of CS2. However, the Rescorla-Wagner model only learns on the basis of the strength of a US and so predicts that no learning should occur for CS2-CS1.

The main limitation of the Rescorla-Wagner model is that it handles learning on a trial-to-trial basis and does not provide a real-time update rule that is more appropriate when considering neural responses. Nonetheless, the learning principles in Eqs 10.1 and 10.2 are preserved in the more detailed temporal difference (TD) reinforcement learning models that have been used to understand brain function.

10.1.1 TD learning

The limitations of the Rescorla-Wagner algorithm are resolved by changing the objective function to learn the expected reward

$$V^*(s_t) = E\{r(t) + \gamma r(t + 1) + \gamma^2 r(t + 1) + \gamma^3 r(t + 3) + ...\} \tag{10.3}$$

To understand how TD works, it is first necessary to appreciate the recursive relationship inherent in this formulation of V^*. First, notice that at time $t + 1$ the world will change so that a new stimulus s_{t+1} will occur, which itself can be used to predict the reward expected from that time onward, so that

$$V^*(s_{t+1}) = E\{r(t + 1) + \gamma r(t + 2) + \gamma^2 r(t + 3) + \gamma^3 r(t + 4) + ...\}. \tag{10.4}$$

From the juxtaposition of Eqs 10.3 and 10.4 it can be seen that

$$V^*(s_t) = E\{r(t) + \gamma V(s_{t+1})\}. \tag{10.5}$$

The power of this formula is that it allows updating to be done on a moment-by-moment basis, not strictly at the end of trials as in the Rescorla-Wagner model. Estimates of V^*, which we again denote by V, should satisfy Eq. 10.5 insofar as they accurately predict future reward. Errors in reward prediction are equal to

$$\delta(t) = r(t) + \gamma V(s_{t+1}) - V(s_t). \tag{10.6}$$

Because $V(t + 1) - V(t)$ is the temporal derivative of V, this error term is called the *temporal difference error* and is the basis of *temporal difference (TD) learning*. There are many variants on TD learning. We will discuss some variations in the remainder of this chapter, but, by and large, neural data are not yet refined enough to warrant venturing beyond the simple error rule in Eq. 10.6. This error term is the basis of the TD(0) algorithm; the "0" indicates that updating is done only on the basis of the immediately preceding stimulus. There is some indication that other prior events are used in learning, but we will not discuss this further (see [4]).

As with Rescorla-Wagner learning, the prediction error term in Eq. 10.6 is used to update value estimates. The form of the update rule in TD(0) is exactly the same as indicated by Eq. 10.2, above.

10.1.2 An example experiment

To better illustrate how TD reinforcement learning works, and to facilitate the discussion of how TD relates to neuroscience data, we will refer to an experimental design that has been run repeatedly, with minor modifications, in monkeys and humans. For modeling, we borrow the particular design used by Hollerman and Schultz [5]. In this experiment, a monkey saw two visual stimuli, each over a corresponding response bar. During the experiment the monkey learned that one visual stimulus predicted a juice reward at a fixed time interval (1 s) after pressing its associated response lever.

In order to model this experiment, we treat the stimulus space as consisting of two relevant features. The first feature is the reward-predicting visual cue and the second feature is the act of pressing the lever. As shown in Fig. 10.1, the visual cue (stimulus) occurs some time prior to the response, which is itself centered at time zero. The liquid reward occurs at 1 s.

For the model, we treat the state at any time s_t to indicate how far into the past each of the two features occurred, if they have occurred. This method of representing prior events is called a "tapped delay line" and has been used previously to model neural data [6]. There is an ongoing debate about whether the tapped delay line method is supported by neural data or not, but it is beyond the scope of this chapter to discuss it here [4,7–9]. For all simulations presented, time is discretized into intervals of 0.02 s. We also only model trials in which the correct response is made. Incorrect responses would have separate associated reward predictions; the model outcomes should be easy to intuit by extrapolating from the effects in rewarded, correct trials.

The performance of the model during the course of learning is shown in Fig. 10.1. We initialized reward predictions to zero, so on the first trial the model makes no predictions and the occurrence of reward elicits a prediction error of the same size as the reward. After this first trial, $s_{t=1}$ is updated according to Eq. 10.2 so that its new value becomes α (since the prediction error is equal to 1 and the previous value was 0). The importance

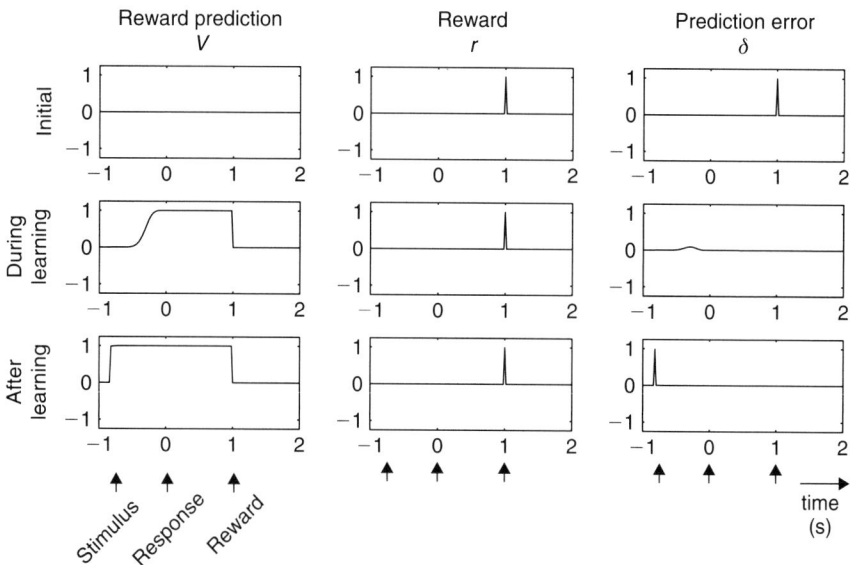

Figure 10.1 Stages in temporal difference learning during example experiment. Reward prediction, reward delivery, and reward prediction error are shown during the first trial of learning, in the late stages of learning, and after learning is complete.

of Eq. 10.6 is apparent on the second training trial. In the time step immediately pre-ceding reward delivery (call time here $t = 1 - \Delta$), $V(s_{t=1-\Delta}) = 0$, but $V(s_{t=1}) = \alpha$. So Eq. 10.6 gives a prediction error equal to $0 + \gamma\alpha - 1 = \gamma\alpha$. Because the prediction error is positive, the value at $t = 1 - \Delta$ gets increased despite the fact that no reward is deliv-ered at this time. The propagation of reward prediction errors back in time continues in this manner until the earliest predictive stimulus (in this case the visual cue) predicts the full value of the future reward. We have plotted the model predictions in the late stages of learning in the middle row of Fig. 10.1. The prediction error is small and distributed over numerous time steps but eventually translates to the stimulus. For the model we have used a learning rate $\alpha = 0.2$ and a discount factor $\gamma = 1$. If γ were less than 1, then the value function, V, would increase exponentially between the time of the stimulus and the reward.

10.1.3 Neural implementation

In a wonderfully peripatetic series of experiments in the early- to mid-1990s, Wolfram Schultz and colleagues provided the first definitive connection between TD learning and brain activity. They recorded from single dopamine neurons in awake, behaving macaque monkeys. Most of the recordings were from dopamine neurons in the substantia nigra pars compacta (SNc), but the reports also include responses from dopamine neurons in the ventral tegmental area (VTA; see Chapter 1 for discussion of relevant anatomy). At the time of the studies, dopamine neurons were broadly associated with several very dif-ferent phenomena of relevance to mental health. Schultz and colleagues began trying to investigate the link between the loss of dopamine neurons and the loss of motor control in Parkinson's disease. Their initial publication reported some weak findings between the firing of dopamine neurons and motor responses in tasks such as that modeled in Fig. 10.1[10]. Instead of movements, the most compelling relationship apparent in dopamin-ergic responses was their relationship with reward.

If a monkey had to reach inside a box to obtain a food reward, then phasic dopamine bursts were apparent when food was present, and pauses in firing were apparent when food was absent [11]. Mirenowicz and Schultz [12] showed that these responses were driven by the unpredictability of the events. When reward is given at predicted times, then dopamine neurons are unresponsive; however, when rewards are delivered unpre-dictably, then phasic bursts occur reliably. Furthermore, trained conditioned stimuli come to evoke responses of equal size as those evoked by unanticipated reward.

This pattern of responding corresponds precisely with the reward prediction error in Eq. 10.6 and illustrated in Fig. 10.1[6]. Discovery of this connection allowed for more direct tests of whether midbrain dopamine neurons truly encode TD prediction errors. The experiment by Hollerman and Schultz [5] described above was a direct test of how positive and negative prediction errors should occur by changing the time of an antici-pated reward delivery (Fig. 10.2). Waelti et al. [13] followed up by confirming the pre-diction of TD models in a blocking procedure. Fiorillo et al. [7] have shown that reward probability is encoded in the amplitude of phasic responses as predicted by the model as well. More recently Kobayashi and Schultz [14] have showed that dopaminergic responses decrease with reward delay as predicted (assuming $\gamma < 1$). Overall, there is now an overwhelming body of data showing that TD prediction errors are an excellent model of the phasic firing of dopamine neurons.

(A) Dopamine neuron

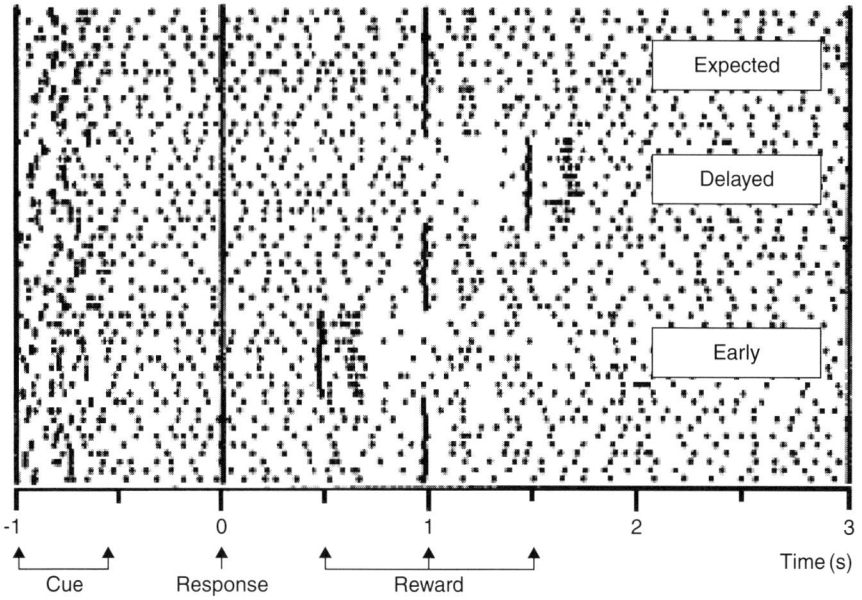

(B) Temporal difference model

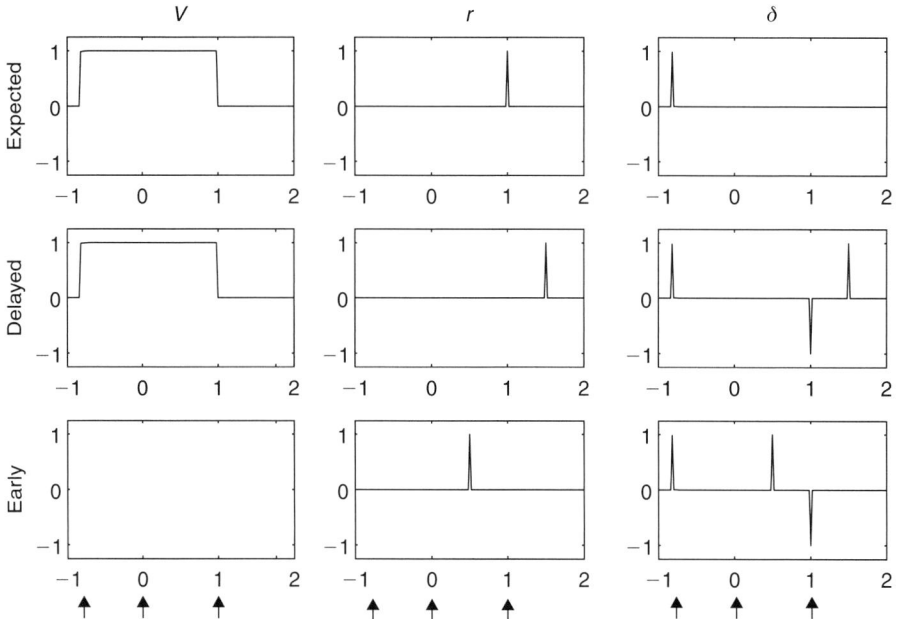

Figure 10.2 Temporal difference model of dopamine neurons. Reward prediction is maintained by a value function *V* that is associated with the earliest predictable cue, in this case a visual indicator of

10.1.4   Reward and reward prediction

The reward prediction error signal is only one component of reinforcement learning algorithms. Most of the extant work on reward learning in neuroscience focuses on this signal, largely because of the work by Schultz and colleagues discussed above. Namely, this component of reinforcement learning has been found in brain activity and so there is good promise in extending these findings. However, knowing the site of the prediction error signal points to candidate sources for other components of reinforcement learning. For example, prediction errors are learning signals to be used to increase or decrease value estimates, in the brain presumably by modulating synaptic weights. There is a high density of dopamine terminals in the striatum, which makes this a reasonable site to look for changes in synaptic weights, and in fact there is good evidence that dopamine serves this hypothesized function in the striatum [15, see Chapter 3]. Of course, this implies that value signals should also be stored in the striatum so that when a stimulus is presented, the activity of striatal neurons should scale with expected value. This too has been observed [16]. The remaining major variable, reward value, has not been as well studied. There are excellent reviews elsewhere that speculate on the source of many other variables important in reinforcement learning [17]. For our purposes here, it is sufficient that we focus on reward prediction error signals.

10.1.5   Variations on TD(0)

Formally, TD(0) is a model most appropriate for Pavlovian conditioning. When actions are considered, then values need to consider the action taken as well as environmental stimuli (such as the nature of visual cues in the example experiment). In reinforcement learning, incorporating actions amounts to learning the value of state-action pairs, that is, learning how valuable an action given some current state of the world. State-action values are usually abbreviated by $Q(s,a)$. The objective in learning Q-values is, again, to accurately predict the discounted sum of all future rewards (i.e., Eq. 10.3). However, future rewards depend on the actions to be taken, and so this quantity is not well defined. Instead, there are two ways to structure Q-values: Either the value should predict the reward expected given the actions that are actually taken (the basis for the SARSA reinforcement learning algorithm), or the value should predict on the basis of the best possible future actions (the basis for Q-learning; see [18] for a review of both algorithms). There is some support for both of these variations in neuronal recordings from dopamine neurons [19,20].

All of the preceding discussion has related to rapid changes in the firing of dopamine neurons. When tonic activity (given by baseline neuronal firing) of dopamine neurons is considered, dopamine seems to be computing errors in the prediction of reward relative

---

Figure 10.2 (*continued*)
which of two buttons delivers a juice reward. After learning, V fully predicts the time of reward, and a prediction error (δ) is positive only at the time of the initial cue. When reward is delayed beyond the expected time, a negative prediction error occurs at the predicted time and is seen as a decrease in firing in the dopamine neuron in panel A. A positive prediction error also occurs at the time of (delayed) reward delivery. Early delivery of reward has similar predicted (panel B) effect, although the decreased firing in the dopamine neuron is not as apparent as for the delayed reward deliver.
Source: Panel A adopted from Hollerman and Schultz (1998) [5].

to average outcomes over a period of time [21,22]. A variation of TD learning known as R-learning [23] accounts for this property. In short, R-learning learns both the average rate of rewards expected to be earned in an environment and how good each action or stimulus is relative to this average.

TD(0) is the simplest of many reinforcement learning algorithms used in machine learning, and several of the properties of more complex algorithms have been related to details of brain function. Critically, none of these variations changes the prediction errors caused by delaying rewards, as depicted in Fig. 10.2. This has important implications for the discussion below; specifically, using this design should evoke prediction error signals that are largely insensitive to the exact structure of reinforcement learning algorithm implemented in the brain. As will be discussed briefly, some specific hypotheses about the nature of learning can be and have been tested in humans (see [24,25]), but additional work in this area is certainly to be expected.

10.2   Human studies of reward processing

There are numerous neuroimaging technologies available for studying reward learning in people (see Chapters 6 & 7). The bulk of our discussion will be restricted to functional magnetic resonance imaging (fMRI) and the blood oxygenation level-dependent (BOLD) signal. However, this is not intended to discount work in other domains. Some excellent research has related the error-related negativity (ERN) measured with EEG to prediction error signals [26]. There is some debate as to how closely associated this signal is to dopaminergic activity [27]. However, the close relationship between the ERN and the feedback-response negativity (FRN; [28]), together with the close relationship of the FRN to prediction error signals like those in Fig. 10.2, indicate that EEG is a very useful tool for measuring aspects of reinforcement learning in people.

The limitation of EEG is that signals are difficult to localize and are limited to the cortex. For the study of reward learning this is particularly problematic since dopamine neurons are located in the brainstem and the vast majority of dopaminergic terminals are found in the basal ganglia. These areas are largely inaccessible using EEG. Positron emission tomography (PET) is another possible method, and it has some very valuable attributes that will be discussed further below. However, PET scanning has poor temporal resolution that makes identification of fast prediction error signals impossible. There have been numerous studies of reward processing using PET [29]; however, the bulk of advances in human studies of reinforcement learning have employed fMRI BOLD imaging.

10.2.1   Computational neuroimaging

Several critical assumptions must be made in order to perform computational neuroimaging. If the end goal is to map the values taken by model parameters to brain activity, then the intervening transformations between computational process and recordable signal must be well understood. Establishing this association is very challenging even for single-neuron recordings. In the preceding discussion we made the implicit assumption that reward prediction error value is represented by the rate of firing of individual neurons. This is certainly a reasonable assumption, but is in no way certain to be true. Neurons are capable of very precise firing [30], which provides feasibility for theories that posit that values are encoded in the precise timing of spikes [31]. Nevertheless, temporal coding schemes are commonly difficult to distinguish from rate codes, and so this first assumption that value correlates with neuronal activity is well supported.

A second important assumption for computational neuroimaging lies in the transformation between neuronal activity and the measured BOLD signal. We will review this relationship in reasonable detail in the next section, but it is worth noting at the outset that the connection is still only imprecisely understood. There is clearly a strong correlation between regional measurements of neuronal activity and BOLD responses, but how the former cause the latter still remains only speculation. This is a strong reason for skepticism regarding fMRI results generally and may even be perceived to be an overwhelming obstacle for progress. However, progress has been made despite this. There are even instances where fMRI has revealed potentially important signals in brain areas previously unrelated to the property of interest. Regions of the posterior cingulate cortex are regularly identified in fMRI studies of reward [32]. Based on this, Michael Platt and colleagues [66] have performed a series of experiments investigating this relationship at the level of individual neurons. When fMRI has identified signals that have profitably led to more direct and more invasive studies, then we feel that skepticism based on tenuous understanding of the source of the BOLD signal is unproductive.

The BOLD response

The BOLD response depends on the local ratio of deoxygenated hemoglobin and oxygenated hemoglobin [33] and closely tracks changes in the cerebral metabolic rate of oxygen consumption and the concomitant changes in cerebral blood flow that accompany neuronal activation [34]. As mentioned above, the BOLD response has been shown to closely track neuronal activity [35–37]. Concurrent measures of neuronal activity and BOLD signals have shown that the BOLD response correlates more strongly with the local field potential (LFP) than it does with measures of neuronal spiking [35]. This strongly suggests that the BOLD response encodes local synaptic current, or a measure of the input to and intraregional processing within a brain area. In spite of this seemingly simple idea that the BOLD response encodes input and local processing, interpretations of how the BOLD response maps onto neuronal function are not straightforward, particularly in cortex [37]. In addition, the BOLD response is incapable of resolving the effects of neuromodulation and whether processing is top-down, bottom-up, or function-specific [37].

A common assumption made during the interpretation of fMRI data is that the transform between the underlying neuronal activity and the BOLD response is linear. There are two consequences to this assumption. First, serial presentation of a stimulus (or different stimuli) should elicit BOLD responses that are the sum of the responses to the stimuli presented individually. This assumption is easily tested using fMRI and seems to hold as long as the rate at which stimuli are presented is modest (roughly no faster than once every 4 s; [38]). For rapidly presented stimuli, the BOLD signal quickly becomes sublinear, which would wreak havoc on data analyses performed using standard general linear model techniques.

The second assumption underlying linearity is that the BOLD signal itself is linearly dependent on underlying neuronal activity. This is probably impossible to determine [37]. Neuronal recordings have shown that signal amplitude changes not only the firing rate of individual neurons but also the number of neurons recruited. Since hemodynamic responses reflect the activity of large neuronal populations, the relationship between the firing of an individual neuron can never be related to the BOLD signal independent of changes in the population of recruited neurons.

One final common complaint about the BOLD response is that while its spatial resolution is the best possible with human neuroimaging (~2 mm), it is still extremely crude. There are many tens of thousands of neurons in individual voxels and it seems unreasonable to expect that the average activity of so many neurons (each of which may have a different and precise function) indicates anything meaningful. This point is particularly relevant since fMRI papers frequently refer to single-neuron studies in order to support their findings. How can studies that average over a hundred or so neurons based on specific, highly variable properties be used to support signals that average over many cubic millimeters of brain tissue, interneurons, and glial cells together?

This question can be easily reversed. What does the activity of individual neurons tell us about the function of a brain region? When the properties of individual neurons are highly consistent across recorded neurons, which is true for dopamine neurons in the SN and VTA, then the relationship is direct. Similarly, for brain areas in the visual cortex in which neurons have consistent properties, if different tuning to stimulus parameters, then again the function of the brain area is clear. The common property is a reasonable summary of the brain region. However, for many brain areas involved in reward processing, and probably other cognitive processes, the variability across neurons is much more problematic. Consider, for example, the work by Padoa-Schioppa and Assad [39] in the orbitofrontal cortex (OFC). All reported neurons in this study had some relationship to the value of the presented options. However, some neurons were related to the reward to be chosen, some to a specific outcome independent of whether it would be chosen, others to the nature of the reward, and still other relationships. To summarize the function of the OFC, the only conclusion is that it is somehow related to reward processing, but the exact function is impossible to pinpoint because different neurons respond to almost every conceivable computation involved in the choice. In cases like this, averaging over a large number of neurons probably captures the function of the region well. Overall, this analysis indicates that the resolution offered by fMRI may be quite revealing. When the function of a region is consistent across neurons, as is true for dopamine neurons, then the averaging produced by fMRI accurately summarizes the function of the brain area. For brain areas related to more complex cognitive processes, such as in the OFC, then averaging over large numbers of neurons loses information but still provides an accurate summary of the function of a region.

In summary, the BOLD response is a surrogate signal for the activity of many neurons, and directly mapping changes in the BOLD response to underlying neuronal activity is difficult, to say the least. However, fMRI is nonetheless an incredibly valuable technique for studying brain function, especially when combined with animal models and other brain function measurement modalities.

Dopamine and the BOLD response

It is worth commenting additionally on what is known about the relationship between dopamine release and the BOLD response. As stated previously, the BOLD response is thought to reflect synaptic activity as opposed to neuronal firing and thus BOLD responses in brain areas where dopamine neurons are known to project are thought to reflect the actions of dopamine. Recent physiological data suggest that such a straightforward interpretation of the BOLD response in brain areas innervated by dopamine, specifically in prefrontal cortex (PFC), is premature (see [40] for review). In the PFC, dopamine is known to affect postsynaptic activity through second messenger receptors [67]. Second messenger receptors utilize effector proteins commonly located in the cell membrane to alter the chemistry of the post-synaptic cell; dopamine uses G-protein coupled receptors in PFC [40]. Effects through second messenger mechanisms occur on the order of seconds, while effects of other neurotransmitters occur on a sub-second timescale (Attwell and Iadecola, 2002). Dopamine clearance at the synapse is much slower in the PFC than in the striatum, and dopamine is thought to work through volume transmission in the PFC [40]. Additionally, dopamine is known to have a widespread effect on the blood flow to brain areas that are targeted by dopaminergic projections (Attwell, 2002). Certain properties of the BOLD response, namely, that it is delayed in time because of the sluggish hemodynamic response and is somewhat spatially blurred compared to the origin of neuronal activity [41], compensate for the slow timescale of dopamine modulation in target structures (specifically the PFC) and for dopamine's widespread modulatory effects. Measuring a BOLD response from brainstem regions containing dopamine nuclei circumvents issues of slow transmission and widespread modulatory effects.

10.2.2   Reward prediction errors in dopamine target regions

The majority of studies of reward learning in people have focused on recordings in the striatum. There are several reasons for this, but the common underlying factor is ease of implementation. The striatum is large, so that recording at a standard resolution of $3 \times 3 \times 3 \, mm^3$ gives many parallel recordings from regions within the striatum. Additionally, the striatum is proximate to the anterior commissure and so registration algorithms used to normalize data across study participants produces good a good match within the striatum. Finally, and most importantly, dopamine afferents are extremely dense in the striatum. Roughly 80% of all of the brain's dopamine terminals are in the striatum [42]. Since fMRI BOLD responses are likely generated at synaptic terminals, then the striatum is an accessible region that is highly likely to be the site of robust dopamine-related signals.

Dopamine-related signals have also been reported in other brain regions that receive dense dopaminergic input. Most notable among these are the ventromedial prefrontal cortex (VMPFC) and OFC. These brain regions pose problems experimentally due to the strong susceptibility artifacts that reduce signal quality. Special acquisition protocols are able to limit these problems, but their existence seems to have restricted the number of reports identifying the VMPFC and OFC in reward studies. Nonetheless, there are numerous reports of prediction error-like BOLD signals in the VMPFC and OFC [43–45]. By and large, for studies that specifically aim to elicit reward prediction error signals, responses in the VMPFC, OFC, and ventral striatum have been found to be largely consistent. If we switch freely between studies reporting these areas, this is why. There are some interesting differences between the reward signals in these brain regions, but they are not clearly understood at this point (but see [46,47]).

The first study to directly induce reward prediction errors in an fMRI experiment was performed by Berns et al. [48]. They gave participants sequences of juice and water squirts in either unpredictable or predictable patterns. Since both juice and water are primary rewards, the predictability of the sequence should modulate the size of related BOLD responses at steady state. More specifically, for the predictable sequence in which juice and water were alternated and delivered at a regular time interval, participants should learn both when and what is coming next. Therefore, after some time, reward deliveries should become fully predicted and neural responses should concomitantly decline to zero. For the unpredictable sequence, the order of juice and water squirts was randomized, as was the time interval between reward deliveries. In this condition neural responses should remain elevated throughout the trial. Berns et al. reported significantly

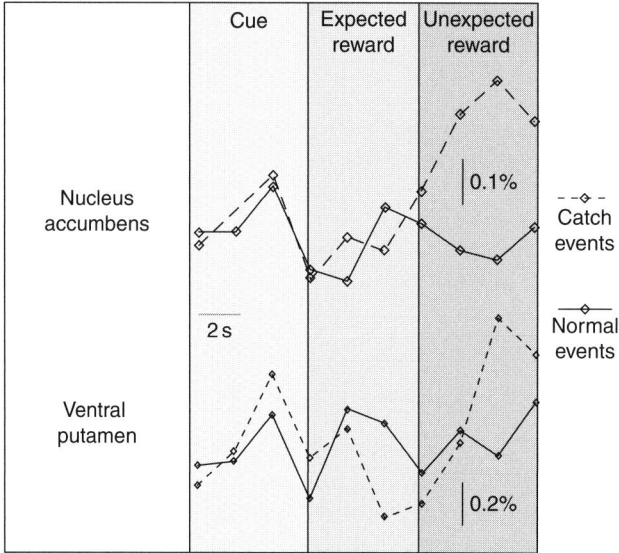

Figure 10.3 Reward prediction errors in human striatum. As in Fig. 10.2, delaying the onset of an expected reward in catch events elicits an elevated BOLD response to the reward delivery. This is apparent in both the nucleus accumbens and in the ventral putamen. The putamen also shows a significant decrease in BOLD response to the omission of reward – the negative prediction error. *Source*: Adapted from McClure et al. (2003) [64].

greater responses in the ventral striatum and VMPFC during the unpredictable sequence relative to the predictable sequence, exactly as would be predicted.

A more precise test of reward prediction errors used the same design as in the experiment by Hollerman and Schultz discussed previously (Fig. 10.2). Participants were conditioned to expect a squirt of juice at a fixed time interval following a conditioned light stimulus. After ample training, several catch events were given (corresponding to the delayed rewards in Fig. 10.2A,B). For the catch events, reward delivery was delayed an additional 4 s beyond the 6 s training time following the CS. As in the response of dopamine neurons, delaying reward delivery elicited two signals in the BOLD responses in the ventral striatum (Fig. 10.3). The most prominent of these signals was a positive prediction error to the delayed delivery of reward. This was apparent in both the nucleus accumbens and in the ventral putamen. A negative prediction error signal following the omission of the expected reward was also observed. However, this signal was apparent only in a limited region within the ventral putamen. The reason for this smaller signal for the negative prediction error signal is unclear. One possibility is that it reflects the limited dynamic range of dopamine firing below its very low baseline firing rate. However, as can be seen in Fig. 10.3, the observed BOLD signals are noisy, and hence it is difficult to come to any strong conclusions due to overall limits on statistical power.

We have focused on our study largely because it is a near replication of the experiment performed by Hollerman and Schultz [5]. However, numerous other experiments have identified reward prediction errors in the striatum and VMPFC [44,49–51]. Together, this work provides a very important demonstration that computational neuroimaging is feasible despite the many lingering questions about the intervening steps between computations and BOLD signals. We have successfully traversed from equations describing reinforcement learning algorithms to BOLD signals in the ventral striatum. The tendency has been to use this success to extend theories of human reward learning. In some cases, this has proven very successful, and we will discuss briefly some of the successes of fMRI in this regard below. However, there are important problems with using fMRI as a tool to extend theories of reward learning, which we will illustrate with a particularly contentious example.

One open question in the study of dopamine neurons is whether they signal rewarding events *per se*, or whether they respond to all behaviorally relevant signals [52]. A prominent theory of dopamine function posits that dopamine is particularly important for directing attention [53], perhaps to indicate that events are motivationally salient [54]. Consistent with this theory is the finding that putative dopamine neurons in the VTA and SN respond to aversive or stressful events [53, 68]). A particularly clean test of this thesis was conducted by Zink and colleagues [55], who showed that BOLD responses in the ventral striatum are equal for salient, non-rewarding events and rewarding events.

The problem with using fMRI in this manner hinges on the distant relationship between dopamine activity and measured BOLD signal. In particular, it is reasonable to expect that dopamine release in the striatum may produce a measurable response, but it is also reasonable to expect that any of the myriad other striatal afferents may also produce a response. The majority of dopamine terminals are in the striatum, but the ventral striatum is also densely innervated by other monoaminergic systems, including the raphe serotonin input and locus coeruleus noradrenergic input. The striatum also has dense glutamatergic inputs from the cortex, thalamus, and elsewhere. In sum, it is reasonable to expect that dopamine activity may produce a striatum BOLD response, but it is unreasonable to make any conclusions about dopamine activity solely on the basis of a BOLD signal. There may be other sources of the signal that are wholly independent of the dopamine systems and the production or reward prediction error signals. Even a lack of signal does not indicate a lack of dopaminergic activity; inhibition of other signal sources may balance signal increases from dopamine neurons. In the case of responses to salient events, norepinephrine is known to respond to these signals and would be expected to produce signals in the striatum such as those recorded [56]. Additionally, more recent work in rodents has shown that dopamine neurons do not respond to aversive events [57]. Instead, another population of neurons, known as tertiary cells [58], in the VTA and SN that are not dopaminergic seems to respond to these events.

So what does this mean for the value of computational neuroimaging? If fMRI can only be used to show commonalities between animal studies and human reward learning, then it is severely limited in its utility. There are several rejoinders to this dilemma.

First, it is probably the case that the questions for which fMRI is an appropriate measurement technique may be only a subset of those related to reinforcement learning. However, the set is certainly not empty. One theory about dopamine function is that is does not relate to reward value in an absolute manner, but instead is modulated by reward value relative to a running average of earned reward. That is, responses to a reward of some magnitude should be small when rewards have been coming at a high rate relative to when they have been scarce. For this problem, fMRI has proven extremely useful [25]. BOLD signals can be made equivalent for winning a sizeable amount of money and earning nothing simply by changing the context of rewards in the experiment [24]. The critical difference for this experiment compared to those related to salience is that this study did not attempt to establish the domain over which prediction error signals apply. Instead, it aimed to establish parameters that govern reinforcement learning. This is still a rich and important domain for understanding human reinforcement learning.

Second, the relationship between a BOLD signal and underlying dopamine signaling may be strengthened with pharmacological manipulations. A recent study by Pessiglione et al. [59] demonstrated that dopamine antagonists both inhibit learning and abolish striatal BOLD responses. If salience-related responses in the striatum were caused by a different neural system than dopamine, then this method would have revealed this.

Third, and related to the previous point, PET scanning may be a very important parallel tool to accompany fMRI. PET has several limitations that have made fMRI the preferred methodology overall for cognitive neuroscience. Most important of these are spatial and temporal resolution. However, PET offers the ability to target specific neurotransmitter systems, including dopamine [60]. One powerful approach may be to conduct an fMRI study while running a second group of participants with PET imaging. Results showing a signal restricted to the striatum, VMPFC, and OFC that supports a particular theory could then be strengthened by a parallel demonstration that dopamine is released as predicted during the task (albeit with coarser spatiotemporal filtering).

Finally, fMRI studies may be redirected at a different anatomical target than the striatum and VMPFC. Recording directly from dopaminergic nuclei in the midbrain would enable direct measurement of the signals that govern the activity of dopamine neurons. The VTA and SN are much more uniform in function than the striatum, even with the tertiary cells mentioned above. BOLD signals in the VTA and SN are still not direct measurements of dopamine function, but they would be a much more precise an indicator of dopamine function than recording in the striatum and PFC.

10.2.3   Direct measurement in the human VTA

As desirable as recording directly from dopamine nuclei is, the technical challenges to acquiring them are equally strong. The brainstem is a very inhospitable environment from the standpoint of fMRI. There are large arteries and draining veins that lie adjacent to the ventral midbrain, where dopamine nuclei are located. Cardiac activity causes large pulsations in these arteries, leading to movement on the order of the resolution of scanning. This is particularly problematic since the brainstem is composed of numerous small nuclei; the VTA is only roughly $3 \times 3\,mm^2$ in an axial plane (Fig. 10.4A), so that movement on the order of a couple of millimeters can easily cause the VTA to move in and out of a recording location.

The best method to account for these motion artifacts is to acquire images at a regular time within the cardiac cycle. The midbrain will still move substantially, but structures will remain at a constant location in each functional scan. To achieve this, a pulse oximeter gates BOLD image acquisition. Since the time between heartbeats is also variable, functional images are most reliable when they are fully acquired in the time between beats. This, of course, means that there is very little time available to acquire individual functional scans (less than a second unless the human participant is in excellent shape), which limits the spatial extent of scans to roughly the height of the midbrain for high resolution images.

With cardiac gating, the remaining technical challenge is to visualize the VTA and SN. There is little variation in T1 relaxation times across midbrain nuclei, so standard T1-weighted anatomical images used in fMRI are ineffective for identifying the VTA or SN. Other pulse sequences create the desired contrast, including proton density-weighted images (Fig. 10.4A; [61]). Finally, a new brainstem normalization algorithm must be used to allow direct comparison of data across subjects [62]. With all of these techniques, strong, spatially specific BOLD responses can be found in the VTA to reward prediction errors.

D'Ardenne et al. [63] conducted two studies using these methodologies. First, they implemented a design that closely approximates Hollerman and Schultz [5] and McClure

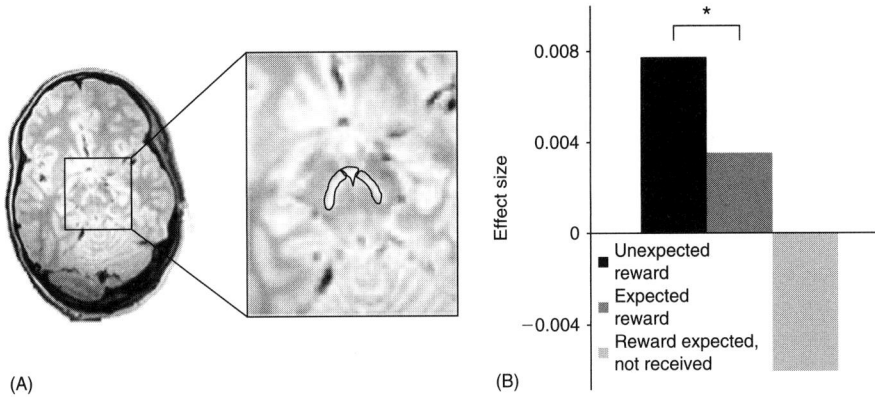

Figure 10.4 BOLD responses in human VTA. (A) The SN and VTA are clearly visible in proton density images. They are outlined in black with the SN flanking the VTA that is located on the midline. (B) Focused recording from the midbrain allows for the identification of both positive and negative prediction errors in the VTA. *Source*: Adapted from D'Ardenne et al. (2008) [63].

et al. [64]. Participants were trained to expect liquid rewards at fixed times (6 s) following visual cues. Delayed reward activity then produced a positive prediction error at the time of reward delivery. A negative prediction error observed in the ventral putamen (cf. Fig. 10.3), but did not replicate in the midbrain. There was a trend for a negative going signal following the omission of expected reward (Fig. 10.4B), but this was not significant.

A second experiment supported the finding that negative prediction errors do not produce appreciable signal changes in the VTA. Participants performed a simple guessing task in which a number between 0 and 10 was presented and they had to guess whether a second number from the same range would be greater or less than the first number (they were never equal). Correct guesses were rewarded with $1 and incorrect guesses resulted in the loss of $1. Since the first number determines the probability of winning (50% for "5" and greater probability for numbers away from 5), reward prediction errors can be estimated for each trial. The VTA was found to correlate directly with this signal when only winning outcomes were included in the analysis. Losses did not elicit responses in the VTA. These findings are consistent with the finding that dopamine neurons do not emit phasic responses to aversive events [57]. Additionally, it indicates that dopaminergic signals scale with the probability of the outcome at the level of the VTA, contrary to other findings [46], but again consistent with dopamine neuron recordings [67]. Finally, and most importantly for the current discussion, these findings indicate that BOLD imaging is sufficiently precise to allow for targeted imaging, even from small structures in inhospitable environments. Signals from these regions scale as predicted by computational models, indicating that fMRI is a powerful method for tracking individual computational processes in the brain.

10.3 Conclusions

Various neuroimaging methods have been used to test computational models of brain function. However, not until the advent of fMRI have these methods offered the spatiotemporal resolution necessary to measure at the level of specific neural structures. The method is not perfect: The spatiotemporal resolution is reasonable for some purposes, but is crude from the perspective of individual neurons. Additionally, the sources of the BOLD signal are only imprecisely known, and so there is reason for concern about what the recording may actually mean. Nevertheless, BOLD responses do scale with neural activity to a reasonable approximation, and, despite reasonable lingering skepticism, the method has proven amazingly powerful. This is particularly apparent for the example experiment that courses through this chapter. When reward delivery is delayed in a conditioning experiment, reward prediction errors may be estimated computationally. This signal is apparent in dopamine neurons [5], BOLD signals in dopamine target regions [43,64], and in BOLD responses in midbrain dopamine nuclei [63]. Moving beyond this, fMRI has already contributed to extending models of reinforcement learning in people [25]. With a critical eye toward what may be concluded on the basis of BOLD responses, we feel that the future is bright for computational neuroimaging with fMRI.

References

[1] E.L. Thorndike, Animal Intelligence, The Macmillan Company, New York, 1911.

[2] R.A. Rescorla, A.R. Wagner, A theory of Pavlovian conditioning: variations in the effectiveness of reinforcement and nonreinforcement, in: A.H. Black, W.F. Prokasy (Eds.), Classical Conditioning II: Current Research and Theory, Appleton-Century-Crofts, 1972.

[3] R.R. Miller, R.C. Barnet, N.J. Grahame, Assessment of the Rescorla-Wagner model, Psychol. Bull. 117 (1995) 363–386.

[4] W.X. Pan, R. Schmidt, J.R. Wickens, B.I. Hyland, Dopamine cells respond to predicted events during classical conditioning: evidence for eligibility traces in the reward-learning network, J. Neurosci. 25 (2005) 6235–6242.

[5] J.R. Hollerman, W. Schultz, Dopamine neurons report an error in the temporal prediction of reward during learning, Nat. Neurosci. 1 (1998) 304–309.

[6] P.R. Montague, P. Dayan, T.J. Sejnowski, A framework for mesencephalic dopamine systems based on predictive Hebbian learning, J. Neurosci. 16 (1996) 1936–1947.

[7] C.D. Fiorillo, P.N. Tobler, W. Schultz, Discrete coding of reward probability and uncertainty by dopamine neurons, Science 299 (2003) 1898–1902.

[8] Y. Niv, M.O. Duff, P. Dayan, Dopamine, uncertainty and TD learning, Behav. Brain Funct. 1 (2005) 6.

[9] N.D. Daw, J.P. O'Doherty, P. Dayan, B. Seymour, R.J. Dolan, Cortical substrates for exploratory decisions in humans, Nature 441 (2006) 876–879.

[10] W. Schultz, Responses of midbrain dopamine neurons to behavioral trigger stimuli in the monkey, J. Neurophysiol. 56 (1986) 1439–1461.

[11] R. Romo, W. Schultz, Dopamine neurons of the monkey midbrain: contingencies of responses to active touch during self-initiated arm movements, J. Neurophysiol. 63 (1990) 592–606.

[12] J. Mirenowicz, W. Schultz, Importance of unpredictability for reward responses in primate dopamine neurons, J. Neurophysiol. 72 (1994) 1024–1027.

[13] P. Waelti, A. Dickinson, W. Schultz, Dopamine responses comply with basic assumptions of formal learning theory, Nature 412 (2001) 43–48.

[14] S. Kobayashi, W. Schultz, Influence of reward delays on responses of dopamine neurons, J. Neurosci. 28 (2008) 7837–7846.

[15] J.N. Reynolds, B.I. Hyland, J.R. Wickens, A cellular mechanism of reward-related learning, Nature 413 (2001) 67–70.

[16] O. Hikosaka, Y. Takikawa, R. Kawagoe, Role of the basal ganglia in the control of purposive saccadic eye movements, Physiol. Rev. 80 (2000) 953–978.

[17] K. Doya, Metalearning and neuromodulation, Neural Netw. 15 (2002) 495–506.

[18] R.S. Sutton, A.G. Barto, Reinforcement Learning, MIT Press, Cambridge, MA, 1998.

[19] G. Morris, A. Nevet, D. Arkadir, E. Vaadia, H. Bergman, Midbrain dopamine neurons encode decisions for future action, Nat. Neurosci. 9 (2006) 1057–1063.

[20] M.R. Roesch, D.J. Calu, G. Schoenbaum, Dopamine neurons encode the better option in rats deciding between differently delayed or sized rewards, Nat. Neurosci. 10 (2007) 1615–1624.

[21] N.D. Daw, D.S. Touretzky, Long-term reward prediction in TD models of the dopamine system, Neural Comput. 14 (2002) 2567–2583.

[22] N.D. Daw, S. Kakade, P. Dayan, Opponent interactions between serotonin and dopamine, Neural Netw. 15 (2002) 603–616.

[23] Schwartz, A. (1993). A reinforcement learning method for maximizing undiscounted rewards. In proceedings of the Tenth International Conference on Machine Learning, San Mateo, CA.

[24] S. Nieuwenhuis, D.J. Heslenfeld, N.J. von Geusau, R.B. Mars, C.B. Holroyd, N. Yeung, Activity in human reward-sensitive brain areas is strongly context dependent, Neuroimage 25 (2005) 1302–1309.

[25] B. Seymour, S.M. McClure, Anchors, scales and the relative coding of value in the brain, Curr. Opin. Neurobiol. 18 (2008) 173–178.

[26] C.B. Holroyd, M.G. Coles, The neural basis of human error processing: reinforcement learning, dopamine, and the error-related negativity, Psychol. Rev. 109 (2002) 679–709.

[27] N. Yeung, M.M. Botvinick, J.D. Cohen, The neural basis of error detection: conflict monitoring and the error-related negativity, Psychol. Rev. 111 (2004) 931–959.

[28] W.H. Miltner, C.H. Baum, M.G. Coles, Event-related potentials following incorrect feedback in a time-estimation task: evidence for a generic neural system for error detection, J. Cogn. Neurosci. 9 (1997) 788–798.

[29] M.J. Koepp, R.N. Gunn, A.D. Lawrence, V.J. Cunningham, A. Dagher, T. Jones, D.J. Brooks, C.J. Bench, P.M. Grasby, Evidence for striatal dopamine release during a video game, Nature 393 (1998) 266–268.

[30] Z.F. Mainen, T.J. Sejnowski, Reliability of spike timing in neocortical neurons, Science 268 (1995) 1503–1506.

[31] F. Theunissen, J.P. Miller, Temporal encoding in nervous systems: a rigorous definition, J. Comput. Neurosci. 2 (1995) 149–162.

[32] S.M. McClure, D.I. Laibson, G. Loewenstein, J.D. Cohen, Separate neural systems value immediate and delayed monetary rewards, Science 306 (2004) 503–507.

[33] S. Ogawa, T.M. Lee, A.R. Kay, D.W. Tank, Brain magnetic resonance imaging with contrast dependent on blood oxygenation, Proc. Natl. Acad. Sci. USA 87 (1990) 9868–9872.

[34] S. Ogawa, T.M. Lee, A.S. Nayak, P. Glynn, Oxygenation-sensitive contrast in magnetic resonance image of rodent brain at high magnetic fields, Magn. Reson. Med. 14 (1990) 68–78.

[35] N.K. Logothetis, J. Pauls, M. Augath, T. Trinath, A. Oeltermann, Neurophysiological investigation of the basis of the fMRI signal, Nature 412 (2001) 150–157.

[36] A. Viswanathan, R.D. Freeman, Neurometabolic coupling in cerebral cortex reflects synaptic more than spiking activity, Nat. Neurosci. 10 (2007) 1308–1312.

[37] N.K. Logothetis, What we can do and what we cannot do with fMRI, Nature 453 (2008) 869–878.

[38] S.A. Huettel, Non-linearities in the blood-oxygenation-level dependent (BOLD) response measured by functional magnetic resonance imaging (fMRI), Conf. Proc. IEEE. Eng. Med. Biol. Soc. 6 (2004) 4413–4416.

[39] C. Padoa-Schioppa, J.A. Assad, Neurons in the orbitofrontal cortex encode economic value, Nature 441 (2006) 223–226.

[40] C.C. Lapish, S. Kroener, D. Durstewitz, A. Lavin, J.K. Seamans, The ability of the mesocortical dopamine system to operate in distinct temporal modes, Psychopharmacology (Berl) 191 (2007) 609–625.

[41] N.K. Logothetis, B.A. Wandell, Interpreting the BOLD signal, Annu. Rev. Physiol. 66 (2004) 735–769.

[42] F.M. Zhou, C.J. Wilson, J.A. Dani, Cholinergic interneuron characteristics and nicotinic properties in the striatum, J. Neurobiol. 53 (2002) 590–605.

[43] J.P. O'Doherty, P. Dayan, K. Friston, H. Critchley, R.J. Dolan, Temporal difference models and reward-related learning in the human brain, Neuron 38 (2003) 329–337.

[44] A.N. Hampton, R. Adolphs, M.J. Tyszka, J.P. O'Doherty, Contributions of the amygdala to reward expectancy and choice signals in human prefrontal cortex, Neuron 55 (2007) 545–555.

[45] A.N. Hampton, P. Bossaerts, J.P. O'Doherty, The role of the ventromedial prefrontal cortex in abstract state-based inference during decision making in humans, J. Neurosci. 26 (2006) 8360–8367.

[46] B. Knutson, J. Taylor, M. Kaufman, R. Peterson, G. Glover, Distributed neural representation of expected value, J. Neurosci. 25 (2005) 4806–4812.

[47] T.A. Hare, J. O'Doherty, C.F. Camerer, W. Schultz, A. Rangel, Dissociating the role of the orbitofrontal cortex and the striatum in the computation of goal values and prediction errors, J. Neurosci. 28 (2008) 5623–5630.

[48] G.S. Berns, S.M. McClure, G. Pagnoni, P.R. Montague, Predictability modulates human brain response to reward, J. Neurosci. 21 (2001) 2793–2798.

[49] J. O'Doherty, P. Dayan, J. Schultz, R. Deichmann, K. Friston, R.J. Dolan, Dissociable roles of ventral and dorsal striatum in instrumental conditioning, Science 304 (2004) 452–454.

[50] B. Seymour, J.P. O'Doherty, P. Dayan, M. Koltzenburg, A.K. Jones, R.J. Dolan, K.J. Friston, R.S. Frackowiak, Temporal difference models describe higher-order learning in humans, Nature 429 (2004) 664–667.

[51] J. Reuter, T. Raedler, M. Rose, I. Hand, J. Glascher, C. Buchel, Pathological gambling is linked to reduced activation of the mesolimbic reward system, Nat. Neurosci. 8 (2005) 147–148.

[52] J.C. Horvitz, Mesolimbocortical and nigrostriatal dopamine responses to salient non-reward events, Neuroscience 96 (2000) 651–656.

[53] P. Redgrave, T.J. Prescott, K. Gurney, Is the short-latency dopamine response too short to signal reward error? Trends Neurosci. 22 (1999) 146–151.

[54] K.C. Berridge, T.E. Robinson, Parsing reward, Trends Neurosci. 26 (2003) 507–513.

[55] C.F. Zink, G. Pagnoni, M.E. Martin, M. Dhamala, G.S. Berns, Human striatal response to salient nonrewarding stimuli, J. Neurosci. 23 (2003) 8092–8097.

[56] G. Aston-Jones, J.D. Cohen, Adaptive gain and the role of the locus coeruleus-norepinephrine system in optimal performance, J. Comp. Neurol. 493 (2005) 99–110.

[57] M.A. Ungless, P.J. Magill, J.P. Bolam, Uniform inhibition of dopamine neurons in the ventral tegmental area by aversive stimuli, Science 303 (2004) 2040–2042.

[58] D.L. Cameron, M.W. Wessendorf, J.T. Williams, A subset of ventral tegmental area neurons is inhibited by dopamine, 5-hydroxytryptamine and opioids, Neuroscience 77 (1997) 155–166.

[59] M. Pessiglione, B. Seymour, G. Flandin, R.J. Dolan, C.D. Frith, Dopamine-dependent prediction errors underpin reward-seeking behaviour in humans, Nature 442 (2006) 1042–1045.

[60] N.D. Volkow, G.J. Wang, J.S. Fowler, J. Logan, D. Schlyer, R. Hitzemann, J. Lieberman, B. Angrist, N. Pappas, R. MacGregor, et al. Imaging endogenous dopamine competition with [11C]raclopride in the human brain, Synapse 16 (1994) 255–262.

[61] H. Oikawa, M. Sasaki, Y. Tamakawa, S. Ehara, K. Tohyama, The substantia nigra in Parkinson disease: proton density-weighted spin-echo and fast short inversion time inversion-recovery MR findings, AJNR. Am. J. Neuroradiol. 23 (2002) 1747–1756.

[62] V. Napadow, R. Dhond, D. Kennedy, K.K. Hui, N. Makris, Automated Brainstem Co-registration (ABC) for MRI, Neuroimage 32 (2006) 1113–1119.

[63] K. D'Ardenne, S.M. McClure, L.E. Nystrom, J.D. Cohen, BOLD responses reflecting dopaminergic signals in the human ventral tegmental area, Science 319 (2008) 1264–1267.

[64] S.M. McClure, G.S. Berns, P.R. Montague, Temporal prediction errors in a passive learning task activate human striatum, Neuron 38 (2003) 339–346.

[65] D. Attwell, C. Iadecola, The neural basis of functional brain imaging signals, Trends Neurosci. 25 (2002) 621–625.

[66] A.N. McCoy, J.C. Crowley, G. Haghighian, H.L. Dean, M.L. Platt, Saccade reward signals in posterior cingulated cortex, Neuron 40 (5) (2003) 1031–1040.

[67] U.S. Bhalla, R. Iyengar, Emergent properties of networks of biological signaling pathways, Science 283 (5400) (1999) 381–387.

[68] J. Mirenowicz, W. Schultz, Preferential activation of dopamine neurons by appetitive rather than aversive stimuli, Nature 379 (6564) (1996) 449–451.

Part Three

Brain Disorders Involving Dysfunctions of Reward and Decision Making Processes

11 Can models of reinforcement learning help us to understand symptoms of schizophrenia?

G.K. Murray and P.C. Fletcher

Department of Psychiatry, Box 189, University of Cambridge, Addenbrooke's Hospital, Cambridge CB2 2QQ, United Kingdom

Abstract

We aim to show that the principles and empirical observations relating to reward and reinforcement learning may be useful in considering schizophrenia. Though this is a complex illness in which the primary symptoms are expressed in terms of bizarre beliefs and perceptions, there is reason to suppose that the underlying deficits reside in brain systems known to be linked to learning, reward, and motivational processes.

We consider two very different symptoms that are characteristic of schizophrenia. The first, delusions, refers to apparently irrational beliefs that arise and are held with extraordinary tenacity in the face of contradictory evidence. There is emerging evidence that such beliefs emerge due to abnormal associative processes perhaps arising as a consequence of disturbed dopaminergic function. The second symptom, anhedonia, refers to the apparent lack of enjoyment in life. In fact, there is now good evidence that anhedonia may relate more to a motivation deficit and, as such, can be considered in the context of the same system as that implicated in delusions.

We highlight the evidence in favour of these perspectives, showing that reinforcement learning may be key to understanding schizophrenia.

Key points

1. Schizophrenia is a chronic and disabling illness characterized by positive symptoms (including the bizarre and frightening beliefs termed delusions) and negative symptoms (including a flattening of responses and an apparent lack of motivation towards goals and rewards, often termed anhedonia).

2. While the illness is not conventionally diagnosed or conceptualized in terms of reward or reinforcement learning, there is growing work suggesting that this area may provide a useful framework for understanding schizophrenia.

3. As a starting point, there is good circumstantial evidence that the brain systems implicated by neuroscientific studies in reinforcement learning overlap with those implicated by clinical studies in schizophrenia.

4. We review more direct evidence, focusing on dopamine, reward learning, and prediction error, suggesting the reinforcement learning system shows evidence of disruption in schizophrenia.

5. Finally, we consider whether this framework may help us to link the underlying physiological changes that accompany the illness to the specific symptoms that characterize it.

11.1 Introduction

Schizophrenia can be a profoundly disabling condition. It is more common than many people think, having an estimated lifetime prevalence of 0.7–1% [1]. It might seem rather odd to include a consideration of schizophrenia in a book such as this one because the condition has not traditionally been linked directly to reward processing. In the main [2], it is defined and diagnosed according to the presence of certain experiences such as hallucinations (perceptions in the absence of stimuli; e.g., the sufferer may hear voices talking critically about him) and delusions (bizarre beliefs; e.g., he may come to believe that he is the victim of intrigue and conspiracy, even to the extent that his life is in danger). It is also accompanied by so-called negative symptoms, which are essentially defined by the absence of desirable functions or behaviors. For example, thinking may be disturbed and disorganized, making communication very difficult. Motivation may be markedly reduced and the sufferer may become isolated and withdrawn. Furthermore, one of the key negative symptoms refers to a reduction in enjoyment (anhedonia). Thus, while the diagnostic process does not invoke notions of disordered reward processing directly, nor is a consideration of reward-processing explicitly within the compass of standard treatments, there are nevertheless a number of aspects of psychopathology in schizophrenia that can fruitfully be considered within the framework of reward and reinforcement learning developed elsewhere in this book. Moreover, given extensive evidence from molecular imaging studies implicating dysregulated striatal dopamine in schizophrenia and other psychoses, combined with the evidence linking striatal dopamine to reinforcement learning and motivation, there are reasons, beyond descriptive considerations of the signs and symptoms, for suggesting that reinforcement learning is worth scrutinizing in psychosis.

We aim to show here that the principles and insights that have emerged from considerations of reward processing in animals and humans may be very important in coming to understand schizophrenia. We will illustrate this with respect to one characteristic positive symptom (delusional beliefs) and one negative symptom (anhedonia). We will begin by reviewing the history of empirical and theoretical observations of reward processing in schizophrenia before relating this to current neuroscientific insights into the brain and the possible neurochemical bases for such processing. We will consider how these observations relate to neurochemically based explanations of schizophrenia, specifically those invoking disruptions of dopaminergic and glutameteric circuitry, together with the possibility that the illness may arise from an impaired interaction between these two systems. We will then develop ideas of how disruptions in reward processing may provide an explanation for delusional beliefs and for anhedonia.

11.2 Theories of altered reward processing in schizophrenia

While, as we have noted above, the traditional conceptualization of schizophrenia has not focused primarily on reward or reinforcement learning, in fact, both motivational deficits and dysfunction of associative learning (closely related to reinforcement learning) were proposed in schizophrenia long before the discovery of dopamine. For example,

Bleuler described avolition and loosening of associations (due to a failure of any unifying concept of purpose or goal) as core features of schizophrenia [3].

Robbins proposed reinforcement learning abnormalities in schizophrenia when he drew parallels between stereotyped behaviors in stimulant-treated rats and schizophrenic stereotyped patterns of thought and behavior [4]. He argued that stereotypy-inducing properties of stimulants were related to their reinforcement enhancing properties, and argued the case for such stimulant-induced behavior as a model for psychotic illness. In the same year, 1976, Miller proposed that dopamine disruption in the striatum could lead to abnormal associative learning processes, which in turn could lead to psychotic symptoms. Miller considered early evidence suggesting that recognition of the association of related features in the environment by humans and animals occurred in the basal ganglia by a dopamine-dependent process. Furthermore, he argued that basal ganglia dopamine overactivity in schizophrenia could lead the lowering of the required threshold for acceptance of conclusions [5]. This is eminiscent of more recent arguments that schizophrenia patients "jump to conclusions" in probabilistic reasoning tasks [6]. Over the course of the 1970s, 1980s, and 1990s, in a series of theoretical articles, Miller developed his theory of the dopaminergic basis of positive psychotic symptoms acting via disruption of mesostriatal reward learning processes, in order to address specific psychotic and manic symptoms, and developments in the understanding of different dopamine receptors classes [7–10].

Meanwhile, Gray, Hemsley, and colleagues were working on a related theory, one that focused more directly on associative aspects of learning rather than on the rewarding and motivational aspects [11–14]. Gray drew on emerging evidence from studies of experimental animals that interactions between the hippocampus and the meso-accumbens pathway are critical in allowing organisms to ignore irrelevant stimuli. While the importance of mismatches ("prediction error"; see [15]) between expectation and outcome has now been recognized in work on associative and reinforcement learning, this was not a component explicitly recognized in the models of Gray and his colleagues. However, in emphasizing the likelihood of a central dopamine-dependent cognitive disturbance in psychosis and in considering how this could contribute to a failure in "the integration of past regularities of experience with current stimulus recognition, learning and action," they clearly posited a model which might now be discussed in terms of a disruption in prediction error signaling.

Gray and Hemsley focused particularly on the classical behavioral associative learning paradigms of latent inhibition [16] and Kamin blocking [17]. They proposed that "Disruption of LI or KB would have the effect that, in accounting for the occurrence of a significant event (a US [unconditioned stimulus]), a schizophrenia patient would be likely to attribute causal efficacy to stimuli that normal individuals would ignore, either because they were familiar and had previously occurred without being followed by a significant event, or because the event was already predicted by other associations" [14]. One of the very attractive features of Gray's model, particularly to those who feel frustrated by the fact that a number of models of psychosis are very narrow in their focus, is that it encompassed four levels of explanation – neuroanatomy, chemistry, cognitive process, and symptoms. This is an important attribute in generating hypotheses that are testable and in providing an explanation that bridges the gaps between the physiological and the mental. Indeed, it foreshadows the development of cognitive neuropsychiatry, which adheres to this principle [18,19] and which has flourished in the last two decades.

The important work of these researchers sets the background for a number of fruitful avenues of research. Common to these developments is the drive to appeal to advances in cognitive neuroscience of learning and reward-processing in order to inspire and constrain theories of schizophrenia. Later in this chapter, we will consider the importance of these developments with regard to delusions and anhedonia, but it is worth noting at this stage that one very good example of this approach was exemplified by the work of Shitij Kapur [20], who drew on contemporary models of reward processing [21] to propose an influential model of how the bizarre beliefs that characterize schizophrenia might be considered in terms of disrupted incentive salience. We return to this below but first make some relevant background observations.

11.3   Dopamine, schizophrenia, and reinforcement learning

Subcortical monoamine function is important in both motivation and learning of goal-directed associations [22,23]. Perhaps dysfunction of this system could explain certain features of schizophrenia. It was previously thought that noradrenaline was the key neurotransmitter mediating these reward-related processes, and Stein and Wise were, as far as we are aware, the first to propose that damage to the noradrenergic reward system could explain the core symptoms of schizophrenia together with its progressive and worsening course [24]. However, as evidence has subsequently demonstrated the importance of another monoamine transmitter, dopamine, as opposed to noradrenaline, in reward processing, and as there is extensive evidence implicating dopamine dysfunction in schizophrenia, then the ascending dopamine system is a much more promising candidate. We now briefly and selectively review the extensive, and sometimes contradictory, literature on dopamine dysfunction in schizophrenia.

There is good evidence that a change in dopamine regulation explains, at least in part, the clinical picture associated with schizophrenia. Drugs that upregulate dopamine function (such as amphetamines, which enhance the release of dopamine and block its reuptake and breakdown) can lead to delusions and hallucinations in apparently healthy people. It seems likely that it is the dopaminergic effects of amphetamines that produce these symptoms because, in animals, the key effects of amphetamine administration (hyperactivity followed by stereotypy) are also produced by pure dopamine agonists. Furthermore, pure dopamine agonists in humans (e.g., L-dopa treatment in Parkinson's disease) can produce psychosis. On the other hand, drugs that block dopamine (as is the case with all established antipsychotic drugs) can dampen and remove the symptoms [25]. Furthermore, Creese et al. (1976) [94] and Seeman and colleagues [26,27] showed a very strong correlation (0.9) between the typical daily dose used to treat psychosis and the dose required to block a dopamine agonist (that is, drugs that need a large dose to block the dopamine agonists also require a large dose to produce an antipsychotic effect). While there is a clear correlation between a drug's antipsychotic dose and its dopamine-blocking properties, no such relationship exists with its serotonin-, noradrenaline-, or histamine-blocking properties. Also relevant is that the antipsychotic drug Flupenthixol has two forms; the alpha-isomer (which blocks dopamine) produces a significantly better reduction in the symptoms of schizophrenia than does the beta-isomer (which does not block dopamine) [28].

These observations have led to the dopamine hypothesis of schizophrenia, which, simply stated, is that schizophrenia is caused by upregulation of dopamine. The dopamine hypothesis has been one of the major route maps in guiding research into schizophrenia and has engendered many experiments and observations. Unfortunately, the direct evidence in favor of the hypothesis is difficult to collect and does not lead to straightforward conclusions. A review of this evidence goes beyond the scope of the current paper but is very well reviewed by McKenna [29], by Abi-Dargham [30,31], by Guillin et al. [32], and by Toda and Abi-Dargham [33]. It does seem that there is little in the way of direct evidence for increased levels of dopamine or its metabolites. An alternative view, that the upregulation is caused not by increased levels of the neurotransmitter but by increased sensitivity of the receptors, also lacks clear support. With the advent of positron emission tomography (PET), the possibility has arrived of *in vivo* measures of D2 receptor binding. Of the two main initial studies, however, one [34] showed evidence that D2 receptor density was greater in schizophrenia; the other [35] did not. Laruelle and colleagues [36] review imaging evidence and report an approach capitalizing on competition between injected radiotracers and endogenous transmitters. This is done through amphetamine administration, which leads to dopamine release, leading to displacement of binding potential of a radiotracer ($[^{123}I]$iodobenzamide [IBZM] or $[^{11}C]$Raclopride) binding to D_2 receptors. Using this approach, they showed a more than twofold increase in dopamine response to amphetamine in patients with schizophrenia, suggesting increased dopamine release in this group. Although abnormalities of presynaptic dopamine function have now been confirmed by several research teams, using various radioligands to assess differing stages of presynaptic dopamine pathways, nevertheless, in each study, while there have been group differences between patients and controls, the overlap with the measurements in the healthy population suggests that whatever is abnormal about dopamine in schizophrenia, it is not straightforward.

11.4   The possible importance of glutamate

It is generally accepted that the symptoms of schizophrenia are unlikely to be explained by a single neurotransmitter deficit. Attention has also focused on glutamate, the major excitatory transmitter of the brain [37,38]. When we block glutamatergic action through one of its key receptors – the NMDA receptor – we can produce in healthy subjects a set of symptoms that resemble schizophrenia [39] and, in patients, a worsening of the particular symptoms that tend to trouble them most when they are ill. The effects of NMDA blockade have been observed in recreational users of phencyclidine ("PCP" or "angel dust") and in people who have received the dissociative anesthetic ketamine. Such observations have been important in the emergence of the NMDA receptor hypofunction model of schizophrenia [40].

There are clear interactions between glutamate (via NMDA) and dopamine systems. Laruelle [36] proposes that glutamate exerts dual NMDA-dependent control of mesocortical and mesolimbic dopamine firing. This consists of an "Activating System" involving direct stimulation of dopamine neurons projecting from the ventral tegmental area (VTA) back to cortex together with bisynaptic stimulation of dopamine neurons projecting from VTA to the ventral striatum (projecting to ventral striatum). It is complemented by a "brake system" in which glutamatergic stimulation of GABAergic inhibitory interneurons or GABA striatotegmental neurons produces an overall inhibitory effect on mesolimbic dopamine. In short, there appears to be a state of glutamate-dopamine balance. One can imagine that disruptions in this balance may lead to dysregulated mesocortical and mesolimbic dopamine firing and may appreciably reduce information flow between cortex and subcortical structures. Again, this is likely to be a simplistic model but one worth exploring. For example, administration of ketamine does indeed upregulate dopamine [41]. A fuller model recognizes that dopamine neurons modulate the NMDA effects on GABAergic neurons (as in the "brake system" alluded to above) and that this modulation differs for D1 and D2 receptors. Thus, D1 facilitates NMDA transmission on GABAergic neurons. D2, on the other hand, has an inhibitory effect. Laruelle points out that this has connotations for both the pathophysiology and the treatment of schizophrenia. Excess D2 receptor stimulation in schizophrenia would inhibit glutamate participation in the ventral striatal "brake system." If glutamate function is already reduced, excess D2 activity would worsen this situation. Together, these two factors would appreciably reduce information flow between cortex and subcortical structures.

In short, a working hypothesis at present is that schizophrenia symptoms emerge from perturbed interaction between glutamatergic and dopaminergic systems. However, as has been compellingly argued [18], the extent to which this observation constitutes an explanation for the condition itself is questionable. After all, a person with schizophrenia expresses the signs and symptoms of his illness at a complex level, a level that feels far removed from neurochemistry. How does increased dopamine produce a strange belief? Why might life feel flat and unexciting as a consequence of the sorts of neurochemical perturbations described above? We believe that both of these apparently disparate phenomena may be understood in terms of reward/reinforcement learning. The growing understanding of the role of these two key neurotransmitter systems – dopaminergic and glutamatergic – in reinforcement learning may provide us with a firmer footing on which to base our cognitive understanding of the symptoms of schizophrenia. In the following sections we try to show how this may be so by considering these two apparently disparate symptoms of the disease – anhedonia and delusions-and by examining the emerging evidence that they could arise from deficits in the brain systems underpinning reinforcement learning. We begin by considering the evidence for a reinforcement processing deficit in schizophrenia before speculating on how the presence of such a deficit might help to explain the emergence and nature of these symptoms.

11.5 Studies of reward processing/reinforcement learning in psychosis: behavioral studies

We now review evidence for whether there are reinforcement learning deficits in psychotic illness. One of the main challenges in answering this question is the lack of available behavioral measures to assess reward processing and incentive motivational processes in humans; the consequence has been that, to date, such processes have only been addressed indirectly in behavioral studies. Patients with schizophrenia display a range of abnormalities of classic associative learning phenomena, including Kamin blocking and latent inhibition [14,42], and these abnormalities are responsive to short-term neuroleptic treatment, which would be consistent with a dopaminergic mechanism. In addition, reward-based decision-making on the Iowa Gambling Test (IGT) has been shown to be impaired in psychosis [43], and this effect also is sensitive to medication status [44]. However, there have been some failures to replicate the case-control difference [45], and it should be remembered the IGT requires several cognitive processes in addition to reward sensitivity.

Generally, in the 1980s and 1990s, the cognitive focus in studies of schizophrenia tended toward processes such as attention, executive function, and memory, while the study of reward processing and motivation was relatively neglected. However, before this, in the 1950s and 1960s, a considerable number of studies examined the effects of either reward or punishment on patients with schizophrenia; however, the focus of these studies was rather different from studies in the modern era. As reviewed by Buss and Lang [46], an important question at the time was whether what today we would call cognitive deficits (or neuropsychological or neurocognitive deficits) in schizophrenia were purely the results of motivational deficits such that patients failed to engage with the experimenter, and therefore any impairments in performance in comparison to a control group could be attributed to the motivational state of patients as opposed to reflecting genuine impairments in functioning. In order to examine this question, a number of studies were conducted by various authors, in which, for example, reaction times were measured without reinforcement. In contrast, reaction time

(RT) performance did improve after electric shock [48]. In a study that could be considered an early fore-runner of work [49] examining sensitivity to positive and negative reinforcement, Garmezy [50] showed that schizophrenia patients were differentially sensitive to verbal punishment (WRONG) and reward (RIGHT). In fact, Skinner himself, together with Ogden Lindsley, conducted conditioning experiments in patients with psychosis over a number of years [51,52]. Then the effect of adding reinforcement, either positive or negative verbal reinforcement, or typically, electric shock, white noise, or money was examined. It should be remembered that these studies were conducted in the era prior to the use of modern diagnostic criteria. For example, Topping and O'Connor [47] found that whilst healthy controls improved on a "serial anticipation task," patients with paranoid schizophrenia worsened and other patients with schizophrenia were unchanged in performance.

More recently, Cutmore and Beninger [53] studied avoidance learning in 20 outpatients with schizophrenia using a paradigm in which participants had to learn to control their rates of button presses to avoid financial punishments. They showed that neuroleptic-treated patients with schizophrenia made fewer correct avoidance responses in comparison to control subjects, though this finding is hard to interpret as neuroleptic-treated healthy controls have also been shown (in a separate study) to make fewer correct responses on the same task. The authors performed a further experiment in another sample of patients with schizophrenia (26 inpatients, 24 of whom were taking dopamine receptor antagonists) and argued that medication may have played a role in the impaired performance of patients, as prolactin levels (prolactin levels are raised by dopamine blockage) explained a significant proportion of patients' variance in performance.

In recent years, Gold and colleagues have been at the forefront of behavioral studies of reward processing in schizophrenia. They have focused on studies of patients with chronic schizophrenia, almost all of whom are taking antipsychotic medication, and attempted to link behavioral deficits in reward processing to negative symptoms. A recent review of Gold's work describes eight studies in this area and concludes that patients do show deficits in rapid learning on the basis of trial to trial feedback, as shown by tasks such as reversal learning [54,55]. This is consistent with previous studies of such learning in schizophrenia [56,57], and with a recent study of our own, using a comparable manipulation, in first-episode psychosis. We observed that in early psychosis, deficits were subtle and modestly correlated with negative symptoms [58]. Perhaps surprisingly, Gold's studies do point to evidence of comparatively intact sensitivity to reward, but document impairments in decision-making in relation to attainment of reward [55,59–60]. We also consider this work in relation to anhedonia below. Gold and colleagues conclude that the deficits that they have observed cannot solely account for the presence of motivational problems and other negative symptoms in their patient groups [55]. One limitation of these studies in patients with chronic schizophrenia is that nearly all the patients are taking antipsychotic medication, and such dopamine antagonist medication has been shown to affect reward processing in healthy volunteers [61,62]. Another recent study of ours showed a failure to modulate behavior in response to a motivational manipulation in patients with first-episode psychosis [63]. Importantly, when we carried out an analysis restricted to a subset of patients – those free from dopamine antagonist medication – the deficits was still observed.

11.6   Studies of reward processing/reinforcement learning in psychosis: neuroimaging studies

As noted above, one of the difficulties in studying reward processing in humans has been the difficulty of finding appropriate behavioral tests with which to investigate the processes

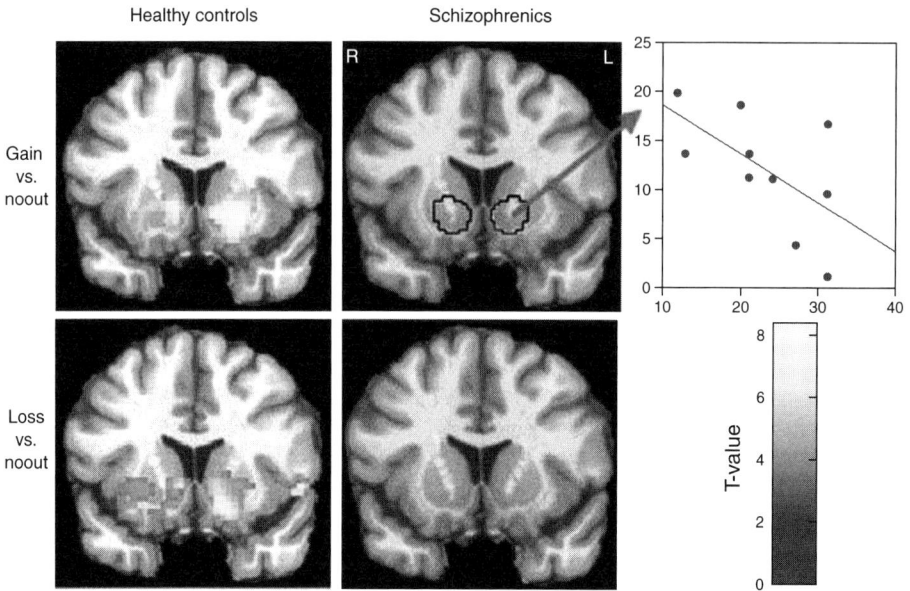

Figure 11.1 Ventral striatal activations in controls and patients performing a reward-processing task. As can be seen, there is reduced ventral striatal response in patients. The graph shows that the degree of reduction across patients is predictive of negative symptoms. See Plate 14 of Color Plate section. *Source*: Taken from Juckel et al. (2006) [64].

that are subtle and often indirectly expressed in terms of attendant behavior. To a large extent, the advent of functional neuroimaging has reinvigorated this area of research. This is partly because the dependent measure, brain activation, may under certain circumstances offer a more sensitive and specific index reward-related processing, and of learning, than behavioral measures. The first functional magnetic resonance imaging (fMRI) study of reward processing in a psychotic disorder came from Juckel et al., who examined 14 unmedicated schizophrenia patients as they performed the Monetary Incentive Delay Task, which, in controls, produces robust ventral striatal activation in the anticipation of reward (when compared to the anticipation of neural feedback). As shown in Fig. 11.1, patients recruited ventral striatum to a significantly smaller extent than did controls, and this failure correlated moderately and significantly with negative symptoms, and moderately but nonsignificantly with positive symptoms [64]. The same group have gone on to show that this difference is partially normalized by adding olanzapine [65,66]. This could explain why Abler and colleagues, who used a different reward processing task, showed that schizophrenia patients taking atypical antipsychotic medication had striatal activations in anticipation of reward that could not be differentiated from controls. The picture is made more complicated and intriguing by the fact that manic patients taking antipsychotic medication did show abnormal striatal activations compared with controls [67].

In a recent fMRI study of reward learning, we showed that brain responses correlating with reward prediction error in the dopaminergic midbrain and in striatal and limbic regions, which are, of course, key targets for dopaminergic projections from this area. In addition, cortical regions such as the dorsolateral prefrontal cortex were abnormal in patients with active psychotic symptoms [68]. Although some patients in the study were taking dopamine receptor antagonist medication, some were not, and the results held in the unmedicated patients, showing that the results could not solely be explained by medication effects. These results are consistent with other studies using different psychological paradigms. Using a largely overlapping sample of patients, we examined causal learning, as opposed to reward learning, in early psychosis, and found abnormal activation in a network of midbrain, striatal, and frontal regions [42]. Interestingly, the severity of the dysfunction of activation in the lateral prefrontal cortex correlated with the severity of delusions. Jensen and colleagues [69] employed an aversive conditioning paradigm, using an unpleasantly loud noise as the unconditioned stimulus. They observed abnormal activation in the ventral striatum in schizophrenia patients, together with a difficulty, as indicated by behavioral measures, in discriminating between motivational salient and neutral stimuli. Specifically, patients activated the ventral striatum more toward neutral (motivationally irrelevant) stimuli than healthy controls.

Taken together, these imaging and behavioral studies provide preliminary evidence for physiological abnormalities in learning about and anticipating rewards and punishments in psychotic illness. This appears to be accompanied by an impaired ability to modulate behavior in response to incentives.

11.7 Can an understanding of reward and dopamine help us to understand symptoms of schizophrenia?

11.7.1 Delusions

Above, we have summarized evidence that reward and reinforcement processing are abnormal in psychosis, perhaps secondary to dopamine, and/or glutamate, dysfunction, which appears to be linked to a network of subcortical (midbrain, striatum, and hippocampus/amygdala) and cortical dysfunction. Here we consider more specifically whether such deficits may relate to, and perhaps explain, one of the key symptoms of schizophrenia: delusions. It is clinically very important to think about whether such abnormalities account for any aspects of patients' mental experience or behavior outside the research laboratory. Patients with psychotic illnesses do not present to their doctor for the first time and complain that their dopamine or glutamate neurotransmitter systems, or indeed their reinforcement learning systems, are dysfunctional. More common is to describe unusual experiences or beliefs, which tend to be accompanied by varying levels of insight. In addition, there is often a decline in occupational, educational, or social function. Thus, the encounter between a patient and a clinician very directly prompts the question of how disturbances at a physiological level relate to disturbances in the mental experience of the patient. This question is important philosophically and scientifically, but also is of very direct relevance to health care, if a mental experience is to be treated with a pharmacological (or, indeed, any other) intervention. As discussed earlier, the first scientist to make the case clearly and repeatedly for relating the emergence of psychotic symptoms to dopamine driven associative and reinforcement learning was Robert Miller. In his 1976 article he wrote [5]:

> *The process of acquiring the associations necessary for learning a conditioned response in an experimental animal depends on the presence of dopamine. In*

> *human schizophrenic patients, an excessive supply of cerebral dopamine may facil-*
> *itate the acquisition of associations between "units of information," to the point*
> *where unrelated features are associated and treated as if they are meaningful com-*
> *binations: this process can be terminated by administering dopamine antagonists.*

Miller's proposition, which has gathered widespread interest in recent years, remains speculative as opposed to definitive, but at the very least it is compatible with subjective reports from patients. One of a number of patients interviewed by McGhie [70] stated, "I had very little ability to sort the relevant from the irrelevant – completely unrelated events became intricately connected in my mind." Similarly, another patient, quoted by Mattusek [71], recounted the experience as follows: "One is much clearer about the relatedness of things, because one can overlook the factuality of things." Another is quoted by Mattusek as reporting: "out of these perceptions came the absolute awareness that my abilities to see connections had been multiplied many times over."

In regard to these quotations, it is well recognized that in many cases, a period of psychosis is preceded by a prodromal period, also known as a pre-delusional state, delusional mood, or delusional atmosphere, in which an individual experiences changes to their thought processes and emotions, but is not frankly ill [72]. A person developing a psychotic illness may feel suspicious, may have a sense that the world is changing in subtle but important ways, or may think he or she is on the verge of making a critically important breakthrough or insight. Such a patient may be feeling a new awareness of such subtleties (a patient previously cared for by one of the authors of this chapter used to refer to his very specific and personal experience of the world, and of detecting subtle changes that others couldn't, as "The Sensitivity"). In these early stages in the development of a psychotic illness, patients frequently experience abnormal thoughts – for example, that a neighbor or the police might be monitoring their behavior – but this thought may initially be no more than a suspicion and is not firmly or completely held. Additionally or alternatively, they may have a sense of seeing the world in a new way, and observing that what appear to be innocuous events actually may have some other hidden but important meaning. As Kurt Schneider [93] stated, "often in these vague delusional moods, perceptions gain this sense of significance not yet defined." For example, one of the patients quoted by Mattusek (above) also stated:

> *At ordinary times I might have taken pleasure in watching the dog, but [previously]*
> *would never have been so captivated by it.*

Such experiences, in the early phase of a disorder, of seeing connections or reading possible meanings into innocuous events, do not represent psychosis but have been termed psychosis-like experiences, or attenuated psychotic symptoms. A parsimonious explanation of the physiology of the early psychotic experience is that it will be closely related, though perhaps of less severity than, the physiology of frank psychosis. Indeed, very recent evidence suggests that patients with such attenuated symptoms, termed an at-risk mental state, do indeed have dopaminergic abnormalities in the striatum similar to patients with established illness, as detected by *in vivo* molecular imaging [73].

In the absence of a firm understanding of how delusions relate to any putative underlying physiological disturbance, it may be easier to conceptualize, at least initially, how physiological abnormalities could lead to the very early, mild symptoms. Indeed, one possibility is that it is a clearer relationship between neurochemical and neurophysiological dysfunction and these initial symptoms than between chronic delusions and the underlying physiological state. After all, a chronic delusion is a belief that has been firmly held for a long time. The delusion may have been *formed* in the context of a profound physiological disturbance, but it is surely possible that it could, like other beliefs, persist long after the physiological (or psychological) precipitants have subsided or faded. An account of the emergence of psychosis appealing to the dysfunction of reinforcement and associative learning can be outlined as follows. Excessive or dysregulated dopamine transmission, where bursts of dopamine release, for example (irrespective of the etiology of the release of dopamine), coincide with unrelated thoughts or perceptions, may result in the coinciding thoughts or perceptions being invested with a sense of value, importance, and association. Extending this idea, and relating it to contemporary view of dopamine's role in normal psychological function, Shitij Kapur [20] appealed to Berridge and Robinson's [21] concept of incentive, or motivational, salience, to explain why an objectively irrelevant experience could, in the mind of a patient with a disturbed dopamine system, become seen as being of the utmost significance. Recall that incentive salience, which is mediated by dopamine, is, according to Berridge and Robinson, that property of an event, object, or thought that captures attention and drives goal-directed behavior because of associations with reward (or punishment). Such feelings of significance in an unusual context would be very likely to preoccupy the mind of the person experiencing them, and would naturally be subjected to a good deal of reflection and possibly rumination. Thus, the speculation that the early symptoms of referential ideas and delusional atmosphere could emerge secondary to or through abnormalities in reward and motivational processing does seem plausible.

The next stage in the argument requires an understanding of how, in time, an unusual thought or experience may become or give rise to an unshakeable false belief – a delusion. How could this happen? Two possibilities have been presented [74]. Under one account, if an experience is unusual enough, then by the exercise of normal reasoning processes, the protagonist may arrive at a delusional belief in order to resolve the uncertainties raised by the unusual and perplexing experiences. This is sometimes known as a "one-stage theory," as it requires only one abnormality – abnormal experience. For example, the experience of hearing a voice in the third person commenting upon one's actions could be explained by the idea that a radio transmitter has been implanted in one's brain or inner ear, and that the voices are radio broadcasts being picked up by such a transmitter. Here, after seeing connections in many events for prolonged periods, eventually a patient may propose a unifying theory to explain a host of otherwise puzzling phenomena. Once an explanation has been reached, it is rewarding to the patient, as it provides relief from anxiety and perplexity [75].

Under an alternative "two-stage" account, an additional "lesion" is required: abnormal reasoning. Proponents of the latter model argue that even if one is subjected to very unusual experiences, such as auditory hallucination, such experiences could be understood in an insightful manner – for example, as being evidence of illness – or one could simply refrain from making any inferences from unusual experiences (and thus, perhaps, remain in a prodromal state without moving to a psychotic state) and that to jump to the conclusion that a transmitter had been implanted in one's brain must indicate a massive failure in the normal process of evaluating evidence to arrive at such a far-fetched belief. Indeed, there is some evidence, though as yet not conclusive, that patients with delusions do jump to conclusions on the basis of little evidence [6,76–78].

One further, though yet preliminary view, is put forward by Fletcher and Frith [92]. Drawing on Bayesian accounts of perception and experience, they suggest that it may be possible to account for the bizarre perceptions, experiences, and beliefs that characterize schizophrenia without the requirement for positing more than one type of disruption. Rather, we can consider our models and inferences about the world in terms of a hierarchy of inferences such that failures of inference at lower levels engender prediction errors which are fed forward and demand inferences at higher levels in order to cope with new or unexpected information. According to this view, a persistent deficit in prediction error-related signaling could lead to the requirement for ever higher and more radical changes in inference, leading to both bizarre experiences when expressed lower in the hierarchy and apparently irrational beliefs at the higher levels.

11.7.2 Anhedonia

The term anhedonia has been used in a number of ways and its use is by no means confined to schizophrenia. Indeed, it is probably more thought of in the context of depressive illness. We should remember, however, that it may affect between one-third and one-half of people with schizophrenia [79]. The term was coined by Ribot [80] (see William James's "The Sick Soul" for a discussion), who saw anhedonia as a decreased capacity for pleasure in a way that is analogous to the decreased capacity for feeling that is found in analgesia. James was graphic in his description of the condition, thinking of it as *passive joylessness and dreariness, discouragement, dejection, lack of taste and zest and spring*. A number of demographic observations with respect to the occurrence of anhedonia in schizophrenia have been made and are worth briefly recounting here. First, it tends to predominate in older patients, where the condition is more long-standing [81,82]. Shoichet and Oakley [83] suggested that it occurs at the early stages, perhaps being progressive, and may also associate with a poor overall prognosis. In an important study, Katsanis et al. [84] used the Chapman anhedonia scale [85] to evaluate patients with schizophrenia, their first-degree relatives, and control subjects. The patients scored more strongly on both social (e.g., "I attach very little importance to having close friends," "There are few things more tiring than to have a long, personal discussion with someone") and physical (e.g., "I have seldom enjoyed any kind of sexual experience," "One food tastes as good as another to me") anhedonia than did relatives or controls. Some would tend to group anhedonia with the negative symptoms of schizophrenia (social withdrawal, apathy, self-neglect), but there is some evidence [79] that the condition dissociates from other negative symptoms. Romney and Candido [86] used a factor analysis in people with schizophrenia and observed that anhedonia, which emerged as trait- rather than state-like, loaded more heavily on depression than other symptoms (positive or negative), although there was a correlation between anhedonia and the negative symptoms of social and emotional withdrawal. In keeping with this, Berenbaum and Oltmanns [87] showed that, in particular, patients who have the so-called blunted affect (i.e., not apparently expressing emotion) showed anhedonia compared to controls. They suggested that we should be wary of confusing anhedonia with emotional blunting, concluding that "Anhedonia is best thought of as a characteristic of depression, whereas affective blunting which encompasses anhedonia is a typical feature of the negative deficit syndrome in schizophrenia."

Clearly, the picture is a confusing one and, added to this, it is worth noting that nowadays the vast majority of people diagnosed with schizophrenia are, or have been, on antipsychotic medicines that have anti-dopaminergic action. The extent to which anhedonia arises from the treatment as opposed to the condition is not clear.

Attempts to understand the underlying causes or mechanisms of anhedonia have had to contend with the fact that it is a somewhat nebulous concept with a usage that can refer to a number of signs and behaviors in patients. Silver and Shlomo [88] have questioned the generally held notion that anhedonia is fundamentally a lack of, or an inability to obtain, pleasure or enjoyment. Using the Snaith Hamilton Pleasure Scale (SHAPS) in patients with schizophrenia, they observed first that about 41% of patients scored normally and, importantly, while there was a moderate positive correlation with negative symptoms (though the mean levels of negative symptoms did not significantly differ between those people with anhedonia and those without), the actual subjective measure scores for lack of enjoyment were less than would be predicted from observations of patients' apparent states of enjoyment and pleasure. In short, it may be that there is an appearance of anhedonia in schizophrenia but that this does not match the subjective state. This is in keeping with the work of Iwase et al. [89] suggesting that patients experience more pleasure in a rewarding stimulus than is shown by their facial expression. Both studies relate to the conclusions of Berenbaum and Oltmanns [87] noted above.

Specifically, it seems that while, when it comes to ostensibly rewarding stimuli, people with anhedonia may not appear so motivated to obtain them and may not show marked signs of their enjoyment, such evidence as there is does not point strongly toward a true reduction in actual enjoyment. At this stage, therefore, it may well be helpful to appeal to the more refined models of reward learning and processing that have emerged from the field of experimental and theoretical neuroscience, just as we have discussed in relation to delusions above. Specifically, there is an important distinction between the anticipation and the consummation of reward (for a discussion of this field, see [90]). Given that dopaminergic function (in particular, that of mesolimbic dopaminergic circuitry) may be important in the anticipation of reward, and perhaps in engendering the motivation for reward and in selecting the actions that may be necessary to attain it, and given the studies cited above, it is worth scrutinizing the possibility that anhedonia in schizophrenia represents a deficit in the anticipation of, and quest for, reward rather than in the pleasure that rewards bring. As we see below, there is some empirical evidence in favor of this.

An important recent observation came from Gard et al. [91], who explicitly distinguished between anticipatory and consummatory pleasure in an elegant study evaluating how people with schizophrenia both predict the future experience of pleasure and enjoy this anticipation. In an initial study, they used an experience-sampling technique in which patients carried a pager and notebook. When paged, they wrote down what they were doing and rated how pleasurable it was. They also noted whether they were anticipating any forthcoming pleasure. The results of this study are shown in Fig. 11.2; they indicate no difference between patients and controls in consummatory pleasure but a clear reduction in anticipatory pleasure. There was also evidence that they tended to be less likely to be engaged in a goal-directed activity at any time. In a complementary experiment, they found comparable results using a scale that measures experience of pleasure more specifically. Their conclusion that anhedonia is actually a failure to anticipate pleasure was supported by the observation that Chapman ratings of anhedonia significantly correlated (negatively) with anticipatory but not consummatory pleasure.

Of course, the anticipation of an event may be useful insofar as it could be important in motivating the behaviors that lead to, or maximize the possibility of, the attainment of that reward. Heerey and Gold [59] showed corroborative evidence that such schizophrenia patients show a mismatch between what they report and how they behave. They used a task in which subjects were able to prolong or decrease exposure, or alter the future likelihood of exposure, to affective slides. While the patients showed the same degree of affective ratings as controls, they did not turn this into actions.

Finally, while there has not been a functional imaging literature that relates directly and primarily to anhedonia in schizophrenia, we believe that observations of disruption in (predominantly dopaminergic) brain systems known to be related to prediction error, reward and learning discussed above (particularly those of Juckel et al. [64,65]) may

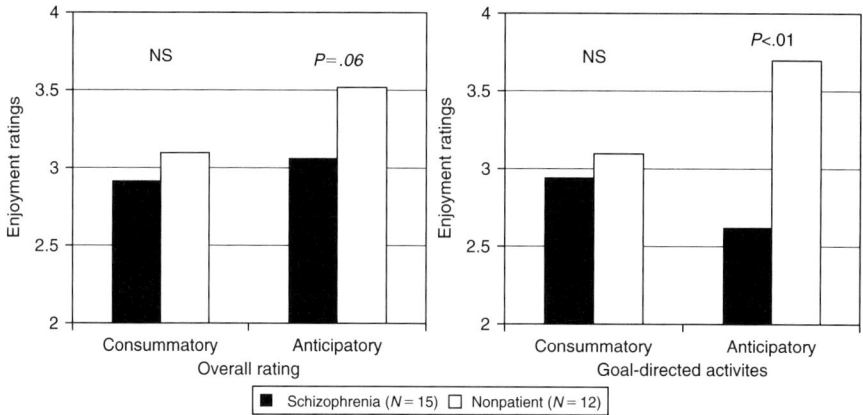

Figure 11.2 Recording so "Consummatory" and "Anticipatory" pleasure for both general and goal-directed activities in patients with schizophrenia and in controls. As can be seen, patients seem to show comparable degrees of consummatory pleasure but less anticipatory pleasure. *Source*: Taken from Gard et al. (2007) [91].

provide important clues that there is a change in motivational function in schizophrenia and that this, coupled with the behavioral observations described above, should lead us to consider anhedonia within the framework of reinforcement learning.

11. 8   Summary

While schizophrenia is not conventionally considered in terms of reward and reinforcement learning, we believe that there are very good grounds for maintaining and adding to the body of work that has brought models of associative learning and rewards processing to psychiatric models of the illness. This is especially relevant now given the advances in our neuroscientific understanding of reward learning and motivation and the consequent development of elegant models of how such processes might be invoked to explain symptoms of schizophrenia [20].

We have tried to show that, given the clear implications of mesolimbic circuitry in particular, the dopaminergic system (and its interactions with the glutamate system) in schizophrenia, are *prima facie* good grounds for supposing that the processes in which this system is most firmly implicated – the learning about and attainment of rewards – are abnormal in schizophrenia. As we have seen, a growing body of empirical evidence supports this possibility.

Furthermore, a consideration of such processes provides a very useful framework in which to consider the emergence of specific symptoms of schizophrenia: notably delusions (one of the key positive symptoms) and anhedonia (a key negative symptom). Once again, the emergent literature suggests that such a framework may be fruitful in linking the symptoms of the illness to the underlying physiological disturbances and, in doing so, helping to bridge the explanatory gap that greatly limits our ability to explain and treat schizophrenia.

Acknowledgements

P.C. Fletcher is supported by the Bernard Wolfe Health Neuroscience Fund and by the Wellcome Trust. G.K. Murray is supported by the Medical Research Council.

References

[1] J. McGrath, S. Saha, D. Chant, J. Welham, Schizophrenia: a concise overview of incidence, prevalence, and mortality, Epidemiol. Rev. (2008).

[2] APA, Diagnostic and Statistical Manual of Mental Disorder-IV, American Psychiatric Association, Washington, DC, 1994.

[3] E. Bleuler, Dementia Praecox or the Group of Schizophrenias, International University Press, New York, 1911/1950.

[4] T.W. Robbins, Relationship between reward-enhancing and stereotypical effects of psychomotor stimulant drugs, Nature 264 (5581) (1976) 57–59.

[5] R. Miller, Schizophrenic psychology, associative learning and the role of forebrain dopamine, Med. Hypotheses 2 (5) (1976) 203–211.

[6] P.A. Garety, D.R. Hemsley, S. Wessely, Reasoning in deluded schizophrenic and paranoid patients: biases in performance on a probabilistic inference task, J. Nerv. Ment. Dis. 179 (4) (1991) 194–201.

[7] R. Miller, Major psychosis and dopamine: controversial features and some suggestions, Psychol. Med. 14 (4) (1984) 779–789.

[8] R. Miller, The time course of neuroleptic therapy for psychosis: role of learning processes and implications for concepts of psychotic illness, Psychopharmacology (Berl) 92 (4) (1987) 405–415.

[9] R. Miller, Striatal dopamine in reward and attention: a system for understanding the symptomatology of acute schizophrenia and mania, Int. Rev. Neurobiol. 35 (1993) 161–278.

[10] G. Chouinard, R. Miller, A rating scale for psychotic symptoms (RSPS): part II: subscale 2: distraction symptoms (catatonia and passivity experiences); subscale 3: delusions and semi-structured interview (SSCI-RSPS), Schizophr. Res. 38 (2–3) (1999) 123–150.

[11] J.A. Gray, J. Feldon, J.N.P. Rawlins, A.D. Smith, The neuropsychology of schizophrenia, Behav. Brain Sci. 14 (1) (1991) 1–19.

[12] J.A. Gray, M.H. Joseph, D.R. Hemsley, A.M. Young, E.C. Warburton, P. Boulenguez, G.A. Grigoryan, S.L. Peters, J.N. Rawlins, C.T. Taib, et al., The role of mesolimbic dopaminergic and retrohippocampal afferents to the nucleus accumbens in latent inhibition: implications for schizophrenia, Behav. Brain Res. 71 (1–2) (1995) 19–31.

[13] J.A. Gray, Dopamine release in the nucleus accumbens: the perspective from aberrations of consciousness in schizophrenia, Neuropsychologia 33 (9) (1995) 1143–1153.

[14] J.A. Gray, Integrating schizophrenia, Schizophr. Bull. 24 (2) (1998) 249–266.

[15] W. Schultz, A. Dickinson, Neuronal coding of prediction errors, Annu. Rev. Neurosci. 23 (2000) 473–500.

[16] R.E. Lubow, Latent inhibition: effects of frequency of nonreinforced preexposure of the CS, J. Comp. Physiol. Psychol. 60 (3) (1965) 454–457.

[17] L.J. Kamin, 'Attention-like' processes in classical conditioning, in: M.R. Jones (Ed.), Miami Symposium on the Prediction of Behavior, 1967: Aversive Stimulation, University of Miami Press, Coral Gables, FL, 1968, pp. 9–31.

[18] C.D. Frith, The Cognitive Neuropsychology of Schizophrenia, Taylor and Francis, Hove, 1992.

[19] A.S. David, A method for studies of madness, Cortex 42 (6) (2006) 921–925.

[20] S. Kapur, Psychosis as a state of aberrant salience: a framework linking biology, phenomenology, and pharmacology in schizophrenia, Am. J. Psychiatry 160 (1) (2003) 13–23.

[21] K.C. Berridge, T.E. Robinson, What is the role of dopamine in reward: hedonic impact, reward learning, or incentive salience? Brain Res. Brain Res. Rev. 28 (3) (1998) 309–369.

[22] L. Stein, Self-stimulation of the brain and the central stimulant action of amphetamine, Fed. Proc. 23 (1964) 836–850.

[23] T.J. Crow, Catecholamine-containing neurones and electrical self-stimulation. 2. A theoretical interpretation and some psychiatric implications, Psychol. Med. 3 (1) (1973) 66–73.

[24] L. Stein, C.D. Wise, Possible etiology of schizophrenia: progressive damage to the noradrenergic reward system by 6-hydroxydopamine, Science 171 (975) (1971) 1032–1036.

[25] S. Kapur, G. Remington, Dopamine D(2) receptors and their role in atypical antipsychotic action: still necessary and may even be sufficient, Biol. Psychiatry 50 (11) (2001) 873–883.

[26] P. Seeman, T. Lee, Antipsychotic drugs: direct correlation between clinical potency and presynaptic action on dopamine neurons, Science 188 (4194) (1975) 1217–1219.

[27] P. Seeman, T. Lee, M. Chau-Wong, K. Wong, Antipsychotic drug doses and neuroleptic/dopamine receptors, Nature 261 (5562) (1976) 717–719.

[28] E.C. Johnstone, T.J. Crow, C.D. Frith, M.W. Carney, J.S. Price, Mechanism of the antipsychotic effect in the treatment of acute schizophrenia, Lancet 1 (8069) (1978) 848–851.

[29] P.J. McKenna, Schizophrenia and Related Syndromes, second ed., Routledge, London, 2007.

[30] A. Abi-Dargham, Do we still believe in the dopamine hypothesis? New data bring new evidence, Int. J. Neuropsychopharmacol. 7 (Suppl 1) (2004) S1–S5.

[31] A. Abi-Dargham, The dopamine hypothesis of schizophrenia, retrieved 14 October 2008 from www.schizophreniaforum.org/for/curr/AbiDargham/default.asp.

[32] O. Guillin, A. Abi-Dargham, M. Laruelle, Neurobiology of dopamine in schizophrenia, Int. Rev. Neurobiol. 78 (2007) 1–39.

[33] M. Toda, A. Abi-Dargham, Dopamine hypothesis of schizophrenia: making sense of it all, Curr. Psychiatry Rep. 9 (4) (2007) 329–336.

[34] D.F. Wong, H.N. Wagner Jr., L.E. Tune, R.F. Dannals, G.D. Pearlson, J.M. Links, C.A. Tamminga, E.P. Broussolle, H.T. Ravert, A.A. Wilson, J.K. Toung, J. Malat, J.A. Williams, L.A. O'Tuama, S.H. Snyder, M.J. Kuhar, A. Gjedde, Positron emission tomography reveals elevated D2 dopamine receptors in drug-naive schizophrenics, Science 234 (4783) (1986) 1558–1563.

[35] L. Farde, F.A. Wiesel, H. Hall, C. Halldin, S. Stone-Elander, G. Sedvall, No D2 receptor increase in PET study of schizophrenia, Arch. Gen. Psychiatry 44 (7) (1987) 671–672.

[36] M. Laruelle, L.S. Kegeles, A. Abi-Dargham, Glutamate, dopamine, and schizophrenia: from pathophysiology to treatment, Ann. NY Acad. Sci. 1003 (2003) 138–158.

[37] J.S. Kim, H.H. Kornhuber, W. Schmid-Burgk, B. Holzmuller, Low cerebrospinal fluid glutamate in schizophrenic patients and a new hypothesis on schizophrenia, Neurosci. Lett. 20 (3) (1980) 379–382.

[38] J.M. Stone, P.D. Morrison, L.S. Pilowsky, Glutamate and dopamine dysregulation in schizophrenia – a synthesis and selective review, J. Psychopharmacol. 21 (4) (2007) 440–452.

[39] E. Pomarol-Clotet, G.D. Honey, G.K. Murray, P.R. Corlett, A.R. Absalom, M. Lee, P.J. McKenna, E.T. Bullmore, P.C. Fletcher, Psychological effects of ketamine in healthy volunteers: phenomenological study, Br. J. Psychiatry 189 (2006) 173–179.

[40] J.H. Krystal, E.B. Perry Jr., R. Gueorguieva, A. Belger, S.H. Madonick, A. Abi-Dargham, T.B. Cooper, L. Macdougall, W. Abi-Saab, D.C. D'Souza, Comparative and interactive human psychopharmacologic effects of ketamine and amphetamine: implications for glutamatergic and dopaminergic model psychoses and cognitive function, Arch. Gen. Psychiatry 62 (9) (2005) 985–994.

[41] L.S. Kegeles, A. Abi-Dargham, Y. Zea-Ponce, J. Rodenhiser-Hill, J.J. Mann, R.L. Van Heertum, T.B. Cooper, A. Carlsson, M. Laruelle, Modulation of amphetamine-induced striatal dopamine release by ketamine in humans: implications for schizophrenia, Biol. Psychiatry 48 (7) (2000) 627–640.

[42] P.R. Corlett, G.K. Murray, G.D. Honey, M.R. Aitken, D.R. Shanks, T.W. Robbins, E.T. Bullmore, A. Dickinson, P.C. Fletcher, Disrupted prediction-error signal in psychosis: evidence for an associative account of delusions, Brain 130 (Pt 9) (2007) 2387–2400.

[43] L.M. Ritter, J.H. Meador-Woodruff, G.W. Dalack, Neurocognitive measures of prefrontal cortical dysfunction in schizophrenia, Schizophr. Res. 68 (1) (2004) 65–73.

[44] R.J. Beninger, J. Wasserman, K. Zanibbi, D. Charbonneau, J. Mangels, B.V. Beninger, Typical and atypical antipsychotic medications differentially affect two nondeclarative memory tasks in schizophrenic patients: a double dissociation, Schizophr. Res. 61 (2–3) (2003) 281–292.

[45] R. Cavallaro, P. Cavedini, P. Mistretta, T. Bassi, S.M. Angelone, A. Ubbiali, L. Bellodi, Basal-corticofrontal circuits in schizophrenia and obsessive-compulsive disorder: a controlled, double dissociation study, Biol. Psychiatry 54 (4) (2003) 437–443.

[46] A.H. Buss, P.J. Lang, Psychological deficit in schizophrenia: I. Affect, reinforcement, and concept attainment, J. Abnorm. Psychol. 70 (1965) 2–24.

[47] G.G. Topping, N. O'Connor, The response of chronic schizophrenics to incentives, Br. J. Med. Psychol. 33 (1960) 211–214.

[48] G. Rosenbaum, W.R. Mackavey, J.L. Grisell, Effects of biological and social motivation on schizophrenic reaction time, J. Abnorm. Psychol. 54 (3) (1957) 364–368.

[49] J.A. Waltz, M.J. Frank, B.M. Robinson, J.M. Gold, Selective reinforcement learning deficits in schizophrenia support predictions from computational models of striatal-cortical dysfunction, Biol. Psychiatry 62 (7) (2007) 756–764.

[50] N. Garmezy, Stimulus differentiation by schizophrenic and normal subjects under conditions of reward and punishment, J. Pers. 20 (3) (1952) 253–276.

[51] O.R. Lindsley, B.F. Skinner, A method for the experimental analysis of the behavior of psychotic patients, Am. Psychol. 9 (1954) 419–420.

[52] O.R. Lindsley, Operant conditioning methods applied to research in chronic schizophrenia, Psychiatr. Res. Rep. Am. Psychiatr. Assoc. 5 (1956) 118–139, discussion, 140–153.

[53] T.R. Cutmore, R.J. Beninger, Do neuroleptics impair learning in schizophrenic patients?, Schizophr. Res. 3 (3) (1990) 173–186.

[54] J.A. Waltz, J.M. Gold, Probabilistic reversal learning impairments in schizophrenia: further evidence of orbitofrontal dysfunction, Schizophr. Res. 93 (1–3) (2007) 296–303.

[55] J.M. Gold, J.A. Waltz, K.J. Prentice, S.E. Morris, E.A. Heerey, Reward processing in schizophrenia: a deficit in the representation of value, Schizophr. Bull. (2008).

[56] R. Elliott, P.J. McKenna, T.W. Robbins, B.J. Sahakian, Neuropsychological evidence for fronto-striatal dysfunction in schizophrenia, Psychol. Med. 25 (3) (1995) 619–630.

[57] C. Pantelis, T.R. Barnes, H.E. Nelson, S. Tanner, L. Weatherley, A.M. Owen, T.W. Robbins, Frontal-striatal cognitive deficits in patients with chronic schizophrenia, Brain 120 (Pt 10) (1997) 1823–1843.

[58] G.K. Murray, F. Cheng, L. Clark, J.H. Barnett, A.D. Blackwell, P.C. Fletcher, T.W. Robbins, E.T. Bullmore, P.B. Jones, Reinforcement and reversal learning in first-episode psychosis, Schizophr. Bull. (2008).

[59] E.A. Heerey, J.M. Gold, Patients with schizophrenia demonstrate dissociation between affective experience and motivated behavior, J. Abnorm. Psychol. 116 (2) (2007) 268–278.

[60] E.A. Heerey, K.R. Bell-Warren, J.M. Gold, Decision-making impairments in the context of intact reward sensitivity in schizophrenia, Biol. Psychiatry 64 (1) (2008) 62–69.

[61] M. Pessiglione, B. Seymour, G. Flandin, R.J. Dolan, C.D. Frith, Dopamine-dependent prediction errors underpin reward-seeking behaviour in humans, Nature 442 (7106) (2006) 1042–1045.

[62] B. Abler, S. Erk, H. Walter, Human reward system activation is modulated by a single dose of olanzapine in healthy subjects in an event-related, double-blind, placebo-controlled fMRI study, Psychopharmacology (Berl) 191 (3) (2007) 823–833.

[63] G.K. Murray, L. Clark, P.R. Corlett, A.D. Blackwell, R. Cools, P.B. Jones, T.W. Robbins, L. Poustka, Incentive motivation in first-episode psychosis: a behavioural study, BMC Psychiatry 8 (2008) 34.

[64] G. Juckel, F. Schlagenhauf, M. Koslowski, T. Wustenberg, A. Villringer, B. Knutson, J. Wrase, A. Heinz, Dysfunction of ventral striatal reward prediction in schizophrenia, Neuroimage 29 (2) (2006) 409–416.

[65] G. Juckel, F. Schlagenhauf, M. Koslowski, D. Filonov, T. Wustenberg, A. Villringer, B. Knutson, T. Kienast, J. Gallinat, J. Wrase, A. Heinz, Dysfunction of ventral striatal reward prediction in schizophrenic patients treated with typical, not atypical, neuroleptics, Psychopharmacology (Berl) 187 (2) (2006) 222–228.

[66] F. Schlagenhauf, G. Juckel, M. Koslowski, T. Kahnt, B. Knutson, T. Dembler, T. Kienast, J. Gallinat, J. Wrase, A. Heinz, Reward system activation in schizophrenic patients switched from typical neuroleptics to olanzapine, Psychopharmacology (Berl) 196 (4) (2008) 673–684.

[67] B. Abler, I. Greenhouse, D. Ongur, H. Walter, S. Heckers, Abnormal reward system activation in mania, Neuropsychopharmacology 33 (9) (2008) 2217–2227.

[68] G.K. Murray, P.R. Corlett, L. Clark, M. Pessiglione, A.D. Blackwell, G. Honey, P.B. Jones, E. T. Bullmore, T.W. Robbins, P.C. Fletcher, Substantia nigra/ventral tegmental reward prediction error disruption in psychosis, Mol. Psychiatry 13 (3) (2008) 239, 267–276.

[69] J. Jensen, M. Willeit, R.B. Zipursky, I. Savina, A.J. Smith, M. Menon, A.P. Crawley, S. Kapur, The formation of abnormal associations in schizophrenia: neural and behavioral evidence, Neuropsychopharmacology 33 (3) (2008) 473–479.

[70] A. McGhie, Attention and perception in schizophrenia, Prog. Exp. Pers. Res. 5 (1970) 1–35.

[71] P. Mattusek, Studies in delusional perception, Archiv für Psychiatrie und Zeitschrift Neurologie 189 (1987) 279–318 (1952). The clinical roots of the schizophrenia concept. J. Cutting and M. Shepherd. Cambridge, Cambridge University Press: 96.

[72] G.E. Berrios, The History of Mental Symptoms: Descriptive Psychopathology since the Nineteenth Century, Cambridge University Press, Cambridge, 1996.

[73] O.D. Howes, A.J. Montgomery, M. Asselin, R.M. Murray, P.M. Grasby, P.K. McGuire, Pre-synaptic striatal dopamine synthesis capacity in subjects at risk of psychosis, Schizophr. Bull. 33 (2) (2007) 371.

[74] R. Langdon, M. Coltheart, The cognitive neuropsychology of delusions, Mind Lang. 15 (1) (2000) 184–218.

[75] B.A. Maher, Delusional thinking and perceptual disorder, J. Indiv. Psychol. 30 (1974) 98–113.

[76] E. Peters, P. Garety, Cognitive functioning in delusions: a longitudinal analysis, Behav. Res. Ther. 44 (4) (2006) 481–514.

[77] C. Fine, M. Gardner, J. Craigie, I. Gold, Hopping, skipping or jumping to conclusions? Clarifying the role of the JTC bias in delusions, Cognit. Neuropsychiatry 12 (1) (2007) 46–77.

[78] M. Menon, R. Mizrahi, S. Kapur, 'Jumping to conclusions' and delusions in psychosis: relationship and response to treatment, Schizophr. Res. 98 (1–3) (2008) 225–231.

[79] G. Loas, P. Boyer, A. Legrand, Anhedonia and negative symptomatology in chronic schizophrenia, Compr. Psychiatry 37 (1) (1996) 5–11.

[80] T.A. Ribot, The Psychology of Emotions, Walter Scott, London, 1897.

[81] M. Harrow, R.R. Grinker, P.S. Holzman, L. Kayton, Anhedonia and schizophrenia, Am. J. Psychiatry 134 (7) (1977) 794–797.

[82] C.G. Watson, L. Jacobs, T. Kucala, A note on the pathology of anhedonia, J. Clin. Psychol. 35 (4) (1979) 740–743.

[83] R.P. Shoichet, A. Oakley, Notes on the treatment of anhedonia, Can. Psychiatr. Assoc. J. 23 (7) (1978) 487–492.

[84] J. Katsanis, W.G. Iacono, M. Beiser, Anhedonia and perceptual aberration in first-episode psychotic patients and their relatives, J. Abnorm. Psychol. 99 (2) (1990) 202–206.

[85] L.J. Chapman, J.P. Chapman, M.L. Raulin, Scales for physical and social anhedonia, J. Abnorm. Psychol. 85 (4) (1976) 374–382.

[86] D.M. Romney, C.L. Candido, Anhedonia in depression and schizophrenia: a reexamination, J. Nerv. Ment. Dis. 189 (11) (2001) 735–740.

[87] H. Berenbaum, T.F. Oltmanns, Emotional experience and expression in schizophrenia and depression, J. Abnorm. Psychol. 101 (1) (1992) 37–44.

[88] H. Silver, N. Shlomo, Anhedonia and schizophrenia: how much is in the eye of the beholder? Compr. Psychiatry 43 (1) (2002) 65–68.

[89] M. Iwase, K. Yamashita, K. Takahashi, O. Kajimoto, A. Shimizu, T. Nishikawa, K. Shinosaki, Y. Sugita, M. Takeda, Diminished facial expression despite the existence of pleasant emotional experience in schizophrenia, Methods Find. Exp. Clin. Pharmacol. 21 (3) (1999) 189–194.

[90] K.C. Berridge, T.E. Robinson, Parsing reward, Trends Neurosci. 26 (9) (2003) 507–513.

[91] D.E. Gard, A.M. Kring, M.G. Gard, W.P. Horan, M.F. Green, Anhedonia in schizophrenia: distinctions between anticipatory and consummatory pleasure, Schizophr. Res. 93 (1–3) (2007) 253–260.

[92] P.C. Fletcher, C.D. Frith, Perceiving is believing: a Bayesian account of the positive symptoms of schizophrenia, Nat. Rev. Neurosci. 10 (2009) 48–58.

[93] K. Schneider, Clinical Psychopathology, Grune and Stratton, New York, 1959.

[94] I. Creese, D.R. Burt, S.H. Snyder, Dopamine receptors and average clinical doses, Science 194 (4264) (1976) 546.

12 Effects of dopamine depletion on reward-seeking behavior: evidence from human and non-human primates

Mathias Pessiglione[1] and Léon Tremblay[2]

[1]Laboratoire INSERM U610, Institut Fédératif de Recherches en Neurosciences, Site Pitié-Salpêtrière, F-75013 Paris, France
[2]Institute of Cognitive Neuroscience, CNRS-5229-University Lyon 1, 67 Bd Pinel 69675 Bron, France

Abstract

Clinical accounts of patients suffering from dopamine depletion, such as in Parkinson's disease, usually report motor symptoms. However, a large body of neuroscientific literature has implicated dopamine in reward processing. Here we review the evidence that dopamine depletion can impair reward-seeking behavior, in both human patients and primate models with Parkinson's disease. We successively envisage different reward-related processes (energization, decision making, and learning), and intend to make a conceptual link between consistent deficits and theoretical functions of dopamine (decoupling, disinhibition, and reinforcement) in fronto-striatal circuitry. We suggest that a primary deficit may concern positive reinforcement of circuits leading to reward, which would fail to facilitate action selection in subsequent choice situations.

Key points

1. Dopamine depletion has little impact on reward-induced behavior energization or on reward-based decision making outside learning contexts.
2. Dopamine depletion does impair reward-based learning but not punishment avoidance.
3. Impaired reward learning could be explained by insufficient dopamine-mediated reinforcement of fronto-striatal pathways.
4. Insufficient reinforcement of fronto-striatal pathways could impede disinhibition of specific approach behaviors when a same rewarded context repeats itself.
5. Dopamine depletion may therefore prevent facilitation of previously rewarded approach behavior.

As evident from other chapters in this book, dopamine has emerged center-stage in reward processing. But what happens when dopamine vanishes from the brain? In this chapter we focus on reward processing dysfunction in situations of dopamine depletion, namely parkinsonism, in both human and non-human primates.

12.1   Preamble: idiopathic Parkinson's disease and the monkey MPTP model

Parkinson's disease (PD) is characterized by a triad of motor symptoms: akinesia, rigidity, and tremor [1]. In past decades, PD patients have often been described as also suffering from cognitive deficits such as dysexecutive syndrome [2–4] and affective disorders such as apathy or depression [5–7]. PD has been attributed to degeneration of dopamine neurons in the substantia nigra [8–10]. Further post-mortem histological studies [11–13] showed that neuronal loss predominates in the dorsal tier of the substantia nigra pars compacta (SNc or A9), with dopamine neurons in the ventral tier, in the area close to the red nucleus (A8) and in the ventral tegmental area (VTA or A10) relatively spared. As a result, dopamine depletion principally affects the dorsal striatum, which is the main target region of the SNc dorsal tier [14–16].

The neurotoxin MPTP (1-methyl-4-phenyl-1,2,3,6-tetrahydropyridine) has been found in a synthesis substance that rendered a group of young drug addicts parkinsonian [17,18]. Systemic injections of MPTP in monkeys can induce a PD-like syndrome with akinesia and rigidity, as well as tremor in certain species such as vervet monkeys [19–21]. In addition, cognitive deficits (notably frontal-like dysexecutive syndrome) have been reported to precede motor symptoms in the course of MPTP intoxication [22–24]. At the histological level, MPTP intoxication replicates the degeneration pattern observed in humans, with drastic dopamine depletion in the dorsal striatum, compared with modest changes in the ventral part, at least in the first stages of disease induction (Fig. 2A) [25–27].

Thus, idiopathic PD in humans and the MPTP model in monkeys appear to be relevant conditions for observing effects of striatal dopamine depletion on reward-seeking behavior. Effects of dopamine depletion in humans are best assessed in withdrawal situations, classically after an overnight off medication. Current medications in PD are metabolic precursor of dopamine (L-DOPA) or dopamine receptor agonists, both of which aim to compensate for dopamine depletion. The control group can be the same patients, or a different patient group, when on medication, as well as healthy subjects matched in terms of age, sex, and level of education. In this review we have chosen not to mention studies comparing directly medicated patients and matched healthy subjects because in such a case it is impossible to know whether the reported deficits are due to dopamine depletion or dopamine replacement medication. In monkeys, we are able to compare pre- and post-intoxication behavior, which is obviously not possible in patients who are already ill when they come to the hospital. In progressive protocols of MPTP injections, we are also able to test for subtle cognitive or affective symptoms in the early stages of parkinsonism, before the onset of gross motor symptoms. The following sections concentrate therefore on studies comparing monkeys in their normal state to MPTP-treated monkeys with nonexistent or mild PD-like motor symptoms.

12.2   Observations: what are the reward-seeking deficits induced by dopamine depletion?

Effects of expected rewards on behavior may be divided into three types:

- energization (exerting more effort when more reward is at stake)
- decision making (choosing the alternative that maximizes reward prediction)
- learning (enhancing the value of context-action association that leads to more reward than predicted)

In this section we review deficits reported in each of these reward-related processes, leaving aside studies of learning, action selection, or decision making not involving rewards.

12.2.1   Energization

Incentive motivation can be construed as a process that translates expected rewards into behavioral activation [28]. This "wanting" process (as observed in approach behavior) may be dissociated from the "liking" process (as observed in consumption behavior) in respect of the same reward [29]. According to Berridge, incentive motivation involves dopamine and ventral basal ganglia circuits, which have been consistently activated in functional neuroimaging studies of reward prediction (for review see references [30–32] and Chapter 7). To assess the integrity of incentive motivation, we need a paradigm that varies the reward at stake and measures the energy of approach behavior. Such a paradigm has been provided in humans and consists in having subjects squeeze a hand grip in order to win different sums of money [33]. Subjects are free to exert as much force as they like, but they know that the harder they squeeze the greater monetary incentive they will win. Like matched healthy subjects, unmedicated PD patients upped the force exerted when more money was at stake (Fig. 1B) [34]. This increase paralleled the increase in skin conductance response to monetary incentive display, which can be taken as an index of autonomous sympathetic arousal [35]. However, both emotional (skin conductance) and motor (grip force) responses to monetary incentives were diminished as compared to control subjects. Consequently, there was no dissociation of liking and wanting processes following dopamine depletion, because emotional evaluation of monetary incentives was correctly translated into motor activation.

A similar finding has been reported in MPTP-treated monkeys, in the context of a study that varied not the quantity but the quality of the reward, while measuring the number and speed of reward-seeking actions initiated by the animal [36]. Reward preferences were controlled in a separate test, where two kinds of food (e.g., cereals and raisins) were available. The food eaten first was considered the preferred one. The different foods were then used as rewards in separate blocks of a visual discrimination task. They were placed in little wells covered by opaque sliding plaques labeled with symbolic cues that monkeys had learned to associate with food prior to MPTP intoxication. The number of attempts and overall speed of food retrieval decreased with MPTP intoxication. Crucially, however, monkeys made more attempts and moved more quickly in blocks proposing their preferred reward than in those proposing the other rewards (Fig. 1A). Incentive motivation, the process whereby behavioral activation is scaled in proportion to expected reward, again appeared to be spared by dopamine depletion. Furthermore, PD-like symptoms appeared less prominent when monkeys were working

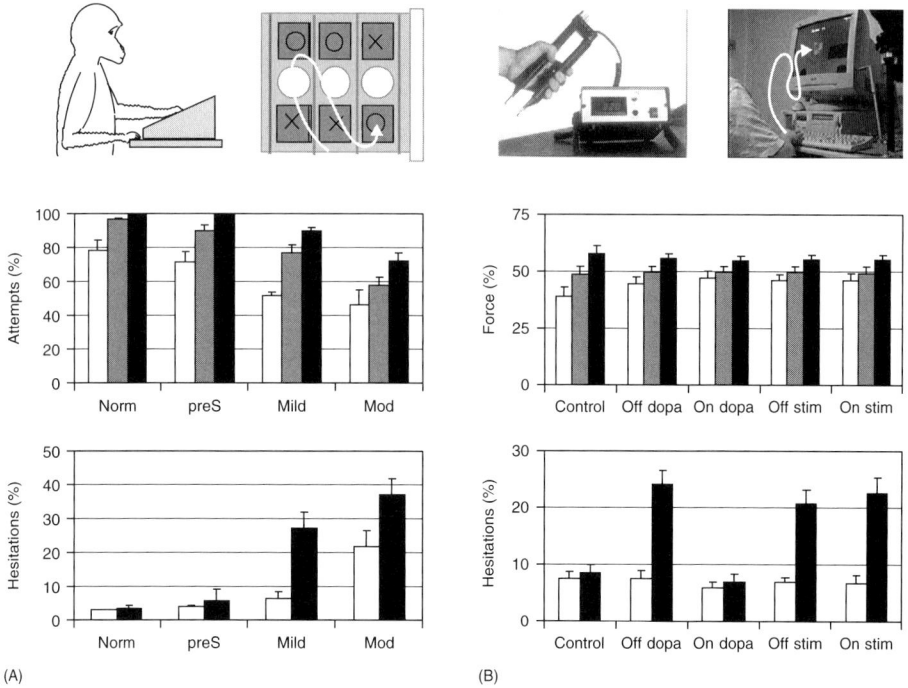

Figure 12.1 Summary of main observations regarding effects of dopamine depletion on energizing behavior (upper panels) and decision making (lower panels). (A) Data from non-human primates [36,50]. Diagrams show successive stages of MPTP-induced parkinsonism: normal, presymptomic, mild, and moderate from left to right. Upper diagram: histograms illustrate percentage of retrieval attempts relative to available rewards. Colors indicate least preferred (white), intermediate (gray), and most preferred rewards (black). Lower diagram: histograms illustrate percentage of hesitations relative to retrieval attempts. A hesitation is a change of reward target during ongoing movement (see food board for illustration). Two levels of uncertainty were contrasted: in the first situation (white) rewards were directly visible, whereas in the other (black) rewards were cued by symbols. (B) Data from human primates [34,60]. Diagrams show different subject groups and treatment conditions: healthy subjects and PD patients on L-DOPA, off L-DOPA, on STN-DBS and off STN-DBS from left to right. Upper diagram: histograms represent the amount of force used to win as much as possible of 1€ (white), 10€ (gray), and 50€ (black). Lower diagram: histograms represent percentage of hesitations relative to initiated movements. A hesitation is a movement back to the keyboard after pointing towards the screen (see image for illustration). Two levels of uncertainty have been contrasted: in the first situation (white) subjects know the associations between cues and rewards, whereas in the other (black) they are facing novel cues the meaning of which they have to learn. Note that the only effect consistently observed under dopamine depletion across species is the exacerbation of overt hesitations in situations of uncertainty (see explanations in main text).

for their preferred reward. This suggests that incentive motivation could help them to overcome motor deficits brought about as a result of dopamine depletion.

According to these results, energization of behavior by potential rewards is still functional in PD. This could be due to relative preservation of dopamine fibers in ventral parts of the basal ganglia, insofar as these ventral (also known as "limbic") circuits connect to reward-related structures such as the orbital and medial prefrontal cortex, anterior cingulate cortex, amygdala, and hippocampus [35,37,38]. Thus, at least in the early stages of PD, apathy would be better characterized as a general difficulty producing behavior, rather than as diminished energization by potential goals or rewards. This difficulty might be secondary to motor and/or cognitive deficits (like akinesia, rigidity, or dysexecutive syndrome) and hence to dopamine depletion in the dorsal parts of basal ganglia circuits. Another possibility is that apathy in PD is not related to dopamine depletion at all, but to degeneration of other modulatory ascending pathways, such as those involving serotonin neurons [39]. It should be noted that apathy is nonetheless responsive to L-DOPA therapy [40–42], which again could reflect a direct effect on reward processing or a consequence of the main therapeutic effects on motor/cognitive symptoms. Some authors [43,44] have even suggested that L-DOPA treatment, while compensating for drastic dopamine depletion in the dorsal striatum, would overdose the relatively spared ventral striatum and impair reward-related processes. Findings relating to this issue are somewhat contradictory, however, and the pathophysiology of apathy in PD is still under debate [7,45,46].

12.2.2 Decision making

Decision making can be defined as a process reducing n alternatives to one. In our context, the criterion for this reduction would be maximization of the cost/benefit ratio. Costs could, for instance, be the delay in reward occurrence or the effort needed to obtain the reward. Benefits can be expressed in terms of rewards (to be obtained) or punishments (to be avoided). To make a decision, the subject has to consider the different options, label them according to the reward (or punishment) prediction and cost estimation, and then select the one that maximizes the cost/benefit ratio. Unfortunately, complex decision-making situations including different levels of delay or effort have not yet been studied in PD patients. In fact, decision making in PD has always been assessed in the context of learning, with the help of paradigms such as the probabilistic classification task [47], probabilistic reversal task [48], Iowa gambling task [42], or transitive inference task [49]. It could be very interesting for further research to assess decisions in paradigms where alternatives are explicitly explained to patients (no learning) and which systematically vary levels of incentives, delays, and efforts.

In monkeys, we were able to investigate simple situations of reward-based decision making [36]. When different kinds of visible rewards were offered, decisions were no different after MPTP treatment than in the normal state: monkeys chose their preferred food first. However, when rewards were hidden under sliding plaques and cued by symbols, as described in the last section, we observed interesting deficits in how decision making (or action selection) was carried out in MPTP-treated monkeys with mild parkinsonism. A first deficit was freezing, that is, the monkey would suddenly stop what it was doing and remain completely immobile for several seconds. A second deficit was hesitation, that is, when it was already in the process of reaching out to take a given reward-associated cue, the monkey would change its mind and reach out for another reward-associated cue instead. Both hesitation and freezing can be interpreted as unresolved selection between competing options. Interestingly, these deficits were rare when the rewards were visible, possibly because they were sufficiently salient in this case (or had sufficient expected value) for the selection process to be completed (Fig. 1A) [50].

We also observed hesitations in human patients, in a paradigm where they were required to choose between touching or not touching a symbolic cue displayed on a computer screen [51]. This particular paradigm (which was adapted from [52]) consists of two cues: the Go cue means patients win a point if they touch it (and otherwise lose), and vice versa for the NoGo cue. At the beginning of a task session, the patient is unaware of these contingencies and has to discover them through trial and error. Once the patient has made at least nine correct responses in a series of 10 trials, the contingencies are automatically reversed and have to be relearned. Hesitations were characterized as a hand moving back and forth between the computer screen and the key the patient had to press to start the next trial. Once again, these hesitations can be interpreted as difficulty selecting between competing options (Go and NoGo responses, in this case). In healthy control subjects hesitations might also have occurred but remained in their head. This suggests that deliberation and execution phases are abnormally coupled in PD, in such a way that hesitations are obvious from behavior. Hesitations were abnormally frequent in patients during the exploration period (prior to discovering and exploiting contingencies), when the expected values of the two options were still uncertain (Fig. 1B). Thus, observing gestures in monkeys and patients revealed that the process of action selection (and not necessarily the final decision) is impaired in PD. However, these results were obtained in situations where rewards were to be retrieved through associations with symbolic cues and might be better characterized as associative learning deficits.

12.2.3 Learning

Here, as with decision making, we consider learning in relation to reward processing, to the exclusion of studies where subjects receive no feedback, as for instance in classical procedural learning paradigms. In feedback-based learning, subjects use previous experience as a basis for predicting the outcome of a given context or action. The outcome may be a judgement ("good" or "correct"), reward (winning points, food, or money) or punishment (losing money or feeling pain). A seminal dissociation was found between PD patients, who were impaired in terms of learning to predict weather from a set of cues but who kept declarative memory of the training episode, and amnesic patients, who could learn the cue-weather associations but then could not remember having been trained [47]. This was the first of a series of experiments showing that, contrary to medial temporal lobe damage (in amnesic patients), striatal dysfunction (in PD patients) impaired gradual associative learning from feedback [53,54]. More specifically, unmedicated patients were impaired in chaining tasks where a sequence of cues leading to a reward is learned step-by-step, from the most proximal to the most distal [55,56]. The suggestion that dopamine makes a specific contribution in this kind of learning is not clear-cut, however, because some deficits were also found under L-DOPA [57].

Another series of experiments used reversal learning tasks, in which associations between cues and outcomes are switched once the subject has met a given performance criterion. One example of such a paradigm was described in the previous section and involves asking subjects to choose between Go and NoGo responses and, in addition to reversals, includes an extinction phase, where both cues give points if not touched. Unmedicated PD patients were found to be impaired in respect of both initial acquisition and reversal of cue-outcome associations, but not in respect of extinction. In the same patients, L-DOPA treatment had no effect on initial acquisition or reversals but did impede extinction. Interestingly, L-DOPA eradicated the hesitations observed in the same paradigm, suggesting that such a decision-making deficit is more closely related to dopamine depletion than learning impairment. Moreover, high frequency stimulation of the subthalamic nucleus (STN-DBS), which is an alternative treatment of PD with similar therapeutical effects on motor symptoms, produced an opposite pattern compared to L-DOPA effects. STN-DBS tended to improve extinction learning [58,59] but did not correct the hesitations observed during decision-making in situations of uncertainty (Fig. 1B) [60].

In a slightly different reversal learning paradigm, where cue-outcome contingencies were probabilistic, unmedicated PD patients were found to perform as well as healthy controls [48,61]. This preserved reversal learning ability has been contrasted with impaired cognitive flexibility and related to striatal denervation pattern, with drastic loss in dorsal and relative sparing in ventral regions. Medication was reported to be detrimental to reversal learning but beneficial to cognitive flexibility, which has been interpreted as an overdose versus compensation effect on the ventral versus dorsal striatum. It should be noted, however, that there was no systematic relationship across studies between reversal learning performance and dopamine depletion/medication, the only consistent result being extinction impediment under L-DOPA. Some of the previously mentioned reversal learning studies also assessed PD patients in the Iowa gambling task [42,58], in which subjects have to choose between decks of cards and work out for themselves that some are advantageous in the long run even if they yield less money at a time. Whether or not they were treated, PD patients were no different from controls in the first assessment but improved less in a second assessment. Such results are nonetheless difficult to interpret, as the Iowa gambling task involves several cognitive processes and personality traits, such as reinforcement learning, rule extraction, risk seeking, and loss aversion.

The idea of separating reward and punishment learning (carrot and stick) proved enlightening. In reversal/extinction tasks, subjects can learn cue-outcome contingencies from either rewards (after correct response) or punishments (after incorrect response). To dissociate the contributions of positive and negative outcomes to reinforcement learning, Frank and colleagues [24] proposed a twofold task. In the training phase, subjects have to choose between two symbolic cues with different probabilities of being correct. They thus have the opportunity to learn from positive feedback that a cue is frequently correct, or from negative feedback that a cue is frequently incorrect. Then, in the probe phase, cues are rearranged in fresh pairs, which subjects have to choose in the absence of feedback. The crucial measure is whether subjects are better at choosing the most rewarded cue or at avoiding the most punished cue, from which it is possible to infer whether they learned by carrot or by stick in the training phase. A double dissociation was found: unmedicated PD patients learned better from negative feedbacks and medicated PD patients from positive feedbacks. This dissociation was specific to the contrast between dopamine depletion versus dopamine replacement medication and was not observed with STN-DBS [62]. The double dissociation has been replicated and extended by two other laboratories in the context of reversal learning [63] and subliminal conditioning (Palminteri et al., in preparation). A differential contribution of dopamine in reward versus punishment learning has also been evidenced in healthy subjects on different dopaminergic drugs [64], or with different dopamine-related genotypes [65]. Furthermore, Frank and colleagues proposed that increased dopamine following positive feedback reinforces approach behavior, and that decreased dopamine following negative feedback reinforces avoidance behavior. This might be why PD patients on medication encounter difficulties with extinction tasks, because too much dopamine impairs reinforcement of avoidance behavior that would normally occur when subjects choose a cue resulting in negative feedback.

12.3   Theories: what is the basal ganglia dysfunction induced by dopamine depletion?

From the last section, the most consistent reward processing deficit after dopamine depletion appears to be a diminished reinforcement of approach behaviors, and consequently difficulty selecting previously rewarded options. The aim of this section is not to describe computational models of the basal ganglia, as described in detail in Chapter 19, but to pinpoint key ideas about the functional impact of dopamine depletion within the fronto-striatal circuits. We think there are three potential functions of dopamine worth mentioning: decoupling, disinhibition, and reinforcement of basal ganglia pathways.

12.3.1 Decoupling

Axon-tracing studies in monkeys have revealed that circuits linking the basal ganglia to the frontal cortex are to some extent segregated [37,66] (see also Chapter 1). According to this view, topography of functional territories is preserved at every stage of the circuitry (principally frontal cortex, striatum, pallidum, and thalamus). The original description distinguished five parallel circuits (motor, oculomotor, dorsolateral prefrontal, lateral orbitofrontal, anterior cingulate) that can be grouped together in three main functional domains (motor, associative, limbic). On a smaller scale, subcircuits can be identified, for instance with respect to somatotopy within the motor circuit [67]. The functional partition of fronto-striatal projection has been confirmed in humans using functional [68] and diffusion tensor imaging [69]. However, several findings argue against complete segregation between parallel circuits. In particular, the drastic reduction in volume between input (striatum) and output (pallidum) structures suggests some degree of convergence between functional circuits. This idea is also borne out by the widespread arborization of pallidal dendrites, enabling them to receive afferences from distant striatal regions [70]. Conversely, there is a degree of divergence in both the cortical afferences and efferences to the basal ganglia, suggesting open interconnected circuits rather than closed loops [38,71].

The degree of functional segregation between basal ganglia circuits could be modulated by dopamine levels, as several electrophysiological approaches have suggested. Passive joint manipulation has been used to define the receptive field of a given neuron within the body map. In the normal state, basal ganglia neurons appeared to be selective of for one joint manipulated in a certain direction. Selectivity was lost after MPTP injections, with neurons responding to different directions and distant joints as if somatotopy was blurred by dopamine depletion. This loss of selectivity was found at the pallidal, thalamic, and cortical levels of basal ganglia circuits [51,72–75]. Disrupted focalization of striato-pallidal transmission was confirmed by microstimulation, a given pallidal neuron responding to several striatal stimulation sites after MPTP treatment, compared to just one in the normal state [76]. Multiple-unit recordings showed that neuronal activities were highly correlated after MPTP-induced dopamine depletion, whereas in the normal state they were quite independent. Once again this was found at the pallidal, thalamic and cortical levels, either at rest or during a Go-NoGo task, and was reversed by administering L-DOPA [51,77–79]. Abnormal correlation was observed between distant electrodes (up to 5 mm) and could be associated or not with rhythmic activities. Synchronized oscillations have also been observed in the STN of human PD patients implanted for deep brain stimulation [80–82]. They have been found to be reduced during movements, to be negatively correlated with motor performance, and to be sensitive to L-DOPA medication, suggesting a link with bradykinesia [83–87]. Thus, on a fine scale, dopamine depletion results in an abnormal correlation between neuronal activities, denoting a difficulty decoupling basal ganglia circuits, such that they can no longer operate in parallel.

12.3.2   Disinhibition

Another influential concept in describing the functional organization of the basal ganglia relates to the so-called direct and indirect pathways [88,89] connecting the striatum to the output structures, namely the substantia nigra pars reticulata (SNr) and globus pallidus pars internalis (GPi). The direct pathway involves one inhibitory synapse, whereas the indirect pathway, which passes through the STN and globus pallidus pars externalis (GPe), includes two successive inhibitory synapses. Because the GPi/SNr projection neurons are again inhibitory, it is suggested that the direct/indirect pathways respectively allow activation/inhibition of their thalamic and hence cortical target. Several authors [90,91] have suggested that the double pathway could be the substrate of a selection device. GPi/SNr neurons exhibit a high spontaneous discharge rate and thus exert an inhibitory tonus on the cortex via the thalamus. It is suggested that the indirect pathway, because of the divergent projection from the STN to the output structures, increases this tonic inhibition, and that, on the contrary, the direct pathway disinhibits a focal target within thalamic, and then cortical, efferent areas. The device would work as a figure/ground extraction: the ground would be secured by the indirect pathway, and the figure delineated by the direct pathway. In the motor domain, this would permit (disinhibit) execution of a desired motor program, while inhibiting the other competing motor programs. There has been some empirical support for such a concept; for instance some degree of striatal stimulation, or SNr inhibition, has been reported to activate thalamic targets and elicit ocular saccades [92,93]. To complete the model, a winner-takes-all mechanism could be implemented at striatal level through inhibitory collaterals to ensure that when a given striato-nigro/pallidal channel is activated the others remain silent.

With this sort of model, dopamine would tune the contrast between direct and indirect pathway activities (that is, between figure and ground). The dopamine receptors D1 and D2 have been localized on different neuronal populations that would participate in direct and indirect pathways, respectively [94]. Because activation of D1 receptors could mediate an excitatory effect, and that of D2 receptors an inhibitory effect [95], dopamine release on striatal neurons would favor the direct pathway to the detriment of the indirect pathway. In parkinsonism, dopamine depletion would then lead to an imbalance in favor of the indirect pathway, resulting in increased inhibition of the thalamus and cortex, blocking movements and hence explaining akinesia. Conversely, sudden excess of dopamine, following L-DOPA intake, would reverse the imbalance, resulting in thalamic and cortical activations that might explain dyskinesia, since pallidal activities have been shown to increase after MPTP intoxication and to decrease after L-DOPA administration [96–98]. The model also offers a rationale for therapeutical effects of STN lesions [99] or high frequency stimulation [100]: it has been suggested that suppression of the excitatory tonus from the STN to the GPi would release the brake on thalamus and cortex and hence alleviate akinesia [101].

The double pathway model has been criticized, however, in respect of both its anatomical assumptions and electrophysiological predictions. Several studies [102,103] have stressed that striatal projection neurons have collaterals that project partly to the GPe (indirect pathway) and partly to the GPi (direct pathway). Furthermore, D1 and D2 receptors have been colocalized on the same neurons [104], which makes it difficult for dopamine to play one pathway against the other. Also, changes in discharge rates predicted by the double pathway model did not always occur [51,74,105]. Finally, the model underestimates the direct projection from the cortex to the STN, the so-called hyperdirect pathway, which could play a key role in basal ganglia processing [75,106,107]. Accordingly, the existence of such a double pathway and the role of dopamine in that context are subject to question, although the general view that the basal ganglia operates as a selection device, increasing signal-to-noise ratio for salient cortical inputs through focal disinhibition, might nonetheless be correct.

12.3.3 Reinforcement

Another line of thinking came from recordings of dopamine neurons activity during conditioned tasks in monkeys. These experiments are largely detailed in Chapter 2, so here we highlight only what is needed to understand the effects of dopamine depletion. Dopamine neurons appeared to encode a reward prediction error; in other words, the difference between an actual and expected reward at a given time [108]. In fact, dopamine neurons are phasically activated by unexpected rewards or novel stimuli [109,110]. During associative learning, the suggestion is that the phasic response increases for a stimulus that predicts the reward and diminishes for actual delivery of the reward [111,112]. After learning, if a reward is announced by a predictive stimulus but then fails to materialize, dopamine neurons are depressed at the expected time of reward delivery [113,114]. They appear, on the contrary, to be insensitive to or even inhibited by unpleasant stimuli or punishments [115,116]. Recent experiments have refined the concept, showing that reward prediction encoding by dopamine neurons is context-dependent [117–119].

The reward prediction error is similiar to the teaching signal used in formal algorithms [120,121] applying some kind of Rescorla-Wagner rule [122] which basically states that the greater the discrepancy between actual and predicted outcomes, the more is learned about the value of the context and/or action. In instrumental learning, for instance, actions leading to more reward than expected would be reinforced, while the others would be weakened. Several authors [123,124] have proposed that such a reinforcement mechanism is implemented in the striatum. Dopamine neurons connect to the neck of striatal dendritic spines, the head of which receives cortical afferences [138]. Dopaminergic axonal terminations are therefore well-placed to modulate the efficacy of cortico-striatal synapses. Moreover, long-term synaptic plasticity [125,126], as well as change in gene expression [127,128] in striatal neurons, have been found to be modulated by dopamine receptor stimulation. Indeed, during instrumental conditioning, striatal activities are shaped by the rewards obtained or missed [129,130].

One way to apply reinforcement learning theory in the striatum involves the actor–critic architecture (Fig. 2B) [131,132]. Depending on the environmental context, the critic system generates a reward prediction while the actor system selects an action. As soon as the outcome is apparent, the difference between the reward predicted by the critic and the reward actually obtained from the environment is computed and sent back as a teaching signal to the critic for improvement of reward prediction and to the actor for improvement of action selection. Functional neuroimaging in humans has yielded some evidence that the role of critic may be played by the ventral striatum, that of actor by the dorsal striatum, and that the reward prediction error (or teaching signal) may be conveyed by dopamine neurons [64,133]. In this context, degeneration of the dopamine axons in the dorsal striatum would suppress the teaching signal needed to reinforce actions leading to more reward than expected.

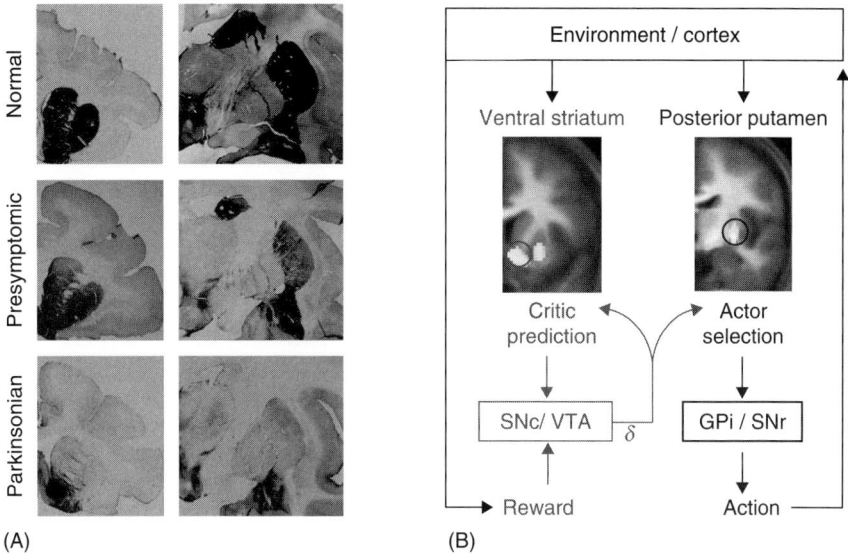

Figure 12.2 Summary of main anatomo-functional concepts underlying the effects of dopamine deple-tion on reward-seeking behavior. (A) Pattern of dopamine fibers degeneration, as revealed by tyro-sine hydroxylase immuno-staining [36]. Successive stages of MPTP-induced parkinsonism are shown from top to bottom. Pictures were taken over frontal sections passing through the anterior (lefthand panels) and posterior (righthand panels) striatum. Note the relative preservation of ventral regions at every stage. (B) Schematic illustration of an actor–critic architecture tentatively implemented in fronto-striatal circuits. Brain images and activations were taken from a functional neuroimaging study in humans [64]. In this model, the posterior putamen plays the role of the actor, selecting an action through focal disinhibition of basal ganglia outputs (via GPi/SNr). The ventral striatum plays the role of the critic, generating a reward prediction based on the contextual information conveyed by cortical inputs. Midbrain dopamine neurons (in the SNc/VTA) compute the difference (δ) between the actual reward coming from the environment and the reward predicted by the critic. Dopamine release would thus be commensurate with reward prediction error and serve as a teaching signal tun-ing the efficacy of fronto-striatal synapses. In the ventral striatum it would improve reward predic-tion, while in the dorsal striatum it would improve action selection. As learning progresses, striatal activities would go less correlated, allowing the various fronto-striatal channels to encode different dimensions (such as reward prediction and action selection) of the behavioral response to the envi-ronmental context. See Plate 15 of Color Plate section.

12.4 Explanations: how can basal ganglia dysfunction account for reward-seeking deficits?

Several network models have found elegant ways of combining the different functional roles considered for striatal dopamine: decoupling, disinhibition, reinforcement [49,134], see also Chapter 19. Although anatomical details of these models are debatable, they share common properties that can provide insight into reward-seeking deficits following dopamine depletion. The key mechanism is reinforcement of cortico-striatal synapses, as a result of dopamine burst that would facilitate pathways producing more reward than expected, whereas the other pathways may be impeded by dopamine dips. If the same context repeats itself, a previously rewarded action would then be more easily selected (or disinhibited). Because different neuronal populations in the dorsal striatum would underpin different actions, their activation in the same context would be progressively de-correlated (decoupled) in the course of learning, possibly with the help of inhibitory collaterals and interneurons. In the case of a Go-NoGo paradigm, for instance, Go and NoGo cells would be equally activated in the first trial, leaving decision-making problematic, that is, with long response times (hesitation) and random output. As learning progresses, contextual cues would activate the appropriate response more easily (Go or NoGo), to the detriment of the other, making decision making fast and accurate.

The most convincing effects of dopamine depletion on reward-seeking behavior were observed during feedback-based Go-NoGo learning paradigms [49,60,62,63]. PD patients are specifically impaired in Go learning from positive feedback; they often fail to choose the most rewarded option, need more trials to attain the performance criterion, and show delayed response times with overt hesitations. These effects are the most convincing because (1) they are reversed by L-DOPA medication but not by STN-DBS, (2) they are also reversed in the case of NoGo learning from negative feedback, which offers perfect control in terms of cognitive demand, and (3) they were observed to some extent in monkeys with dopamine depletion restricted to the dorsal striatum [36,50]. These effects can be accounted for by functional models of the basal ganglia where rewards (positive feedbacks) reinforce a specific pathway underpinning some approach behavior. When dopamine is lacking, the rewarded approaching action is no longer reinforced, and therefore will not be easier to select in the event of future occurrence of the same circumstances. Interestingly, classical symptoms of PD can also be seen as failures in selection mechanisms: co-activation of competing motor programs could lead to akinesia or rigidity. However, the question of whether motor symptoms in PD are due to the same reinforcement deficit as reward-seeking disorders remains to be seen.

12.5   Perspective: dopamine replacement therapy and repetitive behaviors

In this chapter we focused on the effects of dopamine depletion. Nevertheless, the theoretical framework described to account for these effects of dopamine depletion could also apply to the (opposite) effects of dopamine replacement medication. We have already mentioned that L-DOPA can induce disorders in reward-seeking behaviors, such as the inability to extinguish a behavioral response despite negative feedback. Clinically, it has been reported that patients on dopamine replacement medication, particularly with dopamine receptor agonists, are prone to repetitive behavior, such as pathological gambling, compulsive shopping, hypersexuality, or overeating [135–137]. It is tempting to interpret these compulsive forms of behavior as resulting from dopamine-mediated excessive (positive) reinforcement of basal ganglia pathways leading to rewards. This hypothesis is currently under examination.

References

[1] J. Parkinson, An Essay on the Shaking Palsy, Sherwood, Neely and Jones, London, 1817.

[2] B. Dubois, B. Pillon, Cognitive deficits in Parkinson's disease, J. Neurol. 244 (1997) 2–8.

[3] M. Emre, Dementia in Parkinson's disease: cause and treatment, Curr. Opin. Neurol. 17 (2004) 399–404.

[4] D. Muslimovic, B. Post, J.D. Speelman, B. Schmand, Cognitive profile of patients with newly diagnosed Parkinson disease, Neurology 65 (2005) 1239–1245.

[5] S.E. Starkstein, H.S. Mayberg, T.J. Preziosi, P. Andrezejewski, R. Leiguarda, R.G. Robinson, Reliability, validity, and clinical correlates of apathy in Parkinson's disease, J. Neuropsychiatry Clin. Neurosci. 4 (1992) 134–139.

[6] D. Aarsland, J.P. Larsen, N.G. Lim, C. Janvin, K. Karlsen, E. Tandberg, J.L. Cummings, Range of neuropsychiatric disturbances in patients with Parkinson's disease, J. Neurol. Neurosurg. Psychiatry 67 (1999) 492–496.

[7] G.C. Pluck, R.G. Brown, Apathy in Parkinson's disease, J. Neurol. Neurosurg. Psychiatry 73 (2002) 636–642.

[8] C. Tretiakoff, Contribution à l'étude de l'anatomie pathologique du locus niger de Soemmering avec quelques déductions relatives à la pathogénie des troubles du tonus musculaire et de la maladie de Parkinson, Faculté de médecine, 1919.

[9] R. Hassler, Zur pathologie der paralysis agitans und des postenzephalitischen Parkinsonismus, J. Psychol. Neurol. 48 (1938) 387–416.

[10] A. Carlsson, B. Falck, N. Hillarp, Cellular localization of brain monoamines, Acta Physiol. Scand. 56 (1962) 1–28.

[11] E. Hirsch, A.M. Graybiel, Y.A. Agid, Melanized dopaminergic neurons are differentially susceptible to degeneration in Parkinson's disease, Nature 334 (1988) 345–348.

[12] J.M. Fearnley, A.J. Lees, Ageing and Parkinson's disease: substantia nigra regional selectivity, Brain 114 (Pt 5) (1991) 2283–2301.

[13] P. Damier, E.C. Hirsch, Y. Agid, A.M. Graybiel, The substantia nigra of the human brain. II. Patterns of loss of dopamine-containing neurons in Parkinson's disease, Brain 122 (Pt 8) (1999) 1437–1448.

[14] H. Bernheimer, W. Birkmayer, O. Hornykiewicz, K. Jellinger, F. Seitelberger, Brain dopamine and the syndromes of Parkinson and Huntington. Clinical, morphological and neurochemical correlations, J. Neurol. Sci. 20 (1973) 415–455.

[15] I.J. Farley, K.S. Price, O. Hornykiewicz, Dopamine in thelimbic regions of the human brain: normal and abnormal, Adv. Biochem. Psychopharmacol. 16 (1977) 57–64.

[16] S.J. Kish, K. Shannak, O. Hornykiewicz, Uneven pattern of dopamine loss in the striatum of patients with idiopathic Parkinson's disease. Pathophysiologic and clinical implications, N. Engl. J. Med. 318 (1988) 876–880.

[17] G.C. Davis, A.C. Williams, S.P. Markey, M.H. Ebert, E.D. Caine, C.M. Reichert, I.J. Kopin, Chronic Parkinsonism secondary to intravenous injection of meperidine analogues, Psychiatry Res. 1 (1979) 249–254.

[18] J.W. Langston, P. Ballard, J.W. Tetrud, I. Irwin, Chronic Parkinsonism in humans due to a product of meperidine-analog synthesis, Science 219 (1983) 979–980.

[19] R.S. Burns, C.C. Chiueh, S.P. Markey, M.H. Ebert, D.M. Jacobowitz, I.J. Kopin, A primate model of parkinsonism: selective destruction of dopaminergic neurons in the pars compacta of the substantia nigra by N-methyl-4-phenyl-1,2,3,6-tetrahydropyridine, Proc. Natl. Acad. Sci. USA 80 (1983) 4546–4550.

[20] J.D. Elsworth, A.Y. Deutch, D.E. Redmond Jr., J.R. Sladek Jr., R.H. Roth, MPTP-induced parkinsonism: relative changes in dopamine concentration in subregions of substantia nigra, ventral tegmental area and retrorubral field of symptomatic and asymptomatic vervet monkeys, Brain Res. 513 (1990) 320–324.

[21] H. Bergman, A. Feingold, A. Nini, A. Raz, H. Slovin, M. Abeles, E. Vaadia, Physiological aspects of information processing in the basal ganglia of normal and parkinsonian primates, Trends Neurosci. 21 (1998) 32–38.

[22] Y. Stern, J.W. Langston, Intellectual changes in patients with MPTP-induced parkinsonism, Neurology 35 (1985) 1506–1509.

[23] J.S. Schneider, D.P. Roeltgen, Delayed matching-to-sample, object retrieval, and discrimination reversal deficits in chronic low dose MPTP-treated monkeys, Brain Res. 615 (1993) 351–354.

[24] H. Slovin, M. Abeles, E. Vaadia, I. Haalman, Y. Prut, H. Bergman, Frontal cognitive impairments and saccadic deficits in low-dose MPTP-treated monkeys, J. Neurophysiol. 81 (1999) 858–874.

[25] C. Pifl, G. Schingnitz, O. Hornykiewicz, The neurotoxin MPTP does not reproduce in the rhesus monkey the interregional pattern of striatal dopamine loss typical of human idiopathic Parkinson's disease, Neurosci. Lett. 92 (1988) 228–233.

[26] P. Hantraye, M. Varastet, M. Peschanski, D. Riche, P. Cesaro, J.C. Willer, M. Maziere, Stable parkinsonian syndrome and uneven loss of striatal dopamine fibres following chronic MPTP administration in baboons, Neuroscience 53 (1993) 169–178.

[27] C. Jan, M. Pessiglione, L. Tremblay, D. Tande, E.C. Hirsch, C. Francois, Quantitative analysis of dopaminergic loss in relation to functional territories in MPTP-treated monkeys, Eur. J. Neurosci. 18 (2003) 2082–2086.

[28] K.C. Berridge, Motivation concepts in behavioral neuroscience, Physiol. Behav. 81 (2004) 179–209.

[29] K.C. Berridge, T.E. Robinson, Parsing reward, Trends Neurosci. 26 (2003) 507–513.

[30] J.P. O'Doherty, Reward representations and reward-related learning in the human brain: insights from neuroimaging, Curr. Opin. Neurobiol. 14 (2004) 769–776.

[31] B. Knutson, J.C. Cooper, Functional magnetic resonance imaging of reward prediction, Curr. Opin. Neurol. 18 (2005) 411–417.

[32] P.R. Montague, B. King-Casas, J.D. Cohen, Imaging Valuation Models in Human Choice, Annu. Rev. Neurosci. (2006).

[33] M. Pessiglione, L. Schmidt, B. Draganski, R. Kalisch, H. Lau, R.J. Dolan, C.D. Frith, How the brain translates money into force: a neuroimaging study of subliminal motivation, Science 316 (2007) 904–906.

[34] L. Schmidt, B.F. d'Arc, G. Lafargue, D. Galanaud, V. Czernecki, D. Grabli, M. Schupbach, A. Hartmann, R. Levy, B. Dubois, M. Pessiglione, Disconnecting force from money: effects of basal ganglia damage on incentive motivation, Brain 131 (2008) 1303–1310.

[35] H.D. Critchley, Electrodermal responses: what happens in the brain, Neuroscientist 8 (2002) 132–142.

[36] M. Pessiglione, D. Guehl, C. Jan, C. Francois, E.C. Hirsch, J. Feger, L. Tremblay, Disruption of self-organized actions in monkeys with progressive MPTP-induced parkinsonism: II. Effects of reward preference, Eur. J. Neurosci. 19 (2004) 437–446.

[37] G.E. Alexander, M.R. DeLong, P.L. Strick, Parallel organization of functionally segregated circuits linking basal ganglia and cortex, Annu. Rev. Neurosci. 9 (1986) 357–381.

[38] S.N. Haber, The primate basal ganglia: parallel and integrative networks, J. Chem. Neuroanat. 26 (2003) 317–330.

[39] R. Mayeux, J.B. Williams, Y. Stern, L. Cote, Depression and Parkinson's disease, Adv. Neurol. 40 (1984) 241–250.

[40] M.D. Yahr, R.C. Duvoisin, M.J. Schear, R.E. Barrett, M.M. Hoehn, Treatment of parkinsonism with levodopa, Arch. Neurol. 21 (1969) 343–354.

[41] R.G. Brown, C.D. Marsden, N. Quinn, M.A. Wyke, Alterations in cognitive performance and affect-arousal state during fluctuations in motor function in Parkinson's disease, J. Neurol. Neurosurg. Psychiatry 47 (1984) 454–465.

[42] V. Czernecki, B. Pillon, J.L. Houeto, J.B. Pochon, R. Levy, B. Dubois, Motivation, reward, and Parkinson's disease: influence of dopatherapy, Neuropsychologia 40 (2002) 2257–2267.

[43] A.M. Gotham, R.G. Brown, C.D. Marsden, Levodopa treatment may benefit or impair "frontal" function in Parkinson's disease, Lancet 2 (1986) 970–971.

[44] R. Cools, Dopaminergic modulation of cognitive function-implications for L-DOPA treatment in Parkinson's disease, Neurosci. Biobehav. Rev. 30 (2006) 1–23.

[45] D. Aarsland, G. Alves, J.P. Larsen, Disorders of motivation, sexual conduct, and sleep in Parkinson's disease, Adv. Neurol. 96 (2005) 56–64.

[46] K. Dujardin, P. Sockeel, D. Devos, M. Delliaux, P. Krystkowiak, A. Destee, L. Defebvre, Characteristics of apathy in Parkinson's disease, Mov. Disord. 22 (2007) 778–784.

[47] B.J. Knowlton, J.A. Mangels, L.R. Squire, A neostriatal habit learning system in humans, Science 273 (1996) 1399–1402.

[48] R. Cools, R.A. Barker, B.J. Sahakian, T.W. Robbins, Enhanced or impaired cognitive function in Parkinson's disease as a function of dopaminergic medication and task demands, Cereb. Cortex 11 (2001) 1136–1143.

[49] M.J. Frank, L.C. Seeberger, C. O'Reilly R, By carrot or by stick: cognitive reinforcement learning in parkinsonism, Science 306 (2004) 1940–1943.

[50] M. Pessiglione, D. Guehl, E.C. Hirsch, J. Feger, L. Tremblay, Disruption of self-organized actions in monkeys with progressive MPTP-induced parkinsonism. I. Effects of task complexity, Eur. J. Neurosci. 19 (2004) 426–436.

[51] M. Pessiglione, D. Guehl, A.S. Rolland, C. Francois, E.C. Hirsch, J. Feger, L. Tremblay, Thalamic neuronal activity in dopamine-depleted primates: evidence for a loss of functional segregation within basal ganglia circuits, J. Neurosci. 25 (2005) 1523–1531.

[52] E.T. Rolls, J. Hornak, D. Wade, J. McGrath, Emotion-related learning in patients with social and emotional changes associated with frontal lobe damage, J. Neurol. Neurosurg. Psychiatry 57 (1994) 1518–1524.

[53] C.E. Myers, D. Shohamy, M.A. Gluck, S. Grossman, A. Kluger, S. Ferris, J. Golomb, G. Schnirman, R. Schwartz, Dissociating hippocampal versus basal ganglia contributions to learning and transfer, J. Cogn. Neurosci. 15 (2003) 185–193.

[54] D. Shohamy, C.E. Myers, S. Grossman, J. Sage, M.A. Gluck, R.A. Poldrack, Cortico-striatal contributions to feedback-based learning: converging data from neuroimaging and neuropsychology, Brain 127 (2004) 851–859.

[55] H. Nagy, S. Keri, C.E. Myers, G. Benedek, D. Shohamy, M.A. Gluck, Cognitive sequence learning in Parkinson's disease and amnestic mild cognitive impairment: dissociation between sequential and non-sequential learning of associations, Neuropsychologia 45 (2007) 1386–1392.

[56] D. Shohamy, C.E. Myers, S. Grossman, J. Sage, M.A. Gluck, The role of dopamine in cognitive sequence learning: evidence from Parkinson's disease, Behav. Brain Res. 156 (2005) 191–199.

[57] D. Shohamy, C.E. Myers, K.D. Geghman, J. Sage, M.A. Gluck, L-dopa impairs learning, but spares generalization, in Parkinson's disease, Neuropsychologia 44 (2006) 774–784.

[58] V. Czernecki, B. Pillon, J.L. Houeto, M.L. Welter, V. Mesnage, Y. Agid, B. Dubois, Does bilateral stimulation of the subthalamic nucleus aggravate apathy in Parkinson's disease? J. Neurol. Neurosurg. Psychiatry 76 (2005) 775–779.

[59] A. Funkiewiez, C. Ardouin, R. Cools, P. Krack, V. Fraix, A. Batir, S. Chabardes, A.L. Benabid, T.W. Robbins, P. Pollak, Effects of levodopa and subthalamic nucleus stimulation on cognitive and affective functioning in Parkinson's disease, Mov. Disord. 21 (2006) 1656–1662.

[60] M. Pessiglione, V. Czernecki, B. Pillon, B. Dubois, M. Schupbach, Y. Agid, L. Tremblay, An effect of dopamine depletion on decision-making: the temporal coupling of deliberation and execution, J. Cogn. Neurosci. 17 (2005) 1886–1896.

[61] R. Swainson, R.D. Rogers, B.J. Sahakian, B.A. Summers, C.E. Polkey, T.W. Robbins, Probabilistic learning and reversal deficits in patients with Parkinson's disease or frontal or temporal lobe lesions: possible adverse effects of dopaminergic medication, Neuropsychologia 38 (2000) 596–612.

[62] M.J. Frank, J. Samanta, A.A. Moustafa, S.J. Sherman, Hold your horses: impulsivity, deep brain stimulation, and medication in parkinsonism, Science 318 (2007) 1309–1312.

[63] R. Cools, L. Altamirano, M. D'Esposito, Reversal learning in Parkinson's disease depends on medication status and outcome valence, Neuropsychologia 44 (2006) 1663–1673.

[64] M. Pessiglione, B. Seymour, G. Flandin, R.J. Dolan, C.D. Frith, Dopamine-dependent prediction errors underpin reward-seeking behaviour in humans, Nature 442 (2006) 1042–1045.

[65] M.J. Frank, A.A. Moustafa, H.M. Haughey, T. Curran, K.E. Hutchison, Genetic triple dissociation reveals multiple roles for dopamine in reinforcement learning, Proc. Natl. Acad. Sci. USA 104 (2007) 16311–16316.

[66] L.D. Selemon, P.S. Goldman-Rakic, Longitudinal topography and interdigitation of corticostriatal projections in the rhesus monkey, J. Neurosci. 5 (1985) 776–794.

[67] A.W. Flaherty, A.M. Graybiel, Two input systems for body representations in the primate striatal matrix: experimental evidence in the squirrel monkey, J. Neurosci. 13 (1993) 1120–1137.

[68] E. Gerardin, S. Lehericy, J.B. Pochon, S. Tezenas du Montcel, J.F. Mangin, F. Poupon, Y. Agid, D. Le Bihan, C. Marsault, Foot, hand, face and eye representation in the human striatum, Cereb. Cortex 13 (2003) 162–169.

[69] S. Lehericy, M. Ducros, P.F. Van de Moortele, C. Francois, L. Thivard, C. Poupon, N. Swindale, K. Ugurbil, D.S. Kim, Diffusion tensor fiber tracking shows distinct corticostriatal circuits in humans, Ann. Neurol. 55 (2004) 522–529.

[70] J. Yelnik, Functional anatomy of the basal ganglia, Mov. Disord. 17 (Suppl. 3) (2002) S15–S21.

[71] D. Joel, I. Weiner, The organization of the basal ganglia-thalamocortical circuits: open interconnected rather than closed segregated, Neuroscience 63 (1994) 363–379.

[72] M. Filion, L. Tremblay, P.J. Bedard, Abnormal influences of passive limb movement on the activity of globus pallidus neurons in parkinsonian monkeys, Brain Res. 444 (1988) 165–176.

[73] L. Escola, T. Michelet, G. Douillard, D. Guehl, B. Bioulac, P. Burbaud, Disruption of the proprioceptive mapping in the medial wall of parkinsonian monkeys, Ann. Neurol. 52 (2002) 581–587.

[74] J.A. Goldberg, T. Boraud, S. Maraton, S.N. Haber, E. Vaadia, H. Bergman, Enhanced synchrony among primary motor cortex neurons in the 1-methyl-4-phenyl-1,2,3,6-tetrahydropyridine primate model of Parkinson's disease, J. Neurosci. 22 (2002) 4639–4653.

[75] A. Leblois, W. Meissner, E. Bezard, B. Bioulac, C.E. Gross, T. Boraud, Temporal and spatial alterations in GPi neuronal encoding might contribute to slow down movement in Parkinsonian monkeys, Eur. J. Neurosci. 24 (2006) 1201–1208.

[76] L. Tremblay, M. Filion, P.J. Bedard, Responses of pallidal neurons to striatal stimulation in monkeys with MPTP-induced parkinsonism, Brain Res. 498 (1989) 17–33.

[77] A. Nini, A. Feingold, H. Slovin, H. Bergman, Neurons in the globus pallidus do not show correlated activity in the normal monkey, but phase-locked oscillations appear in the MPTP model of parkinsonism, J. Neurophysiol. 74 (1995) 1800–1805.

[78] A. Raz, E. Vaadia, H. Bergman, Firing patterns and correlations of spontaneous discharge of pallidal neurons in the normal and the tremulous 1-methyl-4-phenyl-1,2,3,6-tetrahydropyridine vervet model of parkinsonism, J. Neurosci. 20 (2000) 8559–8571.

[79] G. Heimer, I. Bar-Gad, J.A. Goldberg, H. Bergman, Dopamine replacement therapy reverses abnormal synchronization of pallidal neurons in the 1-methyl-4-phenyl-1,2,3,6-tetrahydropyridine primate model of parkinsonism, J. Neurosci. 22 (2002) 7850–7855.

[80] J.M. Hurtado, C.M. Gray, L.B. Tamas, K.A. Sigvardt, Dynamics of tremor-related oscillations in the human globus pallidus: a single case study, Proc. Natl. Acad. Sci. USA 96 (1999) 1674–1679.

[81] R. Levy, J.O. Dostrovsky, A.E. Lang, E. Sime, W.D. Hutchison, A.M. Lozano, Effects of apomorphine on subthalamic nucleus and globus pallidus internus neurons in patients with Parkinson's disease, J. Neurophysiol. 86 (2001) 249–260.

[82] P. Brown, A. Oliviero, P. Mazzone, A. Insola, P. Tonali, V. Di Lazzaro, Dopamine dependency of oscillations between subthalamic nucleus and pallidum in Parkinson's disease, J. Neurosci. 21 (2001) 1033–1038.

[83] A.G. Androulidakis, C. Brucke, F. Kempf, A. Kupsch, T. Aziz, K. Ashkan, A.A. Kuhn, P. Brown, Amplitude modulation of oscillatory activity in the subthalamic nucleus during movement, Eur. J. Neurosci. 27 (2008) 1277–1284.

[84] A.A. Kuhn, A. Kupsch, G.H. Schneider, P. Brown, Reduction in subthalamic 8-35 Hz oscillatory activity correlates with clinical improvement in Parkinson's disease, Eur. J. Neurosci. 23 (2006) 1956–1960.

[85] A.A. Kuhn, D. Williams, A. Kupsch, P. Limousin, M. Hariz, G.H. Schneider, K. Yarrow, P. Brown, Event-related beta desynchronization in human subthalamic nucleus correlates with motor performance, Brain 127 (2004) 735–746.

[86] G. Foffani, A.M. Bianchi, G. Baselli, A. Priori, Movement-related frequency modulation of beta oscillatory activity in the human subthalamic nucleus, J. Physiol. 568 (2005) 699–711.

[87] M. Weinberger, N. Mahant, W.D. Hutchison, A.M. Lozano, E. Moro, M. Hodaie, A.E. Lang, J.O. Dostrovsky, Beta oscillatory activity in the subthalamic nucleus and its relation to dopaminergic response in Parkinson's disease, J. Neurophysiol. 96 (2006) 3248–3256.

[88] R.L. Albin, A.B. Young, J.B. Penney, The functional anatomy of basal ganglia disorders, Trends Neurosci. 12 (1989) 366–375.

[89] M.R. DeLong, Primate models of movement disorders of basal ganglia origin, Trends Neurosci. 13 (1990) 281–285.

[90] J.W. Mink, The basal ganglia: focused selection and inhibition of competing motor programs, Prog. Neurobiol. 50 (1996) 381–425.

[91] P. Redgrave, T.J. Prescott, K. Gurney, The basal ganglia: a vertebrate solution to the selection problem? Neuroscience 89 (1999) 1009–1023.

[92] G. Chevalier, J.M. Deniau, Disinhibition as a basic process in the expression of striatal functions, Trends Neurosci. 13 (1990) 277–280.

[93] O. Hikosaka, R.H. Wurtz, Modification of saccadic eye movements by GABA-related substances. II. Effects of muscimol in monkey substantia nigra pars reticulata, J. Neurophysiol. 53 (1985) 292–308.

[94] C.R. Gerfen, J.F. McGinty, W.S. Young 3rd, Dopamine differentially regulates dynorphin, substance P, and enkephalin expression in striatal neurons: in situ hybridization histochemical analysis, J. Neurosci. 11 (1991) 1016–1031.

[95] A. Akaike, Y. Ohno, M. Sasa, S. Takaori, Excitatory and inhibitory effects of dopamine on neuronal activity of the caudate nucleus neurons in vitro, Brain Res. 418 (1987) 262–272.

[96] M. Filion, L. Tremblay, Abnormal spontaneous activity of globus pallidus neurons in monkeys with MPTP-induced parkinsonism, Brain Res. 547 (1991) 142–151.

[97] W.D. Hutchison, R. Levy, J.O. Dostrovsky, A.M. Lozano, A.E. Lang, Effects of apomorphine on globus pallidus neurons in parkinsonian patients, Ann. Neurol. 42 (1997) 767–775.

[98] T. Boraud, E. Bezard, D. Guehl, B. Bioulac, C. Gross, Effects of L-DOPA on neuronal activity of the globus pallidus externalis (GPe) and globus pallidus internalis (GPi) in the MPTP-treated monkey, Brain Res. 787 (1998) 157–160.

[99] H. Bergman, T. Wichmann, M.R. DeLong, Reversal of experimental parkinsonism by lesions of the subthalamic nucleus, Science 249 (1990) 1436–1438.

[100] P. Limousin, P. Pollak, A. Benazzouz, D. Hoffmann, J.F. Le Bas, E. Broussolle, J.E. Perret, A.L. Benabid, Effect of parkinsonian signs and symptoms of bilateral subthalamic nucleus stimulation, Lancet 345 (1995) 91–95.

[101] A.L. Benabid, Deep brain stimulation for Parkinson's disease, Curr. Opin. Neurobiol. 13 (2003) 696–706.

[102] A. Parent, L.N. Hazrati, Functional anatomy of the basal ganglia. I. The cortico-basal ganglia-thalamo-cortical loop, Brain Res. Brain Res. Rev. 20 (1995) 91–127.

[103] J. Yelnik, C. Francois, G. Percheron, D. Tande, A spatial and quantitative study of the striat-opallidal connection in the monkey, Neuroreport 7 (1996) 985–988.

[104] O. Aizman, H. Brismar, P. Uhlen, E. Zettergren, A.I. Levey, H. Forssberg, P. Greengard, A. Aperia, Anatomical and physiological evidence for D1 and D2 dopamine receptor colocalization in neostriatal neurons, Nat. Neurosci. 3 (2000) 226–230.

[105] A. Leblois, W. Meissner, B. Bioulac, C.E. Gross, D. Hansel, T. Boraud, Late emergence of synchronized oscillatory activity in the pallidum during progressive Parkinsonism, Eur. J. Neurosci. 26 (2007) 1701–1713.

[106] A. Nambu, A new dynamic model of the cortico-basal ganglia loop, Prog. Brain Res. 143 (2004) 461–466.

[107] A.R. Aron, R.A. Poldrack, Cortical and subcortical contributions to Stop signal response inhibition: role of the subthalamic nucleus, J. Neurosci. 26 (2006) 2424–2433.

[108] W. Schultz, Getting formal with dopamine and reward, Neuron 36 (2002) 241–263.

[109] J. Mirenowicz, W. Schultz, Importance of unpredictability for reward responses in primate dopamine neurons, J. Neurophysiol. 72 (1994) 1024–1027.

[110] R. Romo, W. Schultz, Dopamine neurons of the monkey midbrain: contingencies of responses to active touch during self-initiated arm movements, J. Neurophysiol. 63 (1990) 592–606.

[111] T. Ljungberg, P. Apicella, W. Schultz, Responses of monkey dopamine neurons during learning of behavioral reactions, J. Neurophysiol. 67 (1992) 145–163.

[112] W. Schultz, P. Apicella, T. Ljungberg, Responses of monkey dopamine neurons to reward and conditioned stimuli during successive steps of learning a delayed response task, J. Neurosci. 13 (1993) 900–913.

[113] J.R. Hollerman, W. Schultz, Dopamine neurons report an error in the temporal prediction of reward during learning, Nat. Neurosci. 1 (1998) 304–309.

[114] P. Waelti, A. Dickinson, W. Schultz, Dopamine responses comply with basic assumptions of formal learning theory, Nature 412 (2001) 43–48.

[115] J. Mirenowicz, W. Schultz, Preferential activation of midbrain dopamine neurons by appetitive rather than aversive stimuli, Nature 379 (1996) 449–451.

[116] M.A. Ungless, Dopamine: the salient issue, Trends Neurosci. 27 (2004) 702–706.

[117] H. Nakahara, H. Itoh, R. Kawagoe, Y. Takikawa, O. Hikosaka, Dopamine neurons can represent context-dependent prediction error, Neuron 41 (2004) 269–280.

[118] P.N. Tobler, C.D. Fiorillo, W. Schultz, Adaptive coding of reward value by dopamine neurons, Science 307 (2005) 1642–1645.

[119] H.M. Bayer, P.W. Glimcher, Midbrain dopamine neurons encode a quantitative reward prediction error signal, Neuron 47 (2005) 129–141.

[120] W. Schultz, P. Dayan, P.R. Montague, A neural substrate of prediction and reward, Science 275 (1997) 1593–1599.

[121] R.S. Sutton, A.G. Barto, Reinforcement Learning, MIT Press, Cambridge, MA, 1998.

[122] R.R. Miller, R.C. Barnet, N.J. Grahame, Assessment of the Rescorla-Wagner model, Psychol. Bull. 117 (1995) 363–386.

[123] P.R. Montague, P. Dayan, T.J. Sejnowski, A framework for mesencephalic dopamine systems based on predictive Hebbian learning, J. Neurosci. 16 (1996) 1936–1947.

[124] R.E. Suri, W. Schultz, A neural network model with dopamine-like reinforcement signal that learns a spatial delayed response task, Neuroscience 91 (1999) 871–890.

[125] J.R. Wickens, A.J. Begg, G.W. Arbuthnott, Dopamine reverses the depression of rat corticostriatal synapses which normally follows high-frequency stimulation of cortex in vitro, Neuroscience 70 (1996) 1–5.

[126] D. Centonze, P. Gubellini, B. Picconi, P. Calabresi, P. Giacomini, G. Bernardi, Unilateral dopamine denervation blocks corticostriatal LTP, J. Neurophysiol. 82 (1999) 3575–3579.

[127] C.R. Gerfen, T.M. Engber, L.C. Mahan, Z. Susel, T.N. Chase, F.J. Monsma Jr., D.R. Sibley, D1 and D2 dopamine receptor-regulated gene expression of striatonigral and striatopallidal neurons, Science 250 (1990) 1429–1432.

[128] I. Liste, G. Rozas, M.J. Guerra, J.L. Labandeira-Garcia, Cortical stimulation induces Fos expression in striatal neurons via NMDA glutamate and dopamine receptors, Brain Res. 700 (1995) 1–12.

[129] L. Tremblay, J.R. Hollerman, W. Schultz, Modifications of reward expectation-related neuronal activity during learning in primate striatum, J. Neurophysiol. 80 (1998) 964–977.

[130] M.S. Jog, Y. Kubota, C.I. Connolly, V. Hillegaart, A.M. Graybiel, Building neural representations of habits, Science 286 (1999) 1745–1749.

[131] D. Joel, Y. Niv, E. Ruppin, Actor-critic models of the basal ganglia: new anatomical and computational perspectives, Neural Netw. 15 (2002) 535–547.

[132] K. Doya, Modulators of decision making, Nat. Neurosci. 11 (2008) 410–416.

[133] J. O'Doherty, P. Dayan, J. Schultz, R. Deichmann, K. Friston, R.J. Dolan, Dissociable roles of ventral and dorsal striatum in instrumental conditioning, Science 304 (2004) 452–454.

[134] I. Bar-Gad, H. Bergman, Stepping out of the box: information processing in the neural networks of the basal ganglia, Curr. Opin. Neurobiol. 11 (2001) 689–695.

[135] A.D. Lawrence, A.H. Evans, A.J. Lees, Compulsive use of dopamine replacement therapy in Parkinson's disease: reward systems gone awry? Lancet Neurol. 2 (2003) 595–604.

[136] V. Voon, M.N. Potenza, T. Thomsen, Medication-related impulse control and repetitive behaviors in Parkinson's disease, Curr. Opin. Neurol. 20 (2007) 484–492.

[137] D.A. Gallagher, S.S. O'Sullivan, A.H. Evans, A.J. Lees, A. Schrag, Pathological gambling in Parkinson's disease: risk factors and differences from dopamine dysregulation. An analysis of published case series, Mov. Disord. 22 (2007) 1757–1763.

[138] A.D. Smith, J.P. Bolam, The neural network of the basal ganglia as revealed by the study of synaptic connections of identified neurons, Trends Neurosci 13 (1990) 259–265.

13 A neuropsychological perspective on the role of the prefrontal cortex in reward processing and decision-making

Michael Hernandez, Natalie L. Denburg and Daniel Tranel

Division of Behavioral Neurology and Cogntive Neuroscience, University of Iowa College of Medicine, Iowa City, IA, USA

Abstract

The ventromedial prefrontal cortex (VMPC) in humans plays important roles in cognition and emotion regulation. Damage to the VMPC brain region can produce devastating impairments in higher-order behavioral guidance, social conduct, and emotional regulation, even though functions such as language, movement, and perception are spared. When the VMPC is damaged, patients fail to appreciate and take into account the long-term consequences of their decisions, and they tend to act as if they have "myopia for the future." Lesions of the VMPC also lead to an increase in utilitarian moral judgments and irrational responses to unfair social interactions, both of which have been attributed to emotional dysregulation. Aging has been shown to cause similar decision-making deficits in a substantial subset of older adults, suggesting that the VMPC region can be disproportionately affected by neurological aging.

Key points

1. Lesions of the human ventromedial prefrontal cortex (VMPC) have been shown to impair normal emotional responses and to decrease emotional intelligence.
2. Human VMPC lesions are associated with decision-making deficits in real life and on the Iowa Gambling Task (IGT), a laboratory model of real-world decision-making.
3. Moral judgments can be altered by lesions of the VMPC, so that patients with VMPC damage are *more* willing to choose utilitarian solutions that involve highly aversive personal actions.
4. A substantial subset of ostensibly healthy older adults performs defectively on decision-making tasks such as the Iowa Gambling Task, in a manner reminiscent of neurological patients with VMPC lesions.

5. The VMPC is an important structure for decision-making and emotional regulation, and this sector of the brain may deteriorate disproportionately during aging in some individuals.

13.1 Brief history of neuropsychology

A fundamental goal of this chapter is to highlight insights from the field of neuropsychology into prefrontal brain functions such as reward processing and decision-making. It is appropriate to begin with a brief history [for more in-depth reviews, see [1] or Benton (2000) [27]]. Given the capacity for conscious thought, it seems almost inevitable that a living being will eventually begin to ponder the substrate of this remarkable ability. The quest to discover the biological foundation for our cognitive abilities, including consciousness, is a core endeavor of the entire field of neuropsychology. The search for the corporeal seat of our mind has persisted for nearly two millennia. The earliest hypotheses (c. AD 100–400) suggested that mental functions might be localized along the anterior–posterior axis of the brain or its ventricles. One such theory, put forth by Nemesius (c. AD 390), posited a logical progression from sensory perception in the anterior ventricles, to thinking and reasoning in the third ventricle, and ending with memory in the fourth ventricle. This type of theory fit well with the scientific belief that mental processes resulted from the movement of animal spirits, which could flow freely through the ventricles. Similar theories of ventricular localization were the predominant dogma in the field for centuries to come.

It was not until the seventeenth and eighteenth centuries that the predominant theories about localization of mental functions shifted away from the ventricles into the tissue of the brain. It was during this time (1664) that Thomas Willis wrote his groundbreaking and comprehensive account of neural anatomy, *Cerebri anatome*. Willis utilized comparative anatomy along with clinical observations and existing theories to divide the brain into functional areas. Although many of the specific claims of the researchers of this time period have largely been disproved, the general idea that certain areas of the brain are specialized to perform specific tasks was an important step forward.

The modern science of neuropsychology came into its own during the nineteenth century. During the first half of the nineteenth century, studies with animals demonstrated links between the brain stem and respiration, and showed that ventral and dorsal spinal roots served motor and sensory function respectively. Against this background appeared Franz Joseph Gall (1757–1828), a man with some truly revolutionary ideas. His theory of phrenology held that the cerebrum could be subdivided into a large number of "organs," which were individually responsible for particular personality traits or mental functions. He also proposed that the topography of the cranium was affected by the size of these organs, and that cranioscopic measurements could therefore be used to assess mental abilities.

Although Gall's ideas about localization of function were too specific, they were able to spark some scientific debate, and may have inspired some of the research that followed. A new view of localization was put forth by Jean-Baptiste Bouillaud (1796–1881). Based on autopsy results, Bouillaud reported that lesions of the frontal lobes were capable of causing interruptions in speech. Bouillaud met with formidable opposition against his findings, possibly because of the association of any localizationist thought with phrenology. It was not until the early 1860s, when Paul Broca began to report his findings of language localization in the left hemisphere, that research into the localization of function was able to separate itself from phrenology and become a legitimate field of study. It was around this same time that the scientific community was first introduced to the possible functions of the prefrontal cortex.

13.2   Phineas Gage

Phineas Gage was a nineteenth-century railroad foreman. Laying railroad track in the hilly regions of New England often required the use of explosive charges, the scars of which still mark the roadsides to this day. Holes were drilled, filled with powder, and topped with a fuse and a layer of sand. This was all packed into place with a tamping iron and detonated from a safe distance to excavate any rock that obstructed the desired path of the railroads. On 13 September 1848, this procedure did not go as planned. Gage had filled one such hole with powder and was using his tamping iron to compact it slightly before adding the sand. He turned to look at his men, and this brief distraction was enough to cause him to make contact between the tamping iron and the rock wall inside the hole. The powder exploded, firing the tamping iron like a missile through the front of his head. This particular missile was three feet, seven inches in length, one and one-quarter inch in diameter, and weighed thirteen and quarter pounds. Reports from men working nearby indicated that Gage was blown onto his back and dazed, but was able to speak within a few minutes [25].

Gage was cared for and observed closely by Dr. John M. Harlow for months after the injury. He was given a clean bill of health; however, Harlow promised to discuss the mental manifestations of the patient in a future paper. This promise was fulfilled 20 years later [2], and it laid the groundwork for the idea that behavioral syndromes could be elicited by damage to the frontal lobes. Rather than summarizing his findings, it is informative to read this oft-quoted excerpt from his account:

> His contractors, who regarded him as the most efficient and capable foreman in their employ previous to his injury, considered the change in his mind so marked that they could not give him his place again. He is fitful, irreverent, indulging at times in the grossest profanity (which was not previously his custom), manifesting but little deference for his fellows, impatient of restraint or advice when it conflicts with his desires, at times pertinaciously obstinate, yet capricious and vacillating, devising many plans of future operation, which are no sooner arranged than they are abandoned in turn for others appearing more feasible. In this regard, his mind was radically changed, so decidedly that his friends and acquaintances said he was "no longer Gage."

Phineas Gage died 12 years after his accident, reportedly from complications of seizures. John Harlow was able to get consent from Gage's family to recover his skull 5 years after he had been interred. The request was granted, and the skull of Phineas Gage has been on display, alongside the tamping iron that shot through it, at the Warren Anatomical Medical Museum at Harvard University. The skull rested there undisturbed until a collaborative effort between the University of Iowa and Harvard University brought Phineas Gage back into the spotlight almost 150 years after his famous accident. Damasio and colleagues were able to use computers to recreate Gage's brain in 3D space based on precise measurements and photographs. They were then able to model his brain within the skull (Fig. 13.1) and accurately estimate the areas of the brain that were likely damaged by the tamping iron. The conclusion was that the ventromedial regions of both frontal lobes were damaged, but the dorsolateral regions were spared [3].

The story of Phineas Gage has inspired research into the role of the VMPC in emotional regulation, decision-making, and social behavior. In the current chapter, we will examine findings from each of these lines of research, and then we will introduce a line of

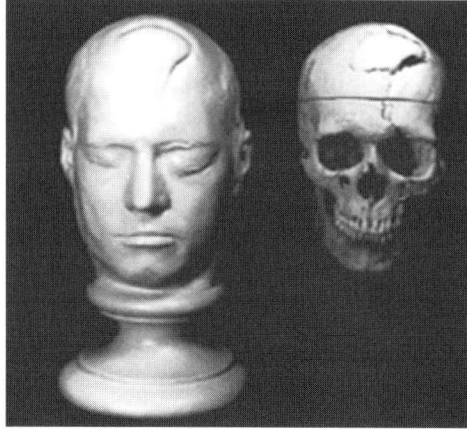

Figure 13.1 The life mask and skull of Phineas Gage [26].

research that attempts to explain all of these deficits within a theoretical framework. The following description of the main underlying hypothesis should help provide a framework for the presentation.

13.3   Somatic marker hypothesis

Many of the problems encountered by patients with VMPC damage have been described previously under the rubric "acquired sociopathy." Although this term is not ideal because of connotations of crime and aggression (which are *not* typical of VMPC patients), the term does help capture the abrupt and astounding changes in personality and behavior that can be elicited by damage to the VMPC. Phineas Gage and patient EVR are prototypical cases of the disorder described in detail by Antonio Damasio [4]. Both men were industrious and successful in their trades, charming and adept at navigating social situations, until sudden brain damage changed them forever. Following lesions to the VMPC, both patients suffered from a similar constellation of deficiencies. They were no longer able to hold gainful employment; they were less responsive to punishment; they tended to present an unrealistically favorable view of themselves; they demonstrated stereotyped but correct manners; they tended to display inappropriate emotional reactions; and their intelligence remained normal. None of these problems appeared to be brewing before the lesion onset, but rather appeared suddenly after damage to the VMPC. The lives of these individuals often pass from one tragic event to the next, from the loss of employment, to disassociation from friends and family, to divorce, leaving them unable to care for themselves and relying on others to support them.

Many of the tragedies that occur in the lives of those with VMPC damage are linked to these major changes in their personality and social functioning. Research has been conducted to enumerate the variety of personality changes that typically result from bilateral damage to the VMPC [5]. Previous studies in this field had been conducted with tools that were not well suited to quantify the variety of neurologically based changes in personality that occur in patients with VMPC damage. The Iowa Scales of Personality Change (ISPC) were developed to overcome the inadequacies of other tests available at the time [6]. The ISPC provides standardized assessment across the wide range of personality changes that can result from common neurological conditions. All personality characteristics included on the instrument are quantified at both current levels as well as levels that existed prior to the neurological insult. Change scores are then calculated for all personality characteristics, regardless of whether a given characteristic is deemed problematic. This instrument utilizes information from informants (e.g., a spouse or family member) who were familiar with the patient before the incident and were in a position to closely observe them in a non-clinical setting subsequent to the event.

The ISPC was used to assess the personality changes associated with bilateral damage to VMPC [5]. Three groups of participants were evaluated: participants who suffered bilateral VMPC damage (PF-BVM), participants with lesions in prefrontal regions that were primarily outside VMPC (PF-NBVM), and participants with lesions outside prefrontal cortices (NPF). The ISPC was used to evaluate changes in personality that occurred in each group subsequent to neurological insult. The mean ratings of the PF-BVM group were significantly higher than the two brain-damaged comparison groups on 14 of 30 personality characteristics.

The authors draw parallels between the constellation of personality disturbances evidenced by the PF-BVM group and features of developmental sociopathy, including shallow affect, irresponsibility, vocational instability, lack of realistic long-term goals, lack of empathy, and poor behavioral control. As noted, the term "acquired sociopathy" is used to convey the similarities of disturbances that occur subsequent to bilateral VMPC damage and lifelong characteristics associated with developmental sociopathy. The similar personality disturbances suggest that VMPC dysfunction underlies developmental sociopathy. This assertion is supported by studies that have shown similar disturbances of psychophysiological functioning among developmental sociopaths and participants with adult-onset lesions in VMPC [5]. Although there are several similarities, substantial differences between developmental and acquired sociopathy have been pointed out. Damage to the VMPC acquired in adulthood is not associated with the need for stimulation, grandiose sense of self-worth, pathological lying, glibness and superficial charm, manipulativeness, and the remorseless abuse of others that is typical of developmental sociopaths (Barrash et al., 1994).

The somatic marker hypothesis, as proposed by Damasio [4], has gained a foothold as an explanation for the impairments in decision-making and emotion-regulation associated with VMPC damage. The hypothesis outlines a neural system of emotion, which is capable of using "somatic markers" to bias decisions at a conscious or nonconscious level. These somatic markers can associate bad feelings with poor decisions or good feelings with advantageous decisions. Lesions of the VMPC deprive patients of these somatic markers, and thereby increase the complexity of the decision-making process. Without somatic markers biasing you toward good decisions, it is easy to get lost in an endless stream of decisions between seemingly equal choices. For example, imagine that you are faced with deciding whether or not to make an extremely risky investment with the promise of a high rate of return. The negative somatic markers associated with the possibility of future financial ruin make you pause and take a closer look at all aspects of the investment.

Damasio has outlined a network of neural structures that play a role in evoking and interpreting somatic markers. There are two main categories of circumstances that may trigger somatic markers. The first set of circumstances involves situations that elicit primary emotions. These are events or objects that seem hardwired to elicit an emotional response virtually from the moment we are born. The bared teeth of a snarling dog or the slithering motion of an approaching cobra are generally fearful stimuli to all people regardless of age or culture. These innately fear-generating situations would likely lead to activation of a limbic structure such as the amygdala. The limbic areas would then be able to activate a variety of neural structures to generate an appropriate body state alteration consistent with the experience of fear.

The second set of emotionally evocative circumstances is somewhat less direct, and can vary widely from one individual to the next. These situations elicit secondary emotions. Imagine that you were asked to recall the day you heard that your first dog passed away. You may feel your heart sink, your gut tighten, and the muscles in your face may turn downward in an expression of sadness. Perhaps you never owned a dog, or maybe you do not even like dogs, in which case you may not feel any of that. The emotional reaction in this case is not innate, but rather based on individual experience. In situations like this, the prefrontal cortices are believed to play an important role. Damasio suggests that pondering emotionally evocative situations first conjures images in early sensory cortices. These images trigger activity in the prefrontal cortices, which has developed associations over your lifetime between emotions and the images that have evoked them in the past. The prefrontal cortices then selectively activate limbic areas including the amygdala or anterior cingulate cortex. As is the case with primary emotions, the limbic structures are able to activate a variety of neural structures to generate a body state alteration consistent with the emotion being experienced.

The preceding paragraphs outline the process of eliciting emotions in response to mental images, but humans can go one step further. For emotions to truly be useful, we have to feel them. An emotional response on its own can be sufficient to initiate avoidance or approach behaviors in a given situation. However, we can have a conscious feeling of the emotion; that is to say, we can be consciously aware of the causal relationship between the mental images and the alterations in our internal body state. This feeling can then be used to create new associations in higher-order cortices to help us plan to avoid unpleasant, or seek out appetitive, experiences in the future. The ongoing mapping of our internal body states takes place in a number of subcortical structures, as well as in insular and parietal cortices. This information must be combined with sensory images in the prefrontal cortices to elicit a feeling.

The VMPC stands out as the heart of neural machinery involved in emotion and feelings. The VMPC receives inputs from all sensory modalities, both internal and external. It is linked with cortical and subcortical motor areas. The VMPC is also able to activate autonomic nervous system effector areas in the hypothalamus and brainstem nuclei. This interconnection allows the VMPC to make associations between external stimuli and the internal body states that they create. Based on previous situations, the VMPC is able to activate autonomic effectors appropriately in novel situations to bias our decisions one way or the other.

13.4   Emotion regulation

Lesions of the VMPC have been shown to blunt normal emotional responses. In a series of studies summarized by Tranel [7], the emotional responses of a group of VMPC patients were examined using psychophysiological techniques. The experimenters tested a group of patients with VMPC damage, a comparison group with brain damage outside of VMPC, and a group of neurologically intact participants. The participants were shown evocative images including social disaster, mutilation, or nudity. As expected, the images elicited high-magnitude skin conductance responses (SCRs) in both the normal and brain-damaged comparison groups. However, the patients with damage to the

VMPC remained unflappable. VMPC patients were able to reliably generate SCRs to unconditioned stimuli, such as a loud noise, but when shown evocative pictures, their SCRs were minimal, or even entirely absent. The lack of SCRs suggests that stimuli that would normally evoke emotional reactions in the general public are no longer evocative subsequent to VMPC damage. Diminished emotional responses can impact everything from social interactions to decision-making. Findings like this open the door to new investigations into the abilities of VMPC patients to reliably regulate and utilize emotional information (Fig. 13.2).

Emotional intelligence is a relatively new field of neuropsychological study. Bar-On et al. [8] set out to determine what areas of the brain constitute the neurological substrate of emotional and social intelligence. To do so, they tested brain-damaged individuals on Bar-On's Emotional Quotient Inventory (EQ-i). The experimental group consisted of six patients with lesions involving the bilateral VMPC, three with damage to the amygdala, and three with damage to the right anterior insula. The experimental group scored significantly lower than the brain-damaged comparison participants, as did each of the anatomical subgroups. Because of the small sample size, and in accord with the proposed circuitry of the somatic marker hypothesis, the results were interpreted for the whole experimental group, rather than analyzed by each anatomical subgroup separately. It is interesting to note, however, that VMPC damage alone was sufficient to significantly

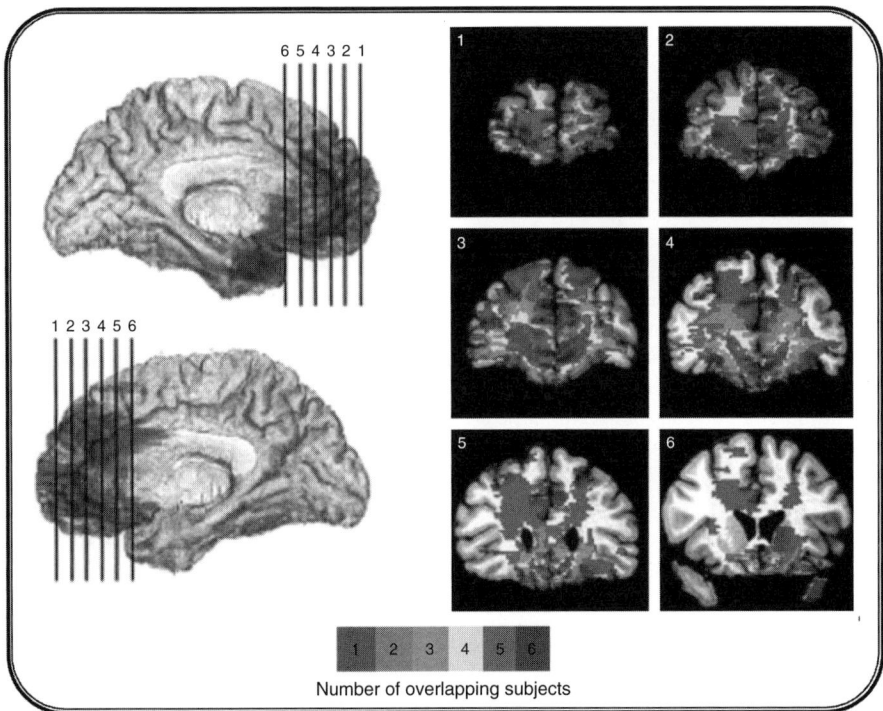

Figure 13.2 Lesion overlap of VMPC patients. Lesions of six VMPC patients displayed in mesial views and coronal slices. The color bar indicates the number of overlapping lesions at each voxel. This lesion overlap map is typical of bilateral VMPC lesion groups used in studies at the University of Iowa. *Source*: Adapted from Koenigs et al. (2007) [12]. See Plate 16 of Color Plate section.

lower EQ-i scores, in spite of the patients having normal scores on tests of cognitive IQ and having demographic characteristics comparable to the comparison groups.

The Bar-On test utilizes a number of subtests, and researchers were able to determine which EQ-i variables were most affected by damage to the neural circuitry of somatic markers. Bar-On lists the patients' problems as "the ability to be aware of oneself and one's emotions, to express oneself and one's feelings, to manage and control emotions, to adapt flexibly to change and solve problems of a personal nature, as well as the ability to motivate oneself and mobilize positive affect." It is easy to see how deficits in this wide range of emotional regulatory processes could lead to problems in everyday life. The lack of insight into their emotions and goals is likely related to many of the reasoning and decision-making deficits that are so pervasive in the lives of these patients.

13.5   Making decisions

Anecdotal descriptions of prefrontal brain damage leading to disruptions in reasoning and goal-directed behavior have existed for a long time. In the work of Bechara et al. [9], the pervasive real-world decision-making disorder of patients with VMPC lesions was finally captured in the laboratory. Patients with VMPC damage (see [4,7] for reviews) were exhibiting obvious deficits in their everyday lives; however, these impairments were extraordinarily elusive in standard neuropsychological testing. It was against this backdrop that Bechara and colleagues [9] developed the test now known as the Iowa Gambling Task (IGT).

The IGT has changed in subtle ways since its original development, so we will explain it as it exists today, and as it has been used most frequently in the literature. The test consists of four decks of cards, A, B, C, and D. Participants are instructed to choose a card from one deck at a time repeatedly until instructed to stop. Each time the participant selects a card, they are told that they have won some money. On some selections, participants encounter monetary losses subsequent to the gain. Participants are informed that some of the decks are better than others and that they can succeed in the game by avoiding the worst decks. The decks are different from each other in three modalities: frequency of punishment, magnitude of gains and losses, and net outcome. Deck A yields a high frequency of punishment, high magnitude of gains and losses, and a negative net outcome. Deck B yields a low frequency of punishment, high magnitude of gains and losses, and a negative net outcome. Deck C yields a high frequency of punishment, low magnitude of gains and losses, and a positive net outcome. Deck D yields a low frequency of punishment, low magnitude of gains and losses, and a positive net outcome. Thus, success can be achieved by making more selections from decks C and D. Participants who acquire this strategy usually report that they succeed by choosing from decks with low initial reward. Participants are asked to stop after completing 100 card selections, and performance has typically been scored as the net advantageous selections [(Selections from C + D) − (Selections from A + B)] in blocks of 20 selections. This scoring allows for visualization of the learning curve that occurs in normal healthy participants.

This laboratory test was able to capture the deficit of reasoning and decision-making that was so obvious in the lives of VMPC patients and yet so indefinable by conventional neuropsychological means. The test was administered to patient EVR and six patients with similar damage to the VMPC. Their results were compared to the performance of a large group of normal, healthy comparison participants. It was found that the comparison participants had no trouble with the task and chose predominantly from decks with advantageous outcomes. The patients with damage to the VMPC were impaired on this task, demonstrating a complete reversal of normal task behavior and making the bulk of their selections from disadvantageous decks. The authors conclude that the VMPC patients were focused on the larger immediate rewards of the disadvantageous decks, and could not take into account the severe delayed punishments associated with these decks. The authors also reversed the reward–punishment order, such that participants encountered immediate punishment and delayed reward, to determine the cause of this effect. The VMPC patients were also impaired on this version of the task, leading the authors to rule out the possibility that the VMPC patients were merely insensitive to punishment. Instead, they concluded that the VMPC patients suffer from a general myopia for the future. From the point of view of the somatic marker hypothesis, this myopia for the future may result from a lack of somatic markers associated with possible future outcomes. The VMPC patients may be able to conjure possible future outcomes, but they would be unable to "mark" them with a positive or negative value, thereby rendering them useless for decision-making [9,10].

Further work with the IGT was conducted to help determine whether or not defective somatic markers play a role in the disruption of the decision-making process. Bechara et al. [10] incorporated recording of SCRs with the administration of their task to evaluate whether or not physiological arousal was involved in biasing decisions. The experimenters also stopped the participants periodically to ask them, "Tell me all you know about what is going on in this game" and "Tell me how you feel about this game." The findings were interesting in both comparison and lesion patients. The normal participants began to make advantageous choices that seemed to be guided by their physiological arousal state before they were consciously aware of the rules of the game. The guidance by physiological arousal was evident in anticipatory SCRs, which were the SCRs generated in the deliberation time before selecting a card. The magnitude of these SCRs was greater in the seconds preceding a selection from a disadvantageous deck than in the moments preceding a selection from an advantageous deck. This signal was apparently able to bias deck selection, that is, decision-making behavior. As soon as the normal comparison participants began to generate discriminatory anticipatory SCRs, they also began to favor selections from the advantageous decks, and all of this happened before they were able to report conscious knowledge of their strategy.

The VMPC patients in this study demonstrated impaired behavioral responses in the task, replicating the findings of Bechara et al. [9]. The new study uncovered a possible reason for this impairment. The anticipatory SCRs that seemed to help guide decision-making in normal comparison participants were significantly diminished in the VMPC patients. Not only was the magnitude of the SCR much lower in VMPC patients, but the SCRs were not able to discriminate between advantageous and disadvantageous decks. It seems plausible that damage to the VMPC precludes the generation of somatic markers to aid in reasoning and decision-making. This work demonstrated that diminished emotional biases due to VMPC dysfunction negatively impacts decision-making. It stands to reason that other aspects of cognition, especially those involved in navigating the social landscape, could be equally impaired by VMPC dysfunction.

13.6   Social interactions and moral judgments

Furtive investigation into the neurological underpinnings of social and moral behavior is a relatively recent phenomenon. This new line of study into the social decision-making capacity of VMPC patients has been advanced by the work of Koenigs and colleagues

[11–13]. Koenigs and Tranel [11] tested patients with VMPC damage with the Ultimatum Game. In the Ultimatum Game, two players are given an amount of money to split, say, $10. One player (the proposer) determines how to split the money and offers a portion to the second player (the responder). The responder then decides whether or not to accept the offer. If the responder accepts the offer, then the players split the money according to the proposal. If the responder rejects the offer, then neither player receives any money. Since any amount of money is better than no money at all, a rational actor would accept any proposed offer. They found that patients with VMPC damage were more likely than normal comparison, or brain-damaged comparison, participants to reject unfair offers. It seems that the VMPC patients are unable to regulate their emotional reaction to the unfair offers as effectively as comparison participants. The authors suggest that intact VMPC functioning may be essential for rationally deciding to accept unfair offers.

In another study, Koenigs et al. [12] investigated the moral judgments of six VMPC patients. The participants in this study were asked to evaluate a set of moral dilemmas and then select the best course of action. Generally, the dilemmas involve making a sacrifice for the greater good (e.g., sacrificing a single life to save several). The experimenters hypothesized that lesions of the VMPC could lead to more utilitarian judgments because the sacrifices would not be as emotionally aversive. The VMPC patients performed no differently from the comparison groups when evaluating low-conflict dilemmas. A low-conflict dilemma is one in which one choice is clearly superior (e.g., transporting a man who is bleeding to death to the hospital even though it will stain your upholstery). The high-conflict dilemmas do not necessarily have an obviously superior choice (e.g., smothering one's baby to save a number of people). Relative to the comparison groups, a larger proportion of the VMPC group chose to engage in the unsavory activity to resolve the high-conflict dilemmas (e.g., smothering the baby). The authors suggest that the damage to the VMPC may eliminate the emotional reaction to the thought of harming others, at which point the participant is more apt to use a utilitarian approach to maximize the aggregate welfare.

It has been found that patients suffering from frontotemporal dementia (FTD) give abnormal responses on a test of moral reasoning. In one study [14], FTD patients were presented with two versions of a classic moral dilemma. In both scenarios, there is a trolley hurtling down the tracks toward a group of five unsuspecting people who will surely die if nothing is done. In the first scenario, the participant has the option of pulling a lever to switch the trolley to a different track where there is only one bystander to be killed. In the second situation, the participant has the option of pushing a large man off of a footbridge and onto the tracks to stop the trolley. In both situations, one person dies if the participant acts, or five people die if the participant takes no action. Classically, healthy people will choose to pull the lever, but will not push a man to his death. The FTD patients in this experiment made no such distinction, endorsing both actions. As the name suggests, FTD primarily involves degradation of brain tissue in the frontal and temporal lobes. It is likely that deterioration within the VMPC contributes to the patients' callous decision-making.

Whether we are checking our email, reading the newspaper, listening to the radio, or walking down the street, advertisers are constantly trying to influence the decisions we make. Koenigs and Tranel [13] investigated whether lesions of the VMPC could interfere with brand biasing. They used the "Pepsi paradox" to test this hypothesis. The paradox is thus: In blind taste tests, Pepsi is reliably preferred over Coke; however, Coke consistently outsells Pepsi. To test the paradox, the experimenters ran a blind and a semi-blind taste test. The blind taste test consists of two plastic cups with no brand information; one contains Pepsi and one contains Coke. The Coke semi-blind taste test involves two cups, one with brand information and one without. The unbranded cup always contains the same soda as the branded cup, but participants are told that it could contain either Coke or Pepsi (in fact, both cups always contain Coke). The Pepsi semi-blind taste test is the same, except that the cups are both filled with Pepsi. In the blind taste tests, VMPC patients and comparison participants alike showed a preference for Pepsi over Coke. The comparison participants chose labeled Coke more than labeled Pepsi in the semi-blind taste tests, reaffirming the Pepsi paradox. However, the VMPC patients chose labeled Pepsi more than labeled Coke in the semi-blind taste test, demonstrating that they were apparently unbiased by the Coke brand. A major goal of commercial advertising is to make positive emotional connections between consumers and specific brands. It seems that the ability to make these associations relies on an intact VMPC.

13.7   The aging VMPC

Acute damage to the VMPC can cause a dramatic and nearly instantaneous change in an individual's ability to regulate emotions and make effective decisions. However, recent research has revealed a much more insidious and pervasive threat to VMPC function—namely, aging. The cognitive neuroscience of aging is a burgeoning field that is beginning to uncover links between the normal aging process and changes in our cognitive abilities. Some of these cognitive changes have been widely recognized for a long time. Older adults are often thought of as more forgetful, and they may not think as quickly as their younger counterparts. However, with age comes wisdom; that is to say, your knowledge base and vocabulary are ever expanding throughout the healthy aging process. While the cognitive neuroscience of aging is interested in discovering the neural underpinnings of these age-related changes, there are some changes that are just recently being linked with aging.

Carstensen [15] has suggested that the normal aging process is sufficient to alter emotional regulation. In her theory of socioemotional selectivity (SES), Carstensen [15] suggests that people's perception of their own lifespan can greatly impact their strategies for emotional regulation. Research based on this theory has shown that older adults demonstrate a positivity bias [16–19]. Thus, older individuals are more likely than their younger counterparts to remember positive experiences, seek out positive social encounters, and pare down their social partners to only those who make them happy. These well-documented changes in motivation, and the emphasis on seeking out emotionally gratifying experiences late in life, suggests that there may be some alteration in VMPC activity associated with the aging process.

Recent work by Denburg and colleagues has begun to investigate whether normal, healthy aging can lead to disruption in the same processes that are disturbed by VMPC lesions [20–22]. This line of research is supported by a body of literature suggesting that the prefrontal cortex is disproportionately vulnerable to the effects of aging. Older adults score significantly worse than younger counterparts on a number neuropsychological tests thought to be sensitive to frontal lobe insults, while matching their performance on non-frontal tests (see [23] for review). Although the volume of the entire brain is reduced with age, the volume of the prefrontal cortex has been shown to decrease more rapidly than other structures (see [23,24] for reviews).

The first of these studies sought to determine if normal healthy aging alone was sufficient to impair the decision-making process [20]. In this study, the IGT was used to evaluate the decision-making ability of a Younger group (aged 26–55 years) and a group of older participants (aged 56–85 years). The younger adults demonstrated superior

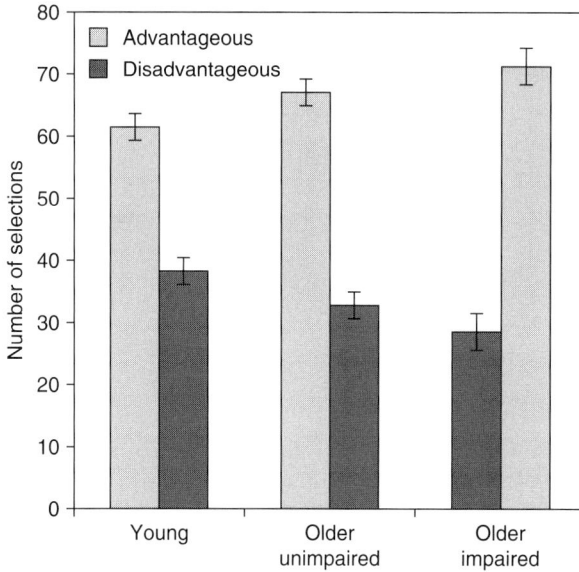

Figure 13.3 Total number of card selections in the Iowa Gambling Task. Data are presented by group (young versus older unimpaired versus older impaired) and by IGT deck selection [advantageous (decks C + D) and disadvantageous (decks A + B)].

performance throughout the task relative to the older adults. The experimenters developed a simple index of performance that they were able to use to classify participants as impaired or unimpaired. Net scores were generated by subtracting bad choices from good choices, and if this value differed significantly from zero (using the binomial test), patients were classified as impaired (significantly less than zero) or unimpaired (significantly greater than zero). Using this index, fewer than 10% of the younger participants qualified as impaired, while over one-third of the older group scored in the impaired range. The impaired older group was compared to the unimpaired older group on a variety of demographic variables and neuropsychological test scores, with no significant differences emerging. This study clearly demonstrated that there is a subset of older adults who are susceptible to decision-making deficits in spite of age-appropriate scores on all manner of neuropsychological tests (Fig. 13.3).

The results of the previous study were replicated and extended to include psychophysiological measurements [21]. This study built on prior work by Bechara et al. [10], which had shown that lesions of the VMPC interfered with participants' ability to generate discriminatory SCRs prior to card selection in the IGT. Denburg et al. [21] sought to determine whether a disruption in the anticipatory SCR might explain the deficit in the subset of older adults who were impaired on the IGT. The results of this study revealed that older adults who were unimpaired on the IGT generated anticipatory SCRs that were capable of discriminating between good and bad decks. The older adults who were impaired on the IGT did not discriminate between good and bad decks. This lack of discriminatory SCRs provides another link between the significant subset of older adults who are impaired on the IGT and patients with stable focal lesions of the VMPC. It is interesting to note that the anticipatory SCRs generated by the unimpaired older adults

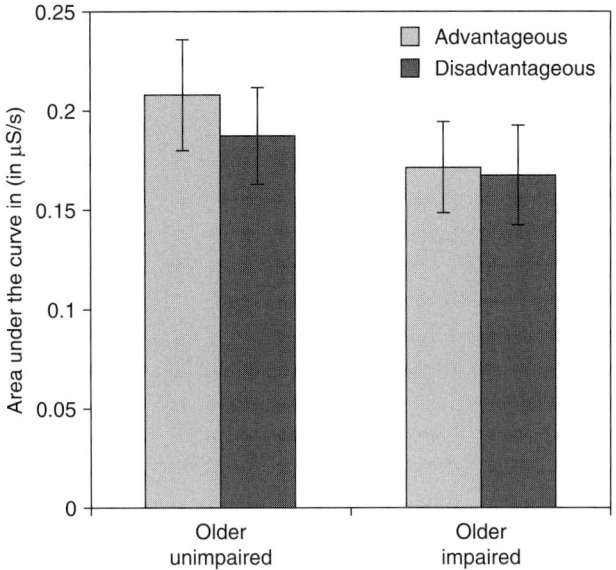

Figure 13.4 Anticipatory skin conductance responses. Data are presented by group (older unimpaired versus older impaired) and by IGT deck selection [advantageous (decks C + D) and disadvantageous (decks A + B)].

[21] were different than those generated by young adults [10]. While younger adults generate higher SCR values in anticipation of selections from the disadvantageous decks, the unimpaired older adults generate higher SCR values prior to selections from the advantageous decks (Fig. 13.4).

From the point of view of the somatic marker hypothesis, it seems plausible that the normal aging process may interfere with the ability to assign somatic markers. The third of older adults who fail the IGT may be failing for the same reason that VMPC patients fail. Aging is apparently capable of eliminating these individuals' ability to assign somatic markers to outcomes altogether. Those older adults who perform well on the IGT do so with apparently reversed somatic markers. Rather than marking the bad decks in a negative way, they are positively marking the good decks to facilitate approach. The use of positive rather than negative somatic markers in later life is in line with research demonstrating a positivity bias associated with older age [16]. Perhaps there is a natural shift in decision-making behavior from avoiding negative stimuli to seeking out positive stimuli. Perhaps this process is disrupted somehow in the impaired older adults such that they are unable to use somatic markers to avoid negative, or seek out positive, stimuli.

Laboratory tests and psychophysiological measures are useful, but ultimately experimenters want to confirm that the results of these techniques translate to real-world situations. Denburg et al. [22] tested the hypothesis that those older adults who were impaired on the IGT would also fail to make appropriate decisions in real-world circumstances. The experimenters devised a test based on a set of real advertisements that had been deemed deceptive by the Federal Trade Commission because they failed to disclose important information about the product. All advertisements were in printed form, as would be found in a magazine or newspaper. A counterpart was created for each of the

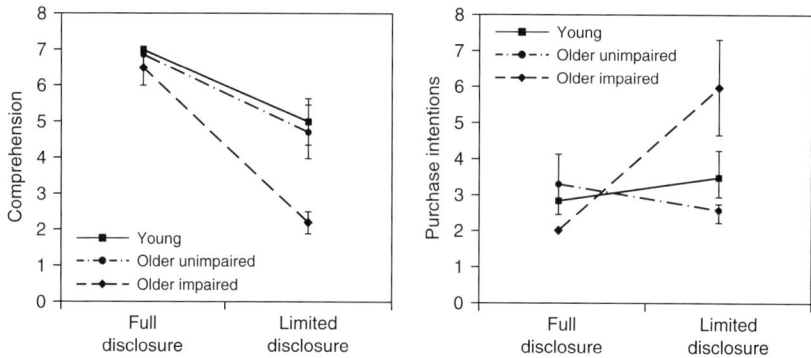

Figure 13.5 Mean comprehension of claims (left panel) and purchase intentions responses (right panel). Data are presented by group (young versus older unimpaired versus older impaired) and by advertisement version (full disclosure versus limited disclosure). *Source*: Preliminary data adapted from Denburg et al. (2007) [22] (note that the data are not analyzed statistically and are not presented in a fully quantitative manner).

deceptive advertisements, which disclosed the important product information that had been withheld. The advertisements were separated into two booklets composed of one half deceptive, or "limited disclosure," ads and the other half non-deceptive, or "full disclosure," ads. The booklets were used to test a group of young (unimpaired) gamblers, and two groups of older gamblers, one impaired and one unimpaired, in such a way that each individual participant was only exposed to one version of each ad (In this context, the term gambler simply refers to the participants' performance on the IGT, and bears no reference to recreational gambling). The experimenters were able to confirm their hypothesis using two separate dependent variables, comprehension and purchase intentions. When viewing full disclosure ads, there were no significant differences in comprehension or purchase intentions. However, when dealing with the limited disclosure ads, older impaired gamblers repeatedly reported lower comprehension and greater purchase intentions. This finding provides evidence for the assertion that these older adults, whose IGT performance is reminiscent of patients with lesions of the VMPC, may demonstrate some of the same real-world deficits in reasoning and decision-making. While this particular study only shows that older impaired gamblers are more susceptible to deceptive advertisements, it leaves open room for future research to determine the full extent of these individuals' disability (Fig. 13.5).

13.8   Conclusions

The ability to make judgments and decisions based on prior experience and projections of possible future outcomes is integral to existence in modern society. This ability seems to rely heavily on the generation of emotions and the integration of these emotions with our memories of people and events. It seems that emotional biases are capable of guiding us away from poor decisions [10], or toward good decisions [21].

It is frightening to think that as we grow older, our capacity for making sound judgments and decisions may be deteriorating just when we need it most. Many older adults are faced with a variety of difficult decisions about managing investments, paying for health care, and dispersing their estate, just to name a few. This age group is also an enticing target for both legitimate and deceptive advertising. As a group, older adults tend to have more disposable income and free time than their younger counterparts, and as such advertisers and con artists will always be looking for ways to tap into that pool of wealth.

If the reader takes nothing else away from this chapter, the message that the VMPC is an integral part of that which makes us human should be clear. Our capacity for future planning, for ruminating on thoughts of loved ones lost, for feeling the moral weight of our decisions all rely on the integrity of the VMPC. Loss of function in this brain area can extract the emotion that colors an individual's life, leaving them living in a bleak, rational world. Lack of emotional biases can make the simplest of decisions seem arduous and overwhelming.

Acknowledgement

This study was supported by NINDS Program Project Grant NS19632 (Daniel Tranel), NIDA R01 DA022549 (Daniel Tranel), and NIA Career Development Award K01 AG022033 (Natalie L. Denburg).

References

[1] S. Finger, History of neuropsychology, Neuropsychology 1–28 (1994).
[2] J.M. Harlow, Recovery after severe injury to the head, Publ. Mass. Med. Soc. 2 (1868) 327–346.
[3] H. Damasio, T. Grabowski, R. Frank, A.M. Galaburda, A.R. Damasio, The return of Phineas Gage: clues about the brain from the skull of a famous patient, Science 264 (1994) 1102–1105.
[4] A.R. Damasio, Descartes' Error, Avon Books, New York, 1994.
[5] J. Barrash, D. Tranel, S.W. Anderson, Acquired personality disturbances associated with bilateral damage to the ventromedial prefrontal region, Dev. Neuropsychol. 18 (2000) 355–381.
[6] J. Barrash, S.W. Anderson, The Iowa Ratings Scales of Personality Change, Department of Neurology, University of Iowa, Iowa City, 1993.
[7] D. Tranel, "Acquired sociopathy": the development of sociopathic behavior following focal brain damage, in: D.C. Fowles, P. Stucker, S.H. Goodman (Eds.), Progress in Experimental Personality & Psychopathology Research, vol. 17, Springer, New York, 1994, pp. 285–311.
[8] R. Bar-On, D. Tranel, N.L. Denburg, A. Bechara, Exploring the neurological substrate of emotional and social intelligence, Brain 126 (2003) 1790–1800.
[9] A. Bechara, A.R. Damasio, H. Damasio, S.W. Anderson, Insensitivity to future consequences following damage to human prefrontal cortex, Cognition 50 (1994) 7–15.
[10] A. Bechara, H. Damasio, D. Tranel, A.R. Damasio, Deciding advantageously before knowing the advantageous strategy, Science 275 (1997) 1293–1295.
[11] M. Koenigs, D. Tranel, Irrational economic decision-making after ventromedial prefrontal damage: evidence from the ultimatum game, J. Neurosci. 27 (2007) 951–956.
[12] M. Koenigs, L. Young, R. Adolphs, D. Tranel, F. Cushman, M. Hauser, A. Damasio, Damage to the prefrontal cortex increases utilitarian moral judgements, Nature 446 (2007) 908–911.
[13] M. Koenigs, D. Tranel, Prefrontal cortex damage abolishes brand-cued changes in cola preference, Soc. Cogn. Affect. Neurosci. 3 (2008) 1–6.

[14] M.F. Mendez, E. Anderson, J.S. Shapira, An investigation of moral judgement in frontotemporal dementia, Cogn. Behav. Neurol. 18 (2005) 193–197.

[15] L.L. Carstensen, Motivation for social contact across the life span: a theory of socioemotional selectivity, Nebr. Symp. Motiv. 40 (1992) 209–254.

[16] L.L. Carstensen, D.M. Isaacowitz, S.T. Charles, Taking time seriously: a theory of socioemotional selectivity, Am. Psychol. 54 (1999) 165–181.

[17] S.T. Charles, M. Mather, L.L. Carstensen, Aging and emotional memory: the forgettable nature of negative images for older adults, J. Exp. Psychol. Gen. 132 (2003) 310–324.

[18] H.H. Fung, L.L. Carstensen, Sending memorable messages to the old: age differences in preferences and memory for advertisements, J. Pers. Soc. Psychol. 85 (2003) 163–178.

[19] G.R. Samanez-Larkin, S.E. Gibbs, K. Khanna, L. Nielsen, L.L. Carstensen, B. Knutson, Anticipation of monetary gain but not loss in healthy older adults, Nat. Neurosci. 10 (2007) 787–791.

[20] N.L. Denburg, D. Tranel, A. Bechara, The ability to decide advantageously declines prematurely in some normal older persons, Neuropsychologia 43 (2005) 1099–1106.

[21] N.L. Denburg, E.C. Recknor, A. Bechara, D. Tranel, Psychophysiological anticipation of positive outcomes promotes advantageous decision-making in normal older persons, Int. J. Psychophysiol. 61 (2006) 19–25.

[22] N.L. Denburg, C.A. Cole, M. Hernandez, T.H. Yamada, D. Tranel, A. Bechara, et al., The orbitofrontal cortex, real-world decision making, and normal aging, Ann. NY Acad. Sci. 1121 (2007) 480–498.

[23] R.L. West, An application of prefrontal cortex function theory to cognitive aging, Psychol. Bull. 120 (1996) 272–292.

[24] C.L. Grady, Cognitive neuroscience of aging, Ann. NY Acad. Sci. 1124 (2008) 127–144.

[25] J.M. Harlow, Passage of an iron rod through the head, 1848, J. Neuropsychiatry Clin. Neurosci. 11 (1999) 281–283.

[26] "The Life Mask and Skull of Phineas Gage," Online image, Countway Rededication Celebration Tour, Warren Anatomical Museum, retrieved 15 August 2008 from www.hms.harvard.edu/countway_tour/phineas.jpg.

[27] A.L. Benton, Exploring the History of Neuropsychology: Selected Papers, Oxford University Press, Oxford, NY, 2000.

[28] J. Barrash, D. Tranel, S.W. Anderson, Assessment of dramatic personality changes after ventromedial frontal lesions, J. Clin. Exp. Neuropsychol. 16 (1994) 66.

Part Four

Genetic and Hormonal Influences on the Reward System

14 Gonadal steroid hormones' influence on reward and decision making processes

Xavier Caldú and Jean-Claude Dreher

Reward and Decision Making Group, Cognitive Neuroscience Center, CNRS-Lyon 1 University, 67 Bd Pinel 69675 Bron, France

Abstract

Current research combining endocrinology and functional neuroimaging starts to unveil the neural influences of gonadal steroid hormones on brain and cognition. This chapter focuses on the effects of gonadal steroid hormones on reward processing and decision making, which critically depend on dopaminergic neurotransmission. Evidence from animal and human studies are reviewed that indicate the important roles played by variations of gonadal steroid hormones on a number of cerebral inter-individual differences (e.g., between men and women, between hypogonadal patients and healthy subjects) and intra-individual differences (e.g., differences across phases of the menstrual cycle or at different stages of the lifespan, such as menopause or andropause). Taken together, these studies help to understand the impact of gonadal steroids on vulnerability to drug abuse, neuropsychiatric diseases with differential expression across males and females, and hormonally mediated mood disorders.

Key points

1. Estrogen and progesterone not only influence ovulation and reproductive behavior but also affect cognitive functions, affective state, and vulnerability to drug abuse.
2. The dopaminergic system is sensitive to circulating gonadal steroid hormones in animals and in humans (evidence from behavioral and neuroimaging experiments).
3. Testosterone modulates reward processing and decision making in men and women.
4. Estradiol and progesterone modulate reward processing and decision making (effects of menstrual cycle and pharmacological manipulations).
5. Hormone replacement therapy affects cognitive functions in women with menopause and in elderly men.

14.1   Introduction

Gonadal steroid hormones modulate the activity of several neurotransmission systems, including the dopaminergic system [1–5]. These effects extend beyond the tuberoinfundibular dopaminergic system, involved in the control of the anterior pituitary and important for reproductive behavior, to the mesolimbic and mesocortical dopaminergic systems, relevant for cognitive activities [6–9], affective state [10–12], and reward processing [13].

Receptors for gonadal steroid hormones have been detected in dopaminergic neurons of the ventral tegmental area and the substantia nigra [5,14,15]. Androgen and estrogen receptors are also expressed in target areas of dopaminergic neurons, such as the amygdala and the prefrontal cortex. Dopamine and circulating estrogens and androgens are known to interact in these brain structures [5,16–18]. In other structures, such as the striatum, autoradiography studies have shown that very few neurons, if any, possess nuclear estrogen receptors [4,17,19]. However, gonadal steroid hormones may also affect dopaminergic activity in the striatum through their action on membrane neuronal G-protein-coupled receptors that activate intracellular signaling systems [1,20]. The striatum has received special attention, because it is a key component of the dopamine-dependent reward system.

In the striatum, there are sexually dimorphic actions of estrogens and progestagens that involve both pro- and antidopaminergic effects that depend on the dose and time of estrogen administration and that are manifested in both the nigrostriatal and mesolimbic dopaminergic systems [21]. For example, estrogen and progesterone exert rapid effects on the amphetamine-induced dopamine increase in the striatum [22]. Also, there is an estrous cycle-dependent variation in the amphetamine-induced increase in striatal dopamine, with greater increases during estrous than during other days of the cycle in rats [23]. After ovariectomy, amphetamine-induced striatal dopamine release is attenuated, but dopamine levels can be restored to normal by repeated administration of estrogen treatment. Similar effects on dopaminergic activity in the striatum have been reported following long-term testosterone treatment in male rats [2]. Moreover, gonadal steroid hormones also influence dopaminergic transmission by affecting the activity and expression of dopamine receptors [24–26].

Gonadal steroid hormone receptors can be activated by other compounds, such as neurotransmitters and growth factors [27]. Indeed, dopamine has been shown to activate gonadal steroid hormone receptors. In particular, dopamine D_1 agonists have been found to mimic the effects of progesterone in facilitating sexual behavior in female rats. This facilitatory effect of dopamine is blocked by administration of progesterone receptor antagonists, indicating that dopamine may regulate behavior by means of cross-talk with steroid receptors in the brain [28,29].

Historically, the study of sex differences has been reduced to sexual behavior, its regulation by gonadal steroid hormones, and their effects on the main brain structure considered responsible for this behavior, that is, the hypothalamus [21]. Today, an increasing amount of data from animal and human studies confute this conception and point toward a more ample vision of between-sex differences, including differences in brain anatomy, chemistry, and function [30]. Sex differences extend far beyond mating behavior and reproduction, and beyond the neural circuits that govern them, to reach the domain of cognition. For instance, it is currently accepted that women outperform men in verbal skills and short-term memory, while men outperform women in spatial abilities [4]. Sex differences are due to a combination of genetic and hormonal events that begin early during development. Behavioral sex differences in humans are also cultural and arise from learning. However, in the sphere of cognitive abilities, the differentiation between nature and nurture becomes less clear. The challenge for researchers is to draw the boundaries between the cultural and biological influences on human behavior and cognition.

One source of biological influence on cognitive performance is gonadal steroid hormones, which, due to their chemical properties, are capable of crossing the blood-brain barrier to exert prominent effects in the brain. Men and women possess the same type of hormones, but their respective amounts are critically different. This has led to the hypothesis that the effects of gonadal steroid hormones, either during early development of the brain or during adulthood, may explain part of the between-sex differences in behavior and cognitive abilities observed in humans. Thus, variations in hormones levels may contribute to the large inter- and intra-individual differences observed during reward processing and decision making [31,32]. Comparing cognitive performance and brain function across or between conditions associated with different levels of gonadal steroid hormones may not only help explain inter-individual differences (e.g., between men and women, between men with different levels of testosterone, or women with different levels of estrogen, etc.) but also intra-individual differences that result from different hormonal status experienced through life (e.g., menstrual cycle, menopause, andropause, etc.).

Since dysfunction of the dopaminergic system seriously impairs reward processing, motivation, and decision making in many neurological and psychiatric disorders (e.g., pathological gambling, drug addiction, schizophrenia, Parkinson's disease), a better understanding of the influences of gonadal steroid hormones on human neural functions would have crucial implications for sex-related differences and menstrual cycle effects on prevalence, course, and treatment response characteristics of neuropsychiatric disorders, as well as on vulnerability to drug abuse. For example, such information could elucidate the mechanism by which women experience greater subjective response to both cocaine [33] and amphetamine [34] during the follicular phase of the menstrual cycle as compared with the luteal phase, and by which women with schizophrenia have later disease onset and less severe course of illness than men [35]. These clinical observations provide evidence that neurosteroids modulate the dopaminergic system in women, but they leave open the question of gonadal steroid hormone modulation on the human reward and decision-making neural circuitry.

14.2   Effects of testosterone on cognitive capacities

The testes secrete several male gonadal steroid hormones, including testosterone, dihydrotestosterone, and androstenedione. Of those, testosterone is the most abundant [36]. Besides its androgenic and anabolic effects, testosterone also exerts influence on brain development and functioning, thereby influencing behavior and cognition. In animals, testosterone increases aggressive behavior [37,38]. However, in humans this effect is more controversial and the effects of testosterone on aggressive behavior appear to be positive, but weak [39–43]. It has been suggested that testosterone is related to dominance in humans, that is, the enhancement of one's status over other people's, which does not necessarily involve aggression [37,39,44,45]. The effects of testosterone on aggressive behavior could be mediated by its fear-reducing properties [46,47] and its relation to selective attention to threat [48]. In females, testosterone induces faster responses to angry faces [49] and enhances the responsiveness of the neural circuits of social aggression, which include the amygdala and the hypothalamus [50].

The higher level of performance shown by men compared to women in some cognitive tasks raises the possibility that testosterone might be involved in the development and maintenance of some cognitive abilities. Perhaps the most studied of these male-advanta-geous abilities are spatial abilities. A positive relationship between testosterone levels and performance has been reported in tasks that engage spatial abilities [51–54]. Other stud-ies have assessed the activational effects of testosterone by directly manipulating its physi-ological concentrations. Current data suggest that the relationship between testosterone levels and spatial abilities may follow a nonlinear, inverted U-shaped function [4,55,56]. Thus, higher adult concentrations of testosterone would be associated with better spatial abilities in males, but only to a certain limit. Yet, beyond an optimum concentration, tes-tosterone may diminish spatial abilities. In women, a single administration of testosterone also increases spatial abilities [57,58]. Another approach to study the effects of testoster-one is based on biorhythms in testosterone secretion, since testosterone levels are higher in the morning than in the evening in men [59–61].

14.2.1   Effects of testosterone on reward processing and decision making

Animal studies. The affective rewarding properties of testosterone and its metabo-lites have been demonstrated in animal studies by using the conditioned place prefer-ence paradigm [62–65]. This paradigm allows inferring the rewarding properties of a drug by the observed tendency of the animal to approach an originally neutral environ-mental stimulus that has been paired with the positive affective consequences of drug administration. Further proof of the rewarding effects of a drug can be derived from the extent to which an animal self-administers it. Studies in rodents demonstrate that both males and females self-administer testosterone [66–68]. Two sites where testosterone and its metabolites exert their rewarding effects are the nucleus accumbens and the intramedial preoptic area of the hypothalamus [63,69,70]. As happens with other rewarding drugs, such as amphetamine [71] and morphine [72], dopamine release mediates the rewarding effects of testosterone, with both D_1 and D_2 receptors playing an important role [73].

Human neuroimaging studies. Recently, functional neuroimaging techniques have been used to explore the effects of gonadal steroid hormones on brain activity related to cog-nitive functioning, including the processing of different types of rewarding stimuli. In a positron emission tomography (PET) study carried out in hypogonadal and eugonadal control men, Redouté and colleagues [74] found differences in brain activation while processing sexual stimuli. The right orbitofrontal cortex, the insula, and the claustrum showed higher responses in untreated patients compared with controls and when they were compared to themselves after receiving hormonal replacement therapy (HRT). The left inferior frontal gyrus also showed a differential response, but in this structure a deac-tivation was observed in controls and in patients after treatment. The fact that the activity observed in these brain regions is modulated by testosterone levels supports the view that their activation or deactivation is related to sexual arousal and not merely to a state of general motivational arousal. The activation of the orbitofrontal cortex, a component of the reward system, may be interpreted as the neural correlate of an appraisal proc-ess through which visual stimuli are categorized as sexual incentives. The testosterone dependency of the activation of this structure suggests that testosterone may increase the motivational salience or subjective value of these stimuli.

In healthy men, processing of visual sexual stimuli has also been found to elicit acti-vation in several structures of the reward system, such as the orbitofrontal cortex, the striatum, and the amygdala [75,76]. Also, differences and similarities between men and women in the response to visual sexual stimuli have been reported using functional magnetic resonance imaging (fMRI). Hamann and colleagues [76] found similar patterns of activation in men and women with passive viewing of sexual stimuli, including common activation of the ventral striatum. However, differences were found in the activation of the amygdala and hypothalamus bilaterally, with men displaying greater activity. According to the authors, the amygdala mediates sex differences in responsiveness to appetitive and biologically salient stimuli, and could also mediate the greater role of visual stimuli observed in males. In order to disentangle whether activation of reward structures was driven specifically by the pleasantness of the stimulus or by its salience, Sabatinelli and colleagues [77] compared viewing of pleasant erotic and romantic couples with viewing of equally arousing unpleasant and neutral pictures. They observed an increased activation in the nucleus accumbens and the medial prefrontal cortex related to the visualization of pleasant images, while viewing of equally salient unpleasant or neutral pictures did not produce such an increase. Thus, these data suggest that these brain structures are reactive to the rewarding properties of stimuli and not to their salience [77].

In a recent fMRI study comparing monetary (secondary rewards) and erotic stimuli (primary rewards) in healthy young heterosexual men, we observed, for both types of reward, a common brain network composed of the striatum, the anterior cingulate cortex, the midbrain, and the anterior insula. In addition, we also found an anteroposterior dissociation in the lateral orbitofrontal cortex, monetary gains being specifically represented in the anterior part of the orbitofrontal cortex, while erotic pictures eliciting activation in its posterior part. This result indicates a new functional division within the orbitofrontal cortex, with more recent cortical circuits supporting symbolic representation of goods and evolutionarily more ancient orbitofrontal regions representing subjective value relative to primary rewards. Moreover, the amygdala was more activated for erotic rewards than for monetary gains [78] (see also Chapter 6).

Behavioral studies

Sex differences have been observed in different aspects of reward processing and decision making. The delay-discounting paradigm measures choice behavior when people are presented with a choice between a small immediate reward and a larger delayed reward. Delay discounting provides an account for impulsivity, which is a core deficit in several neuropsychiatric conditions such as attention deficit hyperactivity disorder or addiction. A delay-discounting factor can be estimated by making subjects choose between variable amounts of any reward delivered immediately and a variably higher amount of this reward delivered after a variable delay. In such a task, men show higher delay discounting rates than women for monetary rewards [79,80]. In other words, men devaluate rewards faster as the delay to the reception of reward increases, which leads them to choose more frequently low immediate over higher delayed rewards. These findings are interesting when considering the higher prevalence observed in men of a number of neuropsychiatric illnesses characterized by increased impulsivity [81–84]. Nonetheless, between-sex differences in decision making depend upon the specific paradigm that is tested. For example, Reavis and Overman [85] found that men performed better than women in the Iowa Gambling Task [85]. In this classic task, participants have to repeatedly choose cards from four decks with the goal of maximizing their earnings. Two disadvantageous decks provide immediate large rewards but also substantial money losses. The other two decks are advantageous, since reward is modest but consistent and punishment is low. Thus, consistent choice of cards from the advantageous decks will result in low short-term but high long-term gains, whereas consistent choice of cards from the disadvantageous decks will result in a long-term loss of money. This task has been used in numerous neuropsychological studies showing impaired decision making after orbitofrontal cortex damage [86,87] (see also Chapter 13). The crucial importance of the integrity of the orbitofrontal cortex in decision making is further demonstrated by a number of gambling tasks involving choices between options that differ in terms of size and probabilities of their associated punishments and rewards [88–90].

A direct influence of testosterone on the development and on the decision-making function of the orbitofrontal cortex is demonstrated by a number of animal and human studies. For example, a surge in perinatal testosterone causes the orbitofrontal cortex to mature faster in male monkeys than in females, which is accompanied by better performance in an object reversal task. Also, early-life androgenized female monkeys perform similarly to normal males and better than normal females [91,92]. In adult humans, testosterone levels negatively influence decision making in both men and women [85,93], and an inverted U-shaped relationship has been found between delay discounting of gains and salivary testosterone levels in men [94]. Whether these effects derive from an increased sensitivity to gains, a lower sensitivity to punishment, or a lower sensitivity to future consequences remains unclear.

14.2.2   Testosterone effects on economic decision making

Little is known about the role of testosterone during economic decision making. However, a recent study demonstrates the involvement of testosterone on a decision-making task engaging players in the ultimatum game [95]. In this game, one player (the "proposer") makes an offer to a second player (the "responder") on how to share a certain sum of money. The word "ultimatum" reflects the non-negotiability of the offer, so the only options for the responder are to accept or reject it. If the responder agrees, the sum is divided as proposed. If there is no agreement, none of the players receives any money. The standard economic solution for the game is for the proposer to offer the smallest amount of money possible and for the responder to accept any offer, on the basis that any monetary amount is better than none. However, extensive behavioral data show that responders tend to accept offers that are considered fair (i.e., those splitting the amount around 50%) and that the rate of rejection increases as offers become unfair [96]. Burnham [95] found that men with higher levels of testosterone rejected more low offers than men with lower levels of testosterone. Furthermore, low second to fourth digit ratio, which has been suggested as a marker of high prenatal testosterone exposure [97,98], is associated with higher discount rates and more rejection of unfair offers in men, although this effect seems to be modulated by contextual cues, such as the status position of the responder or the presence of sex-related cues [99,100]. One possible explanation of this effect may relate to the role of testosterone in dominance. Low offers may be interpreted by responders as a challenge and the acceptance of the offers as harmful for their reputation. In the face of such a threat, men with higher levels of testosterone are more prone to react in a way that preserves their reputation and reasserts their dominance, even if this involves an economic cost.

Another behavioral study measured endogenous steroids in male traders under real working conditions [101]. Traders' morning testosterone levels predicted the profitability during the day, and traders' cortisol raised with both the variance of their trading results and the volatility of the market. These data indicate that higher testosterone may contribute to economic return, whereas cortisol is increased by risk. One drawback of this study is that sampling was done over only 8 days and was performed during a period of low volatility. This study suggests that if acutely raised steroids were to persist for several weeks or even increase as volatility rises, they might have cognitive and behavioral consequences, specifically by shifting risk preferences or disturbing the neural basis for rational choice.

The effect of incidental cues on decision making may be mediated, at least in part, by the activation of the nucleus accumbens. Activation of the nucleus accumbens has been found to predict shifts to high-risk options in an investment task [102]. Moreover, activation of the nucleus accumbens has been observed during anticipation of diverse types of rewards [76,77,103,104], so it may be considered as a neural marker of the positive arousal induced by these rewards [105]. Recent fMRI data indicate that viewing erotic stimuli influences risk taking in healthy young men, partially through the activation of the nucleus accumbens [105]. At a behavioral level, presentation of erotic pictures before decision making increased self-reported positive arousal and subsequent high-risk choices and shifts to the high-risk options. At a functional level, presentation of these erotic stimuli increased activity of several brain structures, including the mesial prefrontal cortex and subcortical regions such as the nucleus accumbens and the putamen. The nucleus accumbens activation partially mediated the influence of positive stimuli on shifts to the high-risk option. These results point toward the neural mechanisms through which anticipatory affect induced by incidental, irrelevant stimuli influence decision making.

14.3   Effects of estradiol and progesterone on cognitive capacities

Estrogens and progestagens are the two main gonadal steroid hormones in women. The most important of the estrogens is estradiol, whose functions include causing cellular proliferation and growth of the tissues of the sex organs and of other tissues related to reproduction, as well as development of secondary sexual traits in females. The main progestagen is progesterone, which is secreted by cells from the corpus luteum, which develops from an ovarian follicle during the luteal phase of the menstrual cycle. The corpus luteum is essential for preparing the uterus for ovum implantation and for maintaining pregnancy [36].

One of the prime site mediators of estrogen's effects on cognition in general, and decision making in particular, may be the prefrontal cortex, as revealed by an early PET study in young women under pharmacological ovarian suppression [106], by comparison between menopausal women with and without hormone replacement therapy [107,108], and by the fact that ovarian steroids are potent regulators of dopaminergic innervation to the prefrontal cortex. Ovariectomy reduces, and subsequent estrogen and progesterone replacement restores, the density of axons immunoreactive for tyrosine hydroxylase in monkey dorsolateral prefrontal cortex [8]. Estradiol treatment, which is associated with changes in dorsolateral prefrontal cortex structural plasticity, also reverses age-related impairment in prefrontal cognitive function in ovariectomized monkeys [109].

In women, the levels of estradiol and progesterone fluctuate through the menstrual cycle. Roughly, the first 14 days correspond to the follicular phase and are characterized by constant low levels of progesterone and a sudden increase of estradiol to reach a peak just before ovulation and decrease again to the initial levels. The next 14 days correspond to the luteal phase. Estradiol levels finish their fall at the beginning of this period and then gradually increase until the midluteal phase, when they start to gradually drop to start a new cycle. During the luteal phase, progesterone levels follow a similar fluctuation to estradiol levels, but always at lower quantities [4,110].

There is evidence in animals and humans that the menstrual cycle effects extend beyond those merely related to reproduction. The menstrual cycle phases influence spatial and verbal cognitive abilities [111–113], attention [114], mood [115], and vulnerability to drugs of abuse [34].

14.3.1 Menstrual cycle effects on reward processing and decision making

Animal and human studies have demonstrated the influences of menstrual cycle and of gonadal hormone levels on the psychological effects of stimulants. In rodents, females are more sensitive to these drugs than males, and estradiol seems to be involved in these sex differences [116], enhancing the effects of these stimulants and drug-seeking behavior [3]. There is also evidence for such an effect in humans. In women, the subjective positive response to stimulants is greater during the follicular phase, when estradiol levels are moderate and progesterone levels are minimal, than in the luteal phase, when both estrogen and progesterone levels are relatively high [33,34]. The rewarding properties of estrogen may involve actions at estrogen receptors in the nucleus accumbens [117,118]. In contrast, progesterone has been found to attenuate the subjective effects of stimulants in women [116,119].

We have recently identified, for the first time in humans, the effects of the menstrual cycle phases on the reward system [13]. Using fMRI, healthy young women were scanned during the midfollicular and luteal phases of their menstrual cycle while they performed a monetary reward task that distinguished the neural concomitants of anticipating uncertain rewards from those of reward outcome. In the midfollicular phase, women showed higher activation in the orbitofrontal cortex and the amygdala during anticipation of uncertain rewards, relative to the luteal phase (Fig. 14.1). At the time of reward delivery,

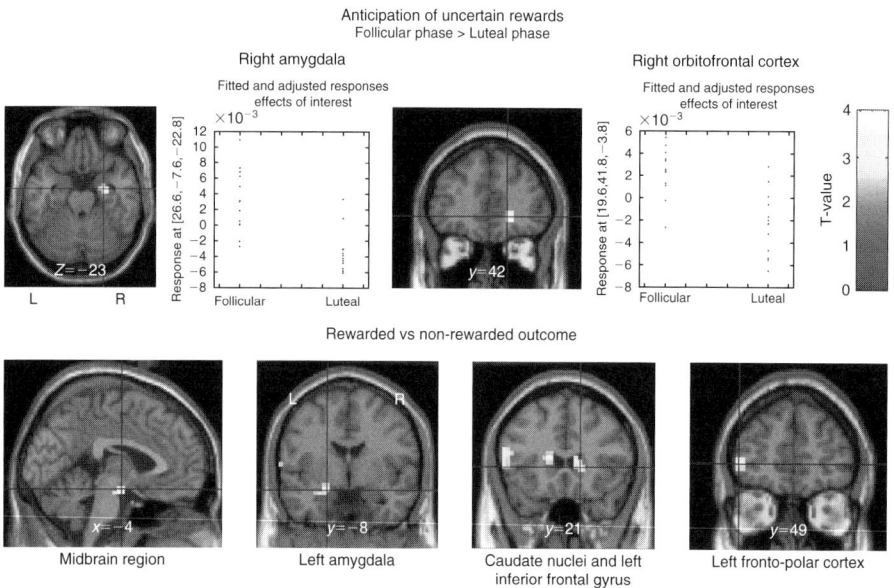

Figure 14.1 Cross-menstrual cycle phase differences in blood oxygen level-dependent (BOLD) response during reward anticipation and at the time of reward delivery. *Top*. During reward anticipation, higher BOLD responses were observed in the follicular phase than in the luteal phase in the right amygdala and orbitofrontal cortex. To the right of each map are shown distributions of BOLD signal response for each woman. *Bottom*. Cross-menstrual cycle phase differences in BOLD response at the time of reward outcome. Greater BOLD response during the follicular phase than during the luteal phase in midbrain, left amygdala, heads of the caudate nuclei, left inferior frontal gyrus, and left fronto-polar cortex [13]. See Plate 17 of Color Plate section.

higher activation was observed in midbrain, striatum, and frontopolar cortex during the follicular phase compared to the luteal phase. These data demonstrate that reactivity of the reward system is heightened in women during the midfollicular phase of the menstrual cycle, when estrogen is unopposed by progesterone. Furthermore, women were compared with a group of men matched for age and level of education. In men, a more robust blood oxygen level-dependent (BOLD) response was observed in the ventral putamen than in women during anticipation of uncertain rewards, whereas women showed stronger activation of the anterior medial prefrontal cortex during reward delivery (Fig. 14.2). Previous neuroimaging studies of reward that grouped men and women together proposed different functions for the ventral striatum and the anterior medial prefrontal cortex, linking the former to reward anticipation and the latter to the time of reward outcome [103]. Extending these reports to anticipation of rewards with maximal uncertainty, we recently found robust ventral striatum activation in a large group of subjects that included both men and women (scanned without monitoring their menstrual cycle) [13]. Our data suggest that these findings may, in part, be driven by sex-specific differences, with men showing higher ventral striatal activity and women exhibiting higher anterior medial prefrontal cortex activity. Thus, reward studies must consider

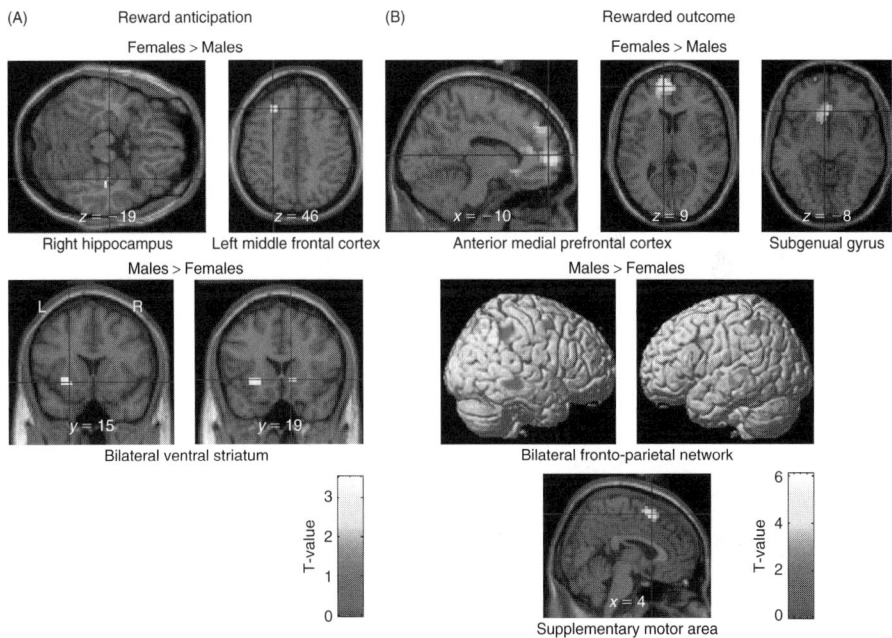

Figure 14.2 Between-sex differences in brain activity during reward anticipation and at the time of reward delivery. (A) During anticipation of uncertain rewards. Statistical maps showing greater right hippocampal and left middle frontal gyrus activity in women than in men, whereas men showed greater activation in bilateral ventral striatum. (B) At the time of reward delivery. Women showed more activation in anterior medial prefrontal cortex and subgenual gyrus compared with men, who, in turn, showed more activation in a bilateral fronto-parietal network, the right inferior temporal cortex, and the supplementary motor area [13].

both sex differences and gonadal steroid actions at the time of testing. Our findings extend to humans the previous observations in animals that the actions of estrogen and progesterone on midbrain dopaminergic projections to the striatum are sexually dimorphic and involve both prodopaminergic and antidopaminergic effects [23].

Finally, brain activity was correlated with gonadal steroid levels, and a positive correlation between activity in the amygdalo-hippocampal complex and estradiol levels was observed regardless of menstrual cycle phase. These results indicate that ovarian steroids modulate reward-evoked neural activity. This modulation may underlie differences observed between sexes and between different phases of the menstrual cycle in women, such as the greater subjective response to addictive drugs observed in women, especially during the follicular phase. The increased reactivity of the reward system during the follicular phase is meaningful also from an evolutionary perspective, since it may underlie the increased availability, receptivity, and desire during the ovulatory period that are thought to facilitate procreation.

Functional neuroimaging studies have also revealed changes in brain activation related to menstrual cycle phase, not only during processing rewarding stimuli but also during processing negative stimuli. In the anterior medial orbitofrontal cortex, activity increases premenstrually and decreases postmenstrually, whereas the lateral orbitofrontal cortex displays the opposite pattern [120]. Moreover, during the follicular phase, a set of areas involved in the response to stress, including the amygdala, the orbitofrontal cortex, and the anterior cingulate gyrus, are more responsive to negative, high arousing stimuli [121]. Although there is more evidence of estradiol modulation on motivational and emotional processes, recent neuroimaging studies also indicate a role for progesterone. For example, the neuroactive metabolite of progesterone, allopregnanolone, modulates memory for faces by influencing amygdala activity [122,123].

Behaviorally, some studies have investigated the menstrual cycle influence on women's social preferences and decision making. For example, women's preference for secondary sexual traits in male faces varies during the menstrual cycle, with women preferring more masculine traits during the follicular phase, when conception is more likely [124–126]. On the other hand, during the midluteal phase, women display higher attraction for apparent health and self-resemblance [126,127]. A woman's preference for testosterone markers on male faces may be influenced by her estrogen/progesterone ratio [128], although recent data suggest that this effect seems to be mediated by progesterone rather than estrogen levels [126,127], and even a role for female testosterone levels has been suggested [129]. Interestingly, similar effects have been reported for voice pitch [130], male odor [131], and male social behavioral displays [132].

These cyclical changes in male trait preferences are meaningful from an evolutionary perspective. More masculine traits are thought to reflect higher resilience to infectious disease but also unwillingness to invest in partners and offspring [128,133]. Thus, these shifts in preferences may represent adaptive trade-offs in mate choice. During ovulation, when chances of conception are high, women may increase their attraction toward men displaying more resistant features and cues to heritable immunity to infectious diseases, so that these positive characteristics may be inherited by the offspring. However, when women's hormonal profile is similar to that during pregnancy or when the body is preparing for pregnancy (e.g., during the luteal phase of the menstrual cycle), women may show stronger preferences for features that might be beneficial at this time, such as social and material support [134].

Some facial cues (e.g., squarer jaws, smaller pupil-to-brow distance) may be interpreted as signaling social dominance (i.e., enhancing one's status and control of resources over conspecifics) and have been suggested to be indicators of a man's potential to achieve a high status [135]. Senior and colleagues studied whether variations in preferences for male traits due to menstrual cycle phases led to differences in decision making [136]. Women participated in a mock job scenario in which they had to assign minimum-, low-, high-, or maximum- status resources to several men previously rated to look either dominant or non-dominant. Women assigned resources of high status to dominant-looking men and resources of low status to non-dominant-looking men. Further analyses showed that during the follicular phase, more high-status resources were allocated to dominant-looking men than to non-dominant-looking men. Thus, the bias due to cyclic hormonal profiles observed in women toward male features that signal phenotypic and genotypic superiority has behavioral effects when making decisions.

Evolutionary psychology proposes that humans have evolved to perceive as attractive those characteristics that are displayed by healthy individuals [128]. These features of what are considered beautiful faces are important biological signals of mate value that motivate behavior in others. Functional neuroimaging studies have demonstrated that viewing beautiful faces activates components of the reward system, such as the ventral striatum and the orbitofrontal cortex, also engaged for different types of rewards, such as drugs and money [137–139]. A classic fMRI study provides an interesting finding for brain processing of facial attractiveness [138]. In this study, subjects were scanned while viewing unfamiliar faces, whose attractiveness they were asked to rate at the end of the session. Strikingly, no region in the brain showed any activation in response to facial attractiveness *per se*. These results led the authors to investigate a possible effect of gaze direction on brain activation related to the processing of facial attractiveness. Interestingly, perceived attractiveness was related to increased activity in the ventral striatum when the eye gaze of the observed person met the eyes of the observer, while when eye gaze was directed away, activity in this region decreased. Thus, the striatum is involved not only in the processing of basic reinforcing stimuli (e.g., food) but also in the evaluation of stimuli with relevance for social interaction. Moreover, the pattern of striatal activity observed in this study is concordant with prediction error signal coding (see Chapters 2 and 6). A returned eye gaze from an attractive face may be considered a better outcome than expected, leading to an increased response. On the other hand, failing to establish eye contact with an attractive face is a disappointing outcome, which leads to reduced striatal activity [138]. In summary, these results suggest that the modulation of the activity of women's reward system by gonadal steroid hormones may also underlie variations similar to those observed regarding other types of motivated behavior.

14.3.2   Dissociating the roles of estrogen and progesterone on reward processing

In our fMRI study mentioned above [13], we scanned women twice, once during the midfollicular phase and once during the luteal phase. However, because both estradiol and progesterone are simultaneously present during the luteal phase, it was not possible to pinpoint the specific effects of estradiol and progesterone on the reward system. This led us to investigate the influence of estradiol and progesterone independently, using fMRI during reward processing in conjunction with an incisive hormonal manipulation paradigm that pharmacologically induces temporary hypogonadism and replaces estrogen and progesterone separately [140]. The temporary hypogonadism was induced by the gonadotropin-releasing harmone (GnRH) agonist Leuprolide Acetate or Lupron. Lupron is used clinically when suppression and/or control of gonadal steroid secretion is the goal, such as in infertility in women and prostate cancer in men. After the second to fourth week of lupron administration, there is a down-regulation of GnRH receptors and an inhibition of pituitary release of gonadotropins, resulting in postmenopausal levels of endogenous gonadal steroid hormones. Young, healthy, regularly-menstruating women, who received no hormonal medication within the preceding 6 months, were scanned during three pharmacologically-controlled hormonal conditions spanning 6 months: ovarian suppression induced by the GnRH agonist, depot leuprolide acetate (Lupron), Lupron plus estradiol replacement, and Lupron plus progesterone replacement. Estradiol and progesterone were administered in a double-blind cross-over design, allowing us to disentangle their respective effects on the activation of the reward system. On each occasion, event-related 3T fMRI scans were performed during presentation of images of slot machines that varied reward probability. Our findings show that different components of the reward system are differentially modulated by temporary menopause induced by Lupron, estradiol replacement, and progesterone replacement. More specifically, during reward anticipation, the ventral striatum activity was more robust in the progesterone replacement condition as compared to the ovarian suppression, while the right amygdalo-hippocampal complex was more robustly activated in the estradiol replacement condition as compared to the ovarian suppression condition. This result is consistent with our previous menstrual cycle findings showing increased amygdalo-hippocampal activity during reward anticipation in the follicular phase, when estradiol is unopposed by progesterone. Taken together, these data demonstrate that different components of the reward system were modulated by temporary hypogonadism, estradiol alone, and progesterone alone.

As mentioned previously, estrogen is also present in males, although in lower quantities than in females, and its effects on males brain and behavior have not been so extensively studied. Recent findings in mice demonstrated that estrogen receptors mediate the facilitatory effects of female cues on male risk taking. Exposure of wild-type male mice to the odor of a novel female mouse enhanced risk taking and reduced avoidance to cat odor. Mice knocked out for either the α or the β estrogen receptors failed to display such a behavior [141]. Since sex-related cues have a parallel effect on decision making and risk taking in human males, who make poorer and riskier decisions in the presence of females or their cues [99,142,143], these results suggest that estrogen receptors may also modulate these behaviors in humans [141].

Dopaminergic dysfunction in aging

Healthy aging is associated with a number of neuroanatomical and neurobiological alterations that result in progressive decline in several cognitive functions dependent upon prefrontal cortex and/or hippocampus, such as working memory and verbal memory, as well as episodic memory, task switching, and processing speed [144–149]. The dopaminergic system is also subject to change during aging. In the striatum, a number of studies have shown an age-related decline of D_2-like receptors, which could be related to a decline in motor and cognitive abilities such as speed of processing and episodic memory [150]. Additionally, Kaasinen and colleagues have shown an extra-striatal decrease of D_2 and D_3 receptors, most pronounced in the prefrontal cortex and anterior cingulate cortex compared to temporal and thalamic regions [151]. However, very little is known about the functional consequences on brain activity of the age-related dopamine decline, because most of the studies on dopamine neurons and receptors have been done post-mortem.

To address this question, we have recently used a multimodal neuroimaging approach, combining 6-[(18)F]FluoroDOPA PET and event-related 3T fMRI in the same subjects. We showed that healthy aging induces functional alterations in the reward system [152]. More precisely, we directly demonstrated a link between midbrain dopamine synthesis and reward-related prefrontal activity in humans, showed that healthy aging induces functional alterations in the reward system (Fig. 14.3), and identified an age-related change in the direction of the relationship (from a positive to a negative correlation) between midbrain dopamine synthesis and prefrontal activity (Fig. 14.4). Our findings provide an important characterization of the interactions between midbrain dopamine function and the reward system in healthy young humans and older subjects, and identify the changes in this regulatory circuit that accompany aging. These results indicate an age-dependent dopaminergic tuning mechanism for cortical reward processing [152].

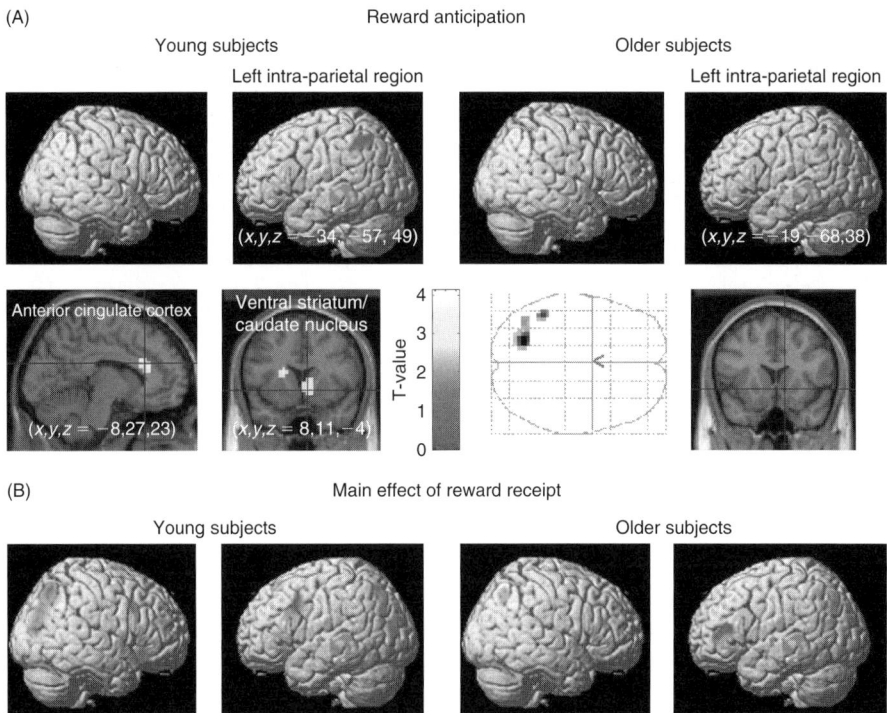

Figure 14.3 Specific brain activation in young and older subjects during reward anticipation and at the time of reward delivery. (A) *Left*. Main effect of anticipating reward in young subjects during the delay period, showing activation in the left intra-parietal cortex, ventral striatum, caudate nucleus, and anterior cingulate cortex. *Right*. Main effect of anticipating reward in older subjects during the delay period, showing activation in the left intra-parietal cortex only. The glass brain and the coronal slice indicate that no ventral striatum activity was observed in older subjects. (B) *Left*. Main effect of reward receipt in young subjects at the time of the rewarded outcome, showing activation in a large bilateral prefronto-parietal network. *Right*. Main effect of reward receipt in older subjects at the time of the rewarded outcome, showing bilateral prefronto-parietal activation [152].

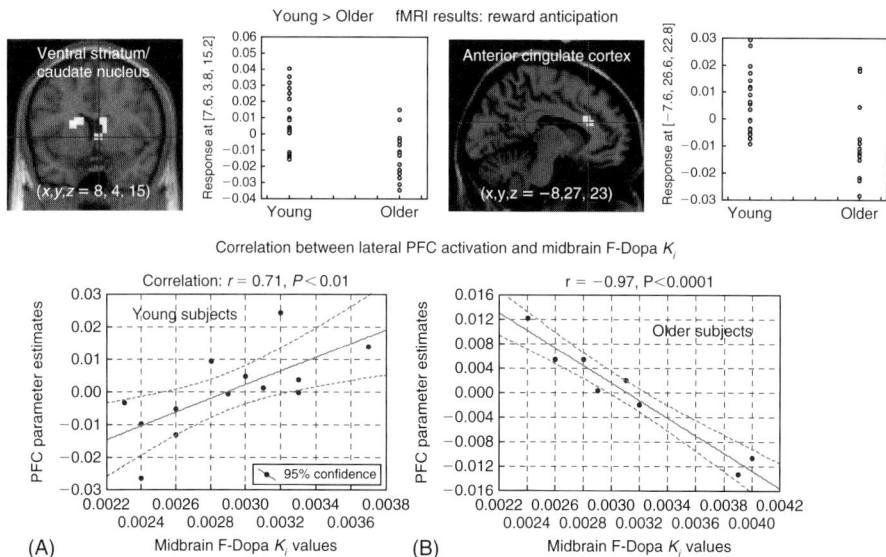

Figure 14.4 *Top.* Between-group comparison during reward anticipation, showing higher ventral striatum and anterior cingulate cortex activation in young subjects. The graphs show parameter estimates in these two brain regions in young and old subjects. *Bottom.* Relationship between midbrain dopamine uptake (K_i) and lateral prefrontal blood oxygen level-dependent (BOLD) signal in young and old adults during reward anticipation. Significant positive correlation of midbrain K_i with BOLD change during reward anticipation in young subjects (x,y,z = 42, 46, 19; Spearman's r = 0.71, $P < 0.01$; regression line with 95% confidence bands) (A) and significant negative correlation of midbrain K_i with BOLD change in older subjects (x,y,z = −23, 30, 15; r = −0.97, $P < 0.0001$) (B). A similar relationship was also observed at the time of reward delivery [152]. See Plate 18 of Color Plate section.

Hormonal replacement therapy (HRT) in aging men and women

Aging is accompanied by gonadal steroid function decline in both men and women, and there is now growing evidence that testosterone and estrogen decline play a role in these aging-related cognitive alterations. It has been proposed that estrogen therapy can reduce or delay the symptoms of Alzheimer's disease and age-related cognitive decline [153–162]. Similar effects have also been reported for testosterone [163–165], although its effects have been less studied. Some studies have reported a beneficial effect of hormone therapy on cognitive decline in women with menopause [166,167]. Current data point toward the existence of a critical window within which estrogen treatment can exert a beneficial effect on the brain [168,169]. Variables such as the time and age at which estrogen is administered and the pattern of administration may predict the clinical outcome [162]. In this sense, for estradiol to exert beneficial effects, it must be administered close to menopause onset and following a pattern of administration that mimics the natural hormonal cycle [162,168,169].

A few studies have started to investigate the influence of HRT in postmenopausal women on different cognitive functions, such as verbal and visuo-spatial abilities, but, to the best of our knowledge, no study to date has investigated decision making or reward processing. For example, HRT-related effects in postmenopausal women who received hormone therapy either with estrogen alone, an estrogen–progestagen combination, or without HRT, showed that estrogen therapy in postmenopausal women can affect visuo-spatial abilities by modulating the functional brain organization [170].

In healthy aged men, moderate exogenous testosterone supplementation improves verbal and spatial memory, while low or large supplementations do not affect cognition [187]. A few neuroimaging studies indicate that HRT enhances brain activity during tasks that examine memory function. For example, women on HRT were found to have better performance on a verbal memory test and greater changes in regional cerebral blood flow during verbal and nonverbal memory tests [188]. Also, men and women on HRT report improvement of their mood and motivation.

14.4   Actions of gonadal steroid hormones in the brain

The actions of gonadal steroid hormones on sex steroid-sensitive brain structures, and the cognitive functions tied to them, have been traditionally divided into organizational and activational [171]. Organizational actions involve the modulation of neuronal development and neuronal circuit formation of a permanent nature [36], leading to sexual dimorphisms. On the other hand, activational effects are considered to be transient and reversible [171]. Although it has long been assumed that organizational effects were restricted to the perinatal period, there is now evidence that permanent neural maturation can occur in adulthood [171,172]. The mechanisms by which gonadal steroid hormones cause sexual dimorphisms in the brain and the consequent differences in cognitive abilities begin to be unveiled. For instance, the rat's hippocampus and the monkey's neocortex transiently express high levels of androgen and estrogen receptors during the first weeks of life [173,174]. Also, the aromatase enzyme that converts testosterone to estradiol has been found in the hippocampus and neocortex during the perinatal period [175,176]. It is possible that early in development androgens are converted to estradiol, which can act on local estrogen receptors and potentially lead to the sexually dimorphic development of brain morphology, neurochemistry, and neurophysiology [4].

Due to ethical (e.g., impossibility to manipulate hormone levels in human fetuses or infants) and methodological (e.g., absence of the technology that permits microscopic analysis of neural organization in living people) limitations, it is difficult to test the organizational hypothesis in humans. However, there is evidence in favor of organizing effects of gonadal steroid hormones coming from subjects exposed to atypical hormone environments during early development, from studies correlating measures of hormone concentrations during hypothetical critical periods and cognitive performance later in life, and from the study of female members of opposite-sex twin pairs. Current data suggest that organizational effects also occur in some aspects of human development, although to a more modest degree than is observed in other species [4].

Unlike sexual behavior, which requires the activating effects of gonadal steroid hormones to be expressed, sexual dimorphisms in cognition do not require these activating effects [177]. However, fluctuations in the levels of circulating gonadal steroid hormones can transiently modify cognitive functioning, as well as the structure and function of the related brain regions. For example, women with reduced estrogen levels due to ovariectomy perform less well on verbal memory tasks than women who begin HRT at the time of the surgery [178]. Indeed, experimental work shows that estrogen can promote neuronal growth processes that result in increased number of dendritic spines, axonal sprouts, and synaptic contacts [158,179,180]. Moreover, the transient nature of these changes is demonstrated by the fact that they are rapidly formed and broken down during natural cyclic variations in estrogen and progesterone in female rats [181].

Many effects of gonadal steroid hormones on human behavior and cognition are probably mediated by their classic actions on the genome. According to the classical model, the effects of gonadal steroid hormones on the brain involve the activation of intracellular receptors that bind to DNA and regulate gene expression. These receptors have been found in several brain regions like the hippocampus, amygdala, cerebral cortex, midbrain, and brainstem [20,36]. The activation of these receptors increases binding of the steroid-receptor complex to steroid receptor binding sites—known as hormones response elements—in the regulatory regions of the target genes, which in turn leads to an alteration of the types and amounts of the mRNA transcripts in the neurons and the consequent change in the production of enzymatic, structural, and receptor proteins [1,36]. For example, estradiol alters the expression of several different enzymes, affecting levels of activity in catecholamine, serotonin, and acetylcholine pathways [4]. These genomic effects are slow, since it takes time for the gonadal steroid hormone to diffuse across the plasma membrane, bind to receptors, and induce the transcriptional changes underlying protein synthesis [36]. However, it is well known that gonadal steroid hormones may produce rapid effects on neuronal excitability [20,36]. For example, estradiol has been found to rapidly excite neurons in the cerebellum, the amygdala, and the CA1 pyramidal neurons of the hippocampus [182–185] by a mechanism that does not seem to involve intracellular estrogen receptors, since these are not found in the responding neurons. Also, estradiol directly potentiates dopamine release in the rat nucleus accumbens [186]. The rapidity of these effects makes it unlikely that they are mediated by a genomic mechanism [21]. The most plausible explanation is that these effects are mediated by membrane receptors or even by novel types of receptors [20,21].

14.5   Conclusions

There is now compelling evidence that gonadal steroid hormones, through cellular and molecular mechanisms of action in the brain, influence behavioral and physiological processes that go beyond their traditional role in the regulation of hypothalamic activity and reproduction. These actions begin during gestation and may produce organizational, long-lasting, structural changes leading to sexual dimorphisms. Later in life, gonadal steroid hormones continue to exert activating, transient effects on specific brain regions. They influence the activity of neurons in brain regions important for cognitive processes, such as the hippocampus and the striatum, even if these structures are practically devoid of specific nuclear receptors. The effects of gonadal steroid hormones in these brain regions may be explained by the powerful trans-synaptic influence on other cells of a small number of neurons containing receptors, or by the action on non-nuclear receptors and second messengers activation [20]. By modulating the neuronal activity of these structures, gonadal steroid hormones influence important cognitive functions and behaviors such as memory, learning, reward processing, and decision making.

Yet one important remaining question is to know why gonadal steroid hormones affect cognition and brain functioning during lifetime. What is the benefit of displaying a better cognitive performance in some functions during periods of life in which estrogen is higher? Unlike women living in modern societies, who go through many cycles of estrogen and progesterone through their lifetimes, it is believed that pregnancy and motherhood was the most common life state of our female ancestors. Thus, it has been suggested that variations in estrogen and progesterone during pregnancy and lactation and their effects on several cognitive functions have been selected because they improved adaptive behaviors during these epochs. For instance, a better memory function may help nest building and location, pup recognition and retrieval, and foraging for food [4]. In parallel, variations in reward processing and decision-making abilities may also confer some advantages for procreation and selection of genetically best-fitted partners [13,128,133].

References

[1] D.R. Rubinow, P.J. Schmidt, Androgens, brain, and behavior, Am. J. Psychiatry 153 (1996) 974–984.

[2] I. Thiblin, A. Finn, S.B. Ross, C. Stenfors, Increased dopaminergic and 5-hydroxytryptaminergic activities in male rat brain following long-term treatment with anabolic androgenic steroids, Br. J. Pharmacol. 126 (1999) 1301–1306.

[3] W.J. Lynch, M.E. Roth, J.L. Mickelberg, M.E. Carroll, Role of estrogen in the acquisition of intravenously self-administered cocaine in female rats, Pharmacol. Biochem. Behav. 68 (2001) 641–646.

[4] J.B. Becker, S.M. Breedlove, D. Crews, M.M. McCarthy, Behavioral endocrinology, second ed., MIT Press, Cambridge, MA, 2002.

[5] L.M. Creutz, M.F. Kritzer, Mesostriatal and mesolimbic projections of midbrain neurons immunoreactive for estrogen receptor beta or androgen receptors in rats, J. Comp. Neurol. 476 (2004) 348–362.

[6] J.S. Janowsky, B. Chavez, E. Orwoll, Sex steroids modify working memory, J. Cogn. Neurosci. 12 (2000) 407–414.

[7] P. Barnes, V. Staal, J. Muir, M.A. Good, 17-Beta estradiol administration attenuates deficits in sustained and divided attention in young ovariectomized rats and aged acyclic female rats, Behav. Neurosci. 120 (2006) 1225–1234.

[8] M.F. Kritzer, A. Brewer, F. Montalmant, M. Davenport, J.K. Robinson, Effects of gonadectomy on performance in operant tasks measuring prefrontal cortical function in adult male rats, Horm. Behav. 51 (2007) 183–194.

[9] S. Schoning, A. Engelien, H. Kugel, S. Schafer, H. Schiffbauer, P. Zwitserlood, E. Pletziger, P. Beizai, A. Kersting, P. Ohrmann, R.R. Greb, W. Lehmann, W. Heindel, V. Arolt, C. Konrad, Functional anatomy of visuo-spatial working memory during mental rotation is influenced by sex, menstrual cycle, and sex steroid hormones, Neuropsychologia 45 (2007) 3203–3214.

[10] A.J. Gregoire, R. Kumar, B. Everitt, A.F. Henderson, J.W. Studd, Transdermal oestrogen for treatment of severe postnatal depression, Lancet 347 (1996) 930–933.

[11] A.J. Ahokas, S. Turtiainen, M. Aito, Sublingual oestrogen treatment of postnatal depression, Lancet 351 (1998) 109.

[12] C.N. Soares, O.P. Almeida, H. Joffe, L.S. Cohen, Efficacy of estradiol for the treatment of depressive disorders in perimenopausal women: a double-blind, randomized, placebo-controlled trial, Arch. Gen. Psychiatry 58 (2001) 529–534.

[13] J.-C. Dreher, P.J. Schmidt, P. Kohn, D. Furman, D. Rubinow, K.F. Berman, Menstrual cycle phase modulates reward-related neural function in women, Proc. Natl. Acad. Sci. USA 104 (2007) 2465–2470.

[14] M.F. Kritzer, Selective colocalization of immunoreactivity for intracellular gonadal hormone receptors and tyrosine hydroxylase in the ventral tegmental area, substantia nigra, and retrorubral fields in the rat, J. Comp. Neurol. 379 (1997) 247–260.

[15] S.W. Mitra, E. Hoskin, J. Yudkovitz, L. Pear, H.A. Wilkinson, S. Hayashi, D.W. Pfaff, S. Ogawa, S.P. Rohrer, J.M. Schaeffer, B.S. McEwen, S.E. Alves, Immunolocalization of estrogen receptor beta in the mouse brain: comparison with estrogen receptor alpha, Endocrinology 144 (2003) 2055–2067.

[16] S.K. Finley, M.F. Kritzer, Immunoreactivity for intracellular androgen receptors in identified subpopulations of neurons, astrocytes and oligodendrocytes in primate prefrontal cortex, J. Neurobiol. 40 (1999) 446–457.

[17] J.E. Donahue, E.G. Stopa, R.L. Chorsky, J.C. King, H.M. Schipper, S.A. Tobet, J.D. Blaustein, S. Reichlin, Cells containing immunoreactive estrogen receptor-alpha in the human basal forebrain, Brain Res. 856 (2000) 142–151.

[18] T. Ravizza, A.S. Galanopoulou, J. Veliskova, S.L. Moshe, Sex differences in androgen and estrogen receptor expression in rat substantia nigra during development: an immunohistochemical study, Neuroscience 115 (2002) 685–696.

[19] Y. Zhou, D.M. Dorsa, Estrogen rapidly induces c-jun immunoreactivity in rat striatum, Horm. Behav. 28 (1994) 376–382.

[20] B. McEwen, Estrogen actions throughout the brain, Recent Prog. Horm. Res. 57 (2002) 357–384.

[21] B.S. McEwen, S.E. Alves, Estrogen actions in the central nervous system, Endocr. Rev. 20 (1999) 279–307.

[22] J.B. Becker, C.N. Rudick, Rapid effects of estrogen or progesterone on the amphetamine-induced increase in striatal dopamine are enhanced by estrogen priming: a microdialysis study, Pharmacol. Biochem. Behav. 64 (1999) 53–57.

[23] J.B. Becker, J.H. Cha, Estrous cycle-dependent variation in amphetamine-induced behaviors and striatal dopamine release assessed with microdialysis, Behav. Brain Res. 35 (1989) 117–125.

[24] J. Demotes-Mainard, E. Arnauld, J.D. Vincent, Estrogens modulate the responsiveness of in vivo recorded striatal neurons to iontophoretic application of dopamine in rats: role of D1 and D2 receptor activation, J. Neuroendocrinol. 2 (1990) 825–832.

[25] D. Guivarc'h, P. Vernier, J.D. Vincent, Sex steroid hormones change the differential distribution of the isoforms of the D2 dopamine receptor messenger RNA in the rat brain, Neuroscience 69 (1995) 159–166.

[26] M. Febo, L.A. Gonzalez-Rodriguez, D.E. Capo-Ramos, N.Y. Gonzalez-Segarra, A.C. Segarra, Estrogen-dependent alterations in D2/D3-induced G protein activation in cocaine-sensitized female rats, J. Neurochem. 86 (2003) 405–412.

[27] J.D. Blaustein, Progestin receptors: neuronal integrators of hormonal and environmental stimulation, Ann. NY Acad. Sci. 1007 (2003) 238–250.

[28] S.K. Mani, J.M. Allen, J.H. Clark, J.D. Blaustein, B.W. O'Malley, Convergent pathways for steroid hormone- and neurotransmitter-induced rat sexual behavior, Science 265 (1994) 1246–1249.

[29] S.K. Mani, J.D. Blaustein, B.W. O'Malley, Progesterone receptor function from a behavioral perspective, Horm. Behav. 31 (1997) 244–255.

[30] L. Cahill, Why sex matters for neuroscience, Nat. Rev. Neurosci. 7 (2006) 477–484.

[31] C. Trepel, C.R. Fox, R.A. Poldrack, Prospect theory on the brain? Toward a cognitive neuroscience of decision under risk, Brain Res. Cogn. Brain Res. 23 (2005) 34–50.

[32] X. Caldú, J.-C. Dreher, Hormonal and genetic influences on processing reward and social information, Ann. NY Acad. Sci. 1118 (2007) 43–73.

[33] S.M. Evans, M. Haney, R.W. Foltin, The effects of smoked cocaine during the follicular and luteal phases of the menstrual cycle in women, Psychopharmacology (Berl) 159 (2002) 397–406.

[34] A.J. Justice, H. de Wit, Acute effects of d-amphetamine during the follicular and luteal phases of the menstrual cycle in women, Psychopharmacology (Berl) 145 (1999) 67–75.

[35] H. Hafner, Gender differences in schizophrenia, Psychoneuroendocrinology 28 (Suppl. 2) (2003) 17–54.

[36] M. Kawata, Roles of steroid hormones and their receptors in structural organization in the nervous system, Neurosci. Res. 24 (1995) 1–46.

[37] A. Mazur, A. Booth, Testosterone and dominance in men, Behav. Brain Sci. 21 (1998) 353–363 discussion 363–397.

[38] A.S. Book, K.B. Starzyk, V.L. Quinsey, The relationship between testosterone and aggression: a meta-analysis, Aggress Viol Behav 6 (2001) 579–599.

[39] K. Christiansen, R. Knussmann, Androgen levels and components of aggressive behavior in men, Horm. Behav. 21 (1987) 170–180.

[40] D.B. O'Connor, J. Archer, W.M. Hair, F.C. Wu, Exogenous testosterone, aggression, and mood in eugonadal and hypogonadal men, Physiol. Behav. 75 (2002) 557–566.

[41] D.B. O'Connor, J. Archer, F.C. Wu, Effects of testosterone on mood, aggression, and sexual behavior in young men: a double-blind, placebo-controlled, cross-over study, J. Clin. Endocrinol. Metab. 89 (2004) 2837–2845.

[42] I. van Bokhoven, S.H. van Goozen, H. van Engeland, B. Schaal, L. Arseneault, J.R. Seguin, J.M. Assaad, D.S. Nagin, F. Vitaro, R.E. Tremblay, Salivary testosterone and aggression, delinquency, and social dominance in a population-based longitudinal study of adolescent males, Horm. Behav. 50 (2006) 118–125.

[43] E.F. Coccaro, B. Beresford, P. Minar, J. Kaskow, T. Geracioti, CSF testosterone: relationship to aggression, impulsivity, and venturesomeness in adult males with personality disorder, J. Psychiatr. Res. 41 (2007) 488–492.

[44] V.J. Grant, J.T. France, Dominance and testosterone in women, Biol. Psychol. 58 (2001) 41–47.

[45] R. Rowe, B. Maughan, C.M. Worthman, E.J. Costello, A. Angold, Testosterone, antisocial behavior, and social dominance in boys: pubertal development and biosocial interaction, Biol. Psychiatry 55 (2004) 546–552.

[46] J. van Honk, J.S. Peper, D.J. Schutter, Testosterone reduces unconscious fear but not consciously experienced anxiety: implications for the disorders of fear and anxiety, Biol. Psychiatry 58 (2005) 218–225.

[47] E.J. Hermans, P. Putman, J.M. Baas, H.P. Koppeschaar, J. van Honk, A single administration of testosterone reduces fear-potentiated startle in humans, Biol. Psychiatry 59 (2006) 872–874.

[48] J. van Honk, A. Tuiten, R. Verbaten, M. van den Hout, H. Koppeschaar, J. Thijssen, E. de Haan, Correlations among salivary testosterone, mood, and selective attention to threat in humans, Horm. Behav. 36 (1999) 17–24.

[49] J. van Honk, A. Tuiten, E. Hermans, P. Putman, H. Koppeschaar, J. Thijssen, R. Verbaten, L. van Doornen, A single administration of testosterone induces cardiac accelerative responses to angry faces in healthy young women, Behav. Neurosci. 115 (2001) 238–242.

[50] E.J. Hermans, N.F. Ramsey, J. van Honk, Exogenous testosterone enhances responsiveness to social threat in the neural circuitry of social aggression in humans, Biol. Psychiatry 63 (2008) 263–270.

[51] K. Christiansen, R. Knussmann, Sex hormones and cognitive functioning in men, Neuropsychobiology 18 (1987) 27–36.

[52] N. Neave, M. Menaged, D.R. Weightman, Sex differences in cognition: the role of testosterone and sexual orientation, Brain Cogn. 41 (1999) 245–262.

[53] I. Silverman, D. Kastuk, J. Choi, K. Phillips, Testosterone levels and spatial ability in men, Psychoneuroendocrinology 24 (1999) 813–822.

[54] C.K. Hooven, C.F. Chabris, P.T. Ellison, S.M. Kosslyn, The relationship of male testosterone to components of mental rotation, Neuropsychologia 42 (2004) 782–790.

[55] S.D. Moffat, E. Hampson, A curvilinear relationship between testosterone and spatial cognition in humans: possible influence of hand preference, Psychoneuroendocrinology 21 (1996) 323–337.

[56] D.B. O'Connor, J. Archer, W.M. Hair, F.C. Wu, Activational effects of testosterone on cognitive function in men, Neuropsychologia 39 (2001) 1385–1394.

[57] S.H. Van Goozen, P.T. Cohen-Kettenis, L.J. Gooren, N.H. Frijda, N.E. Van de Poll, Gender differences in behaviour: activating effects of cross-sex hormones, Psychoneuroendocrinology 20 (1995) 343–363.

[58] A. Aleman, E. Bronk, R.P. Kessels, H.P. Koppeschaar, J. van Honk, A single administration of testosterone improves visuospatial ability in young women, Psychoneuroendocrinology 29 (2004) 612–617.

[59] S.J. Winters, A. Brufsky, J. Weissfeld, D.L. Trump, M.A. Dyky, V. Hadeed, Testosterone, sex hormone-binding globulin, and body composition in young adult African American and Caucasian men, Metabolism 50 (2001) 1242–1247.

[60] M.J. Diver, K.E. Imtiaz, A.M. Ahmad, J.P. Vora, W.D. Fraser, Diurnal rhythms of serum total, free and bioavailable testosterone and of SHBG in middle-aged men compared with those in young men, Clin. Endocrinol. (Oxf) 58 (2003) 710–717.

[61] D.A. Granger, E.A. Shirtcliff, C. Zahn-Waxler, B. Usher, B. Klimes-Dougan, P. Hastings, Salivary testosterone diurnal variation and psychopathology in adolescent males and females: individual differences and developmental effects, Dev. Psychopathol. 15 (2003) 431–449.

[62] G.M. Alexander, M.G. Packard, M. Hines, Testosterone has rewarding affective properties in male rats: implications for the biological basis of sexual motivation, Behav. Neurosci. 108 (1994) 424–428.

[63] M.G. Packard, A.H. Cornell, G.M. Alexander, Rewarding affective properties of intra-nucleus accumbens injections of testosterone, Behav. Neurosci. 111 (1997) 219–224.

[64] M.T. Arnedo, A. Salvador, S. Martinez-Sanchis, E. Gonzalez-Bono, Rewarding properties of testosterone in intact male mice: a pilot study, Pharmacol. Biochem. Behav. 65 (2000) 327–332.

[65] J.C. Jorge, K.T. Velazquez, D.L. Ramos-Ortolaza, I. Lorenzini, J. Marrero, C.S. Maldonado-Vlaar, A testosterone metabolite is rewarding to ovariectomized female rats, Behav. Neurosci. 119 (2005) 1222–1226.

[66] L.R. Johnson, R.I. Wood, Oral testosterone self-administration in male hamsters, Neuroendocrinology 73 (2001) 285–292.

[67] J.L. Triemstra, R.I. Wood, Testosterone self-administration in female hamsters, Behav. Brain Res. 154 (2004) 221–229.

[68] R.I. Wood, L.R. Johnson, L. Chu, C. Schad, D.W. Self, Testosterone reinforcement: intravenous and intracerebroventricular self-administration in male rats and hamsters, Psychopharmacology (Berl) 171 (2004) 298–305.

[69] B.E. King, M.G. Packard, G.M. Alexander, Affective properties of intra-medial preoptic area injections of testosterone in male rats, Neurosci. Lett. 269 (1999) 149–152.

[70] C.A. Frye, M.E. Rhodes, R. Rosellini, B. Svare, The nucleus accumbens as a site of action for rewarding properties of testosterone and its 5alpha-reduced metabolites, Pharmacol. Biochem. Behav. 74 (2002) 119–127.

[71] N. Hiroi, N.M. White, The amphetamine conditioned place preference: differential involvement of dopamine receptor subtypes and two dopaminergic terminal areas, Brain Res. 552 (1991) 141–152.

[72] A.S. Schwartz, P.L. Marchok, Depression of morphine-seeking behaviour by dopamine inhibition, Nature 248 (1974) 257–258.

[73] J.P. Schroeder, M.G. Packard, Role of dopamine receptor subtypes in the acquisition of a testosterone conditioned place preference in rats, Neurosci. Lett. 282 (2000) 17–20.

[74] J. Redouté, S. Stoleru, M. Pugeat, N. Costes, F. Lavenne, D. Le Bars, H. Dechaud, L. Cinotti, J.F. Pujol, Brain processing of visual sexual stimuli in treated and untreated hypogonadal patients, Psychoneuroendocrinology 30 (2005) 461–482.

[75] J. Redouté, S. Stoleru, M.C. Gregoire, N. Costes, L. Cinotti, F. Lavenne, D. Le Bars, M.G. Forest, J.F. Pujol, Brain processing of visual sexual stimuli in human males, Hum. Brain Mapp. 11 (2000) 162–177.

[76] S. Hamann, R.A. Herman, C.L. Nolan, K. Wallen, Men and women differ in amygdala response to visual sexual stimuli, Nat. Neurosci. 7 (2004) 411–416.

[77] D. Sabatinelli, M.M. Bradley, P.J. Lang, V.D. Costa, F. Versace, Pleasure rather than salience activates human nucleus accumbens and medial prefrontal cortex, J. Neurophysiol. 98 (2007) 1374–1379.

[78] G. Sescousse, J.-C. Dreher, Coding of reward type along an antero-posterior gradient in the human orbitofrontal cortex, in: Exciting Biologies meeting, Biology of Cognition, Chantilly, France, 2008.

[79] K.N. Kirby, N.N. Marakovic, Delay-discounting probabilistic rewards: rates decrease as amounts increase, Psychon. Bull Rev 3 (1996) 100–104.

[80] N.M. Petry, K.N. Kirby, H.R. Kranzler, Effects of gender and family history of alcohol dependence on a behavioral task of impulsivity in healthy subjects, J. Stud. Alcohol. 63 (2002) 83–90.

[81] M. Gaub, C.L. Carlson, Gender differences in ADHD: a meta-analysis and critical review, J. Am. Acad. Child Adolesc. Psychiatry 36 (1997) 1036–1045.

[82] P. Moran, The epidemiology of antisocial personality disorder, Soc. Psychiatry Psychiatr. Epidemiol. 34 (1999) 231–242.

[83] J. Rehm, R. Room, W. van den Brink, L. Kraus, Problematic drug use and drug use disorders in EU countries and Norway: an overview of the epidemiology, Eur. Neuropsychopharmacol. 15 (2005) 389–397.

[84] J. Rehm, R. Room, W. van den Brink, F. Jacobi, Alcohol use disorders in EU countries and Norway: an overview of the epidemiology, Eur. Neuropsychopharmacol. 15 (2005) 377–388.

[85] R. Reavis, W.H. Overman, Adult sex differences on a decision-making task previously shown to depend on the orbital prefrontal cortex, Behav. Neurosci. 115 (2001) 196–206.

[86] A. Bechara, H. Damasio, D. Tranel, A.R. Damasio, Deciding advantageously before knowing the advantageous strategy, Science 275 (1997) 1293–1295.

[87] A. Bechara, D. Tranel, H. Damasio, Characterization of the decision-making deficit of patients with ventromedial prefrontal cortex lesions, Brain 123 (Pt 11) (2000) 2189–2202.

[88] R.D. Rogers, A.M. Owen, H.C. Middleton, E.J. Williams, J.D. Pickard, B.J. Sahakian, T.W. Robbins, Choosing between small, likely rewards and large, unlikely rewards activates inferior and orbital prefrontal cortex, J. Neurosci. 19 (1999) 9029–9038.

[89] H. Fukui, T. Murai, H. Fukuyama, T. Hayashi, T. Hanakawa, Functional activity related to risk anticipation during performance of the Iowa Gambling Task, Neuroimage 24 (2005) 253–259.

[90] G. Northoff, S. Grimm, H. Boeker, C. Schmidt, F. Bermpohl, A. Heinzel, D. Hell, P. Boesiger, Affective judgment and beneficial decision making: ventromedial prefrontal activity correlates with performance in the Iowa Gambling Task, Hum. Brain Mapp. 27 (2006) 572–587.

[91] P.S. Goldman, H.T. Crawford, L.P. Stokes, T.W. Galkin, H.E. Rosvold, Sex-dependent behavioral effects of cerebral cortical lesions in the developing rhesus monkey, Science 186 (1974) 540–542.

[92] A.S. Clark, P.S. Goldman-Rakic, Gonadal hormones influence the emergence of cortical function in nonhuman primates, Behav. Neurosci. 103 (1989) 1287–1295.

[93] J. van Honk, D.J. Schutter, E.J. Hermans, P. Putman, A. Tuiten, H. Koppeschaar, Testosterone shifts the balance between sensitivity for punishment and reward in healthy young women, Psychoneuroendocrinology 29 (2004) 937–943.

[94] T. Takahashi, K. Sakaguchi, M. Oki, S. Homma, T. Hasegawa, Testosterone levels and discounting delayed monetary gains and losses in male humans, Neuro Endocrinol. Lett. 27 (2006) 439–444.

[95] T.C. Burnham, High-testosterone men reject low ultimatum game offers, Proc. Biol. Sci. 274 (2007) 2327–2330.

[96] A. Henrich, R. Boyd, S. Bowles, C. Camerer, E. Fehr, H. Gintis, R. McElreath, In search of Homo economicus: behavioral experiments in 15 small-scale societies, Am. Econ. Rev. 91 (2001) 73–78.

[97] J.T. Manning, D. Scutt, J. Wilson, D.I. Lewis-Jones, The ratio of 2nd to 4th digit length: a predictor of sperm numbers and concentrations of testosterone, luteinizing hormone and oestrogen, Hum. Reprod. 13 (1998) 3000–3004.

[98] S. Lutchmaya, S. Baron-Cohen, P. Raggatt, R. Knickmeyer, J.T. Manning, 2nd to 4th digit ratios, fetal testosterone and estradiol, Early Hum. Dev. 77 (2004) 23–28.

[99] B. Van den Bergh, S. Dewitte, Digit ratio (2D:4D) moderates the impact of sexual cues on men's decisions in ultimatum games, Proc. Biol. Sci. 273 (2006) 2091–2095.

[100] K. Millet, S. Dewitte, A subordinate status position increases the present value of financial resources for low 2D:4D men, Am. J. Hum. Biol. 20 (2008) 110–115.

[101] J.M. Coates, J. Herbert, Endogenous steroids and financial risk taking on a London trading floor, Proc. Natl. Acad. Sci. USA 105 (2008) 6167–6172.

[102] C.M. Kuhnen, B. Knutson, The neural basis of financial risk taking, Neuron 47 (2005) 763–770.

[103] B. Knutson, C.M. Adams, G.W. Fong, D. Hommer, Anticipation of increasing monetary reward selectively recruits nucleus accumbens, J. Neurosci. 21 (2001) RC159.

[104] K. Preuschoff, P. Bossaerts, S.R. Quartz, Neural differentiation of expected reward and risk in human subcortical structures, Neuron 51 (2006) 381–390.

[105] B. Knutson, G.E. Wimmer, C.M. Kuhnen, P. Winkielman, Nucleus accumbens activation mediates the influence of reward cues on financial risk taking, Neuroreport 19 (2008) 509–513.

[106] K.F. Berman, P.J. Schmidt, D.R. Rubinow, M.A. Danaceau, J.D. Van Horn, G. Esposito, J.L. Ostrem, D.R. Weinberger, Modulation of cognition-specific cortical activity by gonadal steroids: a positron-emission tomography study in women, Proc. Natl. Acad. Sci. USA 94 (1997) 8836–8841.

[107] P.A. Keenan, W.H. Ezzat, K. Ginsburg, G.J. Moore, Prefrontal cortex as the site of estrogen's effect on cognition, Psychoneuroendocrinology 26 (2001) 577–590.

[108] S.M. Resnick, P.M. Maki, Effects of hormone replacement therapy on cognitive and brain aging, Ann. NY Acad. Sci. 949 (2001) 203–214.

[109] J. Hao, P.R. Rapp, A.E. Leffler, S.R. Leffler, W.G. Janssen, W. Lou, H. McKay, J.A. Roberts, S.L. Wearne, P.R. Hof, J.H. Morrison, Estrogen alters spine number and morphology in prefrontal cortex of aged female rhesus monkeys, J. Neurosci. 26 (2006) 2571–2578.

[110] A. Lacreuse, Effects of ovarian hormones on cognitive function in nonhuman primates, Neuroscience 138 (2006) 859–867.

[111] M. Hausmann, D. Slabbekoorn, S.H. Van Goozen, P.T. Cohen-Kettenis, O. Gunturkun, Sex hormones affect spatial abilities during the menstrual cycle, Behav. Neurosci. 114 (2000) 1245–1250.

[112] D.F. Halpern, U. Tan, Stereotypes and steroids: using a psychobiosocial model to understand cognitive sex differences, Brain Cogn. 45 (2001) 392–414.

[113] L. Rosenberg, S. Park, Verbal and spatial functions across the menstrual cycle in healthy young women, Psychoneuroendocrinology 27 (2002) 835–841.

[114] J. Beaudoin, R. Marrocco, Attentional validity effect across the human menstrual cycle varies with basal temperature changes, Behav. Brain Res. 158 (2005) 23–29.

[115] D.R. Rubinow, P.J. Schmidt, Gonadal steroid regulation of mood: the lessons of premenstrual syndrome, Front. Neuroendocrinol. 27 (2006) 210–216.

[116] S.M. Evans, The role of estradiol and progesterone in modulating the subjective effects of stimulants in humans, Exp. Clin. Psychopharmacol. 15 (2007) 418–426.

[117] C.A. Frye, M.E. Rhodes, Administration of estrogen to ovariectomized rats promotes conditioned place preference and produces moderate levels of estrogen in the nucleus accumbens, Brain Res. 1067 (2006) 209–215.

[118] A.A. Walf, M.E. Rhodes, J.R. Meade, J.P. Harney, C.A. Frye, Estradiol-induced conditioned place preference may require actions at estrogen receptors in the nucleus accumbens, Neuropsychopharmacology 32 (2007) 522–530.

[119] S.M. Evans, R.W. Foltin, Exogenous progesterone attenuates the subjective effects of smoked cocaine in women, but not in men, Neuropsychopharmacology 31 (2006) 659–674.

[120] X. Protopopescu, H. Pan, M. Altemus, O. Tuescher, M. Polanecsky, B. McEwen, D. Silbersweig, E. Stern, Orbitofrontal cortex activity related to emotional processing changes across the menstrual cycle, Proc. Natl. Acad. Sci. USA 102 (2005) 16060–16065.

[121] J.M. Goldstein, M. Jerram, R. Poldrack, T. Ahern, D.N. Kennedy, L.J. Seidman, N. Makris, Hormonal cycle modulates arousal circuitry in women using functional magnetic resonance imaging, J. Neurosci. 25 (2005) 9309–9316.

[122] G. van Wingen, F. van Broekhoven, R.J. Verkes, K.M. Petersson, T. Backstrom, J. Buitelaar, G. Fernandez, How progesterone impairs memory for biologically salient stimuli in healthy young women, J. Neurosci. 27 (2007) 11416–11423.

[123] G.A. van Wingen, F. van Broekhoven, R.J. Verkes, K.M. Petersson, T. Backstrom, J.K. Buitelaar, G. Fernandez, Progesterone selectively increases amygdala reactivity in women, Mol. Psychiatry 13 (2008) 325–333.

[124] P. Frost, Preference for darker faces in photographs at different phases of the menstrual cycle: preliminary assessment of evidence for a hormonal relationship, Percept. Mot. Skills 79 (1994) 507–514.

[125] I.S. Penton-Voak, D.I. Perrett, D.L. Castles, T. Kobayashi, D.M. Burt, L.K. Murray, R. Minamisawa, Menstrual cycle alters face preference, Nature 399 (1999) 741–742.

[126] B.C. Jones, A.C. Little, L. Boothroyd, L.M. Debruine, D.R. Feinberg, M.J. Smith, R.E. Cornwell, F.R. Moore, D.I. Perrett, Commitment to relationships and preferences for femininity and apparent health in faces are strongest on days of the menstrual cycle when progesterone level is high, Horm. Behav. 48 (2005) 283–290.

[127] L.M. DeBruine, B.C. Jones, D.I. Perrett, Women's attractiveness judgments of self-resembling faces change across the menstrual cycle, Horm. Behav. 47 (2005) 379–383.

[128] B. Fink, I.S. Penton-Voak, Evolutionary psychology of facial attractiveness, Curr. Dir. Psychol. Sci. 11 (2002) 154–158.

[129] L.L. Welling, B.C. Jones, L.M. DeBruine, C.A. Conway, M.J. Law Smith, A.C. Little, D.R. Feinberg, M.A. Sharp, E.A. Al-Dujaili, Raised salivary testosterone in women is associated with increased attraction to masculine faces, Horm. Behav. 52 (2007) 156–161.

[130] D.A. Puts, Mating context and menstrual phase affect women's preferences for male voice pitch, Evol. Hum. Behav. 26 (2005) 388–397.

[131] J. Havlicek, S.C. Roberts, J. Flegr, Women's preference for dominant male odour: effects of menstrual cycle and relationship status, Biol. Lett. 1 (2005) 256–259.

[132] S.W. Gangestad, J.A. Simpson, A.J. Cousins, C.E. Garver-Apgar, P.N. Christensen, Women's preferences for male behavioral displays change across the menstrual cycle, Psychol. Sci. 15 (2004) 203–207.

[133] S.W. Gangestad, J.A. Simpson, The evolution of human mating: trade-offs and strategic pluralism, Behav. Brain Sci. 23 (2000) 573–587 discussion 587–644.

[134] B.C. Jones, L.M. DeBruine, D.I. Perrett, A.C. Little, D.R. Feinberg, M.J. Law Smith, Effects of menstrual cycle phase on face preferences, Arch. Sex. Behav. 37 (2008) 78–84.

[135] U. Mueller, A. Mazur, Facial dominance in Homo sapiens as hones signaling of male quality, Behav. Ecol. 8 (1997) 569–579.

[136] C. Senior, A. Lau, M.J. Butler, The effects of the menstrual cycle on social decision making, Int. J. Psychophysiol. 63 (2007) 186–191.

[137] I. Aharon, N. Etcoff, D. Ariely, C.F. Chabris, E. O'Connor, H.C. Breiter, Beautiful faces have variable reward value: fMRI and behavioral evidence, Neuron 32 (2001) 537–551.

[138] K.K. Kampe, C.D. Frith, R.J. Dolan, U. Frith, Reward value of attractiveness and gaze, Nature 413 (2001) 589.

[139] A. Ishai, Sex, beauty and the orbitofrontal cortex, Int. J. Psychophysiol. 63 (2007) 181–185.

[140] J.-C. Dreher, P. Schmidt, E. Baller, P. Kohn, D. Rubinow, D. Furman, K.F. Berman, Modulation of the reward system by gonadal steroids: a combined pharmacological/fMRI study in healthy young women, in: Society for Neuroscience, Washington DC, 2008.

[141] M. Kavaliers, N. Devidze, E. Choleris, M. Fudge, J.A. Gustafsson, K.S. Korach, D.W. Pfaff, S. Ogawa, Estrogen receptors alpha and beta mediate different aspects of the facilitatory effects of female cues on male risk taking, Psychoneuroendocrinology 33 (2008) 634–642.

[142] M. Wilson, M. Daly, Do pretty women inspire men to discount the future? Proc. Biol. Sci. 271 (Suppl. 4) (2004) S177–S179.

[143] D. Ariely, G. Loewenstein, The heat of the moment: the effect of sexual arousal on sexual decision making, J. Behav. Decis. Making 19 (2006) 87–98.

[144] R.L. Buckner, A.Z. Snyder, A.L. Sanders, M.E. Raichle, J.C. Morris, Functional brain imaging of young, nondemented, and demented older adults, J. Cogn. Neurosci. 12 (Suppl. 2) (2000) 24–34.

[145] B. Rypma, M. D'Esposito, Isolating the neural mechanisms of age-related changes in human working memory, Nat. Neurosci. 3 (2000) 509–515.

[146] R. Cabeza, Hemispheric asymmetry reduction in older adults: the HAROLD model, Psychol. Aging 17 (2002) 85–100.

[147] S.L. Thompson-Schill, J. Jonides, C. Marshuetz, E.E. Smith, M. D'Esposito, I.P. Kan, R.T. Knight, D. Swick, Effects of frontal lobe damage on interference effects in working memory, Cogn. Affect. Behav. Neurosci. 2 (2002) 109–120.

[148] V.S. Mattay, F. Fera, A. Tessitore, A.R. Hariri, K.F. Berman, S. Das, A. Meyer-Lindenberg, T.E. Goldberg, J.H. Callicott, D.R. Weinberger, Neurophysiological correlates of age-related changes in working memory capacity, Neurosci. Lett. 392 (2006) 32–37.

[149] F. Sambataro, V.P. Murty, J.H. Callicott, H.Y. Tan, S. Das, D.R. Weinberger, V.S. Mattay, Age-related alterations in default mode network: impact on working memory performance, Neurobiol. Aging (2008).

[150] N.D. Volkow, J. Logan, J.S. Fowler, G.J. Wang, R.C. Gur, C. Wong, C. Felder, S.J. Gatley, Y.S. Ding, R. Hitzemann, N. Pappas, Association between age-related decline in brain dopamine activity and impairment in frontal and cingulate metabolism, Am. J. Psychiatry 157 (2000) 75–80.

[151] V. Kaasinen, H. Vilkman, J. Hietala, K. Nagren, H. Helenius, L. Olsson, L. Farde, J. Rinne, Age-related dopamine D2/D3 receptor loss in extrastriatal regions of the human brain, Neurobiol. Aging 21 (2000) 683–688.

[152] J.-C. Dreher, A. Meyer-Lindenberg, P. Kohn, K.F. Berman, Age-related changes in midbrain dopaminergic regulation of the human reward system, Proc. Natl. Acad. Sci. USA 105 (2008) 15106–15111.

[153] D. Kimura, Estrogen replacement therapy may protect against intellectual decline in postmenopausal women, Horm. Behav. 29 (1995) 312–321.

[154] M.X. Tang, D. Jacobs, Y. Stern, K. Marder, P. Schofield, B. Gurland, H. Andrews, R. Mayeux, Effect of oestrogen during menopause on risk and age at onset of Alzheimer's disease, Lancet 348 (1996) 429–432.

[155] C. Kawas, S. Resnick, A. Morrison, R. Brookmeyer, M. Corrada, A. Zonderman, C. Bacal, D.D. Lingle, E. Metter, A prospective study of estrogen replacement therapy and the risk of developing Alzheimer's disease: the Baltimore Longitudinal Study of Aging, Neurology 48 (1997) 1517–1521.

[156] S.M. Resnick, E.J. Metter, A.B. Zonderman, Estrogen replacement therapy and longitudinal decline in visual memory: a possible protective effect? Neurology 49 (1997) 1491–1497.

[157] D.M. Jacobs, M.X. Tang, Y. Stern, M. Sano, K. Marder, K.L. Bell, P. Schofield, G. Dooneief, B. Gurland, R. Mayeux, Cognitive function in nondemented older women who took estrogen after menopause, Neurology 50 (1998) 368–373.

[158] D.W. Pfaff, N. Vasudevan, H.K. Kia, Y.S. Zhu, J. Chan, J. Garey, M. Morgan, S. Ogawa, Estrogens, brain and behavior: studies in fundamental neurobiology and observations related to women's health, J. Steroid Biochem. Mol. Biol. 74 (2000) 365–373.

[159] M.C. Carlson, P.P. Zandi, B.L. Plassman, J.T. Tschanz, K.A. Welsh-Bohmer, D.C. Steffens, L.A. Bastian, K.M. Mehta, J.C. Breitner, Hormone replacement therapy and reduced cognitive decline in older women: the Cache County study, Neurology 57 (2001) 2210–2216.

[160] P.M. Maki, A.B. Zonderman, S.M. Resnick, Enhanced verbal memory in nondemented elderly women receiving hormone-replacement therapy, Am. J. Psychiatry 158 (2001) 227–233.

[161] P.P. Zandi, M.C. Carlson, B.L. Plassman, K.A. Welsh-Bohmer, L.S. Mayer, D.C. Steffens, J.C. Breitner, Hormone replacement therapy and incidence of Alzheimer disease in older women: the Cache County study, JAMA 288 (2002) 2123–2129.

[162] T. Siegfried, Neuroscience: it's all in the timing, Nature 445 (2007) 359–361.

[163] S.D. Moffat, A.B. Zonderman, E.J. Metter, M.R. Blackman, S.M. Harman, S.M. Resnick, Longitudinal assessment of serum free testosterone concentration predicts memory performance and cognitive status in elderly men, J. Clin. Endocrinol. Metab. 87 (2002) 5001–5007.

[164] S.D. Moffat, A.B. Zonderman, E.J. Metter, C. Kawas, M.R. Blackman, S.M. Harman, S.M. Resnick, Free testosterone and risk for Alzheimer disease in older men, Neurology 62 (2004) 188–193.

[165] V.W. Henderson, E. Hogervorst, Testosterone and Alzheimer disease: is it men's turn now? Neurology 62 (2004) 170–171.

[166] S.R. Rapp, M.A. Espeland, S.A. Shumaker, V.W. Henderson, R.L. Brunner, J.E. Manson, M.L. Gass, M.L. Stefanick, D.S. Lane, J. Hays, K.C. Johnson, L.H. Coker, M. Dailey, D. Bowen, Effect of estrogen plus progestin on global cognitive function in postmenopausal women: the Women's Health Initiative Memory Study: a randomized controlled trial, JAMA 289 (2003) 2663–2672.

[167] S.A. Shumaker, C. Legault, S.R. Rapp, L. Thal, R.B. Wallace, J.K. Ockene, S.L. Hendrix, B.N. Jones III, A.R. Assaf, R.D. Jackson, J.M. Kotchen, S. Wassertheil-Smoller, J. Wactawski-Wende, Estrogen plus progestin and the incidence of dementia and mild cognitive impairment in postmenopausal women: the Women's Health Initiative Memory Study: a randomized controlled trial, JAMA 289 (2003) 2651–2662.

[168] P.M. Maki, Hormone therapy and cognitive function: is there a critical period for benefit? Neuroscience 138 (2006) 1027–1030.

[169] J.H. Morrison, R.D. Brinton, P.J. Schmidt, A.C. Gore, Estrogen, menopause, and the aging brain: how basic neuroscience can inform hormone therapy in women, J. Neurosci. 26 (2006) 10332–10348.

[170] U. Bayer, M. Hausmann, Estrogen therapy affects right hemisphere functioning in postmenopausal women, Horm. Behav. (2008).

[171] A.P. Arnold, S.M. Breedlove, Organizational and activational effects of sex steroids on brain and behavior: a reanalysis, Horm. Behav. 19 (1985) 469–498.

[172] R.D. Romeo, Puberty: a period of both organizational and activational effects of steroid hormones on neurobehavioural development, J. Neuroendocrinol. 15 (2003) 1185–1192.

[173] A.S. Clark, N.J. MacLusky, P.S. Goldman-Rakic, Androgen binding and metabolism in the cerebral cortex of the developing rhesus monkey, Endocrinology 123 (1988) 932–940.

[174] J.A. O'Keefe, Y. Li, L.H. Burgess, R.J. Handa, Estrogen receptor mRNA alterations in the developing rat hippocampus, Brain Res. Mol. Brain Res. 30 (1995) 115–124.

[175] N.J. MacLusky, A.S. Clark, F. Naftolin, P.S. Goldman-Rakic, Estrogen formation in the mammalian brain: possible role of aromatase in sexual differentiation of the hippocampus and neocortex, Steroids 50 (1987) 459–474.

[176] N.J. MacLusky, M.J. Walters, A.S. Clark, C.D. Toran-Allerand, Aromatase in the cerebral cortex, hippocampus, and mid-brain: ontogeny and developmental implications, Mol. Cell. Neurosci. 5 (1994) 691–698.

[177] C.L. Williams, A.M. Barnett, W.H. Meck, Organizational effects of early gonadal secretions on sexual differentiation in spatial memory, Behav. Neurosci. 104 (1990) 84–97.

[178] B.B. Sherwin, Estrogenic effects on memory in women, Ann. NY Acad. Sci. 743 (1994) 213–230 discussion 230–211.

[179] C.S. Woolley, B.S. McEwen, Estradiol mediates fluctuation in hippocampal synapse density during the estrous cycle in the adult rat, J. Neurosci. 12 (1992) 2549–2554.

[180] V.G. VanderHorst, G. Holstege, Estrogen induces axonal outgrowth in the nucleus retroambiguus-lumbosacral motoneuronal pathway in the adult female cat, J. Neurosci. 17 (1997) 1122–1136.

[181] C.S. Woolley, E. Gould, M. Frankfurt, B.S. McEwen, Naturally occurring fluctuation in dendritic spine density on adult hippocampal pyramidal neurons, J. Neurosci. 10 (1990) 4035–4039.

[182] J. Nabekura, Y. Oomura, T. Minami, Y. Mizuno, A. Fukuda, Mechanism of the rapid effect of 17 beta-estradiol on medial amygdala neurons, Science 233 (1986) 226–228.

[183] S.S. Smith, B.D. Waterhouse, D.J. Woodward, Sex steroid effects on extrahypothalamic CNS. I. Estrogen augments neuronal responsiveness to iontophoretically applied glutamate in the cerebellum, Brain Res 422 (1987) 40–51.

[184] M. Wong, R.L. Moss, Electrophysiological evidence for a rapid membrane action of the gonadal steroid, 17 beta-estradiol, on CA1 pyramidal neurons of the rat hippocampus, Brain Res. 543 (1991) 148–152.

[185] M. Wong, R.L. Moss, Long-term and short-term electrophysiological effects of estrogen on the synaptic properties of hippocampal CA1 neurons, J. Neurosci. 12 (1992) 3217–3225.

[186] T.L. Thompson, R.L. Moss, Estrogen regulation of dopamine release in the nucleus accumbens: genomic- and nongenomic-mediated effects, J. Neurochem. 62 (1994) 1750–1756.

[187] M.M. Cherrier, A.M. Matsumoto, J.K. Amory, M. Johnson, S. Craft, E.R. Peskind, M.A. Raskind, Characterization of verbal and spatial memory changes from moderate to supraphysiological increases in serum testosterone in healthy older men, Psychoneuroendocrinology 32 (2007) 72–79.

[188] S.M. Resnick, P.M. Maki, S. Golski, M.A. Kraut, A.B. Zonderman, Effects of estrogen replacement therapy on PET cerebral blood flow and neuropsychological performance, Horm. Behav. 34 (1998) 171–182.

15 Hormone effects on specific motivational states and underlying CNS arousal

Mihaela Stavarache[1], Donald Pfaff[1] and Justine Schober[1,2]

[1]Laboratory of Neurobiology and Behavior, The Rockefeller University, 1230 York Avenue, New York 10065
[2]Hamot Medical Center, 201 State Street, Erie, PA 16550

Abstract

Sex drive is discussed not only in the context of the performance of mating behaviors, but also as a product of more fundamental, primitive CNS arousal processes. These have been conceived as a "generalized arousal" force that depends on dopaminergic systems as well as several other transmitters and peptides. We have studied how generalized arousal transmitters affect ventromedial hypothalamic neurons that serve sexual arousal. Finally, we review the generation of sexual arousal at three different levels of the neuraxis.

Key points

1. Specific motivated behaviors are linked to states of CNS arousal, which are, in turn, fueled by a primitive, fundamental, generalized CNS arousal force.
2. Sources of sexual arousal are distributed up and down the neuraxis, from genital sensory inputs to hypothalamic hormone-sensitive neurons.

With respect to drive reduction and need reduction theories of reward, this chapter will focus on what causes increased drive, following increased bodily needs, to begin with. In the case of sex drive, the hormonal antecedents have been clearly established.

First, for females: After sufficient priming with estrogenic hormones, progesterone injections greatly elevate the female's state of sexual motivation and, subsequently, sexual behavior [1]. For four-footed laboratory animals, the lordosis behavior, a standing posture coupled with vertebral dorsiflexion, permits fertilization. We have worked out its neuronal circuit and have identified several genes whose transcription is increased by estrogens and whose gene products foster lordosis behavior [1].

For males, testosterone action on neurons in the preoptic area is necessary and sufficient for the facilitation of mounting, but peripheral actions of testosterone are also required for normal penile penetration and ejaculation. A crucial mediator of testosterone effects on male-type sex behavior is dopamine (DA) signaling on preoptic neurons [2].

For both females and males, hormonal "drives" on sexual behavior are not limited to consummatory responses themselves. Animals show increased motivation, as proven by their courtship behaviors, conditioned place preferences, willingness to learn arbitrarily chosen operants, and to suffer pain in order to gain access to the mating partner.

15.1 CNS arousal underlying the activation of motivated behaviors

The ability of sex hormones to increase the performance of sexual behaviors when all other aspects of the experiment are held constant is proof of the ability of these sex hormones to increase sexual motivation. For both experimental animals and for human behavior, motivational states are subdivided into their specific aspects (e.g., sex, hunger, thirst, fear, etc.) and their general aspects (accounting for the activation of *any* behavior). These general aspects usually go under the name "arousal," which in turn can be subdivided into specific forms (leading to alertness, attention, etc.) and general forms (including but not limited to the sleep/wake cycle).

We are studying the most primitive, elementary form of arousal, called "generalized arousal," which has been given the following operational definition [3]:

A more aroused animal or human being

   a.   is more responsive to sensory stimuli in all modalities,
   b.   emits more voluntary motor activity, and
   c.   is more reactive, emotionally.

Ascending neuroanatomical systems supporting generalized CNS arousal are well known, and include noradrenergic (NA), dopaminergic, histaminergic, serotonergic, and cholinergic systems, augmented by the actions of orexin/hypocretin. Because of the emphasis of this book on decision and reward, we will describe dopaminergic systems as previously reviewed [3].

Dopamine (DA). Dopaminergic axons course from the brainstem toward the forebrain via two predominant routes. From the substantia nigra they go forward to innervate a huge subcortical motor control region of the forebrain called the "striatum" because of its histological appearance. This forebrain region interests me because current research suggests it may do many things beyond simple motor control. A second DA system arises in a loosely formed cell group in the midbrain called the ventral tegmental area (VTA). These DA neurons are famous for innervating the phylogenetically ancient cortex called the "limbic system," known to be important for controls over motivational states and moods. Notably, some of these DA axons reach the prefrontal cortex, where they synapse on neurons which coordinate the left and right sides of the frontal cortex. This is important in part because the two sides of this region of cortex have opposite effects on arousal and mood: Heightened activity on the right side is associated with lousy feelings in humans, but on the left side, good positive feelings. Just as important: Some of these prefrontal cortical neurons project back to the VTA. This emphasizes the bipolar, bidirectional feature of arousal systems highlighted in the previous review [3].

These DA projections can be distinguished functionally from the NA axonal trajectories by DA's tendency to synapse in more anterior regions of the cerebral cortex, those associated with motor activity. This can be contrasted to more posterior (except for occipital cortex) trajectories of NA axons, associated with sensory processing.

DA clearly contributes to the maintenance of a waking state. When the concentration of DA in the synaptic cleft is elevated by knocking out the gene for the DA transporter protein which would efficiently remove it, the resultant mice have remarkable behavioral hyperactivity in novel environments, making them look like animals on psychostimulants. This may be due to DA terminations in the shell of a basal forebrain region called nucleus accumbens. Disorders of DA physiology have been claimed to contribute to schizophrenia, and some of the animal pharmacology intended to test this idea has implicated the dopamine D2 receptor.

Among the five genes that code for DA receptors, not all are alike. Most striking are the antagonisms between the biochemical effects of D2 as opposed to D1 receptors. In fact, even the different isoforms of D2 receptor gene products have distinct functions. A long form is mainly postsynaptic and a short form is primarily presynaptic. We are just beginning to understand how these molecular differences serve neurophysiological functions controlling behavior.

Most exciting for my lab are the findings that DA terminations in the basal forebrain foster sexual arousal. Elaine Hull and her colleagues have made a compelling case that DA release in the preoptic area fuels sexual arousal and pursuit of females by males. In females as well, dopaminergic function is important. Cheryl Frye and her colleagues have shown that progesterone metabolites acting in VTA can influence arousal through mechanisms in the basal forebrain, perhaps related to the fact that Jill Becker reported sex hormone actions on DA-sensitive systems there. These experiments showed strong hormonal and DA effects on movement control, including the kinds of locomotion involved in female courtship behaviors. Sexual arousal puts forth a well-understood set of mechanisms illustrating how arousal can work. In the words of Professor Susan Iversen, at Oxford, the DA systems are "integral to motivational arousal."

We propose a significant revision of DA theory as I consider the projections of VTA neurons to the nucleus accumbens. This nucleus has obvious connections to the phenomenon of reward. As a result, DA terminations there were interpreted merely as coding reward. I think things are actually a bit more complicated and subtle. A strong line of research from Jon Horvitz at Boston College demonstrated that the salience of stimuli, *per se*, would be the critical requirement for activating DA neurons rather than reward, *per se*. Put another way, the reward value of a stimulus is just one way for that stimulus to gain salience. Destroying DA systems markedly slows responses to salient stimuli and leads to the omission of responses. Continuing on this theme, DA neurons are not necessarily sensitive to reward itself but instead seem to signal anticipations and predictions of future rewarding events. Fluctuations of DA levels in nucleus accumbens during rewarded acts are consistent with the following, new point of view: DA projections to nucleus accumbens signal excitement and arousal, not simply reward.

Further, two prominent features of DA neurobiology tie its arousing power to information theory. First, the *salience* of a stimulus depends exactly upon unpredictable and uncertain change. This maximizes information transfer according to the math presented in Chapter 2. Second, it is the variation in *predictability* of a reward that engages DA systems. Thus, informatic calculations provide the concepts and the metric fundamental to DA and arousal neurobiology [3].

Of course, mesolimbic DA projections participate in both positive reward phenomena and in fear motivation. According to the results of Kent Berridge's lab [4], these different affective states are mediated by DA actions at different rostral/caudal levels in the shell of nucleus accumbens.

15.2   Estrogens and CNS arousal

The definition and quantification of elementary arousal on CNS, fundamental to all cognitive functions and beyond, reaching the level of emotional and sexual behaviors, had been for quite some time the center of interest to neuroscientists worldwide. Its complex structure and the multiple hormonal influences such as estrogen, orexin, and so on raised a series of challenges to the goal of working out a reliable, reproducible paradigm that will allow a detailed study of CNS arousal.

Knowing that estrogenic effects on behaviors reflecting arousal, including sexual arousal, have an autonomic component, we have developed an array of techniques for simultaneous brain activity recordings (EEG), heart rate recordings (ECG), neck muscular tonus (EMG), and behavioral recordings in free-moving conscious mice, and we defined a series of external stimuli to be applied during monitoring, which allowed us to quantify the arousal of CNS and the role of estrogen in its activation (Fig. 15.1). A step farther, considering the new formulation of CNS arousal introduced by Garey et al. [5], in which female mice without functional estrogen receptor alpha genes were markedly deficient in an assay of generalized arousal, we addressed our question in genetically altered mice, lacking the estrogen receptor alpha gene.

We analyzed our results by separately looking at each type of recording we conducted in our animals (Fig. 15.2), but also by integrating all three sets of results and searching for possible correlations among them.

The experiments performed in genetically wild-type (WT) mice brought to our attention few interesting findings. As expected, hormonal treatment influenced all three recordings by bringing out a higher activity in estrogen treated animals. Hormonally induced changes in different brain waves were significant especially in response to olfactory and vestibular stimuli. Heart rate was increased in the estrogen-treated group both before and after applying a stimulus (Fig. 15.2), but it reached a statistically significant level only in the post-stimulus period, showing that estrogen made the animals more reactive to external stimuli. Neck muscular activity and behavior also showed changes consistent with our EEG and ECG findings.

The last interesting finding was the estrogen influence on the degree of correlation among measures (Fig. 15.3). Based on the theory that a generalized arousal function [5] would dominate the animals' responses in this experimental situation, we predicted a high degree of correlation among arousal measurements, but, surprisingly, estrogen treatment seamed to de-correlate these measurements.

According to a previous report [5], estrogen receptor alpha seems to have an important role in mediating estrogen's role on CNS arousal, its deletion reducing the generalized arousal. We applied a similar experimental paradigm on genetically altered mice. WT males, with or without estrogen treatment, were compared to estrogen receptor-alpha null deletion mice (ER-alpha gene knockouts, KO). We did not notice as expected a simple shift in all our measures following hormonal treatment in neither group. However, with a higher dose of estrogen, treated WT males exhibited a higher pre-stimulus heart rate than KO males in all three sensory stimulus modalities, a finding consistent with previous reports [6].

Surprisingly, a constant finding in our data was the remarkable brain asymmetry, as expressed by the brain waves' distribution along the frequency power spectra of left versus right side EEG recordings, consisting in less power in the theta frequency range on the right side (before and after application of the stimuli) and in the beta and gamma frequency range on the left side (opposite to the finding in the pre-stimulus state).

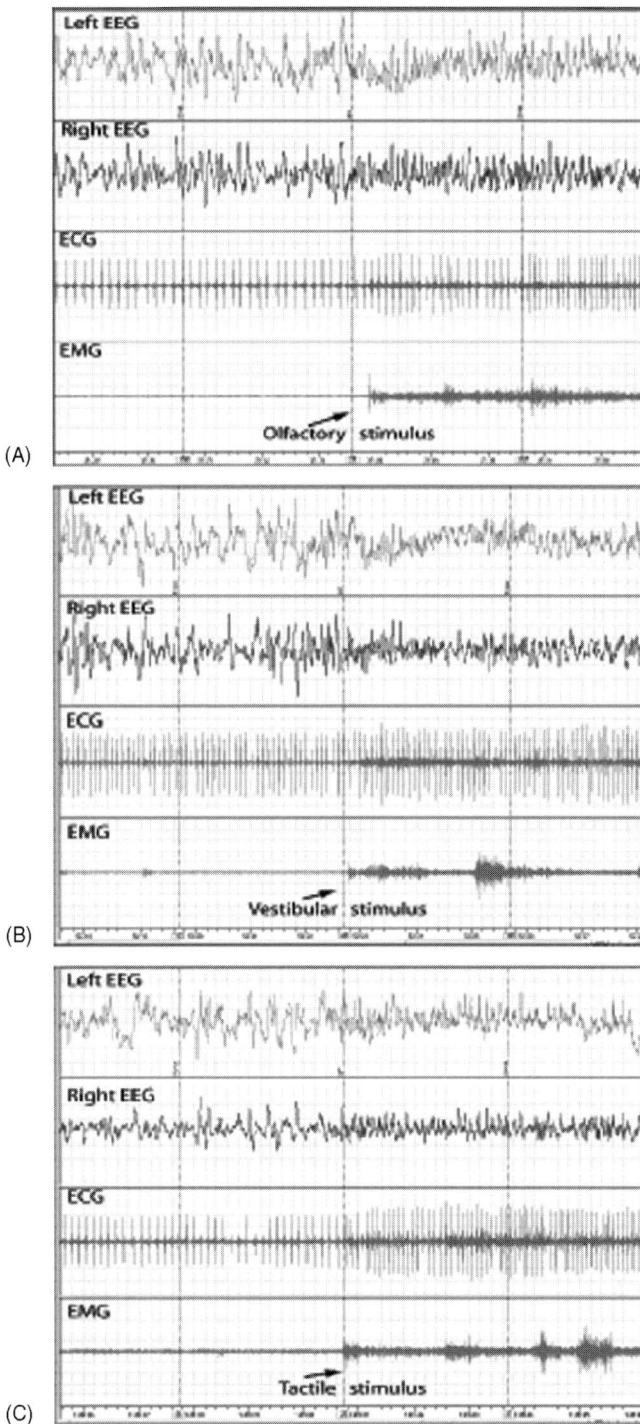

Figure 15.1 Examples of raw data. Recordings of EEG, ECG, and EMG before and after (A) the olfactory stimulus, (B) vestibular stimulus, and (C) tactile stimulus in C57/Bl/J6 animals. Time line: the vertical dotted black lines are separated by 3 s.

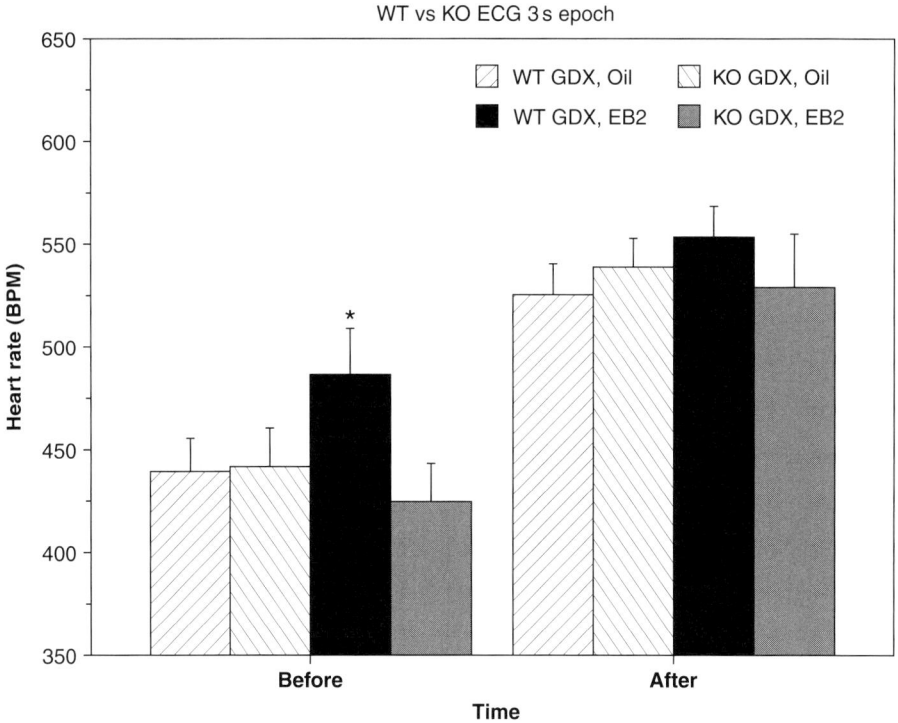

Figure 15.2 Across stimuli averaged heart rate in ER alpha WT and ER alpha KO mice 3s before and after applying the stimuli under oil and estrogen (higher dose) treatment. *$P < 0.05$. WT GDX, Oil – gonadectomized ER alpha WT oil treated; WT GDX, EB2 – gonadectomized ER alpha WT estrogen treated; KO GDX, Oil – gonadectomized ER alpha KO oil treated; KO GDX, EB2 – gonadectomized ER alpha KO estrogen treated.

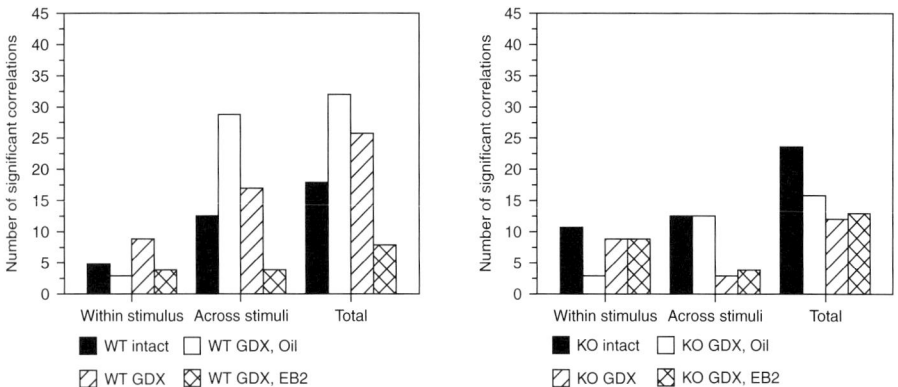

Figure 15.3 Number of significant correlations across and within stimuli in ER alpha WT mice (left) and ER alpha KO mice (right) before applying the stimuli. WT GDX, Oil – gonadectomized ER alpha WT oil treated; WT GDX, EB2 – gonadectomized ER alpha WT estrogen treated; KO GDX, Oil – gonadectomized ER alpha KO oil treated; KO GDX, EB2 – gonadectomized ER alpha KO estrogen treated.

Interestingly, while the pre-stimulus changes were noted in all groups, the post-stimuli changes were observed in intact animals and more frequently post estrogen treatment.

A constant finding in our data is the strong tendency for hormonal treatment to *de-correlate* measures associated with arousal in WT animals. This was noted in both intact and estrogen-treated castrated animals. Furthermore, a higher estrogen dose markedly reduced the number of correlations among arousal measures, specifically before sensorial stimulus application.

In KO animals, the degree of correlation among arousal measures was drastically decreased after castration compared to the similar change process in WT animals. The ability of estrogen to de-correlate was decreased but not absent in the absence of estrogen receptor alpha.

In summary, there are complex relations among different physiological measures related to arousal of CNS; estrogen, one of the many factors influencing its level of activation, depends on the gene coding for estrogen receptor alpha in its modulation of generalized arousal.

15.3   Sources of sexual arousal

Sex hormones act on at least three levels of the neuraxis to increase sexual arousal. The first to be discovered was in the hypothalamus/preoptic area [1]. Interestingly, while estrogenic hormonal actions in the ventromedial hypothalamus increase sexual arousal, neurons in the preoptic area have exactly the opposite effect—they inhibit female-typical behaviors. Instead, following testosterone administration, they increase male sexual arousal.

Second, sex hormones act on the ascending monoaminergic systems to increase activity fostering generalized arousal, and these transmitters in turn affect ventromedial hypothalamic neurons, for example, which govern female sex behavior. In our lab, patchclamp recording techniques have been used to show how histamine [7] and norepinephrine [8] mediate the signaling from generalized arousal pathways to facilitate specific sexual behaviors.

Third, we have begun to use immunocytochemical techniques to analyze how estrogenic hormones could affect the epithelium of the female genitalia, obviously one of the most arousing regions of the skin on the surface of the body [9–13]. Tactile stimulation of the vulvar epithelium initiates changes that suggest complex integrative mechanisms. Influences of skin temperature, hormonal environment, mechanical compliance of the tissue, and inflammation, as well as large number of transmitters and neuropeptides involved in peripheral pathways serving female sexual arousal, speak of a direct sensory role [9]. Genital epithelial cells may actively participate in sensory function to initiate sexual arousal by expressing receptors and releasing neurotransmitters in response to stimuli, resulting in epithelial-neuronal interactions.

In the human female, ERα nuclear staining was found to be present in the stroma of the labia minora, close to the clitoris, and basal and suprabasal in epidermal cells membrane restricted to superficial sections of the labia minora. ERβ was found in the stroma of the labia minora, closer to the clitoris and in superficial sections, in the basal epidermal cells membrane and apocrine glandular epithelial cells membrane. Cell membrane stain was observed in basal and suprabasal epithelial cells and fibroblasts in lamina propria [10].

Arousing properties of genital epithelium may come from both direct and indirect effects of hormones, related to estrogen receptivity, and neural patterns within dermatomes. In mice, ERα was observed in the epithelium of the glans of the clitoris as well as in the glandular tissue, preputial, and apocrine glans. ERα was observed in the nuclei of stromal cells around the cavernous tissue and near the epithelium of the clitoris. Cytoplasm localization of ERα was detected in few cells in an area ventral to the clitoral glans. Nuclear staining was also observed in the connective tissue cells surrounding the clitoris. ERβ immunostaining in the clitoris, adjacent tissue, along with nuclear staining in the vessels of the cavernous tissue of the clitoris, was noted. nNOS immunostaining within the clitoris, the preputial glans, and adjacent connective tissue support the epithelial sensorial role [11]. With regard to neural connectivity, in the mouse, distal genital innervation came from three nerve bundles: one related to the perineal region, one through the corpus cavernosus, and the third between the dorsal part of the clitoris and the urethra. Communicating nerve fibers were identified between perineal, corpus cavernosus nerve, and the dorsal nerve of the clitoris. Immunostaining for neuronal nitric oxide synthase (nNOS) showed that the corpus cavernous nerve sends nNOS positive fibers to join the dorsal nerve of the clitoris. In the same distal area of the clitoris, the connecting branches between the perineal nerve and the dorsal nerve of the clitoris are also nNOS positive [12]. A rich network of nerve bundles and terminal branches was identified and associated with nNOS immunostaining in the cavernous tissue of the body of clitoris. Nitric oxide control of vasodilation and neuronal signaling between the corpus cavernous nerve and the dorsal nerve of the clitoris could contribute to the engorgement and subsidence of clitoral tissue, but may also support the initiation of sexual arousal by tactile stimuli. Again in a mouse model, neuronal tracing studies support an epithelial initiation of arousal by subcutaneous injection of the clitoral epithelium that follows an afferent pattern of labeling in the spinal cord consistent with pudendal and hypogastric innervation of external genitalia and clitoris [13]. We have shown that WGA-HRP was carried via primary sensory afferents, labeling terminal projections in the spinal cord. The distribution extended from S1 to L2 with no labeling seen in the L3 spinal cord, caudally in levels S1 through L4, and rostrally in L2. The greatest density of labeling for nerve fibers from the clitoris was noted in the L5/L6 spinal cord, with very sparse labeling caudally in the sacral spinal cord and rostrally in L2. This study establishes the link between the hormonally receptive tissue of genital/clitoral epithelium and ascending sensory systems.

15.4   Future directions

Progress in understanding the hormonal, neuroanatomical, biophysical, and molecular underpinnings of sexual motivation has been so remarkable that we now can turn back to certain intellectual problems in the field and look at them with a new view. Perhaps the most important is the distinction between appetitive behaviors (AB) and consummatory behaviors (CB). Clearly, the CNS arousal systems described above serve both. Because generalized arousal is essential for the activation of *any* behavior, it is easy to see, for example, in the case of male mating behavior, that a high level of CNS arousal is required for the male to search for and find a female; but then, of course, it is also required to support mounting, erection, and ejaculation. Many neuroendocrinologists subscribe to the AB/CB distinction (e.g., see [14]). The classical ethologists such as Konrad Lorenz and Niko Tinbergen found it useful because, for a wide variety of animals, it provided "terminology to organize many behavioral phenomena for causal analysis" ([14], p. 307). On the other hand, Professor Benjamin Sachs [15] criticized the distinction (a) because he finds it difficult to identify a clear boundary between AB and CB, and (b) because in a long chain of behaviors an individual response might be the CB of a foregoing behavior and the AB or a subsequent behavior. This conceptual dilemma must be sorted out with respect to its application to hormonally controlled sex behaviors. In any case, it is clear that preoptic neurons regulate both AB and CB for male sexuality [16]. In some animals, more rostral preoptic region cell groups affect AB, and more caudal, CB [16]. It is a sign of high accomplishment in this field that scientists can turn to this type of question with considerable cellular and molecular data that bear on the issue.

References

[1] D.W. Pfaff, Drive: Neurobiological and Molecular Mechanisms of Sexual Motivation, MIT Press, Cambridge, MA, 1999.

[2] E.M. Hull, R.L. Meisel, B.D. Sachs, Male sexual behavior, in: D.W. Pfaff, A.P. Arnold, A.M. Etgen, S.E. Fahrbach, R.T. Rubin (Eds.), Hormones, Brain, and Behavior, Academic Press, San Diego, CA, 2002.

[3] D.W. Pfaff, Brain Arousal and Information Theory: Neural and Genetic Mechanisms, Harvard University Press, Cambridge, MA, 2006.

[4] A. Faure, S.M. Reynolds, J.M. Richard, K.C. Berridge, Mesolimbic dopamine in desire and dread: enabling motivation to be generated by localized glutamate disruptions in nucleus accumbens, J. Neurosci. 28 (28) (2008) 7184–7192.

[5] J. Garey, A. Goodwillie, J. Frohlich, M. Morgan, J.A. Gustafsson, O. Smithies, K.S. Korach, S. Ogawa, D.W. Pfaff, Genetic contributions to generalized arousal of brain and behavior, Proc. Natl. Acad. Sci. USA 100 (19) (2003) 11019–11022.

[6] J. Pamidimukkala, B. Xue, L.G. Newton, D.B. Lubahn, M. Hay, Estrogen receptor-alpha mediates estrogen facilitation of baroreflex heart rate responses in conscious mice, Am. J. Physiol. Heart Circ. Physiol. 288 (3) (2005) H1063–H1070.

[7] J. Zhou, A.W. Lee, N. Devidze, Q. Zhang, L.M. Kow, D.W. Pfaff, Histamine-induced excitatory responses in mouse ventromedial hypothalamic neurons: ionic mechanisms and estrogenic regulation, J. Neurophysiol. 98 (6) (2007) 3143–3152.

[8] A.W. Lee, A. Kyrozis, V. Chevaleyre, L.M. Kow, N. Devidze, Q. Zhang, A.M. Etgen, D.W. Pfaff, Estradiol modulation of phenylephrine-induced excitatory responses in ventromedial hypothalamic neurons of female rats, Proc. Natl. Acad. Sci. USA 105 (20) (2008) 7333–7338.

[9] N. Martin-Alguacil, J. Schober, L.M. Kow, D. Pfaff, Arousing properties of the vulvar epithelium, J. Urol. 176 (2) (2006) 456–462.

[10] N. Martin-Alguacil, D.W. Pfaff, L.M. Kow, J.M. Schober, Oestrogen receptors and their relation to neural receptive tissue of the labia minora, BJU Int. 101 (11) (2008) 1401–1406.

[11] N. Martin-Alguacil, J.M. Schober, L.M. Kow, D.W. Pfaff, Oestrogen receptor expression and neuronal nitric oxide synthase in the clitoris and prepucial gland structures of mice, BJU Int. 102 (11) (2008) 1719–1723.

[12] N. Martin-Alguacil, D.W. Pfaff, D.N. Shelley, J.M. Schober, Clitoral sexual arousal: an immunocytochemical and innervation study of the clitoris, BJU Int. 101 (11) (2008) 1407–1413.

[13] N. Martin-Alguacil, J.M. Schober, D.R. Sengelaub, D.W. Pfaff D.N. Shelley, Clitoral sexual arousal: neuronal tracing study from the clitoris through the spinal tracts, J. Urol. 180 (4) (2008) 1241–1248.

[14] G.F. Ball, J. Balthazart, How useful is the appetitive and consummatory distinction for our understanding of the neuroendocrine control of sexual behavior? Horm. Behav. 53 (2) (2008) 307–311 author reply 315–318.

[15] B.D. Sachs, A contextual definition of male sexual arousal, Horm. Behav. 51 (5) (2007) 569–578.

[16] J. Balthazart, G.F. Ball, Topography in the preoptic region: differential regulation of appetitive and consummatory male sexual behaviors, Front. Neuroendocrinol. 28 (4) (2007) 161–178.

16 The genetic basis of individual differences in reward processing and the link to addictive behavior

Juliana Yacubian and Christian Büchel

NeuroImage Nord, Department of Systems Neuroscience, University Medical Center Hamburg-Eppendorf, Martinistr. 52, 20246 Hamburg, Germany

Abstract

Dopaminergic neurotransmission is widely recognized to be critical to the neurobiology of reward, motivation, and addiction. Genetic variation in several key dopaminergic subsystems, presumably resulting in altered central dopaminergic tone and neurotransmission, has been associated with various aspects of personality and temperament as well as susceptibility to addiction. However, enthusiasm for the potential of such genetic variation to addiction has been tempered by inconsistent results and failed attempts to replicate specific associations. Such inconsistency may reflect the underlying biological nature of the relationship between allelic variants in dopamine-related genes, each of presumably slight effect, and observable behaviors that as a rule reproduce complex functional interactions. This chapter focuses on advances made to date in an effort to link genetic individual variations and reward processing as a possible basis for addictive behaviors.

Key points

1. Dopaminergic reward system and addictive behavior.
2. Pathological gambling: model for addiction without a substance.
3. Individual differences and vulnerability to addictive behaviors.
4. Candidate gene studies of dopamine transmission: DAT and COMT.
5. Imaging genetics of the DAT/COMT interaction and reward sensitivity.

Converging evidence from animal and human studies has revealed that reward processing depends on dopaminergic neurotransmission and that dopamine is a critical neuromodulator in the generation and regulation of reward responses [1,2]. Genetic variation in several key dopaminergic subsystems, presumably resulting in altered central dopaminergic tone and neurotransmission, has been associated with various aspects of personality and temperament [3] as well as susceptibility to addiction [4,5]. However, enthusiasm for the potential of such genetic variation to addiction has been tempered by inconsistent results and failed attempts to replicate specific associations [6]. Such inconsistency may reflect the underlying biological nature of the relationship between allelic variants in dopamine-related genes, each of presumably slight effect, and observable behaviors that as a rule reproduce complex functional interactions.

Taking into account that the biological impact of variation in a gene travels across a progressively complex way from neurons to neural networks until behavior, the activity of brain regions involved in reward processes in humans (e.g., tegmental ventral area, ventral striatum, prefrontal cortex) represents a "window" to observe how genes influence behavior. Therefore, functional polymorphisms in dopamine-related genes might have marked influence upon the functionality of these underlying neural systems and intermediate their final effect on behavior.

16.1   Dopaminergic reward system and addictive behavior

Any activity, substance, object, or behavior that has become the major focus of a person's life to the exclusion of other activities, or that has begun to harm the individual or others physically, mentally, or socially is considered an addictive behavior [7]. Drug addiction and addictive behavior place a significant burden on society through their impact on health, social cohesion, crime, and comorbidity with neuropsychiatric disorders. In the last decades, major advances in genetics and molecular and cell biology have led to the identification and cloning of many of the primary targets of addictive behavior [8,9], and there has been a critical discussion on the role of dopamine in addiction [10,11]. Generally, it is now accepted that dopamine is crucial in the development and persistence of addiction. However, its precise role in the relationship between reward and addictive behaviors remains a major challenge.

Several studies have shown that dopamine is important in experiencing reward and in the motivational aspects of drug use such as craving. Many drugs of abuse, including amphetamine, cocaine, heroin, nicotine, cannabis, and alcohol, while having very different primary molecular targets, all have the common action of increasing dopamine neurotransmission in the ventral striatum (nucleus accumbens) [12–14]. This commonality of action has led to the widely held view that the mesolimbic dopaminergic system plays a general role in the reinforcing effects of drugs, perhaps stemming from a more general role in mediating aspects of natural reward [2,15].

Most studies addressing the role of dopamine in reward processes have been conducted in animal models. Recordings in freely moving animals have shown that dopamine neuron activity peaks right before animals engage in heroin self-administration behavior [16]. Similarly, dopamine release increases immediately prior to responding for cocaine as well as after presentation of a drug-related cue and the drug itself [17–20]. In general, these findings suggest that an increase in dopamine transmission facilitates drug-associated behaviors.

Pharmacological studies also substantiate the idea that dopamine is important in addiction-related behaviors. Drugs that decrease dopaminergic transmission generally produce a decrease in drug reward. Accordingly, the systemic administration of the GABA agonist baclofen, which inhibits the activity of the dopaminergic system, has been shown to reduce self-administration of psychostimulants and opiates under different schedules of reinforcement [21–23]. Similar findings were reported after direct infusion of baclofen into the ventral tegmental area [24,25], indicating that these effects are probably specific to the decreases in activity of dopaminergic neurons.

Even though the studies above indicate a relationship between increased dopaminergic tone and addiction, there is also abundant evidence for decreases in dopamine being related to addiction [26]. Withdrawal from long-term use of addictive drugs can lead to a hypodopaminergic state, resulting in a chronic state of anhedonia. As a consequence, drugs are used to stimulate the dopamine activity in the striatum and orbitofrontal cortex in an attempt to alleviate this state. This can be regarded as a "need for dopamine" [27], and it has been argued that this state could decrease an individual's interest in stimuli that are not related to drugs and promote the search for drugs, so as to counteract the decrease in dopaminergic tone [26,28,29]. These views are not incompatible; a dual role for dopamine in drug craving has been proposed, where drug craving and relapse in the addicted individual could be the result of two separate phenomena. Chronic craving would be the result of a reduced dopaminergic tone; in this case, the individual would take drugs to alleviate this hypodopaminergic state [26,29]. Instant craving, instead, would be caused by a temporary increase in dopaminergic transmission, which would act like a trigger to precipitate relapse [30,31].

Several human imaging studies have demonstrated that endogenous dopamine release in the striatum is correlated with the experience of pleasure (drug-induced euphoria) evoked by different categories of drugs [32–36]. For instance, Barrett et al. [37] showed that the hedonic effects of cigarette smoking are associated with increased dopaminergic activity in the dorsal striatum. Furthermore, a study using single photon emission computed tomography (SPECT) in combination with a dopamine D2/D3 radiotracer showed that the magnitude of the decrease in dopamine D2 receptor availability was significantly associated with the self-reported positive reinforcing effects of amphetamine [38]. Moreover, Oswald et al. [39] found that amphetamine administration resulted in striatal dopamine release, which was positively correlated with self-reported drug-liking. However, there are also studies showing drug-induced dopamine release in the striatum, but which failed to find associations with hedonic effect. For example, Boileau et al. [40] found that an oral dose of alcohol promotes dopamine release in the brain, with a preferential effect in the ventral striatum, and Leyton et al. [30] found that amphetamine released dopamine in the ventral striatum, but in both studies a relation with subjective hedonic effects was not found.

In spite of some studies [30,40] that fail to demonstrate a relation between hedonic effects and drug-induced release of dopamine in striatum, a great number of studies investigating the role of dopamine in the experience of pleasure in humans are compatible with the view that dopamine release and high levels of extracellular dopamine in the ventral striatum are associated with the pleasurable effects of drugs of abuse. Conversely, Berridge [41] disentangles the hedonic effect produced by substances of abuse from dopamine release and emphasizes the dissociation between the hedonic effects of drugs ("liking") and its incentive value ("wanting"), so that the dopamine system becomes supersensitized to both the direct effects of the drug and associated stimuli that are not directly attributable to the drug. This phenomenon may be responsible for pathologic wanting independently of withdrawal symptoms or hedonic effects, and may produce compulsive drug-seeking behavior. In the development of drug addiction, although the hedonic effects ("liking") progressively decrease, drugs become pathologically wanted (craving).

16.2   Pathological gambling: model for addiction without a substance

In contrast to drug addiction, in which a determined substance is used to induce pleasure, addictive behaviors, such as gambling, are characterized by the engagement in a behavior to bring about excitement [42]. One model proposed for pathological gambling is as an addiction without the drug [43]. Pathological gambling and substance use disorders share many features: an intense desire to satisfy a need, loss of control over the substance use or behavior, periods of abstinence and tolerance, thoughts about the use of the substance or related activities, and continued engagement in the behavior despite significant social and occupational problems related to it [7].

A pathological gambler's desire to bet may be analogous to cravings experienced by substance abusers. A study of a large sample of substance abusers and pathological gamblers suggested that pathological gamblers had more difficulties resisting gambling urges than substance abusers had resisting drug cravings [44]. Approximately one-third of pathological gamblers experience irritability, psychomotor agitation, difficulties concentrating, and other somatic complaints following periods of gambling, features that share similarities with withdrawal symptoms [45].

Pathological gamblers often increase the frequency of their bets or the amount of money they gamble to achieve the desired level of excitement. This behavior is suggestive of drug tolerance. Pathological gamblers may become preoccupied only with gambling-related activities despite negative domestic, professional, financial, and social consequences of their gambling [46].

Further support for the categorization of pathological gambling as a non-substance related addiction is emerging from brain imaging data suggesting that similar components of the mesolimbic pathway are involved in pathological gambling and substance-related addictive behaviors [47–49]. Taking this into consideration, pathological gambling is a perfect model for studying the function/dysfunction of reward pathways in addiction without direct influence of a substance.

The advent of modern neuroimaging techniques like positronen-emissions-tomographie (PET) and functional Magnetic Resonance Imaging (fMRI) allows investigation of the mechanisms behind pathological gambling.

In an early study 12 pathological gamblers and 12 closely matched healthy controls were investigated using fMRI and a guessing task known to robustly activate the ventral striatum [50]. During the scanning, the subjects had to choose a playing card by pressing a button. They won €1 if the color of the chosen card was red; otherwise they lost €1. First, it was verified that the task robustly activated the ventral striatum. A significantly greater activity during winning than during losing was observed in the ventral striatum in both groups. A direct comparison of the two groups showed significantly lower activation of the right ventral striatum in pathological gamblers than in controls (Fig. 16.1A). In addition, pathological gamblers showed significantly weaker activation in the ventromedial prefrontal cortex (vmPFC) (Fig. 16.1C). A regression analysis trying to correlate signal changes in the ventral striatum with the severity of gambling in each patient showed that the severity of gambling in pathological gamblers (as assessed with a gambling questionnaire) showed a negative correlation with the response in the right ventral striatum and the response in the vmPFC (Fig. 16.1B and 16.1D).

These findings showed that pathological gamblers, compared with control subjects, showed less ventral striatal activation than did controls, and gambling severity correlated inversely with ventral striatal activation [50]. Similarly, adults with alcohol dependence versus those without have been found to activate ventral striatum less robustly in anticipation of working for monetary reward, and similar findings have been observed in subjects' family history positive for alcoholism versus negative family histories [51]. Diminished ventral striatal activation in individuals who suffer from an addiction also appears relevant to craving states, as above described in animal experiments. In a study

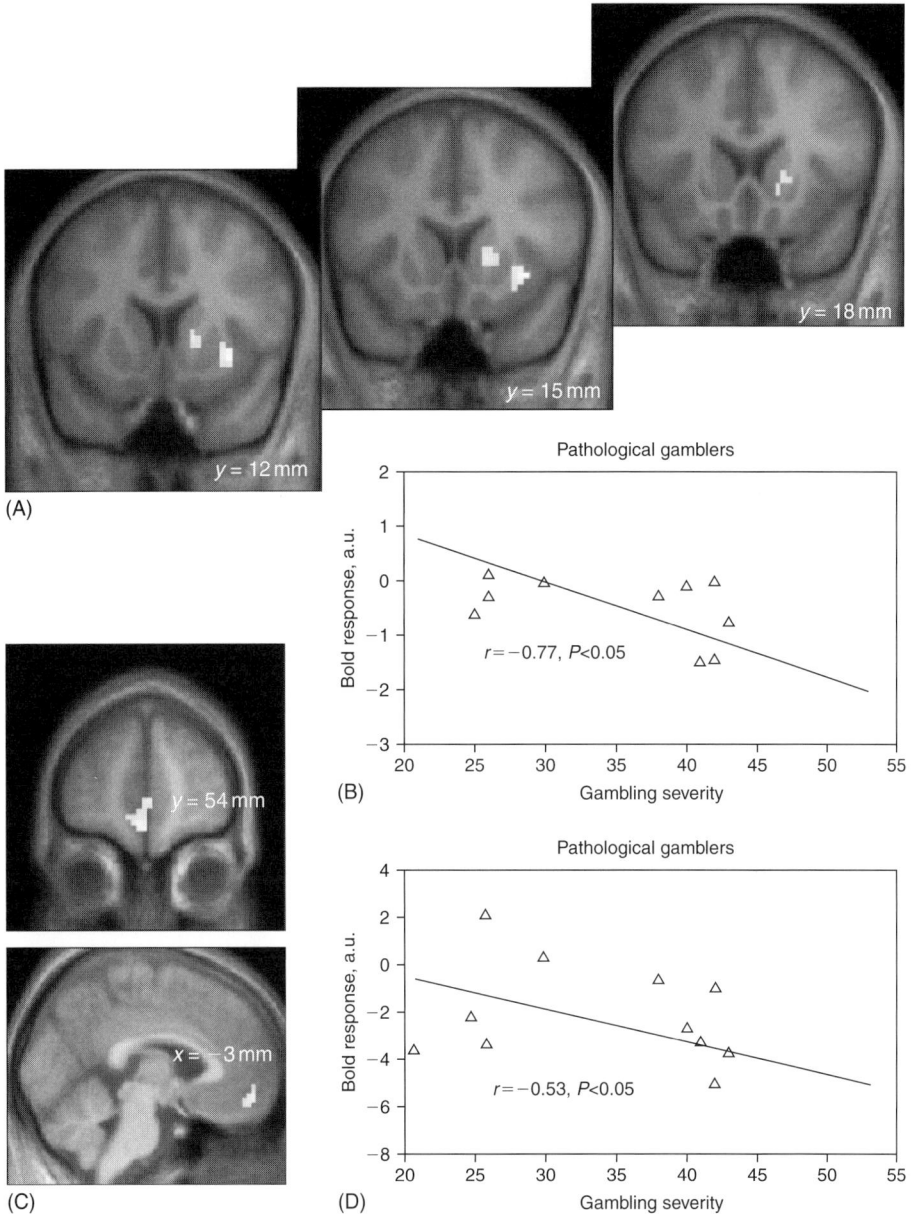

Figure 16.1 Differences in activation between the controls and the pathological gamblers. (A) Lower activation in the right ventral striatum of pathological gamblers compared with controls at $P < 0.001$ masked with the contrast winning > losing at $P < 0.001$. Activity within this area was negatively correlated with gambling severity of individual pathological gamblers (B). (C) Pathological gamblers also showed less activation in the ventromedial prefrontal cortex. Again, activation was negatively correlated with gambling severity (D). The y axes in B and D represent parameter estimates from the single-subject analysis and are directly related to BOLD signal change. See Plate 19 of Color Plate section.

of gambling urges in pathological gambling and cocaine cravings in cocaine dependence, diminished activation of ventral striatum similarly distinguished addicted from control subjects during viewing of the respective gambling or drug videotapes [52].

Moreover, decreased activation of vmPFC has been observed in pathological gamblers during the presentation of gambling cues [48] or performance of the Stroop Color–Word Interference Task [47]. Diminished activation of left vmPFC similarly distinguished pathological gambling and bipolar subjects from controls during Stroop performance [47,53], and diminished activation of this region has been associated with impulsive aggression in depressed subjects [54]. These findings suggest that vmPFC is involved in impulse regulation across a spectrum of diagnostic disorders. vmPFC has been implicated as a critical component of decision-making circuitry in risk–reward assessment, with abnormal function demonstrated in association with substance use disorders [55,56].

By analogy to drug addiction, it has been speculated that pathological gambling might also be related to a deficiency of the mesolimbic dopaminergic reward system [57]. The reward deficiency model supports the idea that a hypodopaminergic state is one of the main causes that triggers drug seeking and taking, even after prolonged abstinence periods, perpetuating the vicious cycle [26]. In addiction, albeit reduced in its activity, the system remains hyperresponsive to substances of abuse, fostering chronic vulnerability to the system. This model is consistent with the imaging results [50] that confirmed a diminished activation of areas involved in reward processing.

16.3 Individual differences and vulnerability to addictive behaviors

In the last few decades, the identification of the factors that determine individual differences in propensity for addiction has become one of the major challenges of drug abuse research. Drug abuse vulnerability is a complex trait with strong genetic influences documented in classic family and twins genetic studies [58]. Moreover, emerging data from both clinical and animal experiments suggest that there exist "vulnerable" phenotypes and genotypes that are more predisposed to drug abuse [59].

Distinctive differences in the subjective effects of drugs in humans have been frequently recorded [38,60,61]. For example, volunteers who preferred the effects of amphetamine to placebo showed increased scores of euphoria and positive mood, compared to anxiety and depression in subjects who preferred the effects of placebo over amphetamine [60].

Findings from imaging studies have shed further light on the neural correlates of these subjective differences. Volkow et al. (1999) showed that the intensity of the euphoria ("high") induced by methylphenidate was significantly correlated with levels of released dopamine. Subjects who had the greatest dopamine increase described the most intense high [34]. Additionally, the magnitude of decrease in D2 receptor availability was significantly associated with the positive reinforcing effects of the methylphenidate [35]. In another report, a correlation between the release of dopamine in response to amphetamine and self-reports of "drug wanting" and the personality trait of novelty seeking was shown [30]. In support of these findings, rhesus monkeys with extensive cocaine self-administration history showed significant decreases in D2 receptor densities throughout the striatum compared to monkeys with a history of food reinforcement [62]. Recently, Gilman et al. [63] showed in an fMRI study that self-ratings of alcohol intoxication correlated with striatal activation, suggesting that striatal activation may contribute to the subjective experience of pleasure and reward during intoxication.

These findings suggest that differences between subjects in the rate of dopamine release, catabolism, and D2 receptor distribution might play a role in the predisposition to drug abuse. The nature of these individual differences is currently unclear but may involve, among others, interindividual genetic variations.

16.4   Candidate gene studies of dopamine transmission: DAT and COMT

Analyses of genes expressed in dopamine neurons that play important roles in drug reward have been allowed the identification of various candidate genes for interindividual differences in drug abuse vulnerability [64]. In this context, important target genes are those involved in the mechanisms to remove and regulate synaptic dopamine and terminate the signaling produced by this neurotransmitter.

Among others, two major proteins take part in terminating the action of dopamine in the brain: catechol-O-methyl transferase (COMT) and the dopamine transporter (DAT). Most of the dopamine released into the synaptic cleft is transported back into the presynaptic cell by the DAT that belongs to the family of catecholamine reuptake pumps. The regional distribution of DAT includes mesostriatal, mesolimbic, and mesocortical pathways, and its action is blocked selectively by drugs such as cocaine. COMT is a major enzyme in dopamine catabolism that influences cortical dopamine flux, especially in prefrontal cortex (PFC) as a result of the paucity of DAT in this region [65]. Disturbances of this system, for example, by fluctuation in COMT enzyme activity or availability of DAT, are expected to affect brain reward processes with possible impact on susceptibility to psychiatric diseases.

Studies in transgenic mouse models have shown that altered expression of these specific dopaminergic genes can substantially influence drug abuse vulnerability. These studies support the importance of the plasma membrane DAT and COMT enzyme. Giros et al. [66] found that the disruption of mice DAT gene results in spontaneous hyperlocomotion despite major adaptive changes such as decreases in neurotransmitter and receptor levels. In homozygous mice, dopamine persisted at least 100 times longer in the extracellular space, providing a biochemical explanation of the hyperdopaminergic phenotype and demonstrating the critical role of the transporter in regulating neurotransmission. This authors noted that the DAT is an obligatory target of cocaine and amphetamine, as demonstrated by the fact that these psychostimulants had no effect on locomotor activity or dopamine release and uptake in mice lacking the transporter. Additionally, mice overexpressing the DAT showed significantly greater cocaine preference than control mice [67]. On the other hand, COMT-disrupted mice clearly show behavioral disturbances, especially increased anxiety and aggression, which supports a possible link between abnormalities of COMT function and psychiatric disorders [68]. However, apart from behavioral abnormalities, the COMT-deficient mice are able to develop fairly normally, suggesting the existence of compensatory mechanisms to overcome the lack of COMT.

The level of COMT enzyme activity is genetically polymorphic in humans and leads to a variation in enzymatic activity. One common polymorphism is a guanine to adenosine substitution at codon 158, resulting in a change in amino acids from valine to methionine (COMT, Val-158-Met) [69]. The Met-containing COMT (Met/Met) enzyme has 25% of the activity of Val-containing COMT (Val/Val), leading to a marked reduction in dopamine metabolism for the Met/Met COMT enzyme and, consequently, a prolonged presence of dopamine. Indeed, COMT appears to play a primary role in dopamine metabolism in the prefrontal cortex but not in other brain regions such as the striatum.

For example, in COMT knock-out mice, dopamine levels are elevated by over 200% in frontal cortex but not in striatum [68,70].

Human studies of COMT functional alleles in polysubstance abusers and nonusers provide a provisional association of a functional gene variant with substance abuse vulnerability. Vandenbergh et al. [71] reported that the proportion of substance abusers with the high-enzyme-activity Val/Val genotype was substantially more frequent than in drug-free controls. The COMT gene has also been implicated in novelty-seeking [72] and heroin addiction [73]. Recently, Puls et al. [74] demonstrated an association between epistatic effects of COMT and glutamate receptor (mGluR3) genotypes and hippocampal volume in alcohol-dependent patients.

The DAT human gene displays a polymorphic 40-base pair (bp) variable number of tandem repeat, of which alleles of nine and ten repeats (9R and 10R) are the most common in Caucasians [75]. The 10R allele has been related to higher levels of expression of the gene [76–80], although other studies have reported higher levels of transcription associated with the 9R allele [81] or no association between this polymorphism and DAT density [82]. In spite of these conflicting results, it is likely that this DAT genotype contributes to differences in the ability of the DAT to remove dopamine from the synapse. Some studies support the notion that this genotype alters an individual's positive and negative responses to psychostimulants. Cocaine users with the 9R genotype appear more susceptible to cocaine-induced paranoia than those with the 10R genotype [83]. Strikingly, Lott et al. [84] reported that healthy volunteers with the 9R genotype have a diminished responsiveness to acute amphetamine injections on measures of global drug effect, dysphoria, feeling high, anxiety, and euphoria, suggesting that the DAT gene is a fundamental contributor to individual variability in response to stimulants. This is consistent with the finding in children with attention deficit hyperactivity disorder (ADHD) who show decreased therapeutic response to methylphenidate in the 9R genotype [85,86]. Taken together, these results point to a "protective" effect of the 9R allele from developing psychostimulant abuse, since the subjects with 9R allele may experience few subjective effects of psychostimulants. However, DAT polymorphisms have not clearly been identified as a risk factor for the development of alcoholism [76], but it has been associated with the development of severe alcohol withdrawal symptoms [87]. The role of DAT polymorphisms in nicotine addiction has also been investigated. Most studies suggest that the 9R allele of the DAT is related to a decreased likelihood of being smoker [88–90]; however, there have been conflicting reports on such a relationship [91].

16.5 Imaging genetics of the DAT/COMT interaction and reward sensitivity

Despite the potential influence of genetic variations in dopamine function on reward processing, the underlying neurobiological correlates of this functional relationship remain unknown. Because the physiological response of the dopaminergic reward system is influenced by the termination of the dopamine signaling that anticipates the subjective experience of rewarding, the COMT and DAT genotype variations may have an obvious impact at the level of reward sensitivity.

In studies of normal genetic polymorphisms, fMRI is in a strong position to support important explanatory links between genetic brain function and behavior. Thus, fMRI can be a helpful tool to confirm and extend the association between genes and specific networks involved in the reward processing and motivational behavior.

On the basis of the fact that the hemodynamic responses to reward anticipation in the ventral striatum is an indirect index of dopamine release, the association between individual variations in COMT and DAT genes influencing the reward processing was investigated [92]. Using a guessing task sensitive to reward-related activation [93], it was demonstrated that during reward anticipation, a gene–gene interaction between COMT and DAT influenced the neural responses of the ventral striatum (Fig. 16.2A). This epistatic interaction explained interindividual differences in ventral striatal sensitivity for reward value: Most genotype combinations exhibited increased striatal activity with more likely and larger rewards, except two genotype combinations (COMT Met/Met DAT 10R and COMT Val/Val DAT 9R), which were associated with decreased responses (Fig. 16.2C–F). Particularly interesting was that when sorting genotypes from COMT Met/Met DAT 10R allele to COMT Val/Val DAT 9R allele, it originated an inverted U-shape (Fig. 16.2H) relationship between genotype and ventral striatal blood oxygen level dependency (BOLD) response, interpreted as consistent with the notion that dopaminergic tone is regulated by the interaction between COMT and DAT [92]. In line with these findings, Dreher et al. [94] confirmed that interactions between COMT and DAT genotype influenced the BOLD signal in the ventral striatum during reward anticipation. Moreover, these authors also described an effect on BOLD responses in the right lateral and orbital areas of the prefrontal cortex and in the midbrain during reward delivery.

Nevertheless, this striatal blunted response in the COMT Met/Met DAT 10R and COMT Val/Val DAT 9R combinations to anticipated reward is not necessarily equal to reduced behavioral reactivity. Actually, blunted neuronal response to anticipated reward may provoke increased reward-seeking behavior as a means of compensating for relatively low levels of ventral striatum activation [95]. Scheres et al. [96] showed an association between low ventral striatum activation and symptoms of impulsivity/hyperactivity in children with ADHD; based on the association of impulsivity, reward-seeking behavior, and addiction, these authors concluded that diminished neural reward anticipation may contribute as a risk factor for addictive behaviors [96].

In order to answer the question if the observed gene–gene interaction in the fMRI study was behaviorally relevant, the average individual sensation-seeking scores for individual genotypes were plotted into the same coordinate system as the BOLD responses of the ventral striatum. This plot also revealed a nonlinear relationship (Fig. 16.2I), with the genotypes linked to BOLD decreases in the ventral striatum exhibiting the highest sensation-seeking scores. This underlines the behavioral relevance of the genetic and neurophysiological analysis and suggests that a genetically modulated dysfunction in neural reward processing could possibly predisposes to addiction [97,98].

Importantly, these results provide neural evidence to support the hypothesis that the response to anticipated rewards is influenced by determined genotype combinations and that some individuals, depending on their genotype, could present a diminished response to anticipated rewards in ventral striatum, which has been described as a possible vulnerability factor for addiction [33,50]. As drug intake is seen to compensate for this altered sensitivity [99], it is worth mentioning that recent data have shown that nicotine can evoke significantly more ventral striatal dopamine release in volunteers with the DAT 9R or COMT Val/Val genotype [100]. In the above-mentioned fMRI study, these are exactly the genotypes that, in an epistatic fashion, exhibit a blunted response to more likely and greater rewards.

16.6 Looking forward

Taken together, these results are a starting point to identify specific neural correlates of genetic interactions that affect reward sensitivity and behavior and possibly render individuals vulnerable to addictive behavior.

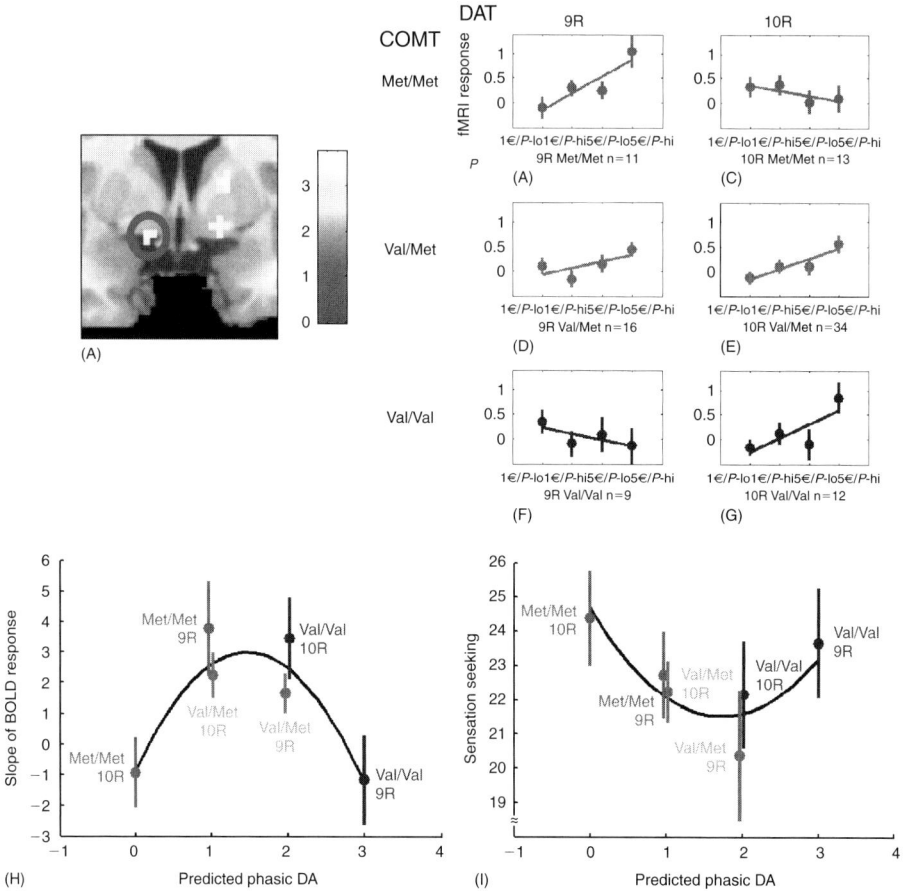

Figure 16.2 Functional gene–gene interactions between the COMT and DAT genotypes in the left ventral striatum. (A) Coronal section shows the average ventral striatal fMRI response to reward anticipation across all subjects overlaid on a template high-resolution MR image. (B–G) Individual fMRI responses from the left ventral striatum (peak x, y, z: -15, 9, -9mm) as a function of reward probability, magnitude, and genotype. The activation increase related to more probable and greater rewards depends on a gene–gene interaction between the COMT and DAT genotypes. A positive slope (B, D, E, and G) indicates more activation for €5 high-probability (P-hi) trials as compared with €1 low-probability (P-low) trials. In some combinations of the COMT and DAT genotypes (C and F), the slope is blunted, presumably reflecting suboptimal neural encoding of reward. (H) Relationship between genotype using COMT as the major grouping factor and the slope of the individuals' left ventral striatal (peak x, y, z: -15, 9, -9mm) activation increase with increasing reward, and (I) the individuals' sensation-seeking scores as indexed by a trait questionnaire. Fitting a second-order polynomial (U-shaped) to the data was significant [left ventral striatum, $T(89) = 3.1$; sensation seeking, $T(89) = 1.8$; all $P < 0.05$].

Mechanisms underlying addiction are individual, genetic, and environmental factors that can modulate the reinforcing effects of the first contact with addictive behaviors, including substances of abuse. Genetic differences can make this "first contact" more or less pleasurable or aversive to a particular individual and can affect the toxicity of a substance, the intensity of psychoactive effects, and the likelihood of different aspects of dependence. In the search for the primal mechanisms of these gene–functional–environmental interactions, two perspectives will be useful in guiding future work. The first perspective is the analysis of genetic factors, including the investigation of whether environmental factors could alter epigenetic programming of dopamine genes, as occurs for other genes [101], and whether these genetic factors have functional consequences at the neural level, such as leading to alterations in activation or in structural morphology of networks that regulate reward processing and finally behavior. The second perspective will have to address how behavioral interventions may counterbalance the vulnerability that may stem from either genetic predispositions or exposure to unfavorable gene–environment interactions.

References

[1] W. Schultz, Predictive reward signal of dopamine neurons, J. Neurophysiol. 80 (1998) 1–27.
[2] R.A. Wise, P.P. Rompre, Brain dopamine and reward, Annu. Rev. Psychol. 40 (1989) 191–225.
[3] R.A. Depue, P.F. Collins, Neurobiology of the structure of personality: dopamine, facilitation of incentive motivation, and extraversion, Behav. Brain Sci. 22 (3) (1999) 491–517.
[4] R. Wise, Addiction becomes a brain disease, Neuron 26 (2000) 27–33.
[5] T.E. Robinson, K.C. Berridge, Addiction, Annu. Rev. Psychol. 54 (2003) 25–53.
[6] D. Ball, Addiction science and its genetics, Addiction 103 (2008) 360–367.
[7] World Health Organization, International Statistical Classification of Diseases and Related Health Problems, tenth rev., World Health Organization, Geneva, 1992.
[8] E.J. Nestler, Molecular mechanisms of drug addiction, J. Neurosci. 12 (1992) 2439–2450.
[9] E.J. Nestler, Molecular mechanisms of drug addiction in the mesolimbic dopamine pathway, Semin. Neurosci. 5 (1993) 369–376.
[10] T.E. Robinson, K.C. Berridge, The neural basis of drug craving: an incentive-sensitization theory of addiction, Brain Res. Brain Res. Rev. 18 (1993) 247–291.
[11] R.A. Wise, Dopamine, learning and motivation, Nat. Rev. Neurosci. 5 (2004) 483–494.
[12] G. Di Chiara, A. Imperato, Drugs abused by humans preferentially increase synaptic dopamine concentrations in the mesolimbic system of freely moving rats, Proc. Natl. Acad. Sci. USA 85 (1988) 5274–5278.
[13] H.O. Pettit, J.B. Justice Jr., Dopamine in the nucleus accumbens during cocaine self-administration as studied by in vivo microdialysis, Pharmacol. Biochem. Behav. 34 (1989) 899–904.
[14] F. Weiss, Y.L. Hurd, U. Ungerstedt, A. Markou, P.M. Plotsky, G.F. Koob, Neurochemical correlates of cocaine and ethanol self-administration, Ann. NY Acad. Sci. 654 (1992) 220–241.
[15] G. Di Chiara, The role of dopamine in drug abuse viewed from the perspective of its role in motivation, Drug Alcohol Depend. 38 (1995) 95–137.
[16] E.A. Kiyatkin, G.V. Rebec, Impulse activity of ventral tegmental area neurons during heroin Impulse activity of ventral tegmental area neurons during heroin self-administration in rats, Neuroscience 102 (2001) 565–580.
[17] P.E. Phillips, G.D. Stuber, M.L. Heien, R.M. Wightman, R.M. Carelli, Subsecond dopamine release promotes cocaine seeking, Nature 422 (2003) 614–618.
[18] G.D. Stuber, R.M. Wightman, R.M. Carelli, Extinction of cocaine self-administration reveals functionally and temporally distinct dopaminergic signals in the nucleus accumbens, Neuron 46 (2005) 661–669.
[19] F. Weiss, R. Martin-Fardon, R. Ciccocioppo, T.M. Kerr, D.L. Smith, O. Ben-Shahar, Enduring resistance to extinction of cocaine-seeking behavior induced by drug-related cues, Neuropsychopharmacology 25 (2001) 361–372.
[20] R. Ito, J.W. Dalley, T.W. Robbins, B.J. Everitt, Dopamine release in the dorsal striatum during cocaine-seeking behavior under the control of a drug-associated cue, J. Neurosci. 22 (2002) 6247–6253.

[21] K. Brebner, A.R. Childress, D.C. Roberts, A potential role for GABA(B) agonists in the treatment of psychostimulant addiction, Alcohol Alcohol. 37 (2002) 478–484.

[22] K. Brebner, R. Phelan, D.C. Roberts, Effect of baclofen on cocaine self-administration in rats reinforced under fixed-ratio 1 and progressive-ratio schedules, Psychopharmacology 148 (2000) 314–321.

[23] P. Di Ciano, B.J. Everitt, The GABA(B) receptor agonist baclofen attenuates cocaine- and heroin-seeking behavior by rats, Neuropsychopharmacology 28 (2003) 510–518.

[24] Z.X. Xi, E.A. Stein, Baclofen inhibits heroin self-administration behavior and mesolimbic dopamine release, J. Pharmacol. Exp. Ther. 290 (3) (1999) 1369–1374.

[25] P. Di Ciano, B.J. Everitt, Contribution of the ventral tegmental area to cocaine-seeking maintained by a drug-paired conditioned stimulus in rats, Eur. J. Neurosci. 19 (2004) 1661–1667.

[26] M. Melis, S. Spiga, M. Diana, The dopamine hypothesis of drug addiction: hypodopaminergic state, in: R.J. Bradley, A.R. Harris, P. Jenner (Eds.), International Review of Neurobiology, 63, Academic Press, San Diego, CA, 2005, pp. 102–131.

[27] C.A. Dackis, M.S. Gold, D.R. Sweeney, The physiology of cocaine craving and "crashing", Arch. Gen. Psychiatry 44 (3) (1987) 298–300.

[28] A. Imperato, A. Mele, M.G. Scrocco, S. Puglisi-Allegra, Chronic cocaine alters limbic extracellular dopamine. Neurochemical basis for addiction, Eur. J. Pharmacol. 212 (1992) 299–300.

[29] N.D. Volkow, J.S. Fowler, G.J. Wang, R.Z. Goldstein, Role of dopamine, the frontal cortex and memory circuits in drug addiction: insight from imaging, Neurobiol. Learn. Mem. 78 (3) (2002) 610–624.

[30] M. Leyton, I. Boileau, C. Benkelfat, M. Diksic, G. Baker, A. Dagher, Amphetamine-induced increases in extracellular dopamine, drug wanting, and novelty seeking: a PET/[11C]raclopride study in healthy men, Neuropsychopharmacology 27 (6) (2002) 1027–1035.

[31] L.M. Oswald, D.F. Wong, Y. Zhou, A. Kumar, J. Brasic, M. Alexander, W. Ye, H. Kuwabara, J. Hilton, G.S. Wand, Impulsivity and chronic stress are associated with amphetamine-induced striatal dopamine release, Neuroimage 36 (1) (2007) 153–166.

[32] M. Laruelle, A. Abi-Dargham, C.H. van Dyck, W. Rosenblatt, Y. Zea-Ponce, S.S. Zoghbi, R.M. Baldwin, D.S. Charney, P.B. Hoffer, H.F. Kung, SPECT imaging of striatal dopamine release after amphetamine challenge, J. Nucl. Med. 36 (1995) 1182–1190.

[33] N.D. Volkow, G.J. Wang, M.W. Fischman, R.W. Foltin, J.S. Fowler, N.N. Abumrad, S. Vitkun, J. Logan, S.J. Gatley, N. Pappas, R. Hitzemann, C.E. Shea, Relationship between subjective effects of cocaine and dopamine transporter occupancy, Nature 386 (1997) 827–830.

[34] N.D. Volkow, G.J. Wang, J.S. Fowler, J. Logan, S.J. Gatley, A. Gifford, R. Hitzeman, Y-S. Ding, N. Pappas, Prediction of reinforcing response to psychostimulants in humans by brain dopamine D2 receptor levels, Am. J. Psychiatry 156 (1999) 1440–1443.

[35] N.D. Volkow, G.J. Wang, J.S. Fowler, J. Logan, S.J. Gatley, C. Wong, R. Hitzeman, N. Pappas, Reinforcing effects of psychostimulants in humans are associated with increases in brain dopamine and occupancy of D2 receptors, J. Pharmacol. Exp. Ther. 291 (1999) 409–415.

[36] W.C. Drevets, C. Gautier, J.C. Price, D.J. Kupfer, P.E. Kinahan, A.A. Grace, J.L. Price, C.A. Mathis, Amphetamine-induced dopamine release in human ventral striatum correlates with euphoria, Biol. Psychiatry 49 (2) (2001) 81–96.

[37] S.P. Barrett, I. Boileau, J. Okker, R.O. Pihl, A. Dagher, The hedonic response to cigarette smoking is proportional to dopamine release in the human striatum as measured by positron emission tomography and [(11)C]raclopride, Synapse 54 (2004) 65–71.

[38] A. Abi-Dargham, L.S. Kegeles, D. Martinez, R.B. Innis, M. Laruelle, Dopamine mediation of positive reinforcing effects of amphetamine in stimulant naive healthy volunteers: results from a large cohort, Eur. Neuropsychopharmacol. 13 (2003) 459–468.

[39] L.M. Oswald, D.F. Wong, M. McCaul, Y. Zhou, H. Kuwabara, L. Choi, J. Brasic, G.S. Wand, Relationships among ventral striatal dopamine release, cortisol secretion, and subjective responses to amphetamine, Neuropsychopharmacology 30 (2005) 821–832.

[40] I. Boileau, J.M. Assaad, R.O. Pihl, C. Benkelfat, M. Leyton, M. Diksic, R.E. Tremblay, A. Dagher, Alcohol promotes dopamine release in the human nucleus accumbens, Synapse 49 (2003) 226–231.

[41] K.C. Berridge, The debate over dopamine's role in reward: the case for incentive salience, Psychopharmacology 191 (3) (2007) 391–431.

[42] C. Holden, "Behavioral" addictions: do they exist? Science 294 (5544) (2001) 980–982.

[43] M.N. Potenza, The neurobiology of pathological gambling, Semin. Clin. Neuropsychiatry 6 (2001) 217–226.

[44] B. Castellani, L. Rugle, A comparison of pathological gamblers to alcoholics and cocaine misusers on impulsivity, sensation seeking, and craving, Int. J. Addict. 30 (3) (1995) 275–289.

[45] I. Wray, M. Phil, M.G. Dickerson, Cessation of high frequency gambling and "withdrawal" symptoms, Br. J. Addict. 76 (1981) 401–405.

[46] H.R. Lesieur, R.J. Rosenthal, Pathological gambling: a review of the literature (prepared for the American Psychiatric Association Task Force of DSM-IV Committee on Disorders of Impulse Control Not Elsewhere Classified), J. Gambl. Stud. 7 (1991) 5–39.

[47] M.N. Potenza, H.C. Leung, H.P. Blumberg, B.S. Peterson, R.K. Fulbright, C.M. Lacadie, An fMRI Stroop task study of ventromedial prefrontal cortical function in pathological gamblers, Am. J. Psychiatry 160 (2003) 1990–1994.

[48] M.N. Potenza, M.A. Steinberg, P. Skudlarski, R.K. Fulbright, C.M. Lacadie, M.K. Wilber, Gambling urges in pathological gambling: a functional magnetic resonance imaging study, Arch. Gen. Psychiatry 60 (2003) 828–836.

[49] D. Crockford, B. Goodyear, J. Edwards, J. Quickfall, N. el-Guebaly, Cue-induced brain activity in pathological gamblers, Biol. Psychiatry 58 (10) (2005) 787–795.

[50] J. Reuter, T. Raedler, M. Rose, I. Hand, J. Glascher, C. Buchel, Patholgical gambling is linked to reduced activation of the mesolimbic reward system, Nat. Neurosci. 8 (2005) 147–148.

[51] D. Hommer, J.M. Bjork, B. Knutson, D. Caggiano, G. Fong, C. Danube, Motivation in children of alcoholics, Alcohol. Clin. Exp. Res. 28 (2004) 22A.

[52] M.N. Potenza, C. Gottschalk, P. Skudlarski, et al., Neuroimaging Studies of Behavioral and Drug Addictions: Gambling Urges in Pathological Gambling and Cocaine Cravings in Cocaine Dependence, American Psychiatric Association, New York, 2004.

[53] H.P. Blumberg, H.C. Leung, P. Skudlarski, et al., A functional magnetic resonance imaging study of bipolar disorder: state- and trait-related dysfunction in ventral prefrontal cortices, Arch. Gen. Psychiatry 60 (2003) 601–609.

[54] R.S. Dougherty, T. Deckersbach, C. Marci, et al., Ventromedial prefrontal cortex and amygdala dysfunction during an anger induction positron emission tomography study in patients with major depressive disorder with anger attacks, Arch. Gen. Psychiatry 61 (2004) 795–804.

[55] E.D. London, M. Ernst, S. Grant, K. Bonson, A. Weinstein, Orbitofrontal cortex and human drug abuse: functional imaging, Cereb. Cortex 10 (2000) 334–342.

[56] A. Bechara, Risky business: emotion, decision-making, and addiction, J. Gambl. Stud. 19 (2003) 23–51.

[57] K. Blum, J.G. Cull, E.R. Braverman, D.E. Comings, Reward deficiency syndrome, Am. Scientist 84 (1996) 132–145.

[58] N. Risch, K. Merikangas, The future of genetic studies of complex human diseases, Science 273 (5281) (1996) 1516–1517.

[59] P.V. Piazza, V. Deroche-Gamonent, F. Rouge-Pont, M. Le Moal, Vertical shifts in self-administration dose-response functions predict a drug-vulnerable phenotype predisposed to addiction, J. Neurosci. 20 (11) (2000) 4226–4232.

[60] H. de Wit, E.H. Uhlenhuth, C.E.F. Johanson, Individual differences in the reinforcing and subjective effects of amphetamine and diazepam, Drug Alcohol Depend. 16 (1986) 341–360.

[61] D.M. Fergusson, L.J. Horwood, M.T. Lynskey, P.A. Madden, Early reactions to cannabis predict later dependence, Arch. Gen. Psychiatry 60 (2003) 1033–1039.

[62] M.A. Nader, J.B. Daunais, T. Moore, S.H. Nader, R.J. Moore, H.R. Smith, D.P. Friedman, L.J. Porrino, Effects of cocaine self-administration on striatal dopamine systems in rhesus monkeys: initial and chronic exposure, Neuropsychopharmacology 27 (2002) 35–46.

[63] J.M. Gilman, V.A. Ramchandani, M.B. Davis, J.M. Bjork, D.W. Hommer, Why we like to drink: a functional magnetic resonance imaging study of the rewarding and anxiolytic effects of alcohol, J. Neurosci. 28 (2008) 4583–4591.

[64] D. Goldman, G. Oroszi, F. Ducci, The genetics of addictions: uncovering the genes, Nat. Rev. Genet. 6 (7) (2005) 521–532.

[65] J. Chen, B.K. Lipska, N. Halim, Q.D. Ma, M. Matsumoto, S. Melhem, B.S. Kolachana, T.M. Hyde, M.M. Herman, J. Apud, M.F. Egan, J.E. Kleinman, D.R. Weinberger, Functional analysis of genetic variation in catechol-O-methyltransferase (COMT): effects on mRNA, protein, and enzyme activity in postmortem human brain, Am. J. Hum. Genet. 75 (2004) 807–821.

[66] B. Giros, M. Jaber, S.R. Jones, R.M. Wightman, M.G. Caron, Hyperlocomotion and indifference to cocaine and amphetamine in mice lacking the dopamine transporter, Nature 379 (1996) 606–612.

[67] D.M. Donovan, L.L. Miner, M.P. Perry, R.S. Revay, L.G. Sharpe, S. Przedborski, V. Kostic, R.M. Philpot, C.L. Kirstein, R.B. Rothman, C.W. Schindler, G.R. Uhl, Cocaine reward and MPTP toxicity: alteration by regional variant dopamine transporter overexpression, Brain Res. Mol. Brain Res. 73 (1999) 37–49.

[68] J.A. Gogos, M. Morgan, V. Luine, M. Santha, S. Ogawa, D. Pfaff, M. Karayiorgou, Catechol-O-methyltransferase-deficient mice exhibit sexually dimorphic changes in catecholamine levels and behavior, Proc. Natl. Acad. Sci. USA 95 (1998) 9991–9996.

[69] H.M. Lachman, D.F. Papolos, T. Saito, Y.M. Yu, C.L. Szumlanski, R.M. Weinshilboum, Human catechol-O-methyltransferase pharmacogenetics: description of a functional polymorphism and its potential application to neuropsychiatric disorders, Pharmacogenetics 6 (1996) 243–250.

[70] L. Yavich, M.M. Forsberg, M. Karayiorgou, J. Gogos, P.T. Männistö, Site-specific role of catechol-O-methyltransferase in dopamine overflow within prefrontal cortex and dorsal striatum, J. Neurosci. 27 (2007) 10196–10209.

[71] D.J. Vandenbergh, L.A. Rodriguez, I.T. Miller, G.R. Uhl, H.M. Lachman, High-activity catechol-O-methyltransferase allele is more prevalent in polysubstance abusers, Am. J. Med. Genet. 74 (1997) 439–442.

[72] J. Benjamin, Y. Osher, M. Kotler, I. Gritsenko, L. Nemanov, R.H. Belmaker, R.P. Ebstein, Association between tridimensional personality questionnaire (TPQ) traits and three functional polymorphisms: dopamine receptor D4 (DRD4), serotonin transporter promoter region (5-HTTLPR), and catechol-O-methyltransferase (COMT), Mol. Psychiatry 5 (2000) 96–100.

[73] R. Horowitz, A. Shufman, S. Aharoni, S. Aharoni, I. Kremer, H. Cohen, R.P. Ebstein, Confirmation of an excess of the high enzyme activity COMT val allele in heroin addicts in a family-based haplotype relative risk study, Am. J. Med. Genet. 96 (2000) 599–603.

[74] I. Puls, J. Mohr, J. Wrase, J. Priller, J. Behr, W. Kitzrow, N. Makris, H.C. Breiter, K. Obermayer, A. Heinz, Synergistic effects of the dopaminergic and glutamatergic system

on hippocampal volume in alcohol-dependent patients, Biol. Psychol. 79 (2008) 126–136 doi:10.1016/j.biopsycho.2008.03.001.

[75] A. Kang, M.A. Palmatier, K.K. Kidd, Global variation of a 40-bp VNTR in the 3′-untranslated region of the dopamine transporter gene (SLC6A3), Biol. Psychiatry 46 (1999) 151–160.

[76] A. Heinz, D. Goldman, D.W. Jones, R. Palmour, D. Hommer, J.G. Gorey, K.S. Lee, M. Linnoila, D.R. Weinberger, Genotype influences in vivo dopamine transporter availability in human striatum, Neuropsychopharmacology 22 (2000) 133–139.

[77] L.K. Jacobsen, J.K. Staley, S.S. Zoghbi, J.P. Seibyl, T.R. Kosten, R.B. Innis, J. Gelernter, Prediction of dopamine transporter binding availability by genotype: a preliminary report, Am. J. Psychiatry 157 (2000) 1700–1703.

[78] S. Fuke, S. Suo, N. Takahashi, H. Koike, N. Sasagawa, S. Ishiura, The VNTR polymorphism of the human dopamine transporter (DAT1) gene affects gene expression, Pharmacogenomics J. 1 (2001) 152–156.

[79] J. Mill, P. Asherson, C. Browes, U. D'Souza, I. Craig, Expression of the dopamine transporter gene is regulated by the 3′ UTR VNTR: evidence from brain and lymphocytes using quantitative RT-PCR, Am. J. Med. Genet. 114 (2002) 975–979.

[80] S.H. VanNess, M.J. Owens, C.D. Kilts, The variable number of tandem repeats element in DAT I regulates in vitro dopamine transporter density, BMC Genet. 6 (2005) 55.

[81] C.H. Van Dyck, R.T. Malison, L.K. Jacobsen, J.P. Seibyl, J.K. Staley, M. Laruelle, R.M. Baldwin, R.B. Innis, J. Gelernter, Increased dopamine transporter availability associated with the 9-repeat allele of SLC6A3 gene, J. Nucl. Med. 46 (2005) 745–751.

[82] D. Martínez, J. Gelernter, A. Abi-Dargham, C.H. Van Dyck, L. Kegeles, R.B. Innis, M. Laruelle, The variable number of tandem repeats polymorphism of the dopamine transporter gene is not associated with significant change in dopamine transporter phenotype in humans, Neuropsychopharmacology 24 (2001) 553–560.

[83] J. Gelernter, H.R. Kranzler, S. Satel, P.A. Rao, Genetic association between dopamine transporter alleles and cocaine-induced paranoia, Neuropsychopharmacology 11 (1994) 195–200.

[84] D.C. Lott, S.J. Kim, E.H. Cook Jr., H. de Wit, Dopamine transporter gene associated with diminished subjective response to amphetamine, Neuropsychopharmacology 30 (2005) 602–609.

[85] E.H. Cook Jr., M.A. Stein, M. Krasowski, et al., Association of attention-deficit disorder and the dopamine transporter gene, Am. J. Med. Genet. 56 (1995) 993–998.

[86] M.A. Stein, I.D. Waldman, C.S. Sarampote, K.E. Seymour, A.S. Robb, C. Conlon, S.J. Kim, E.H. Cook, Dopamine transporter genotype and methylphenidate dose response in children with ADHD, Neuropsychopharmacology 30 (2005) 1374–1382.

[87] L.G. Schmidt, T. Sander, Genetics of alcohol withdrawal, Eur. Psychiatry 15 (2000) 135–139.

[88] C. Lerman, N.E. Caporaso, J. Audrain, et al., Evidence suggesting the role of specific genetic factors in cigarette smoking, Health Psychol. 18 (1999) 14–20.

[89] S.Z. Sabol, M.L. Nelson, C. Fisher, et al., A genetic association for cigarette smoking behavior, Health Psychol. 18 (1999) 7–13.

[90] D.S. Timberlake, B.C. Haberstick, J.M. Lessem, A. Smolen, M. Ehringer, J.K. Hewitt, C. Hopfer, An association between the DAT1 polymorphism and smoking behavior in young adults from the National Longitudinal Study of Adolescent Health, Health Psychol. 25 (2) (2006) 190–197.

[91] A.F. Jorm, A.S. Henderson, P.A. Jacomb, et al., Association of smoking and personality with a polymorphism of the dopamine transporter gene: results from a community survey, Am. J. Med. Genet. 96 (2000) 331–334.

[92] J. Yacubian, T. Sommer, K. Schroeder, J. Gläscher, R. Kalisch, B. Leuenberger, D.F. Braus, C. Büchel, Gene-gene interaction associated with neural reward sensitivity, Proc. Natl. Acad. Sci. USA 104 (2007) 8125–8130.

[93] J. Yacubian, J. Gläscher, K. Schroeder, T. Sommer, D.F. Braus, C. Büchel, Dissociable systems for gain- and loss-related value predictions and errors of prediction in the human brain, J. Neurosci. 26 (2006) 9530–9537.

[94] J.C. Dreher, P. Kohn, B. Kolachana, D.R. Weinberger, K.F. Berman, Variation in dopamine genes influences responsivity of the human reward system, Proc. Natl. Acad. Sci. USA, 106 (2009) 617–622.

[95] T.W. Robbins, B.J. Everitt, Drug addiction: bad habits add up, Nature 398 (1999) 567–570.

[96] A. Scheres, M.P. Milham, B. Knutson, F.X. Castellanos, Ventral striatal hyporesponsiveness during reward anticipation in attention-deficit/hyperactivity disorder, Biol. Psychiatry 61 (5) (2007) 720–724.

[97] D.E. Comings, K. Blum, Reward deficiency syndrome: genetic aspects of behavioral disorders, Prog. Brain Res. 126 (2000) 325–341.

[98] G.F. Koob, M. Le Moal, Drug addiction, dysregulation of reward, and allostasis, Neuropsychopharmacology 24 (2001) 97–129.

[99] T.E. Wilens, Impact of ADHD and its treatment on substance abuse in adults, J. Clin. Psychiatry 65 (2004) 38–45.

[100] A.L. Brody, M.A. Mandelkern, R.E. Olmstead, D. Scheibal, E. Hahn, S. Shiraga, E. Zamora-Paja, J. Farahi, S. Saxena, E.D. London, J.T. McCracken, Gene variants of brain dopamine pathways and smoking-induced dopamine release in the ventral caudate/nucleus accumbens, Arch. Gen. Psychiatry 63 (2006) 808–816.

[101] I.C. Weaver, N. Cervoni, F.A. Champagne, et al., Epigenetic programming by maternal behavior, Nat. Neurosci. 7 (2004) 847–854.

17 Catechol-*O*-methyltransferase (COMT) genotype effects on brain activation elicited by affective stimuli and cognitive tasks

Andreas Heinz and Imke Puls

Department of Psychiatry and Psychotherapy, Charité Campus Mitte, Charité – University Medical Center, Schumannstr. 20–21, 10117 Berlin, Germany

Abstract

The catechol-O-methyltransferase (COMT) gene has been extensively studied with respect to its effects on prefrontal and limbic activation. COMT is the most relevant dopamine degrading enzyme in the prefrontal cortex, strongly influencing the amount of dopamine available. Several studies evaluated the effects on cerebral activation of the common val158met polymorphism. The met158 allele, which is presumably linked to higher synaptic dopamine levels as a result of decreased enzyme activity, was associated with better working memory performance but also increased brain activation on presentation of aversive stimuli. It was associated with increased ventro-striatal activation during anticipation of loss. Although a major effect of this genetic variant on cognitive and affective processing and hence an increased susceptibility to various psychiatric symptoms is plausible, many well designed studies produced inconsistent results. Subsequent studies therefore focused on haplotype analysis and epistatic gene–gene interactions. In this chapter, we will give an overview of studies of imaging genetics in COMT.

Key points

1. Imaging genetics provide a useful tool for understanding genotype–phenotype interactions and their potential role in psychiatric disorders.
2. Genetic variants of COMT, particularly the common val158met polymorphism, have a strong impact on brain activation that is much more prominent than their influence on psychiatric diseases.
3. Epistatic gene interactions have been found between dopaminergic and glutamatergic genes, but also between different dopaminergic genes.

17.1 Introduction

Heritability, that is, the variance in a trait that is due to genetic effects [1], is relatively high for several psychiatric disorders; however, it is often difficult to test for gene effects due to the weak and sometimes inconsistent association between genetic variance and the observed behavior. The catechol-O-methyltransferase gene (COMT) on chromosome 22q11 has been extensively studied. COMT is one of the principal enzymes that metabolizes the neurotransmitters dopamine, norepinephrine, and epinephrine, and the COMT gene contains an evolutionarily recent G to A missense mutation, that results into a substitution of methionine (met) for valine (val) at codon 158 (val[158]met), cataloged as single nucleotide polymorphism (SNP) rs4680 [2]. The enzyme containing met[158] is unstable at 37°C and only reaches one-third to one-fourth of the activity of the enzyme containing the val[158] allele [3,4]. The alleles are co-dominant, and therefore heterozygous individuals have enzyme activity that is midway between homozygote individuals [5]. Studies in COMT-knockout mice revealed increased DA levels in the prefrontal cortex (PFC), where DATs are expressed in low numbers and not within synapses and hence dopamine degradation via COMT regulates extracellular dopamine concentrations, whereas no COMT effect was found on dopamine levels in the DAT-rich striatum [6–9].COMT effects on norepinephrine and dopamine may modulate processing of affective stimuli, because norepinephrine is of utmost importance for the function of limbic structures such as the amygdala, hippocampus, and the thalamus [10]. The majority of noradrenergic neurons is located in the locus coeruleus (pons) and project to multiple cortical and subcortical areas such as the hippocampus, amygdala, and thalamus, which are crucial for processing of emotions and memory [11].

In spite of this rather strong effect of COMT genotype on prefrontal dopamine metabolism, effects on dopamine-related clinical behavior were rather weak: carriers of the met[158] allele showed a 4% reduction in perseverative errors in an executive function task that involves PFC function [12], a finding that was replicated in several [13–15] but not all studies [16]. Behavioral genetics also revealed an effect of the COMT val[158]met genotype on negative mood states [17]. Likewise, not more than 4% of the variance in trait anxiety were explained by a functional SNP in the regulatory region of the serotonin transporter gene [18]. Such weak associations between gene effects and overt behavior may easily escape replication [19]. Therefore, it has been suggested that so-called intermediate phenotypes such as *in vivo* receptor or transporter availability measured with positron emission tomography (PET) or stimulus-evoked brain activation measured with functional magnetic resonance imaging (fMRI) may be more directly affected by genetic variation and therefore can be used to assess genotype effects and gene–gene interactions.

17.2   COMT effects on brain activation elicited by working memory and executive control

A series of brain imaging studies focused on working memory, the ability to keep information "online," to manipulate it and to shift hypotheses, and frequently used the Wisconsin Card Sorting Test (WCST). In this task, healthy volunteers activate a network involving the prefrontal, superior parietal, and medial temporal cortices [20]. It has been suggested that prefrontal dopamine concentrations affect task performance and the related neuronal activation, since amphetamine application has been shown to focus task-related regional cerebral blood flow, while reduced dopamine availability in Parkinson's disease was associated with increased blood flow, suggesting an ineffective decrease in the signal-to-noise ratio [21]. Also, in schizophrenia prefrontal dysfunction may at least partially be caused by a deficit in tonic dopamine release, and release of dopamine and other monoamines following amphetamine application increased both working memory performance and signal-to-noise ratio in the PFC of schizophrenic patients [22,23].

COMT genotype has been reported to modulate PFC function during a working memory task in healthy control subjects as well as in schizophrenic patients and their relatives [12]. Patients suffering from schizophrenia performed worse than healthy volunteers; however, a similar relation between COMT genotype and task performance was found in schizophrenic patients, albeit on an altogether lower level of performance. Patients who carried the val[158] allele that rapidly metabolizes dopamine displayed worse performance on the WCST compared with subjects who carry the met[158] that slowly metabolizes extracellular dopamine [12]. Relatives of schizophrenic patients showed intermediate performance and may have additional protective factors that prevent the manifestation of psychotic symptoms. Nevertheless, the effects of COMT on WCST performance were analogous, that is, subjects carrying the genotype with higher dopamine metabolism and presumably lower dopamine concentrations showed increased functional activation of the dorsolateral PFC and anterior cingulate, which was attributed to greater inefficiency of brain activation [12]. Further studies revealed that COMT genotype modulates functional activation of the dorsolateral PFC during information encoding rather than retrieval [24]. A similar effect of the COMT val[158]met polymorphism on task performance and functional activation of the cingulate cortex was observed when attentional control was tested in healthy volunteers: the number of val[158] alleles was associated with poorer task performance and increased brain activation, interpreted as a sign of inefficient information processing [25].

It has been suggested that dopamine concentrations in the PFC affect WM performance following an "inverted U" shaped function, that is, WM performance is best at intermediate dopamine levels and decreases with both too high and too low dopamine availability. In striking accordance with this hypothesis, Mattay et al. [26] observed that subjects carrying the COMT val[158] allele with higher dopamine metabolism, profited from amphetamine application, while this was not the case in subjects carrying the met[158] allele that was associated with (already) high prefrontal dopamine concentrations [26].

Subsequent studies also focused on haplotype analysis of the COMT gene, including several more SNPs in addition to the val[158]met variant. Nackley et al. [27] showed that COMT haplotypes modulate protein expression by altering mRNA secondary structure which implicates more profound information of haplotype analysis based on functional relevance compared to single genetic alterations. Meyer-Lindenberg et al. [28] suggested that functional brain activation elicited by a working memory task is best explained when further COMT polymorphisms are assessed in addition to the well-studied val[158]met SNP: SNP rs2097603 in the P2 promoter region and a SNP in the 3' region (rs165599) interacted with COMT val[158]met effects on prefrontal working memory responses. Homozygous met[158] carriers who are sited near the peak of an inverted U-shaped curve displaying the effect of extracellular dopamine on prefrontal activity are shifted either towards lower or dysfunctionally higher extracellular dopamine levels by further genetic variants modulating COMT enzyme activity [28]. However, the observation that a combination of different genetic markers increases explained variance of functional brain activation does not necessarily mean that modeling genotype effects with more markers is automatically preferable, since models of higher complexity always have a higher capacity for fitting the data well. A researcher is actually interested in the generalization ability of a model, not simply the model fit. To every given dataset one could find an infinite number of models that perfectly fit the data, but do not generalize well. Therefore, a model of exactly the right complexity should be chosen, and future imaging studies will have to assess whether haplotype analysis is actually preferable when explaining, for example, COMT genotype effects on functional brain activation elicited by cognitive or affective paradigms.

17.3   COMT effects and negative mood states

If the COMT val[158] allele has a slight disadvantage for executive function, why is this allele highly prevalent (>50%) in the general population. It has been suggested that the val[158] allele may have compensating advantages, and one of these could be an increased emotional resilience against negative mood states [17,29,30]. The met[158] allele was associated with a higher risk for major depression and bipolar affective disorder [31–34], alcoholism as well as increased alcohol intake in social drinkers and the development of alcohol dependence [35–37]. No relationship was observed between COMT genotype and anxiety disorders taken as a whole [31,32], however, homozygous female met[158] carriers displayed higher levels of dimensionally measured anxiety [17]. Zubieta and coworkers showed that individuals who are homozygous for the COMT met[158] allele displayed higher sensory and affective ratings of pain and higher ratings for negative affect in response to sustained pain [30]. Moreover, the met[158] allele was associated with obsessive-compulsive disorder in males, a disease that belongs to the group of anxiety-related disorders [38]. Some studies found a gene dose effect, so that the association with obsessive-compulsive disorder and alcohol consumption was strongest with the homozygous met[158] genotype [31,37]. A balance of cognitive and behavioral advantages and disadvantages may therefore maintain both functional COMT alleles at high frequencies.

In accordance with the hypothesis that COMT met[158] carriers display an increased risk for negative mood states, healthy volunteers carrying this genotype also displayed increased activation of their amygdala and lateral PFC when they viewed aversive versus neutral stimuli [39] (Fig. 17.1). There was a linear correlation between the number of met[158] alleles and the BOLD fMRI response elicited by aversive stimuli in limbic and prefrontal brain areas; the highest correlations were found in the ventrolateral prefrontal cortex (VLPFC, BA 47), anterior cingulate (BA 33), amygdala, hippocampus, and thalamus. The COMT genotype did not significantly interact with central processing of positive versus neutral stimuli. The VLPFC was also activated during induction of sadness [40] and recall of sad autobiographical memories [41, 42]. Increased activation was also found in patients suffering from major depression [43] and obsessive-compulsive disorder [44–46]. Moreover, a strong impact of genotype on processing of aversive visual stimuli was found in the cognitive subdivision of the anterior cingulate [39], a region that has previously been linked with the regulation of affective states [47]. COMT genotype also interacted with the activation of the left dorsal hippocampus and the thalamus elicited by aversive versus neutral stimuli. The thalamus is involved in controlling attentional processes and the level of activation is modified by norepinephrine [48]. COMT genotype has also been suggested to modulate thalamic endorphin release and the associated pain perception [30]. The hippocampus has been implicated in the inhibition of stress responses via inhibitory connections with many of the subcortical structures involved; it is activated during acute stress [49] and may be crucial for regulation of arousal and affective states [50]. Confrontation with affective cues may thus induce excessive activation of brain areas associated with emotional reactivity and cognitive behavior control and contribute to the lowered resilience against anxiety and further negative mood states in COMT met[158] allele carriers.

The positive correlation between brain activation elicited by aversive stimuli and the number of met[158] alleles suggests that the amplified activation of limbic and prefrontal

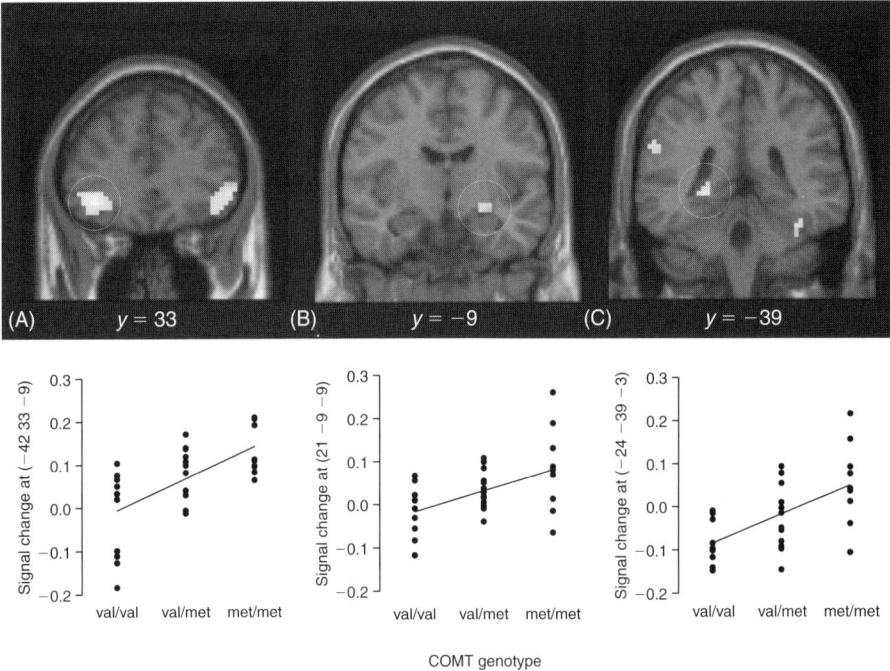

Figure 17.1 Correlation between COMT met[158] allele dosage (0 = val/val, 1 = val/met or 2 = met/met) and activation by aversive stimuli of the (A) ventrolateral PFC, (B) right amygdala, and (C) left dorsal hippocampus. In the upper row, statistical maps are shown ($P < 0.05$ *corrected* for volume of mask, cluster size ≥ 10 voxels). In the lower row, neural responses of individuals are shown as related to COMT genotype, showing an allele-dose dependent effect with heterozygotes having intermediate effects. Individual BOLD responses were extracted from the voxel with the highest T value inside the cluster circled on the left. *Source*: Modified from Smolka et al. (2005) [39]. See Plate 20 of Color Plate section.

areas by emotional stimuli is due to increased levels of dopamine. Studies in COMT-deficient mice revealed increased dopamine levels in the PFC [51]. Therefore, the observed effects in the PFC could be due to increased dopamine availability in COMT met[158] allele carriers, which may represent one possible contribution to the decreased emotional resilience of this genotype. First studies on gene–gene interactions suggested that COMT val[158]met effects on functional brain activation elicited by aversive stimuli interact with the genetic constitution of a transcriptional control region upstream of the serotonin transporter gene, and that the genetic effects on functional limbic activation are additive [52]. This finding emphasizes the role of serotonergic neurotransmission in affective processing and suggests that genetic imaging can be used to assess gene–gene interactions.

Additive genotype effects were also observed on prefrontal activation during working memory performance. In the frontal cortex, extracellular dopamine concentrations are regulated by both enzyme degradation via COMT and reuptake via DATs. A 3′ variable number tandem repeat (VNTR) polymorphism in the DAT gene had previously been observed to modulate *in vivo* transporter availability, thus presumably affecting dopamine reuptake capacity and hence extracellular dopamine concentrations [53]. Therefore, both COMT and

DAT genotypes may affect dopamine-dependent prefrontal function. Indeed, additive effects of COMT and DAT genotype were observed on neuronal activity elicited by a working memory task as measured with fMRI [54, 55].

17.4   Epistatic gene–gene interactions modulating dopamine and glutamate interactions

Genetic variation of the mGluR3 gene has been associated with individual differences in glutamatergic signaling, and both COMT val[158]met and mGluR3 genotype have been suggested to influence prefrontal signal-to-noise ratios. When gene–gene interactions were assessed in a working memory paradigm, Tan et al. [24] observed an epistatic interaction between the two genes, with COMT met[158] homozygotes mediating against the effect of the mGluR3 genotype putatively associated with suboptimal glutamatergic signaling. Epistatic gene effects have also been found when a novel method for detecting associations between a set of genetic markers and phenotypical measurements based on machine learning techniques was applied on volumetric data in alcohol-dependent patients and healthy controls: hippocampal volume was found to be associated with epistatic effects of the COMT and mGluR3 genes in alcohol-dependent patients but not in controls [56]. These data are in line with prior studies supporting a role for dopamine–glutamate interaction in modulation of alcohol dependence [57].

If COMT genotype interacts with hippocampal volume, can it also influence memory performance? A study by Bertolino et al. [54] suggested that the COMT val[158] allele was associated with relatively poorer performance at memory retrieval, and also with reduced recruitment of neuronal resources in the hippocampus and increased activation of the VLPFC during both memory encoding and retrieval. Behavioral accuracy during retrieval was predicted by functional coupling between the hippocampus and VLPFC [54,55]. Again, an epistatic gene–gene interaction was observed when the effects of both the COMT val[158]met and the DAT 3′ VNTR polymorphisms were assessed on hippocampal function during memory tasks: presence of the DAT 9-repeat allele with reduced *in vivo* availability of DATs [53] modulated activity in the hippocampus in the opposite direction of homozygous DAT 10-repeat alleles depending on COMT val[158]met genotype [58]. This finding emphasizes the need to assess interactions between genes that directly or indirectly modulate dopamine availability.

17.5   COMT effects in the brain reward system

Neuronal processing of reward anticipation and reception depends on dopaminergic neurotransmission in ventral striatum (for review see also Chapter 16). While the common COMT val[158]met polymorphism has been shown to substantially influence extracellular dopamine concentrations in the cortex where DATs are relatively rare, the direct effect of COMT on dopamine in the DAT-rich striatum may be limited. Nevertheless, COMT val[158]met and the previously mentioned VNTR polymorphism of the DAT have been shown to interact with reward-associated activation of the ventral striatum [59]: comparable to studies on limbic brain activation elicited by affective stimuli, met[158] homozygous individuals with presumably greater dopamine availability displayed greater brain activation in the ventral striatum and PFC. An epistatic gene–gene interaction between COMT and DAT was suggested by the study of Yacubian et al. [59]: subjects with a COMT and DAT

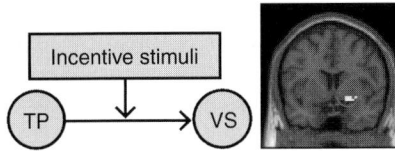

Figure 17.2 Modulation of connectivity between the anterior temporal cortex and the ventral striatum by reward related cues. During the anticipation of both monetary gain (and loss) the right temporal pole (TP) showed an enhanced connectivity to the ventral striatum (VS). *Source*: Modified from Schmack et al. (2008) [61].

genotype combination that suggested either very high or very low extracellular dopamine showed a blunted ventral striatal response to reward. Dreher et al. [60] also displayed an effect of COMT and DAT genes and their interaction during reward anticipation and delivery: the highest activation was observed in individuals with presumably large amounts of synaptic dopamine available due to their genotypes.

However, why should COMT genotype affect functional activation of the striatum, which is rich in DATs? Indeed, if extracellular dopamine is quickly taken up by DAT, there may be little dopamine left for COMT degradation. A recent functional imaging study suggested that COMT val[158]met genotype interacts with brain activation elicited by the anticipation of loss but not gain in both the ventral striatum and anterior temporal cortex. The anterior temporal cortex has been linked to the coupling of sensory information with emotional contents and showed enhanced connectivity to the ventral striatum during the processing of incentive stimuli [61] (Fig. 17.2). These results suggest that the effect of COMT genotype on striatal reactivity during loss anticipation is driven by a top-down modulation from the cortex and support the evidence that COMT genotype effects are stronger for negative compared with positive affective states.

Altogether, these studies suggest that COMT val[158]met genotype interacts with central processing of aversive stimuli in prefrontal and temporal cortex, and that top-down modulation of limbic brain areas may increase the vulnerability of met[158] carriers for disorders characterized by negative affect, thus potentially balancing improved working memory performance in this genotype. Several studies suggest that gene–gene interactions have to be considered to fully appreciate COMT genotype effects on neuronal and behavioral correlates; however, the advantage of such models still requires to be demonstrated in direct model comparison. Nevertheless, imaging genetics provides a useful tool to further understand genotype–phenotype interactions and their potential role in cognitive and mood disorders in the human brain.

Acknowledgement

This study was supported by the Deutsche Forschungsgemeinschaft (He 2597/4-2).

References

[1] T.K. Rice, I.B. Borecki, Familial resemblance and heritability, Adv. Genet. 42 (2001) 35–44.
[2] H.M. Lachman, D.F. Papolos, T. Saito, Y.M. Yu, C.L. Szumlanski, R.M. Weinshilboum, Human catechol-O-methyltransferase pharmacogenetics: description of a functional polymorphism and its potential application to neuropsychiatric disorders, Pharmacogenetics 6 (1996) 243–250.

[3] T. Lotta, J. Vidgren, C. Tilgmann, et al., Kinetics of human soluble and membrane-bound cat-
     echol O-methyltransferase: a revised mechanism and description of the thermolabile variant of
     the enzyme, Biochemistry 34 (1995) 4202–4210.

[4] R.S. Spielman, R.M. Weinshilboum, Genetics of red cell COMT activity: analysis of thermal
     stability and family data, Am. J. Med. Genet. 10 (1981) 279–290.

[5] R.M. Weinshilboum, D.M. Otterness, C.L. Szumlanski, Methylation pharmacogenetics: cat-
     echol O-methyltransferase, thiopurine methyltransferase, and histamine N-methyltransferase,
     Annu. Rev. Pharmacol. Toxicol. 39 (1999) 19–52.

[6] J.A. Gogos, M. Morgan, V. Luine, et al., Catechol-O-methyltransferase-deficient mice exhibit
     sexually dimorphic changes in catecholamine levels and behavior, Proc. Natl. Acad. Sci. USA
     95 (1998) 9991–9996.

[7] D.A. Lewis, D.S. Melchitzky, S.R. Sesack, R.E. Whitehead, S. Auh, A. Sampson, Dopamine
     transporter immunoreactivity in monkey cerebral cortex: regional, laminar, and ultrastructural
     localization, J. Comp. Neurol. 432 (2001) 119–136.

[8] M.S. Mazei, C.P. Pluto, B. Kirkbride, E.A. Pehek, Effects of catecholamine uptake blockers in
     the caudate-putamen and subregions of the medial prefrontal cortex of the rat, Brain Res. 936
     (2002) 58–67.

[9] J.A. Moron, A. Brockington, R.A. Wise, B.A. Rocha, B.T. Hope, Dopamine uptake through
     the norepinephrine transporter in brain regions with low levels of the dopamine transporter:
     evidence from knock-out mouse lines, J. Neurosci. 22 (2002) 389–395.

[10] J.E. Lisman, A.A. Grace, The hippocampal-VTA loop: controlling the entry of information into
     long-term memory, Neuron 46 (2005) 703–713.

[11] K.L. Phan, T. Wager, S.F. Taylor, I. Liberzon, Functional neuroanatomy of emotion: a meta-
     analysis of emotion activation studies in PET and fMRI, Neuroimage 16 (2002) 331–348.

[12] M.F. Egan, T.E. Goldberg, B.S. Kolachana, et al., Effect of COMT Val108/158 Met genotype
     on frontal lobe function and risk for schizophrenia, Proc. Natl. Acad. Sci. USA 98 (2001)
     6917–6922.

[13] A.K. Malhotra, L.J. Kestler, C. Mazzanti, J.A. Bates, T. Goldberg, D. Goldman, A functional
     polymorphism in the COMT gene and performance on a test of prefrontal cognition, Am. J.
     Psychiatry 159 (2002) 652–654.

[14] R. Joober, J. Gauthier, S. Lal, et al., Catechol-O-methyltransferase Val-108/158-Met gene vari-
     ants associated with performance on the Wisconsin Card Sorting Test, Arch. Gen. Psychiatry
     59 (2002) 662–663.

[15] T.E. Goldberg, M.F. Egan, T. Gscheidle, et al., Executive subprocesses in working memory:
     relationship to catechol-O-methyltransferase Val158Met genotype and schizophrenia, Arch.
     Gen. Psychiatry 60 (2003) 889–896.

[16] B.C. Ho, T.H. Wassink, D.S. O'Leary, V.C. Sheffield, N.C. Andreasen, Catechol-O-methyl
     transferase Val158Met gene polymorphism in schizophrenia: working memory, frontal lobe
     MRI morphology and frontal cerebral blood flow, Mol. Psychiatry 10 (2005) 287–298.

[17] M.A. Enoch, M.A. Schuckit, B.A. Johnson, D. Goldman, Genetics of alcoholism using interme-
     diate phenotypes, Alcohol. Clin. Exp. Res. 27 (2003) 169–176.

[18] K.P. Lesch, D. Bengel, A. Heils, et al., Association of anxiety-related traits with a
     polymorphism in the serotonin transporter gene regulatory region, Science 274 (1996)
     1527–1531.

[19] J. Gelernter, H. Kranzler, J.F. Cubells, Serotonin transporter protein (SLC6A4) allele and hap-
     lotype frequencies and linkage disequilibria in African- and European-American and Japanese
     populations and in alcohol-dependent subjects, Hum. Genet. 101 (1997) 243–246.

[20] A. Heinz, B. Romero, D.R. Weinberger, Functional mapping with single photon emission computed
     tomography (and positron emission tomography), in: S.M. Lawrie, E.C. Johnstone, D.R. Weinberger

(Eds.), Brain Imaging in Schizophrenia. Part II – Functional Neuroimaging/Chapter 8, Oxford University Publications, Oxford, 2004, pp. 167–212.

[21] V.S. Mattay, A. Tessitore, J.H. Callicott, et al., Dopaminergic modulation of cortical function in patients with Parkinson's disease, Ann. Neurol. 51 (2002) 156–164.

[22] D.G. Daniel, D.R. Weinberger, D.W. Jones, et al., The effect of amphetamine on regional cerebral blood flow during cognitive activation in schizophrenia, J. Neurosci. 11 (1991) 1907–1917.

[23] V.S. Mattay, K.F. Berman, J.L. Ostrem, et al., Dextroamphetamine enhances "neural network-specific" physiological signals: a positron-emission tomography rCBF study, J. Neurosci. 16 (1996) 4816–4822.

[24] H.Y. Tan, Q. Chen, S. Sust, J.W. Buckholtz, J.D. Meyers, M.F. Egan, V.S. Mattay, A. Meyer-Lindenberg, D.R. Weinberger, J.H. Callicott, Epistasis between catechol-O-methyltransferase and type II metabotropic glutamate receptor 3 genes on working memory brain function, Proc. Natl. Acad. Sci. USA 104 (2007) 12536–12541.

[25] G. Blasi, V.S. Mattay, A. Bertolino, et al., Effect of catechol-O-methyltransferase val158met genotype on attentional control, J. Neurosci. 25 (2005) 5038–5045.

[26] V.S. Mattay, T.E. Goldberg, F. Fera, et al., Catechol O-methyltransferase val158-met genotype and individual variation in the brain response to amphetamine, Proc. Natl. Acad. Sci. USA 100 (2003) 6186–6191.

[27] A.G. Nackley, S.A. Shabalina, I.E. Tchivileva, K. Satterfield, O. Korchynskyi, S.S. Makarov, W. Maixner, L. Diatchenko, Human catechol-O-methyltransferase haplotypes modulate protein expression by altering mRNA secondary structure, Science 314 (2006) 1930–1933.

[28] A. Meyer-Lindenberg, T. Nichols, J.H. Callicott, J. Ding, B. Kolachana, J. Buckholtz, V.S. Mattay, M. Egan, D.R. Weinberger, Impact of complex genetic variation in COMT on human brain function, Mol. Psychiatry 11 (2006) 867–877.

[29] M.A. Enoch, K. Xu, E. Ferro, C.R. Harris, D. Goldman, Genetic origins of anxiety in women: a role for a functional catechol-O-methyltransferase polymorphism, Psychiatr. Genet. 13 (2003) 33–41.

[30] J.K. Zubieta, M.M. Heitzeg, Y.R. Smith, et al., COMT val158met genotype affects mu-opioid neurotransmitter responses to a pain stressor, Science 299 (2003) 1240–1243.

[31] K. Ohara, M. Nagai, Y. Suzuki, M. Ochiai, K. Ohara, No association between anxiety disorders and catechol-O-methyltransferase polymorphism, Psychiatry Res. 80 (1998) 145–148.

[32] K. Ohara, M. Nagai, Y. Suzuki, K. Ohara, Low activity allele of catechol-O-methyltransferase gene and Japanese unipolar depression, Neuroreport 9 (1998) 1305–1308.

[33] L.A. Mynett-Johnson, V.E. Murphy, E. Claffey, D.C. Shields, P. McKeon, Preliminary evidence of an association between bipolar disorder in females and the catechol-O-methyltransferase gene, Psychiatr. Genet. 8 (1998) 221–225.

[34] D.F. Papolos, S. Veit, G.L. Faedda, T. Saito, H.M. Lachman, Ultra-ultra rapid cycling bipolar disorder is associated with the low activity catecholamine-O-methyltransferase allele, Mol. Psychiatry 3 (1998) 346–349.

[35] J. Tiihonen, T. Hallikainen, H. Lachman, et al., Association between the functional variant of the catechol-O-methyltransferase (COMT) gene and type 1 alcoholism, Mol. Psychiatry 4 (1999) 286–289.

[36] T. Wang, P. Franke, H. Neidt, et al., Association study of the low-activity allele of catechol-O-methyltransferase and alcoholism using a family-based approach, Mol. Psychiatry 6 (2001) 109–111.

[37] J. Kauhanen, T. Hallikainen, T.P. Tuomainen, et al., Association between the functional polymorphism of catechol-O-methyltransferase gene and alcohol consumption among social drinkers, Alcohol. Clin. Exp. Res. 24 (2000) 135–139.

[38] M. Karayiorgou, C. Sobin, M.L. Blundell, et al., Family-based association studies support a sexually dimorphic effect of COMT and MAOA on genetic susceptibility to obsessive-compulsive disorder, Biol. Psychiatry 45 (1999) 1178–1189.

[39] M.N. Smolka, G. Schumann, J. Wrase, et al., Catechol O-methyltransferase *val158-met* genotype affects processing of emotional stimuli in the amygdala and prefrontal cortex, J. Neurosci. 25 (2005) 836–842.

[40] J. Levesque, F. Eugene, Y. Joanette, et al., Neural circuitry underlying voluntary suppression of sadness, Biol. Psychiatry 53 (2003) 502–510.

[41] H.J. Markowitsch, M.M. Vandekerckhovel, H. Lanfermann, M.O. Russ, Engagement of lateral and medial prefrontal areas in the ecphory of sad and happy autobiographical memories, Cortex 39 (2003) 643–665.

[42] M. Pelletier, A. Bouthillier, J. Levesque, et al., Separate neural circuits for primary emotions? Brain activity during self-induced sadness and happiness in professional actors, Neuroreport 14 (2003) 1111–1116.

[43] W.C. Drevets, Neuroimaging studies of mood disorders, Biol. Psychiatry 48 (2000) 813–829.

[44] C.M. Adler, P. McDonough-Ryan, K.W. Sax, S.K. Holland, S. Arndt, S.M. Strakowski, fMRI of neuronal activation with symptom provocation in unmedicated patients with obsessive compulsive disorder, J. Psychiatr. Res. 34 (2000) 317–324.

[45] D. Mataix-Cols, S. Cullen, K. Lange, et al., Neural correlates of anxiety associated with obsessive-compulsive symptom dimensions in normal volunteers, Biol. Psychiatry 53 (2003) 482–493.

[46] S. Saxena, A.L. Brody, M.L. Ho, et al., Differential cerebral metabolic changes with paroxetine treatment of obsessive-compulsive disorder vs major depression, Arch. Gen. Psychiatry 59 (2002) 250–261.

[47] K.L. Phan, D.A. Fitzgerald, P.J. Nathan, et al., Neural substrates for voluntary suppression of negative affect: a functional magnetic resonance imaging study, Biol. Psychiatry 57 (2005) 210–219.

[48] J.T. Coull, Neural correlates of attention and arousal: insights from electrophysiology, functional neuroimaging and psychopharmacology, Prog. Neurobiol. 55 (1998) 343–361.

[49] J.F. Lopez, H. Akil, S.J. Watson, Neural circuits mediating stress, Biol. Psychiatry 46 (1999) 1461–1471.

[50] N. McNaughton, J.A. Gray, Anxiolytic action on the behavioural inhibition system implies multiple types of arousal contribute to anxiety, J. Affect. Disord. 61 (2000) 161–176.

[51] L. Yavich, M.M. Forsberg, M. Karayiorgou, et al., Site-specific role of catechol-O-methyltransferase in dopamine overflow within prefrontal cortex and dorsal striatum, J. Neurosci. 27 (2007) 10196–10209.

[52] M.N. Smolka, M. Bühler, G. Schumann, et al., Gene-gene effects on central processing of aversive stimuli, Mol. Psychiatry 12 (2007) 307–317.

[53] A. Heinz, D. Goldman, D.W. Jones, R. Palmour, D. Hommer, J.G. Gorey, K.S. Lee, M. Linnoila, D.R. Weinberger, Genotype influences in vivo dopamine transporter availability in human striatum, Neuropsychopharmacology 22 (2000) 133–139.

[54] A. Bertolino, G. Blasi, V. Latorre, et al., Additive effects of genetic variation in dopamine regulating genes on working memory cortical activity in human brain, J. Neurosci. 26 (2006) 3918–3922.

[55] A. Bertolino, V. Rubino, F. Sambataro, et al., Prefrontal-hippocampal coupling during memory processing is modulated by COMT val158met genotype, Biol. Psychiatry 60 (2006) 1250–1258.

[56] I. Puls, J. Mohr, J. Wrase, J. Priller, J. Behr, W. Kitzrow, N. Makris, H.C. Breiter, K. Obermayer, A. Heinz, Synergistic effects of the dopaminergic and glutamatergic system on hippocampal volume in alcohol-dependent patients, Biol. Psychol. 79 (2008) 126–136 doi:10.1016/j.biopsycho.2008.03.001.

[57] A. Heinz, M. Schäfer, J.D. Higley, J.H. Krystal, D. Goldman, Neurobiological correlates of the disposition and maintenance of alcoholism, Pharmacopsychiatry 36 (Suppl. 3) (2003) 255–258.

[58] A. Bertolino, A. Di Giorgio, G. Blasi, et al., Epistasis between Dopamine Regulating Genes Identifies a Nonlinear Response of the Human Hippocampus During Memory Tasks, Biol. Psychiatry (2008).

[59] J. Yacubian, T. Sommer, K. Schroeder, J. Glaescher, R. Kalisch, B. Leuenberger, D.F. Braus, C. Buechel, Gene-gene interaction associated with neutral reward sensitivity, Proc. Natl. Acad. Sci. USA 104 (2007) 8125–8130.

[60] J.-C. Dreher, P. Kohn, B. Kolachana, et al., Variation in dopamine genes influences responsivity of the human reward system. www.pnas.org/cgi/doi/10.1073/pnas.0805517105.

[61] K. Schmack, F. Schlagenhauf, P. Sterzer, et al., Catechol-O-methyltransferase val(158)met genotype influences neural processing of reward anticipation, Neuroimage (2008) doi:10.1016/j.neuroimage.2008.06.019.

[62] A. Abi-Dargham, O. Mawlawi, I. Lombardo, et al., Prefrontal dopamine D1 receptors and working memory in schizophrenia, J. Neurosci. 22 (2002) 3708–3719.

[63] J.D. Bremner, J.H. Krystal, S.M. Southwick, D.S. Charney, Noradrenergic mechanisms in stress and anxiety: I. Preclinical studies, Synapse 23 (1996) 28–38.

[64] J.H. Callicott, A. Bertolino, V.S. Mattay, et al., Physiological dysfunction of the dorsolateral prefrontal cortex in schizophrenia revisited, Cereb. Cortex 10 (2000) 1078–1092.

[65] J.H. Callicott, V.S. Mattay, A. Bertolino, et al., Physiological characteristics of capacity constraints in working memory as revealed by functional MRI, Cereb. Cortex 9 (1999) 20–26.

[66] J. Chen, B.K. Lipska, N. Halim, et al., Functional analysis of genetic variation in catechol-O-methyltransferase (COMT): effects on mRNA, protein, and enzyme activity in postmortem human brain, Am. J. Hum. Genet. 75 (2004) 807–821.

[67] A.R. Hariri, V.S. Mattay, A. Tessitore, F. Fera, W.G. Smith, D.R. Weinberger, Dextroamphetamine modulates the response of the human amygdala, Neuropsychopharmacology 27 (2002) 1036–1040.

[68] A.R. Hariri, D.R. Weinberger, Imaging genomics, Br. Med. Bull. 65 (2003) 259–270.

[69] P.J. Lang, M.M. Bradley, B.N. Cuthbert, The International Affective Picture System (IAPS), Center for Research in Psychophysiology, University of Florida, Gainsville, FL, 1999.

[70] P.J. Lang, M.M. Bradley, J.R. Fitzsimmons, et al., Emotional arousal and activation of the visual cortex: an fMRI analysis, Psychophysiology 35 (1998) 199–210.

[71] D.S. Manoach, R.L. Gollub, E.S. Benson, et al., Schizophrenic subjects show aberrant fMRI activation of dorsolateral prefrontal cortex and basal ganglia during working memory performance, Biol. Psychiatry 48 (2000) 99–109.

[72] J.S. Morris, K.J. Friston, C. Buchel, et al., A neuromodulatory role for the human amygdala in processing emotional facial expressions, Brain 121 (Pt 1) (1998) 47–57.

[73] M.L. Phillips, W.C. Drevets, S.L. Rauch, R. Lane, Neurobiology of emotion perception I: The neural basis of normal emotion perception, Biol. Psychiatry 54 (2003) 504–514.

[74] M. Reuter, J. Hennig, Association of the functional catechol-O-methyltransferase VAL158MET polymorphism with the personality trait of extraversion, Neuroreport 16 (2005) 1135–1138.

[75] J.A. Rosenkranz, A.A. Grace, Modulation of basolateral amygdala neuronal firing and afferent drive by dopamine receptor activation in vivo, J. Neurosci. 19 (1999) 11027–11039.

[76] M.B. Stein, M.D. Fallin, N.J. Schork, J. Gelernter, COMT Polymorphisms and Anxiety-Related Personality Traits, Neuropsychopharmacology (2005).

[77] A. Tessitore, A.R. Hariri, F. Fera, et al., Dopamine modulates the response of the human amygdala: a study in Parkinson's disease, J. Neurosci. 22 (2002) 9099–9103.

[78] P. Vuilleumier, J.L. Armony, K. Clarke, M. Husain, J. Driver, R.J. Dolan, Neural response to emotional faces with and without awareness: event-related fMRI in a parietal patient with visual extinction and spatial neglect, Neuropsychologia 40 (2002) 2156–2166.

[79] D.R. Weinberger, Implications of normal brain development for the pathogenesis of schizo-
     phrenia, Arch. Gen. Psychiatry 44 (1987) 660–669.
[80] D.R. Weinberger, K.F. Berman, B.P. Illowsky, Physiological dysfunction of dorsolateral prefron-
     tal cortex in schizophrenia. III. A new cohort and evidence for a monoaminergic mechanism,
     Arch. Gen. Psychiatry 45 (1988) 609–615.
[81] D.R. Weinberger, K.F. Berman, R. Suddath, E.F. Torrey, Evidence of dysfunction of a prefron-
     tal-limbic network in schizophrenia: a magnetic resonance imaging and regional cerebral blood
     flow study of discordant monozygotic twins, Am. J. Psychiatry 149 (1992) 890–897.

Part Five

Computational Models of the Reward System and Decision Making

18 Optimal decision-making theories

Rafal Bogacz

Department of Computer Science, University of Bristol, Bristol BS8
1UB, United Kingdom

Abstract

In case of many decisions based on sensory information, the sensory stimulus or its neural representation are noisy. This chapter reviews theories proposing that the brain implements statistically optimal strategies for decision making on the basis of noisy information. These strategies maximize the accuracy and speed of decisions, as well as the rate of receiving rewards for correct choices. The chapter first reviews computational models of cortical decision circuits that can optimally perform choices between two alternatives. Then, it describes a model of cortico-basal-ganglia circuit that implements the optimal strategy for choice between multiple alternatives. Finally, it shows how the basal ganglia may modulate decision processes in the cortex, allowing cortical neurons to represent the probabilities of alternative choices being correct. For each set of theories their predictions are compared with existing experimental data.

Key points

1. Integrating sensory information over time increases the accuracy of decisions.
2. Optimal decision strategies describe when to stop the integration of information, and they minimize the decision time for any required accuracy.
3. Several models of cortical decision circuits have been proposed that implement the optimal strategy for choice between two alternatives.
4. It has been proposed that the optimal strategy for choice between multiple alternatives is implemented in the cortico-basal-ganglia circuit.
5. In the proposed model, the cortico-basal-ganglia circuit computes the posterior probabilities of alternatives being correct, given the sensory evidence.

18.1 Introduction

Imagine an animal trying to decide if a shape moving behind the leaves is predator or prey. The sensory information the animal receives may be noisy and partial (e.g., occluded by the leaves) and hence need to be accumulated over time to gain sufficient accuracy, but the speed of such choices is also of critical importance. Due to the noisy nature of the sensory information, such decisions can be considered as statistical problems. This chapter reviews theories assuming that during perceptual decisions the brain performs statistically optimal tests, thereby maximizing the speed and accuracy of choices.

The optimal decision-making theories are motivated by an assumption that evolutionary pressure has been promoting animals that make fast and accurate choices. Although optimality is not always achieved, these theories provide interpretation for existing data and further experimental predictions that can guide empirical research. The optimal decision-making strategies are often precisely defined and relatively simple, thus they constrain the parameters of the models of neural decision circuits.

This chapter is organized as follows. Section 18.2 reviews models assuming that cortical decision circuits implement an optimal test for choice between two alternatives. Section 18.3 reviews the model of cortico-basal-ganglia circuit assuming that it implements optimal choice between multiple alternatives; this model is closely related to that described in Chapter 19. Section 18.4 shows how the basal ganglia may modulate the integration of sensory evidence in the cortex and allow cortical neurons represent the probabilities of alternative choices being correct. Section 18.5 discusses open questions. In addition, the Appendices contain essential derivations presented step-by-step (without skipping any calculations) such that they can be understood without extensive mathematical background.

In this chapter we focus on models of decision making in highly practiced task; the models describing task acquisition are discussed in Chapter 19. Throughout this chapter we use population level models describing activities of neuronal populations rather than individual neurons. Although this level of modeling is unable to capture many important details of neural decision circuits, it helps in understanding the essence of computation performed by various populations during decision process.

18.2   Models of optimal decision making in the cortex

In this section we first briefly review the responses of cortical neurons during a choice task; a more detailed review is available in Chapter 8. Next, the statistically optimal decision strategy and its proposed neural implementations are described. Finally, the predictions of the models are compared with experimental data.

18.2.1   Neurobiology of decision processes in the cortex

The neural bases of decision are typically studied in the motion discrimination task, in which a monkey is presented with a display containing moving dots [1]. A fraction of the dots moves left on some trials or right on other trials, while the rest is moving randomly. The task of the animal is to make a saccade (i.e., an eye movement) in the direction of motion of the majority of dots.

One of the areas critically important for this task is the medial temporal (MT) area in the visual cortex. The neurons in area MT respond selectively for a particular directions of motion, thus the MT neurons preferring left motion are more active on trials when the majority of dots move left, while the neurons preferring right motion are more active on trials when the majority of dots move right [1]. However, their activity is also very noisy, as the stimulus itself is noisy.

Let us now consider the decision faced by the areas receiving input from MT. Let us imagine a judge listening to the activity from the two populations of MT neurons, each preferring one of the two directions. The MT neurons produce spikes that can be interpreted as votes for the alternative directions. The task of the judge is to choose the alternative receiving more votes, that is, corresponding to the MT population with higher mean firing rate. Note however that the judge cannot measure the mean firing rate instantaneously, as the spikes are discrete events spread out over time. Thus the judge needs to observe the MT activity for a period of time and integrate the evidence or "count the votes" until it reaches a certain level of confidence.

Indeed, such an information integration process has been observed in the lateral intra-parietal (LIP) area and frontal eye field during the motion coherence task. Neurons in area LIP respond selectively before and during saccades in particular directions. It has been observed that the LIP neurons selective for the chosen direction gradually increase their firing rate during the motion discrimination task [2, 3], and the data indicate that these neurons integrate the input from corresponding MT neurons over time [4–6]. Thus, using the judge metaphor, the LIP neurons "count the votes" and represent the total numbers of votes in their firing rate. The neurons representing integrated evidence have also been observed in other tasks in areas within the frontal lobe [7–10].

18.2.2 Optimal stopping criterion for two alternatives

The analysis still leaves an open question: When should the integration process be stopped and action executed? This subsection first considers this question intuitively, then it presents an optimal stopping criterion formally, and describes in what sense it is optimal.

Stopping criteria. The simplest possible criterion is to stop the integration whenever the integrated evidence, or the total number of votes, for one of the alternatives reaches a threshold. This strategy is known as the race model [11]. Another possibility is to stop the integration when the *difference* between the integrated evidence in favor of the winning and losing alternatives exceeds a threshold. This strategy is referred to as the diffusion model [12–14].

The diffusion model is usually formulated in a different but equivalent way: It includes a single integrator which accumulates the difference between the sensory evidence supporting the two alternatives. A choice is made in favor of the first alternative if the integrator exceeds a positive threshold, or in favor of the second alternative if the integrator decreases below a negative threshold.

As will be demonstrated formally here, the diffusion model provides an optimal stopping criterion. The advantage of diffusion over race models can also be seen intuitively, as the diffusion model allows the decision process to be modulated by the amount of conflict between evidence supporting alternatives on a given trial: Note that decisions will take longer when the evidence for the two alternatives is similar, and importantly, that decisions will be faster when there is little evidence for the losing alternative. By contrast, in the race model the decision time does not depend on the level of evidence for the losing alternative [15].

Statistical formulation. Let us now formalize the decision problem. For simplicity, let us assume that time can be divided into discrete steps. Let $x_i(t)$ denote the sensory evidence supporting alternative i at time t, which in the motion discrimination task corresponds to the firing rate of the MT neurons selective for alternative i at time t. Let y_i denote the evidence for alternative i integrated until time t:

$$y_i = \sum_{\tau=1}^{t} x_i(\tau). \tag{18.1}$$

Gold and Shadlen [16, 17] formulated the decision as a statistical problem in the following way: They assumed that $x_i(t)$ come from a normal distribution with mean μ_i and standard deviation σ. They defined hypotheses H_i stating that the sensory evidence supporting alternative i has higher mean:

$$H_1: \mu_1 = \mu^+, \mu_2 = \mu^-; H_2: \mu_1 = \mu^-, \mu_2 = \mu^+, \tag{18.2}$$

where $\mu^+ > \mu^-$. The optimal procedure for distinguishing between these hypotheses is provided by the sequential probability ratio test (SPRT) [18], which is equivalent to the diffusion model [12], as will be shown. According to SPRT, at each moment of time t, one computes the ratio of the likelihoods of the sensory evidence given the hypotheses:

$$R = \frac{P(x(1..t)|H_1)}{P(x(1..t)|H_2)}, \tag{18.3}$$

where $x(1..t)$ denotes a set of all sensory evidence observed so far [i.e., $x_1(1)$, $x_2(1)$, ..., $x_1(t)$, $x_2(t)$]. If R exceeds a threshold Z_1 or decreases below a lower threshold Z_2, the decision process is stopped and the choice is made (H_1 if $R > Z_1$ or H_2 if $R < Z_2$). Otherwise the decision process continues and another sample of sensory information is observed. Thus note that SPRT observes sensory evidence only for as long as it is necessary to distinguish between the hypotheses.

The relationship between SPRT and the diffusion model is described in Appendix 18A. Its first part shows that R in the SPRT changes in a similar way as the single integrator in the diffusion model (which accumulates the difference between the sensory evidence supporting the two alternatives). Namely, if at a given moment of time t, the sensory evidence supports the first alternative more than the second [i.e., $x_1(t) > x_2(t)$] then R increases; and otherwise R decreases. The second part of Appendix 18A shows that $\log R$ is exactly proportional to the difference between the integrated evidence:

$$\log R = g(y_1 - y_2), \tag{18.4}$$

where g is a constant. Thus according to SPRT, the decision process will be stopped when the difference $(y_1 - y_2)$ exceeds a positive threshold (equal to $\log Z_1/g$) or decreases below a negative threshold (equal to $\log Z_2/g$). Hence the SPRT (with hypotheses of Eq. 18.2) is equivalent to the diffusion model.

Optimality. The SPRT is optimal in the following sense: it minimizes the average decision time for any required accuracy [19]. Let us illustrate this property by comparing the race and the diffusion models. In both models, speed and accuracy are controlled by the height of decision threshold, and there exists a speed-accuracy tradeoff. But if we choose the thresholds in both models giving the same accuracy for a given sensory input, then the diffusion model will on average be faster than the race model.

One can ask if this optimality property could bring benefits to animals. If we consider a scenario in which an animal receives rewards for correct choices, then making fast choices allows an animal to receive more rewards per unit of time. In particular, Gold and Shadlen [17] considered a task in which the animal receives a reward for correct choices, there is no penalty for errors, and there is a fixed delay D between the response and the onset of the next choice trial. In this task the reward rate is equal to the ratio of accuracy AC and the average duration of the trial [17]:

$$RR = \frac{AC}{RT + D}, \tag{18.5}$$

where RT denotes the average reaction time. The reward rate depends on decision threshold. But Appendix 18B shows that the diffusion model with appropriately chosen threshold gives higher or equal reward rate than any other decision strategy. Furthermore, the diffusion model maximizes reward rate not only for the task described above, but also for a wide range of other tasks [20].

18.2.3   Neural implementations

As mentioned in the previous subsection, the optimal decision strategy is to make a choice when the difference between the evidence supporting the two alternatives exceeds a threshold. However, the neurophysiological data suggest that an animal makes a choice when the activity of integrator neurons selective for a given alternative exceeds a fixed threshold [3, 21]. One way to reconcile these two observations is to assume that the firing rate of these neurons represents the difference in evidence supporting the two alternatives. Several models have been proposed that exhibit this property, and they are briefly reviewed in this subsection.

Let us refer to the population of cortical integrator neurons selective for a particular alternative as an integrator. In the model shown in Fig. 18.1A, the integrators directly accumulate the difference between the activities of sensory neurons via feed-forward inhibitory connections [2, 22].

Thus this model is equivalent to the diffusion model. An alternative model shown in Fig. 18.1B assumes that integrators mutually inhibit each other [23]. An analysis of the dynamics of this model reveals that, for certain parameter values, the activity of integrators is approximately proportional to the difference between the integrated evidence, thus it also approximates the diffusion model [20].

In the models shown in Fig. 18.1A and 18.1B, the sensory neurons send both excitatory and inhibitory connections. But in the brain the cortico-cortical connections are only excitatory, thus Fig. 18.1C and 18.1D shows more realistic versions of the models in Fig. 18.1A and 18.1B in which the inhibition is provided by a population of inhibitory inter-neurons (the model in Fig. 18.1D has been proposed in [24]). It is easy to set the parameters of the model shown in Fig. 18.1C so it also integrates the difference between sensory evidence (in particular, the weights of connections between sensory and integrator populations need to be twice as large as the other weights). Similarly Wong and Wang [25] have shown that the model in Fig. 18.1D can also for certain parameters integrate the difference between sensory evidence.

In summary, there are several architectures of cortical decision networks, shown in Fig. 18.1, that can approximate the optimal decision making for two alternatives. Matlab codes allowing simulation and comparison of performance of the models described in this chapter are available http://www.cs.bris.ac.uk/home/rafal/optimal/codes.html

18.2.4   Comparison with experimental data

The diffusion model has been shown to fit the reaction time (RT) distributions from a wide range of choice tasks [26–28]. Furthermore, the diffusion model has been shown to describe the patterns of RTs and the growth of information in neurons involved in the decision process better than the race model [29–31].

The diffusion model has been also used to explain the effect of stimulation of MT and LIP neurons during the motion discrimination task. Ditterich et al. [4] showed that stimulation of MT neurons selective for a particular alternative produced two effects: reduced

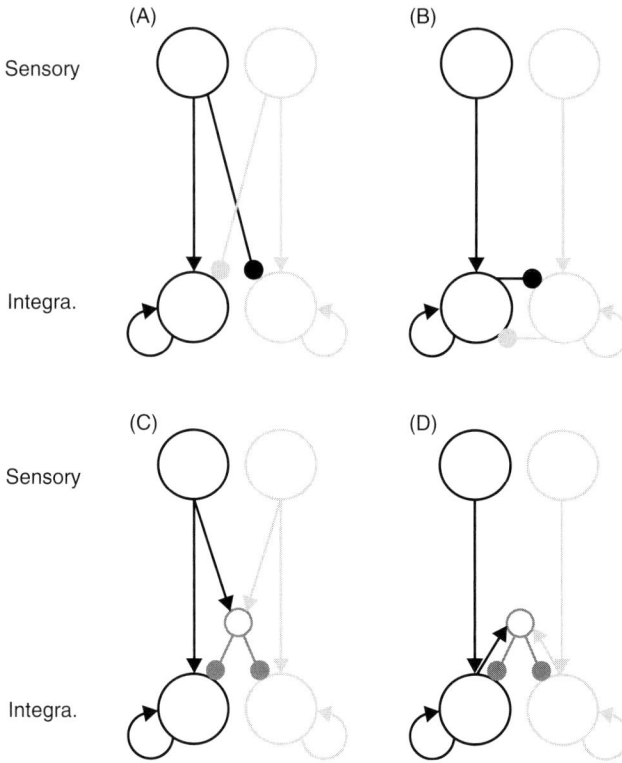

Figure 18.1 Connections between neuronal populations in cortical models of decision making (A) Shadlen and Newsome model, (B) Usher and McClelland model, (C) feed-forward pooled inhibition model, (D) Wang model. Open circles denote neuronal populations. Arrows denote excitatory connections; lines ended with circles denote inhibitory connections. Thus the open circles with self-excitatory connections denote the integrator populations. Black and gray pathways correspond to neuronal populations selective for the two alternative choices. Sensory – sensory cortex encoding relevant aspects of stimuli; Integra. – cortical region integrating sensory evidence.

RTs on trials when this alternative was chosen, and increased RTs when the other alternative was chosen. The second effect suggests that the decision is made on the basis of the difference between integrated evidence, and thus supports the diffusion model over the race model. Hanks et al. [32] compared these effects of MT stimulation with the effects of LIP stimulation. By estimating parameters of the diffusion model, they established that the effect of MT stimulation on RTs is best explained by change in sensory evidence, while the effect of LIP stimulation is best explained by change in the integrated evidence. This analysis supports the model in which the activity of LIP neurons represent the difference between integrated information from MT neurons.

The models shown in Fig. 18.1 can also fit the time-courses of neural activity in LIP neurons during the choice process. In particular, due to the inhibitory connections, the models can describe the decrease in firing rate of LIP neurons representing the losing alternative [22, 24, 33]. However, the current neurophysiological data do not allow us to distinguish which type of inhibition (feed-forward or mutual) is present in the integrator networks. We will come back to this question in Section 18.5.1.

18.3 Model of decision making in the cortico-basal-ganglia circuit

This section reviews a theory [34] suggesting that the cortico-basal-ganglia circuit implements a generalization of SPRT to choice between multiple alternatives, the Multihypothesis SPRT (MSPRT) [35]. This section follows the same organization as Section 18.2.

18.3.1 Neurobiology of decision processes in the basal ganglia

The basal ganglia are a set of nuclei connected with one another, cortex and subcortical regions. Redgrave et al. [36] have proposed that the basal ganglia act as a central switch resolving competition between cortical regions vying for behavioral expression. In the default state the output nuclei of the basal ganglia send tonic inhibition to the thalamus and brain stem, and thus block execution of any actions [37, 38]. To execute a movement, the firing rates of the corresponding neurons in the output nuclei need to decrease [37, 38], thus releasing the corresponding motor plan from inhibition.

Another property of basal ganglia organization relevant to the model is that within each nucleus different neurons are selective for different body parts [39, 40]. On the basis of this observation it has been proposed that basal ganglia are organized into channels corresponding to individual body parts that traverse all nuclei [41]. Two sample channels are shown in two colors in Fig. 18.2.

Furthermore, the connectivity between nuclei is usually within channels [41]; for example, neurons in the motor cortex selective for the right hand project to the neurons in striatum selective for the right hand, etc. The only exception is the subthalamic nucleus (STN) where neurons project more diffusely across channels [43, 44] (Fig. 18.2).

Figure 18.2 shows a subset of basal ganglia connectivity required for optimal decision making [34]. The figure does not show "the indirect pathway" between the striatum and the output nuclei via the globus pallidus (GP). It has been suggested that this pathway is involved in learning from punishments [45] (see Chapter 19) and will not be discussed in this chapter for simplicity, but it can be included in the model and it continues to implement MSPRT [34].

18.3.2 Optimal stopping criterion for multiple alternatives

Let us first describe MSPRT intuitively (a more formal description will follow). As mentioned in Section 18.2.2, to optimize performance, the choice criterion should take into account the amount of conflict in the evidence. Consequently, in the MSPRT, a choice is made when the integrated evidence for one of the alternatives exceeds a certain level, but this level is not fixed; rather it is increased when the evidence is more conflicting:

$$y_i > Threshold + Conflict, \tag{18.6}$$

where *Threshold* is a fixed value. Subtracting *Conflict* from both sides, the criterion for making a choice can be written as:

$$y_i - Conflict > Threshold. \tag{18.7}$$

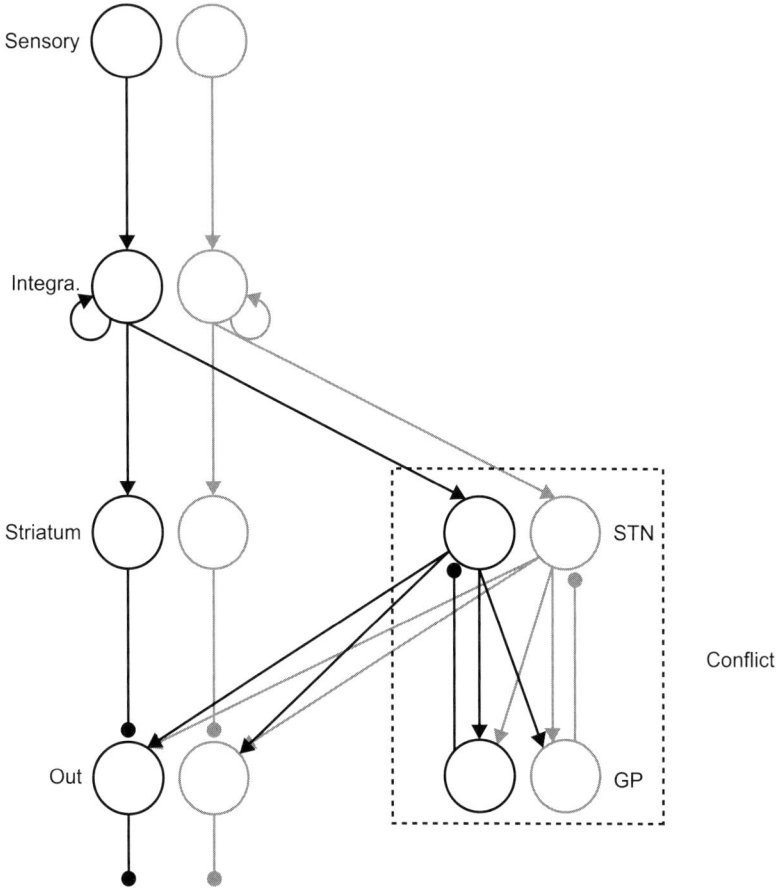

Figure 18.2 A subset of the cortico-basal-ganglia circuit required to implement MSPRT. Connectivity between areas based on Gurney et al. [42]. Pairs of circles correspond to brain areas: Sensory – sensory cortex encoding relevant aspects of stimuli (e.g., MT in motion discrimination task), Integra. – cortical region integrating sensory evidence (e.g., LIP in tasks with saccadic response), STN – subthalamic nucleus, GP – globus pallidus (or its homolog GPe in primates), Out – output nuclei: substantia nigra pars reticulate and entopeduncular nucleus (or its homolog GPi in primates). Arrows denote excitatory connections; lines ended with circles denote inhibitory connections. Black and gray pathways correspond to two sample channels.

In order to implement the MSPRT, *Conflict* needs to take a particular form:

$$Conflict = \log \sum_{j=1}^{N} \exp y_j, \tag{18.8}$$

where N is the number of alternative choices (we use the italicized word *Conflict* to refer to a term defined in Eq. 18.8, and the non-italicized word "conflict" to refer to a general situation where sensory evidence supports more than one alternative). Equation 18.8 is said to express conflict because it involves summation of evidence across alternatives, but it also includes particular nonlinearities, and to understand where they come from, we need to describe MSPRT more formally.

MSPRT is a statistical test between N hypotheses. We can generalize the hypotheses described in Eq. 18.2, so that the hypothesis H_i states that the sensory evidence supporting alternative i has the highest mean:

$$H_i: \mu_i = \mu^+, \mu_{j \neq i} = \mu^-. \tag{18.9}$$

In the MSPRT, at each time t, and for each alternative i, one computes the probability of alternative i being correct given all sensory evidence observed so far; let us denote this probability by P_i:

$$P_i = P(H_i | x(1..t)). \tag{18.10}$$

If for any alternative P_i exceeds a fixed threshold, the choice is made in favor of the corresponding alternative; otherwise the sampling continues. Appendix 18C shows that the logarithm of P_i is equal to:

$$\log P_i = y_i - \log \sum_{j=1}^{N} \exp y_j. \tag{18.11}$$

Equation 18.11 includes two terms: the integrated evidence y_i and *Conflict* defined in Eq. 18.8. Thus MSPRT is equivalent to making a choice when the difference between y_i and *Conflict* exceeds a threshold.

MSPRT has similar optimality property as SPRT; namely, it minimizes the decision time for any required accuracy (which has been shown analytically for accuracies close to 100% [47], and simulations demonstrate that MSPRT achieves shorter decision times than simpler models also for lower accuracies [48]). Thus, given the discussion in Section 18.2.2 and Appendix 18B, MSPRT also maximizes the reward rate.

18.3.3 Neural implementation

Bogacz and Gurney [34] proposed that the circuit of Fig. 18.2 computes the expression $y_i -$ *Conflict* (required for MSPRT). In their model, y_i are computed in cortical integrators accumulating input from sensory neurons (Fig. 18.2), and the *Conflict* is computed by STN and GP (we will describe how it can be computed later). The output nuclei receive inhibition from cortical integrators via the striatum and excitation from STN, thus they compute in the model:

$$OUT_i = -y_i + \textit{Conflict} = -(y_i - \textit{Conflict}). \tag{18.12}$$

Thus the output nuclei in the model represent the negative of the expression that is compared against a threshold in MSPRT (cf. Eq. 18.7). Therefore, in the model the choice is made when the activity of any output channel OUT_i decreases below the threshold, in agreement with selection by disinhibition reviewed in Section 18.3.1.

Frank [49] has also proposed that the conflict is computed in STN (see Chapter 19). STN has a suitable anatomical location to modulate choice process according to the conflict, as it can effectively inhibit all motor programs by its diffuse projections to output nuclei [50]. Studies of patients who receive deep brain stimulation to STN support the idea that STN computes conflict. They suggest that disrupting computations in STN makes patients unable to prevent premature responding in high conflict choices [51, 52] (see Chapter 19 for details).

Bogacz and Gurney [34] showed that input sent by STN to the output nuclei can be proportional to the particular form of *Conflict* defined in Eq. 18.8, if the neurons in STN and GP had the following relationships between their input and the firing rate:

$$STN = \exp{(input)}, \tag{18.13}$$

$$GP = input - \log{(input)}. \tag{18.14}$$

Let us analyze how each term in Eq. 18.8 can be computed. For ease of reading let us restate Eq. 18.8:

$$Conflict = \log \sum_{j=1}^{N} \exp y_j. \tag{18.8}$$

Starting from the right end of Eq. 18.8, the integrated evidence y_i is provided to the STN in the model by a direct connection from cortical integrators (Fig. 18.2). The exponentiation is performed by the STN neurons (cf. Eq. 18.13). The summation across channels is achieved due to the diffuse projections from the STN. In the model, each channel in the output nuclei receives input from all channels in the STN; hence, the input to the output neurons is proportional to the sum of activity in STN channels. The only non-intuitive element of the computation of Eq. 18.8 is the logarithm—it is achieved by the interactions between STN and GP, as shown in Appendix 18D.

18.3.4 Comparison with experimental data

The input-output relationships of Eqs 18.13 and 18.14 form predictions of the model. The first prediction says that the firing rate of STN neurons should be proportional to the exponent of their input. Figure 18.3 shows the firing rate as a function of injected current for seven STN neurons, for which this relationship has been studied precisely [53, 54]. Solid lines show fits of the exponential function to firing rates below 135 Hz, suggesting that up to approximately 135 Hz the STN neurons have an input-output relationship that is very close to exponential.

For the entire range in Fig. 18.3, the input-output relationship seems to be sigmoidal, often used in neural network models, and one could ask how unique the exponential relationship discussed here is, as every sigmoidal curve has a segment with an exponential increase. However, note that typical neurons have much lower maximum firing rate, so even if they had an exponential segment, it would apply to a much smaller range of firing rates. By contrast, the STN neurons have exponential input-output relationship for up to ~135 Hz, and this is approximately the operating range of these neurons in humans during choice tasks [55].

The model also predicts that GP neurons should have approximately linear input-output relationship (because the linear term in Eq. 18.14 dominates for higher *input*).

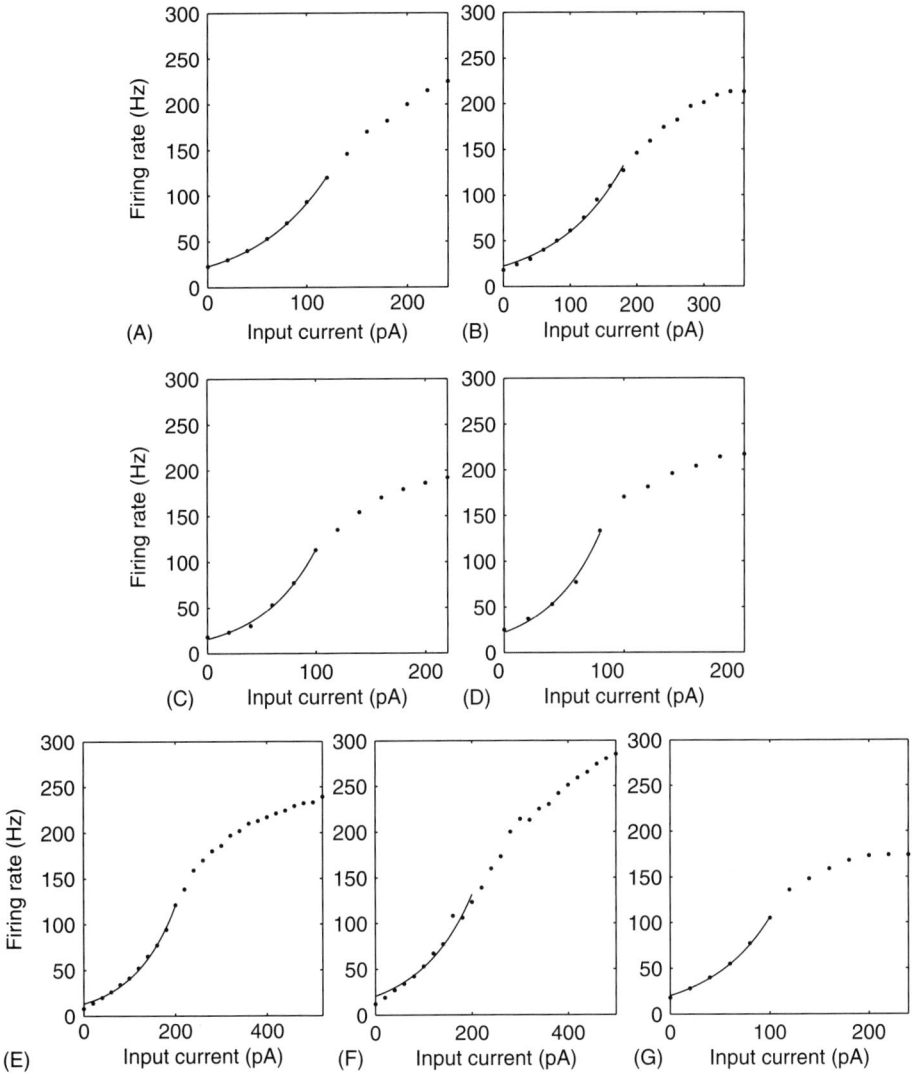

Figure 18.3 Firing rates f of STN neurons as a function of input current I. Panels A–D re-plot data on the firing rate of STN neurons presented in Hallworth et al. [53] in Figures 4b, 4f, 12d, and 13d, respectively (control condition). Panels E–G re-plot the data from STN presented in Wilson et al. [54] in Figures 1c, 2c, and 2f, respectively (control condition). Lines show best fit of the function $f = a \exp(b\,I)$ to the points with firing rates below 135 Hz.

Neurophysiological studies suggest that there are three distinct subpopulations of neurons in GP, and the one which contributes most to the population firing rate has indeed the linear input-output relationship [56, 57].

The model is also consistent with behavioral data from choice tasks. First, for two alternatives the model produces the same behavior as the diffusion model, because then MSPRT reduces to SPRT, thus the model fits all behavioral data that the diffusion model can describe (see Section 18.2.4). Second, the model reproduces the Hick's law, stating that the decision time is proportional to the logarithm of the number of alternatives [34]. Third, Norris [58] has shown that MSPRT describes patterns of RTs during word recognition (which can be interpreted as a perceptual decision with the number of alternatives equal to the number of words known by participants).

18.4   Basal ganglia and cortical integration

This section discusses the relationship between the models presented in the two previous sections, and how the basal ganglia may modulate cortical integration allowing cortical integrators to represent probabilities of corresponding alternatives being correct.

18.4.1   Inhibition between cortical integrators

In the model shown in Fig. 18.2, a cortical integrator accumulates sensory evidence only for the corresponding alternative. This simple model is inconsistent with the observation that integrators representing the losing alternative decrease their firing rate during a choice process [2]; to account for this observation the inhibitory connections need to be introduced, as shown in Fig. 18.1.

Nevertheless, if the simple cortical integration in the model of the cortico-basal-ganglia circuit is replaced by any of the models in Fig. 18.1, the circuit still implements MSPRT [34], as we shall now explain. Note that in the biologically more realistic models of Fig. 18.1C and 18.1D, both integrators receive the same inhibition from a pool of inhibitory neurons. The basal ganglia model has a surprising property that if the same inhibition, *inh*, is applied to all integrators, the activity of output nuclei does not change. Intuitively, this property is desirable for the basal ganglia network because, as we discussed in Section 18.2.2, the optimal choice criterion should be based on differences between integrated evidence for the alternatives, so increasing or decreasing the activity of all integrators should not affect the optimal choice criterion. This property is shown formally in Appendix 18E.

18.4.2   Representing probabilities in integrators' firing rate

Recently a modified version of the cortico-basal-ganglia model has been proposed [46] which only differs from the one described in Section 18.8 in that, the integration is performed via cortico-basal-ganglia-thalamic loops as shown in Fig. 18.4. In this modified model the circuit of STN and GP (represented by a small circle in Fig. 18.4) provides the indirect inhibition to the integrators which is the same for all integrators. Due to the property described in the previous paragraph, the activity of output nuclei in the model of Fig. 18.4 is exactly the same as in the model of Fig. 18.2, thus the former also implements MSPRT [46].

Let us now investigate the properties of the cortical integrators predicted by the model of Fig. 18.4. Let us recall that in the model the activities of output nuclei are equal to (from Eqs 18.8, 18.11, and 18.12):

$$OUT_i = -\log P_i \tag{18.15}$$

(recall that P_i denotes the probability of alternative i being correct given the sensory evidence). The integrators in Fig. 18.4 receive input from the sensory neurons and effective

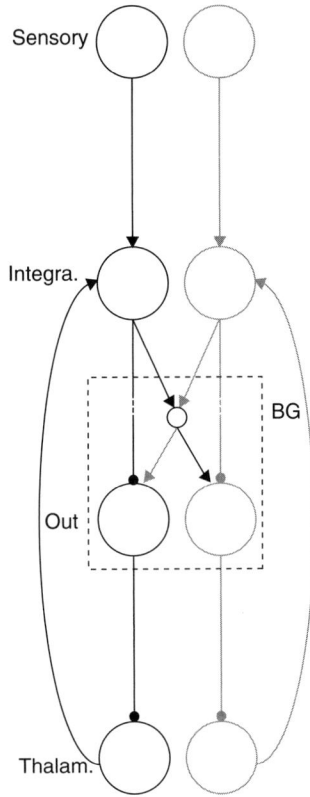

Figure 18.4 Connectivity in the model of integration in cortico-basal-ganglia thalamic loops. Notation as in Figs. 18.1 and 18.2. The dotted rectangle indicates the basal ganglia which are modeled in exactly the same way as in Fig. 18.2, but here for simplicity not all nuclei are shown: small circle represents STN and GP, and cortical integrators send effective inhibition to the output nuclei via the striatum not shown for simplicity.

inhibition from the output nuclei. If there is no sensory evidence coming, the activity of the integrators corresponding to alternative i is proportional to $\log P_i$ (from Eq. 18.15). Thus in this model the cortical integrators represent $\log P_i$ in their firing rate, they update $\log P_i$ according to new sensory evidence, and the basal ganglia continuously renormalizes the cortical activity such that P_i sum up to 1.

18.4.3 Incorporating prior probabilities

Let us now investigate how one can incorporate into the model of Fig. 18.4 the prior probabilities, that is, expectations about correct alternative prior to stimulus onset (e.g., that may arise in perceptual choice task when one stimulus is presented on a greater fraction of trials than others). Before the sensory evidence is provided, P_i are equal to the prior probabilities. Hence, given the discussion in the previous paragraph to utilize the

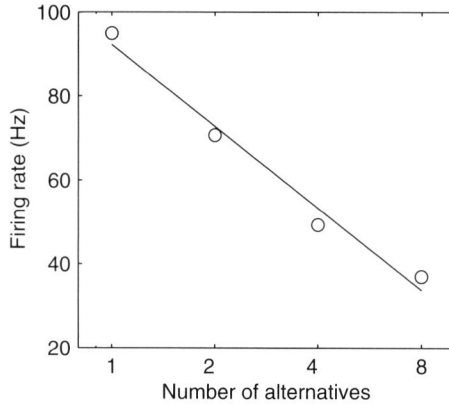

Figure 18.5 Firing rates f of superior colliculus neurons before stimulus onset as a function of the number of alternatives N. The circles correspond to the experimental data taken from Figure 4 of Basso and Wurtz [62] averaged across two time periods (the position of each dot was computed from the heights of bars in the original figure as [black bar $+$ 2 $\times$ gray bar]/3, because the gray bars were showing the average firing rate on two times longer intervals than the black bars). The solid line shows the best fitting logarithmic function $f = a \log N + b$.

prior information in the decision process, the initial values of the integrators (just before stimulus onset) should be equal to the logarithm of the prior probabilities.

18.4.4 Comparison with experimental data

The theory reviewed in this section predicts that the activity of integrator neurons should be proportional to $\log P_i$. Two studies [59, 60] have shown directly that activity of LIP neurons is modulated by P_i prior to and during the decision process respectively. But their published results do not allow us to distinguish if the LIP neurons represent $\log P_i$ or some other function of P_i. Nevertheless, there are two less direct studies supporting the hypothesis that the activity of cortical integrators prior to stimulus onset is proportional to the logarithms of the prior probabilities.

First, Carpenter and Williams [61] have also proposed that the starting point of integration is proportional to the logarithm of the prior probability, on the basis of careful analysis of RTs. In their experiment, participants were required to make an eye movement to a dot appearing on the screen. Carpenter and Williams [61] observed that the median RT to a dot appearing in a particular location was proportional to:

$$\text{median RT} \sim -\log Prior, \tag{18.16}$$

where *Prior* was computed as the fraction of trials within a block in which the dot appears in this location. Now notice that if there were no noise in sensory evidence, then RT would always be constant and proportional to the distance between the starting point (firing rate of integrators at stimulus onset) and the threshold (firing rate at the moment of decision). If the noise is present, RT differs between trials, but the median RT is equal to the distance between the starting point and the threshold (this relation is exact in a particular model used by Carpenter and Williams [61] and approximate in other models):

$$\text{median RT} \sim \textit{Threshold} - \textit{starting point} \tag{18.17}$$

Putting Eqs 18.16 and 18.17 together implies that the starting point is proportional to $\log Prior$.

Second, Basso and Wurtz [62] recorded neural activity in the superior colliculus (a subcortical structure receiving input from cortical integrators) in a task in which the number of alternative choices N differed between blocks. Note that in this task $Prior = 1/N$, and thus $\log Prior = -\log N$. Figure 18.5 shows that the firing rate before stimulus onset in their task was approximately proportional to $-\log N$, and hence to $\log Prior$.

18.5   Discussion

In this chapter we reviewed theories proposing that cortical networks and cortico-basal-ganglia circuit implement optimal statistical tests for decision making on the basis of noisy information. The predictions of these theories have been shown to be consistent with both behavioral and neurophysiological data. We have also reviewed a theory suggesting that the basal ganglia modulate cortical integrators allowing them to represent probabilities of corresponding alternatives being correct. In this section we discuss open questions.

18.5.1   Open questions

Let us discuss four open questions relating to the theories reviewed in this chapter.

1. Is the integration of sensory evidence supported by feedback loops within the cortex (Fig. 18.1) or by the cortico-basal-ganglia-thalamic loops (Fig. 18.4)? These possibilities could be distinguished by deactivation of striatal neurons (in the relevant channels) during a decision task. Then, if information is integrated via the cortico-basal-ganglia-thalamic loops, the gradual increasing firing rates of cortical integrators should no longer be observed.

2. What type of inhibition is present between cortical integrators? In this chapter we reviewed three possible pathways by which cortical integrators can compete and inhibit one another, shown in Figs. 18.1C, 18.1D, and 18.4. It should be possible to distinguish between these models on the basis of future neurophysiological studies. For example, in tasks in which the amount of evidence for the two alternatives can be varied independently, the feed-forward inhibition model predicts that the activity of the integrators should only depend on the difference between sensory evidence, while the mutual-inhibition model predicts that it should also depend on the total input to the integrators [15].

3. What else is represented by the cortical integrators? The theories reviewed in this chapter propose that the integrators encode integrated evidence or the probability of the corresponding alternative being correct. However, it is known that the firing rate of the cortical integrators is also modulated by other factors, for example, motor preparation or general desirability of alternatives [63]. It would be interesting to investigate how these other factors can further optimize decision making.

4. What is the relationship between decision making and reinforcement learning in the basal ganglia? The basal ganglia are also strongly involved in reinforcement learning (see Chapter 19). It would be interesting to integrate reinforcement learning and decision-making theories [46]. Furthermore, it could be interesting to model the role of dopamine during decision process, and how it modulates information processing in the basal ganglia during choice.

18A   Appendix A: Diffusion model implements SPRT

This appendix describes the relationship between SPRT and the diffusion model. First note that if we assume that $x_i(t)$ are sampled independently, then the likelihood of the sequence of samples is equal to the product of the likelihoods of individual samples:

$$P(x(1..t)|H_1) = \prod_{\tau=1}^{t} P(x(\tau)|H_1), \tag{18A.1}$$

where $x(\tau)$ denotes a pair: $x_1(\tau)$, $x_2(\tau)$. Substituting Eq. 18A.1 into Eq. 18.3 and taking the logarithm, we obtain:

$$\log R = \sum_{\tau=1}^{t} \log \frac{P(x(\tau)|H_1)}{P(x(\tau)|H_2)}. \tag{18A.2}$$

We will now illustrate how $\log R$ changes during the choice process. First note that according to Eq. 18A.2, at each time step t, a term is added to $\log R$ which only depends on $x(t)$. This term will be positive if $x_1(t) > x_2(t)$, because then $x(t)$ will be more likely given hypothesis H_1 (stating that $\mu_1 > \mu_2$) than given hypothesis H_2, thus $P(x(t)|H_1) > P(x(t)|H_2)$. Hence in each time step, $\log R$ increases if $x_1(t) > x_2(t)$, and analogously decreases if $x_1(t) < x_2(t)$.

Let us now derive the likelihood ratio given in Eq. 18.3 for the hypotheses of Eq. 18.2. Let us start with the numerator of Eq. 18.3. Hypothesis H_1 states that $x_1(t)$ come from a normal distribution with mean μ^+, while $x_2(t)$ come from a normal distribution with mean μ^- (see Eq. 18.2). Thus denoting the probability density of normal distribution with mean μ and standard deviation σ by $f_{\mu,\sigma}$ Eq. 18A.1 becomes:

$$P(x(1..t)|H_1) = \prod_{\tau=1}^{t} f_{\mu^+,\sigma}(x_1(\tau)) f_{\mu^-,\sigma}(x_2(\tau)). \tag{18A.3}$$

Using the equation for the normal probability density function, we obtain:

$$P(x(1..t)|H_1) = \prod_{\tau=1}^{t} \frac{1}{\sqrt{2\pi}\sigma} \exp\left(-\frac{(x_1(\tau) - \mu^+)^2}{2\sigma^2}\right) \frac{1}{\sqrt{2\pi}\sigma} \exp\left(-\frac{(x_2(\tau) - \mu^-)^2}{2\sigma^2}\right). \tag{18A.4}$$

Performing analogous calculation for the denominator of Eq. 18.3 we obtain very similar expression as in Eq. 18A.4 but with swapped μ^+ and μ^-. Hence, when we write the ratio of the numerator and the denominator, many terms will cancel. First, the constants in front of the exponents will cancel and we obtain:

$$R = \prod_{\tau=1}^{t} \frac{\exp\left(-\dfrac{(x_1(\tau) - \mu^+)^2}{2\sigma^2}\right)\exp\left(-\dfrac{(x_2(\tau) - \mu^-)^2}{2\sigma^2}\right)}{\exp\left(-\dfrac{(x_1(\tau) - \mu^-)^2}{2\sigma^2}\right)\exp\left(-\dfrac{(x_2(\tau) - \mu^+)^2}{2\sigma^2}\right)}. \tag{18A.5}$$

Second, if we expand the squares inside the exponents, and split the exponents using $\exp(a + b) = \exp(a)\exp(b)$, most of the terms will cancel, and we obtain:

$$R = \prod_{\tau=1}^{t} \frac{\exp\left(\dfrac{\mu^+ x_1(\tau)}{\sigma^2}\right)\exp\left(\dfrac{\mu^- x_2(\tau)}{\sigma^2}\right)}{\exp\left(\dfrac{\mu^- x_1(\tau)}{\sigma^2}\right)\exp\left(\dfrac{\mu^+ x_2(\tau)}{\sigma^2}\right)}. \tag{18A.6}$$

Now if we join the terms including $x_1(\tau)$ using $\exp(a)/\exp(b) = \exp(a - b)$, and do the same for the terms including $x_2(\tau)$ we obtain:

$$R = \prod_{\tau=1}^{t} \exp(gx_1(\tau))\exp(-gx_2(\tau)), \quad \text{where } g = \frac{\mu^+ - \mu^-}{\sigma^2}. \tag{18A.7}$$

If we put the product inside the exponent, it becomes a summation, and using Eq. 18.1 we obtain:

$$R = \frac{\exp(gy_1)}{\exp(gy_2)}. \tag{18A.8}$$

In summary, there were many cancellations during the derivation, and comparing Eqs 18.3 and 18A.8 reveals that the only term which remains from $P(x(1..t)|H_i)$ is the exponent of the evidence integrated in favor of alternative i, and the exponentiation comes from the exponent in the normal probability density function. Taking the logarithm of Eq. 18A.8 gives Eq. 18.4.

18B   Appendix B: Diffusion model maximizes reward rate

This appendix shows that the diffusion model with optimally chosen threshold achieves higher or equal reward rate than any other model of decision making. As mentioned in Section 18.2.2, decision-making models exhibit a speed-accuracy tradeoff (controlled by the decision threshold). For a given task, let us denote the average RT of the diffusion model for a given accuracy by $RT_d(AC)$, and the RT of another model by $RT_a(AC)$. The optimality of SPRT implies that for any accuracy level AC:

$$RT_d(AC) \leq RT_a(AC). \tag{18B.1}$$

Similarly, let us denote the reward rates of the diffusion and the other model for a given level of accuracy by $RR_d(AC)$ and $RR_a(AC)$ respectively. Let us denote the accuracy level that maximizes the reward rate of the diffusion model by AC_d, so from this definition for any accuracy level AC:

$$RR_d(AC) \leq RR_a(AC_d). \tag{18B.2}$$

Similarly, let us denote the accuracy maximizing the reward rate of the other model by AC_a. We can now derive the following relationship between the maximum possible reward rates achieved by the two models:

$$RR_a(AC_a) = \frac{AC_a}{RT_a(AC_a) + D} \leq \frac{AC_a}{RT_d(AC_a) + D} = RR_d(AC_a) \leq RR_d(AC_d). \tag{18B.3}$$

In the above derivation, the first inequality comes from Inequality Eq. 18B.1, and the second inequality from Inequality Eq. 18B.2. Thus Inequality Eq. 18B.3 implies that the highest reward rate possible for the diffusion model, $RR_d(AC_d)$, is higher or equal than the highest possible reward rate in any other model, $RR_a(AC_a)$.

18C Appendix C: MSPRT

This appendix shows that the logarithm of the probability P_i defined in Eq. 18.10 is expressed by Eq. 18.11. We can compute P_i from the Bayes theorem:

$$P_i \equiv P(H_i \mid x(1..t)) = \frac{P(x(1..t) \mid H_i)P(H_i)}{P(x(1..t))}. \tag{18C.1}$$

As usual in statistical testing, we assume that one of the hypotheses H_i is correct, thus the probability of sensory evidence $P(x(1..t))$ is equal to the average probability of sensory evidence given the hypotheses (weighted by the prior probabilities of the hypotheses):

$$P_i = \frac{P(x(1..t) \mid H_i)P(H_i)}{\sum_{j=1}^{N} P(x(1..t) \mid H_j)P(H_j)}. \tag{18C.2}$$

Let us for simplicity assume that we do not have any prior knowledge favoring any of the alternatives, so the prior probabilities are equal (Section 18.4.3 shows how the prior probabilities can be incorporated). Then the prior probabilities in Eq. 18C.2 cancel and it becomes:

$$P_i = \frac{P(x(1..t)|\, H_i)}{\sum\limits_{j=1}^{N} P(x(1..t)|\, H_j)}. \tag{18C.3}$$

Now, recall that in Appendix 18A we have already evaluated a very similar ratio for a similar set of hypotheses. Following calculations like those in Appendix 18A, analogous cancellations happen, and Eq. 18C.3 becomes (cf. Eq. 18A.8):

$$P_i = \frac{\exp(gy_i)}{\sum\limits_{j=1}^{N} \exp(gy_j)}, \tag{18C.4}$$

where g is a constant defined in Eq. 18A.7. As we observed in Appendix 18A, the exponentiation of integrated evidence comes from the exponents present in the normal probability density function. If we take the logarithm of Eq. 18C.4, then the division becomes a subtraction:

$$\log P_i = \log \exp(gy_i) - \log \sum\limits_{j=1}^{N} \exp(gy_j). \tag{18C.5}$$

Equation 18C.5 involves two terms: In the first term the logarithm cancels the exponentiation so it becomes the integrated evidence (scaled by constant g), while the second is the *Conflict* in evidence (scaled by g). For simplicity, we ignore the constant g, because its precise value has been shown to be of little importance for performance [34], and then Eq. 18C.5 becomes Eq. 18.11.

18D   Appendix D: STN and GP can compute the optimal conflict

In this appendix, we show that if STN and GP have input-output relationship given by Eqs 18.13 and 18.14, then the sum of the activities of STN channels is equal to *Conflict*. Let us denote the activities of channel i in STN and GP by STN_i and GP_i respectively. The STN receives input from cortical integrators and inhibition from GP, hence

$$STN_i = \exp(y_i - GP_i). \tag{18D.1}$$

Let us denote the sum of activity of all STN channels by Σ:

$$\Sigma = \sum\limits_{j=1}^{N} STN_j. \tag{18D.2}$$

In the model of Fig. 18.2, GP receives input from all STN channels, hence

$$GP_i = \Sigma - \log \Sigma. \tag{18D.3}$$

Substituting Eq. 18D.3 into Eq. 18D.1 gives

$$STN_i = \exp(y_i - \Sigma + \log\Sigma). \tag{18D.4}$$

Using the property of exponentiation $e^{a+b} = e^a e^b$ we obtain:

$$STN_i = \exp(y_i)\exp(-\Sigma)\Sigma. \tag{18D.5}$$

Summing over i and using Eq. 18D.2 we obtain:

$$\Sigma = \sum_{i=1}^{N} \exp(y_i)\exp(-\Sigma)\Sigma. \tag{18D.6}$$

Taking the logarithm of Eq. 18D.6 we get:

$$\log\Sigma = \log\sum_{i=1}^{N}\exp y_i - \Sigma + \log\Sigma. \tag{18D.7}$$

$\log\Sigma$ cancels on both sides in Eq. 18D.7, and moving Σ on the left side we see that the sum of activities of all STN channels is equal to *Conflict*:

$$\Sigma = \log\sum_{i=1}^{N}\exp y_i. \tag{18D.8}$$

18E   Appendix E: Basal ganglia model is unaffected by inhibition of integrators

This appendix shows that if the same inhibition is applied to all cortical integrators projecting to the basal ganglia, the activity of the output nuclei in the model does not change. To see this property, we subtract *inh* from y_i in the first line of Eq. 18E.1 (cf. Eqs 18.8 and 18.12) and observe that *inh* cancels out (last equality in Eq. 18E.1) and the activity of the output nuclei does not change.

$$
\begin{aligned}
OUT_i &= -(y_i - inh) + \log\left(\sum_{j=1}^{N}\exp(y_j - inh)\right) = \\
&= -y_i + inh + \log\left(\left(\sum_{j=1}^{N}\exp y_j\right)\exp(-inh)\right) = \\
&= -y_i + inh + \log\left(\sum_{j=1}^{N}\exp y_j\right) + \log\exp(-inh) = -y_i + \log\left(\sum_{j=1}^{N}\exp y_j\right). \tag{18E.1}
\end{aligned}
$$

Acknowledgement

This work was supported by EPSRC grants EP/C514416/1 and EP/C516303/1. The author thanks Simon Chiu for reading the previous version of the manuscript and for his very useful comments.

References

[1] K.H. Britten, M.N. Shadlen, W.T. Newsome, J.A. Movshon, Responses of neurons in macaque MT to stochastic motion signals, Vis. Neurosci. 10 (1993) 1157–1169.

[2] M.N. Shadlen, W.T. Newsome, Neural basis of a perceptual decision in the parietal cortex (area LIP) of the rhesus monkey, J. Neurophysiol. 86 (2001) 1916–1936.

[3] J.D. Roitman, M.N. Shadlen, Response of neurons in the lateral intraparietal area during a combined visual discrimination reaction time task, J. Neurosci. 22 (2002) 9475–9489.

[4] J. Ditterich, M. Mazurek, M.N. Shadlen, Microstimulation of visual cortex affect the speed of perceptual decisions, Nat. Neurosci. 6 (2003) 891–898.

[5] J.D. Schall, Neural basis of deciding, choosing and acting, Nat. Rev. Neurosci. 2 (2001) 33–42.

[6] J.I. Gold, M.N. Shadlen, The neural basis of decision making, Annu. Rev. Neurosci. 30 (2007) 535–574.

[7] P. Cisek, J.F. Kalaska, Neural correlates of reaching decisions in dorsal premotor cortex: specification of multiple direction choices and final selection of action, Neuron 45 (2005) 801–814.

[8] H.R. Heekeren, S. Marrett, P.A. Bandettini, L.G. Ungerleider, A general mechanism for perceptual decision-making in the human brain, Nature 431 (2004) 859–862.

[9] K.G. Thompson, D.P. Hanes, N.P. Bichot, J.D. Schall, Perceptual and motor processing stages identified in the activity of macaque frontal eye field neurons during visual search, J. Neurophysiol. 76 (1996) 4040–4055.

[10] H.R. Heekeren, S. Marrett, L.G. Ungerleider, The neural systems that mediate human perceptual decision making, Nat. Rev. Neurosci. 9 (2008) 467–479.

[11] D. Vickers, Evidence for an accumulator model of psychophysical discrimination, Ergonomics 13 (1970) 37–58.

[12] D.R.J. Laming, Information Theory of Choice Reaction Time, Wiley, New York, 1968.

[13] R. Ratcliff, A theory of memory retrieval, Psychol. Rev. 83 (1978) 59–108.

[14] M. Stone, Models for choice reaction time, Psychometrika 25 (1960) 251–260.

[15] R. Bogacz, Optimal decision-making theories: linking neurobiology with behaviour, Trends Cogn. Sci. 11 (2007) 118–125.

[16] J.I. Gold, M.N. Shadlen, Neural computations that underlie decisions about sensory stimuli, Trends Cogn. Sci. 5 (2001) 10–16.

[17] J.I. Gold, M.N. Shadlen, Banburismus and the brain: decoding the relationship between sensory stimuli, decisions, and reward, Neuron 36 (2002) 299–308.

[18] A. Wald, Sequential Analysis, Wiley, New York, 1947.

[19] A. Wald, J. Wolfowitz, Optimum character of the sequential probability ratio test, Ann. Math. Stat. 19 (1948) 326–339.

[20] R. Bogacz, E. Brown, J. Moehlis, P. Holmes, J.D. Cohen, The physics of optimal decision making: a formal analysis of models of performance in two-alternative forced choice tasks, Psychol. Rev. 113 (2006) 700–765.

[21] D.P. Hanes, J.D. Schall, Neural control of voluntary movement initiation, Science 274 (1996) 427–430.

[22] M.E. Mazurek, J.D. Roitman, J. Ditterich, M.N. Shadlen, A role for neural integrators in perceptual decision making, Cereb. Cortex 13 (2003) 1257–1269.

[23] M. Usher, J.L. McClelland, The time course of perceptual choice: the leaky, competing accumulator model, Psychol. Rev. 108 (2001) 550–592.

[24] X.J. Wang, Probabilistic decision making by slow reverberation in cortical circuits, Neuron 36 (2002) 955–968.

[25] K.-F. Wong, X.-J. Wang, A recurrent network mechanism of time integration in perceptual decisions, J. Neurosci. 26 (2006) 1314–1328.

[26] R. Ratcliff, R. Gomez, G. McKoon, A diffusion model account of the lexical decision task, Psychol. Rev. 111 (2004) 159–182.

[27] R. Ratcliff, J.N. Rouder, A diffusion model account of masking in two-choice letter identification, J. Exp. Psychol. Hum. Percept. Perform. 26 (2000) 127–140.

[28] R. Ratcliff, A. Thapar, G. McKoon, A diffusion model analysis of the effects of aging on brightness discrimination, Percept. Psychophys. 65 (2003) 523–535.

[29] R. Ratcliff, A. Cherian, M. Segraves, A comparison of macaques behavior and superior colliculus neuronal activity to predictions from models of two-choice decisions, J. Neurophysiol. 90 (2003) 1392–1407.

[30] R. Ratcliff, P.L. Smith, Comparison of sequential sampling models for two-choice reaction time, Psychol. Rev. 111 (2004) 333–367.

[31] P.L. Smith, R. Ratcliff, Psychology and neurobiology of simple decisions, Trends Neurosci. 27 (2004) 161–168.

[32] T.D. Hanks, J. Ditterich, M.N. Shadlen, Microstimulation of macaque area LIP affects decision-making in a motion discrimination task, Nat. Neurosci. 9 (2006) 682–689.

[33] J. Ditterich, Stochastic models of decisions about motion direction: behavior and physiology, Neural Netw. 19 (2006) 981–1012.

[34] R. Bogacz, K. Gurney, The basal ganglia and cortex implement optimal decision making between alternative actions, Neural Comput. 19 (2007) 442–477.

[35] C.W. Baum, V.V. Veeravalli, A sequential procedure for multihypothesis testing, IEEE Trans. Inf. Theory 40 (1994) 1996–2007.

[36] P. Redgrave, T.J. Prescott, K. Gurney, The basal ganglia: a vertebrate solution to the selection problem? Neuroscience 89 (1999) 1009–1023.

[37] G. Chevalier, S. Vacher, J.M. Deniau, M. Desban, Disinhibition as a basic process in the expression of striatal functions. I. The striato-nigral influence on tecto-spinal/tecto-diencephalic neurons, Brain Res. 334 (1985) 215–226.

[38] J.M. Deniau, G. Chevalier, Disinhibition as a basic process in the expression of striatal functions. II. The striato-nigral influence on thalamocortical cells of the ventromedial thalamic nucleus, Brain Res. 334 (1985) 227–233.

[39] A.P. Georgopoulos, M.R. DeLong, M.D. Crutcher, Relations between parameters of step-tracking movements and single cell discharge in the globus pallidus and subthalamic nucleus of the behaving monkey, J. Neurosci. 3 (1983) 1586–1598.

[40] E. Gerardin, S. Lehericy, J.B. Pochon, S.T. Montcel, J.F. Mangin, F. Poupon, Y. Agid, D. Le Bihan, C. Marsault, Foot, hand, face and eye representation in human striatum, Cereb. Cortex 13 (2003) 162–169.

[41] G.E. Alexander, M.R. DeLong, P.L. Strick, Parallel organization of functionally segregated circuits linking basal ganglia and cortex, Annu. Rev. Neurosci. 9 (1986) 357–381.

[42] K. Gurney, T.J. Prescott, P. Redgrave, A computational model of action selection in the basal ganglia. I. A new functional anatomy, Biol. Cybern. 84 (2001) 401–410.

[43] A. Parent, L.N. Hazrati, Anatomical aspects of information processing in primate basal ganglia, Trends Neurosci. 16 (1993) 111–116.

[44] A. Parent, Y. Smith, Organization of efferent projections of the subthalamic nucleus in the squirrel monkey as revealed by retrograde labeling methods, Brain Res. 436 (1987) 296–310.

[45] M.J. Frank, L.C. Seeberger, R.C. O'Reilly, By carrot or by stick: cognitive reinforcement learning in parkinsonism, Science 306 (2004) 1940–1943.

[46] R. Bogacz, optimal decision-making in cortico-basal-ganglia-thalamic loops, forum of European Neuroscience, Geneva, Abstracts, 126.2 (2008).

[47] V.P. Dragalin, A.G. Tertakovsky, V.V. Veeravalli, Multihypothesis sequential probability ratio tests – part I: asymptotic optimality, IEEE Trans. Inf. Theory 45 (1999) 2448–2461.

[48] T. McMillen, P. Holmes, The dynamics of choice among multiple alternatives, J. Math. Psychol. 50 (2006) 30–57.

[49] M.J. Frank, Hold your horses: a dynamic computational role for the subthalamic nucleus in decision making, Neural Netw. 19 (2006) 1120–1136.

[50] J.W. Mink, The basal ganglia: focused selection and inhibition of competing motor programs, Prog. Neurobiol. 50 (1996) 381–425.

[51] M.J. Frank, J. Samanta, A.A. Moustafa, S.J. Sherman, Hold your horses: impulsivity, deep brain stimulation, and medication in parkinsonism, Science 318 (2007) 1309–1312.

[52] M. Jahanshahi, C.M. Ardouin, R.G. Brown, J.C. Rothwell, J. Obeso, A. Albanese, M.C. Rodriguez-Oroz, E. Moro, A.L. Benabid, P. Pollak, P. Limousin-Dowsey, The impact of deep brain stimulation on executive function in Parkinson's disease, Brain 123 (Pt 6) (2000) 1142–1154.

[53] N.E. Hallworth, C.J. Wilson, M.D. Bevan, Apamin-sensitive small conductance calcium-activated potassium channels, through their selective coupling to voltage-gated calcium channels, are critical determinants of the precision, pace, and pattern of action potential generation in rat subthalamic nucleus neurons in vitro, J. Neurosci. 23 (2003) 7525–7542.

[54] C.J. Wilson, A. Weyrick, D. Terman, N.E. Hallworth, M.D. Bevan, A model of reverse spike frequency adaptation and repetitive firing of subthalamic nucleus neurons, J. Neurophysiol. 91 (2004) 1963–1980.

[55] Z.M. Williams, J.S. Neimat, G.R. Cosgrove, E.N. Eskandar, Timing and direction selectivity of subthalamic and pallidal neurons in patients with Parkinson disease, Exp. Brain Res. 162 (2005) 407–416.

[56] H. Kita, S.T. Kitai, Intracellular study of rat globus pallidus neurons: membrane properties and responses to neostriatal, subthalamic and nigral stimulation, Brain Res. 564 (1991) 296–305.

[57] A. Nambu, R. Llinas, Electrophysiology of globus pallidus neurons in vitro, J. Neurophysiol. 72 (1994) 1127–1139.

[58] D. Norris, The Bayesian reader: explaining word recognition as an optimal Bayesian decision process, Psychol. Rev. 113 (2006) 327–357.

[59] M.L. Platt, P.W. Glimcher, Neural correlates of decision variables in parietal cortex, Nature 400 (1999) 233–238.

[60] T. Yang, M.N. Shadlen, Probabilistic reasoning by neurons, Nature 447 (2007) 1075–1080.

[61] R.H. Carpenter, M.L. Williams, Neural computation of log likelihood in control of saccadic eye movements, Nature 377 (1995) 59–62.

[62] M.A. Basso, R.H. Wurtz, Modulation of neuronal activity in superior colliculus by changes in target probability, J. Neurosci. 18 (1998) 7519–7534.

[63] M.C. Dorris, P.W. Glimcher, Activity in posterior parietal cortex is correlated with the relative subjective desirability of action, Neuron 44 (2004) 365–378.

19 The basal ganglia in reward and decision making: computational models and empirical studies

Bradley B. Doll and Michael J. Frank

Department of Cognitive and Linguistic Science and Department of Psychology, Brown University, 190 Thayer St., Providence, RI 02912-1978

Abstract

The basal ganglia (BG) are implicated in a wide variety of motor and cognitive behaviors, making it difficult to extract a unifying function of these brain structures. We review a series of neurocomputational models that focus on the action selection and reinforcement learning functions of the BG, and their modulation by dopamine, as constrained by a broad range of data. We begin with the "basic" model, which forms the core mechanism for later appended models including the roles of norepinephrine, cognitive and affective components of prefrontal cortex, and the interaction between verbal instructions and reinforcement learning. We further review experiments designed to test model predictions as a function of disease, medications, genetics, and behavioral manipulations. Abstract mathematical models that have been used in conjunction with these accounts are also discussed.

Key points

1. Separate "Go" and "NoGo" neuronal populations within the striatum represent positive and negative values of actions, with their relative difference determining the probability that an action is selected.
2. These populations learn from positive and negative decision outcomes via dopaminergic modulation of D1 and D2 receptors.
3. The subthalamic nucleus (STN) additionally modulates the overall decision threshold in proportion to response/reinforcement conflict, and prevents impulsive choice when multiple actions are potentially rewarding.
4. Human experiments support these assertions: Go and NoGo learning are oppositely affected by dopaminergic manipulation, whereas STN stimulation leads to impulsive high-conflict decisions.
5. Appended models include the roles of cortical norepinephrine (NE) for adapting the exploration versus exploitation trade-off, and prefrontal cortical regions for maintaining reward and goal-directed information in working memory.

19.1   Introduction

In recent years, computational models of learning and decision making have become increasingly prevalent in psychology and neuroscience. These models describe brain function across a wide range of levels, from highly detailed models of ion channels and compartments of individual neurons [1], to abstract models that focus on the cognitive machinations the brain appears to produce [2]. Here we focus on the ground gained through the use of neural network models that fall in the middle of this range, constrained by both implementational and functional considerations. These models seek to uncover how learning at the cognitive level arises from core biological principles of the brain, in terms of neuronal function and systems-level interactions between multiple brain areas.

We discuss a series of interrelated models of corticostriatal circuits, the development of which was constrained by a variety of data on multiple levels of analysis, from physiology to behavior. The models have been successful in predicting behavioral outcomes resulting from manipulations of basal ganglia (BG) functionality via medications, diseases, disorders, and genetics. We also discuss how core computational principles can be extracted from complex neural models to develop simplified models in abstract mathematical form, which in turn can be quantitatively fit to behavioral data to test specific hypotheses. Such models are also useful for deriving best-fitting model parameters to correlate with biological signals (e.g., as in functional neuroimaging; see Chapter 10), which can be used for further refinement and development of mechanistic principles.

19.2   BG circuitry and function

The basic network model we describe captures the action selection function of the BG [3–5]. This assembly of deep brain structures receives multiple candidate behaviors from cortex, and performs a critical organizational task by "gating" the most appropriate response while suppressing competing responses [6]. The striatum (including the caudate, putamen, and nucleus accumbens) receives this input and projects output to the globus pallidus (and substantia nigra), which in turn projects to the thalamus [7]. The thalamus projects back to cortex, completing the corticostriatal loop. The anatomy of these structures facilitates action selection along the "direct" and "indirect" pathways which facilitate and inhibit response execution, respectively [8,9]. Many updates to this anatomy have been provided since the basic Albin et al. [9] functional model was conceived (see Chapter 1), many of which are incorporated in the network models we describe below. Nevertheless, the basic segregation of direct and indirect pathways remains a fundamental aspect of many contemporary models and has enormous support.

The effects of striatal activity at the thalamus differ between the direct and indirect pathway by an additional synapse along the indirect pathway. In the direct pathway, striatal activity inhibits the internal segment of the globus pallidus (GPi), which tonically inhibits the thalamus (Fig. 19.1A and 19.1B). Thus, direct pathway activity *disinhibits* the thalamus, allowing an action to be executed. Along the indirect pathway, striatal projection neurons synapse at the external segment of the globus pallidus (GPe). Because the GPe sends inhibitory projections to the GPi [10], striatal inhibition of the GPe allows the tonic activation of the GPi to rise, further inhibiting the thalamus. Anatomical evidence suggests that these striatal projections to GPi and GPe constitute independent "subloops" within the circuit [8].

The counteractive effects of the two pathways constitute the core mechanics of the action selection faculties of the BG. The multitude of independent subloops to and from

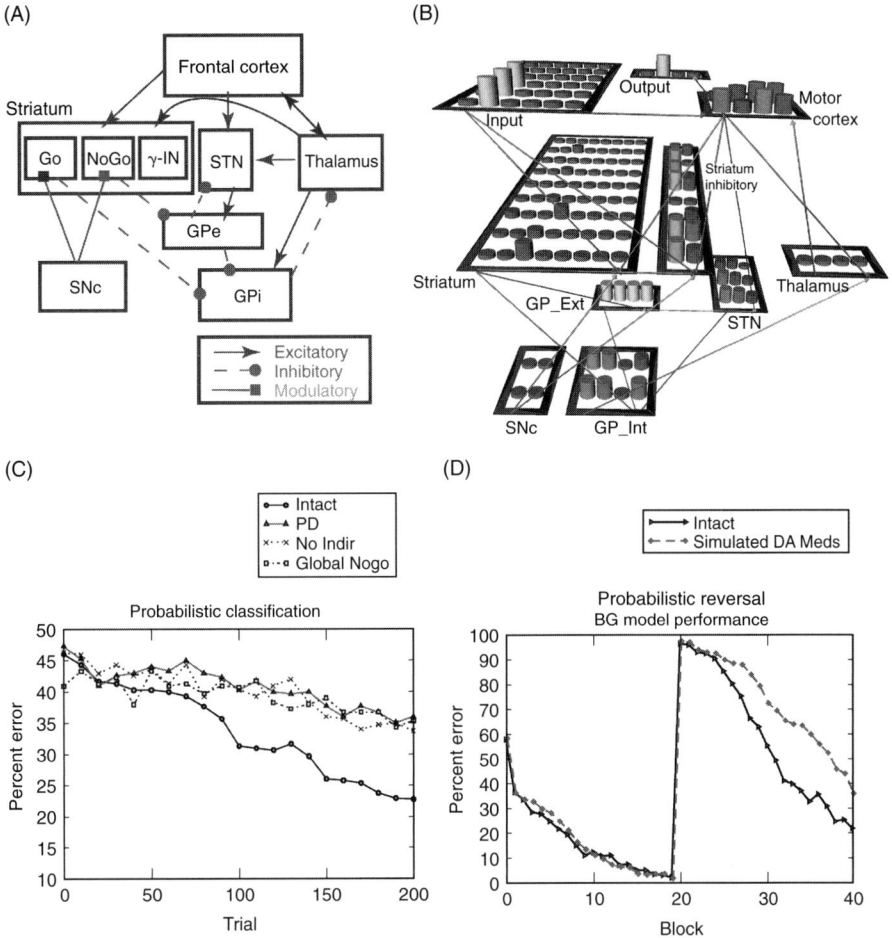

Figure 19.1 (A) Functional anatomy of the BG circuit. In addition to the classic "direct" and "indirect" pathways from striatum to BG output nuclei originating in striatonigral (Go) and striatopallidal (NoGo) cells, respectively, this updated architecture features focused projections from NoGo units to GPe and strong top-down projections from cortex to thalamus. Further, the STN is incorporated as part of a hyperdirect pathway, receiving inputs from frontal cortex and projecting directly to both GPe and GPi. (B) Neural network model of this circuit, with four different responses represented by four columns of motor units, four columns each of Go and NoGo units within striatum, and corresponding columns within GPi, GPe, and thalamus. In this updated model, fast-spiking GABA-ergic interneurons (γ-IN) regulate striatal activity via inhibitory projections. (C) Probabilistic learning, simulating the challenging probabilistic classification "weather prediction" task. Models with simulated PD were impaired at learning to resolve complex probabilistic discriminations [153], as were models without the indirect NoGo pathway, or with only nonspecific "Global" NoGo representations. (D) Model probabilistic reversal learning. Simulated medication, via partial blockade of DA dips, led to selectively impaired reversal, as seen in medicated patients [11]. See Plate 21 of Color Plate section.

different cortical regions allows a single action to be executed, while all other candidate actions are suppressed [6]. Dopaminergic nigrostriatal projections affect this selection process synergistically, as dopamine (DA) excites cells in the direct pathway while inhibiting those in the indirect pathway.

A great deal of research has shown phasic increases in striatal DA upon the appearance of unpredicted rewards (positive prediction errors), and, more controversially, phasic decreases when predicted rewards are not received (negative prediction errors) [12,13]. For simplicity, we do not focus our discussion here on mechanisms upstream of the DA system, which include the amygdala, ventral striatum, and other structures (see Chapter 1 and O'Reilly et al. [14] for a model). In reinforcement learning theory, these structures would all contribute to the "critic" [15], that is, the Pavlovian association of environmental state with value [16]. Instead, given that these phasic DA signals are computed, our models focus on how they drive learning and choice in the downstream "actor."

Phasic DA signals differentially affect activity in the direct and indirect pathways via the excitatory effects of DA at D1 receptors and the inhibitory effects at D2 receptors. While D1 receptors are most prevalent in the direct pathway, D2 receptors predominate in the indirect pathway [17–19]. This localization supports the facilitatory role of DA in action selection, where increases activate the direct pathway and inhibit the indirect pathway [20] and decreases of DA have the opposite effect [19,21].

In addition to modulating activity in the BG, DA also drives learning in the form of synaptic modification in the corticostriatal pathway. Evidence indicates that the presence of DA facilitates long-term potentiation (LTP) at D1 receptors and long-term depression at D2 receptors [22,23]. Our model described below also predicted that during negative prediction errors associated with DA dips [12,13,24,25], there would be LTP in D2-containing neurons in the indirect pathway [21]. Recent studies support this basic assumption of the model, showing that whereas synaptic potentiation in the direct pathway is dependent on D1 receptor stimulation, potentiation in the indirect pathway is dependent on a *lack* of D2 receptor stimulation [26].

19.2.1 *From motor to cognitive actions*

Though classically thought to organize motor behaviors, evidence suggests that this action selection mechanism also facilitates cognitive homologues of motor acts such as decision making and working memory updating [4,5,21,27–29]. Decisions in psychology experiments, like decisions in life, ultimately reduce to discriminations between available behaviors: whether to press the left button or the right button when confronted with a particular stimulus in a particular context; whether to devote time to writing a grant proposal, or spend it conducting experiments. Similarly, internal behaviors must be chosen among: whether to continue to maintain current contents of working memory, or to update with new incoming stimuli; whether to continue focusing on this chapter while screening out less relevant background information, or to attend to the song on the radio and update working memory with the artist's name so you can download it from iTunes. The BG mechanisms we outline here allow the brain to pick between these options.

19.3 Basic model

Though the modified models we describe below feature added structures, all share the same core action selection gating structure of the BG, consistent with the existence of multiple parallel loops linking BG with different parts of frontal cortex [7]. Here, we describe how the basic model maps onto the biology of the BG before turning to novel model predictions and their recent empirical support.

The network models (Fig. 19.1B) are implemented in the Leabra neural simulation framework [30]. Membrane potentials are simulated via differential equations as a function of ionic excitation, inhibition, and leak conductances. A "point neuron" activation function is used to approximate the integrated membrane potential of the neuron and convert it to a single rate-coded activation of the network units with a function that approximates that produced by spiking units[1]. Learning is simulated via changes in synaptic connection strengths among units in the network via Hebbian and contrastive Hebbian principles. Finally, the effects of DA are simulated by modulating relative Go and NoGo activity in the striatum. For mathematical details of the models, please refer to the appendices of Frank [21,31].

The basic BG model is based on the classical direct/indirect pathway model described above, but also includes several anatomical and physiological updates, and explores their dynamics during action selection (within a trial) and as a function of learning/plasticity (across trials). See Cohen and Frank [32] for a detailed discussion of other aspects of BG physiology not discussed here, including the roles of striatal interneurons and other anatomical projections.

The BG model [21] features simulated layers for core structures in the corticostriatal loop (striatum, GPe, GPi, thalamus, premotor cortex, and substantia nigra; Fig. 19.1B). Parameters of the units in these various layers are tuned to match the general properties and excitability of those in the corresponding brain regions (see Frank [31], for parameter values and biological correspondence). Input is received into the BG system via the sensory cortex, and output is produced at the motor cortex. While simpler models might be developed to describe the learning functions of the BG, inclusion of these various layers affords a view into how their interaction produces a dynamic feedback control system for selecting among multiple alternative actions.

By experiencing phasic dopaminergic feedback the basic model can learn the statistics (probabilities of reward for each stimulus–response mapping) of a number of task environments [21,33]. In such environments, an input stimulus appearing in sensory cortex activates units in premotor cortex prior to striatum, in accordance with physiological evidence [6,34,35]. Activity directly induced in the premotor cortex is insufficient to execute a response, and requires additional "bottom-up" support from the BG by way of the thalamus to drive response activity above threshold. Striatal units receive sensory input projections together with information about activated cortical motor representations, and can then evaluate whether or not to "gate" the response currently being considered [21]. Activation of striatal "Go" units in the direct pathway results in inhibition of the GPi, which releases the thalamus from tonic inhibition and allows a given premotor cortical response to surpass threshold. Simultaneously, other responses are suppressed by activation of striatal "NoGo" units in the indirect pathway. This activity has an opposing effect via an extra inhibitory synapse through GPe before projecting to GPi [10], thereby preventing the execution of the corresponding response.

Following response selection, the model receives positive or negative feedback depending on its choice and the programmed task contingencies. The critical components of

---

[1]Note that this rate-coded simplification is used in the majority of our simulations, but spiking units can also be incorporated into the model, without a loss of generality. Preliminary simulations with spiking units, though noisier, are consistent with the rate-coded results we discuss in this chapter. Future work will incorporate these biological details, allowing more detailed examination of spike-timing dependencies (e.g., in plasticity [26]).

this feedback are the phasic DA bursts and dips which accompany positive and negative feedback, respectively. Bursts of simulated DA drive positive weight changes between the stimulus representation in sensory cortex and Go units, just as DA has been shown to facilitate LTP in corticostriatal synapses via D1 receptors [22,26,36–38]. These weight changes increase the efficacy of the input stimulus in eliciting the same Go unit activity the next time it is encountered. In complement, DA dips accompanying negative feedback increase activity of NoGo cells due to the removal of inhibitory effects of DA at D2 receptors [21,26]. This increases the efficacy of the stimulus in eliciting the same NoGo unit activity the next time it is encountered. By these complementary learning mechanisms, the model learns to select stimulus–response conjunctions that have a high probability of yielding reward, and to avoid those with a low probability of reward. In addition to this DA-dependent learning, the model learns along the direct sensory to motor cortex projection. This relatively slower learning ingrains repeatedly selected actions as "habits," and becomes increasingly independent of BG activity over time [21,39,40].

On the surface, parallel Go and NoGo pathways appear superfluous. Either path on its own should be sufficient to learn which behaviors are the most advantageous in any environment (e.g., by simply facilitating the action with highest Go activity). This ostensible redundancy may, however, belie an adaptive choice mechanism. By simultaneously learning positive (Go) and negative (NoGo) probabilistic associations, the contrast between the two can be enhanced beyond what either pathway would learn on its own, making the discrimination easier [32], and resulting in better probabilistic discrimination when both pathways are included (Fig. 19.1C) [21]. Further, the independence of these pathways may actually enhance adaptive responses in complex environments. Suppose a specific response is rewarding in most contexts but punishing in other similar contexts. By learning NoGo associations that link the specific aspects of the negative context to the response, aversive outcomes can be avoided without unlearning the Go associations which are adaptive in other contexts. In the absence of these dual pathways associations would have to be relearned each time the environment changed.

19.4   Empirical support for basic model

The basic model, having been built to account for existing cognitive and physiological data [21], generated a number of predictions subsequently supported by experiments [41–43]. These experiments reinforce the notion that DA dips and bursts drive Go and NoGo learning in probabilistic environments. They also indicate that separable mechanisms govern learning from positive and negative feedback.

To test the model predictions, a probabilistic selection task was designed, in which participants repeatedly choose among three different forced-choice stimulus pairings and receive probabilistic positive and negative feedback (Fig. 19.2A). Upon attaining sufficient accuracy on the individual training pairs, participants are then tested with a novel transfer phase in which all possible pairings of stimuli (some having been rewarded more often than others) are presented without feedback. In this test phase, preference for the most reliably rewarding stimulus is a measure of Go learning. Conversely, avoidance of the most reliably punishing stimulus is a measure of NoGo learning.

If Go and NoGo learning are indeed dissociable, and driven by the differential effects of DA at D1 and D2 receptors as the model suggests, changes in tonic and phasic DA induced by drugs or pathology in humans should produce learning changes similar to those produced by changes in simulated DA in the model. Indeed, in the probabilistic

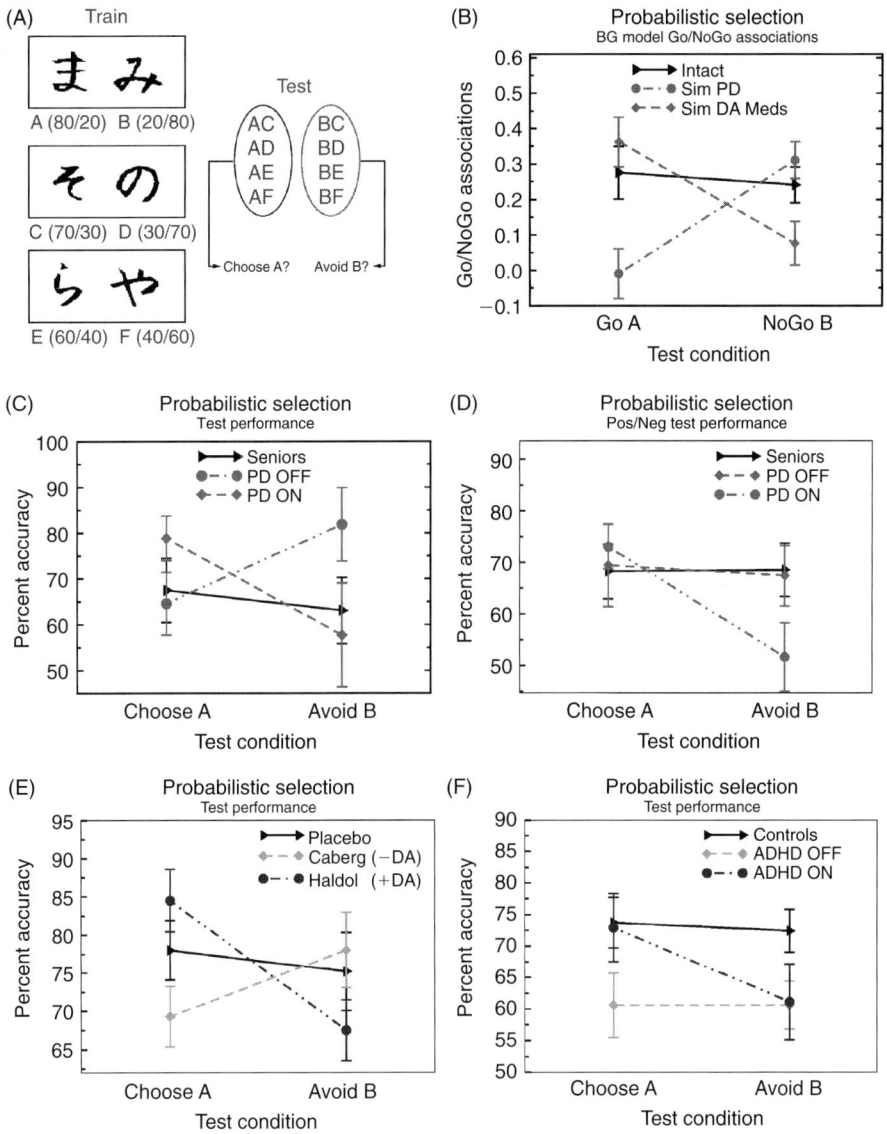

Figure 19.2 (A) Example stimulus pairs (Hiragana symbols) used in the probabilistic selection task, intended to minimize verbal encoding. One pair is presented per trial, selection results in the probabilistic positive/negative feedback shown. At test, all combinations are serially presented and no feedback follows choice. (B) BG model predictions for PD patients in this task, showing relative Go and NoGo striatal activation states when presented with stimulus A and B respectively. Error bars reflect standard error across 25 model runs with random initial weights. (C) Test performance in PD patients and healthy senior controls where choosing A depends on having learned from positive feedback, while avoiding B depends on having learned from negative feedback [41]. (D) Replication in another group of patients, where the most prominent effects were observed in the NoGo learning condition [45]. (E) Similar results in healthy participants on DA agonists and antagonists [42] and (F) adult ADHD participants on and off stimulant medications [44].

selection task, low levels of striatal DA were associated with impaired Go learning, but, if anything, *enhanced* NoGo learning, whereas DA levels tonically elevated by DA medications produced spared or enhanced Go learning, but caused substantial *deficits* in NoGo learning [41–46]. Below, we elaborate how these effects are borne out in the *a priori* model that motivated the experiments in the first place, and their implication for Parkinson's disease (PD) and related disorders.

19.4.1   *PD and medication effects*

PD is marked by the death of dopaminergic cells in the substantia nigra [47]. The resulting reduction in DA produces the rigidity and quiescence characteristic of the disease. PD patients are typically treated with DA replacement medication, such as L-dopa, a DA precursor which elevates spike-dependent phasic DA release [48–51]. It is at present unclear whether L-dopa also elevates tonic DA levels. While this treatment alleviates motor symptoms, over time it often produces unintended motor tics called dyskinesia. Curiously, some PD patients also develop decision-making problems (such as pathological gambling, hypersexuality, compulsive medication consumption, etc.) when taking such medication [52,53]. Simulations of increased and decreased DA levels in the model offer clarification of the mechanisms underlying these behavioral changes in patients.

In the model, PD was simulated by reducing the number of intact DA units in the substantia nigra, and hence both tonic and phasic DA levels. This reduction decreases learning along the direct/Go pathway, due to decreased D1 stimulation, but actually increases learning along the indirect/NoGo pathway [21]. The latter enhancement of NoGo learning is a product of the D2 receptor disinhibition that results from DA reduction. In the healthy brain, DA dips are phasic and accompany negative prediction errors. In contrast, PD results in abnormally low tonic levels of DA, which causes hyperexcitability in NoGo cells [19,54]. Via simple Hebbian principles, the resulting increased activation leads to enhanced potentiation of corticostriatal NoGo units [21]. Both of the above posited effects – reduced Go/D1-dependent synaptic potentiation together with elevated NoGo/D2-dependent potentiation – were recently confirmed experimentally in a mouse model of PD [26]. This mechanism was sufficient to simulate the relatively *enhanced* learning from negative feedback in non-medicated human Parkinson's patients (Fig. 19.2B–19.2D) [41,45].

Although the majority of early cognitive studies in PD tested medicated patients, it is now clear that medication status is a major factor, as it improves some aspects of cognition while impairing others [11,21,51]. Chronic administration of L-dopa (the main DA medication used to treat PD) has been shown to increase expression of *zif-268*, an immediate early gene that has been linked with synaptic plasticity [55], in striatonigral (Go), but not striatopallidal (NoGo) neurons [56]. In the models, DA medication is simulated by increasing DA levels (both tonic and phasic). Because delivery of the pharmacological drug cannot account for time periods in which DA levels *should* be low (i.e., during negative prediction errors), their continual stimulation of D2 receptors leads to inhibition of the NoGo pathway and concomitantly impaired NoGo learning [21]. Again, direct physiological evidence for this mechanism was recently reported, whereby D2 receptor stimulation eliminated synaptic potentiation in the NoGo pathway [25]. Simulations revealed that these effects were sufficient to produce relatively enhanced positive feedback learning but impaired negative feedback learning, as in medicated human patients [41,45] (Fig. 19.2B). Moreover, this same mechanism was originally simulated to account for impaired probabilistic reversal learning in medicated patients (Fig. 19.1D)

[11,21], an effect later confirmed to be due to impaired learning from negative prediction errors [43].

These findings are not restricted to the relatively extreme case of PD. Even in healthy aging, striatal dopaminergic function declines [57–60], accounting for many cognitive deficits seen in older age [61,62]. Nevertheless, according to the model, low levels of striatal DA should actually *facilitate* probabilistic NoGo learning, as in PD. Indeed, it was found that those older than 70 years of age show relatively improved NoGo learning compared with adults between 60 and 70 years of age [63].

Thus far, the majority of work undertaken to test model predictions has utilized forced alternative choice task paradigms, providing mechanisms for how specific decisions are made. However, the same model also predicts that the *speed* at which responses are made should also vary as a function of relative Go and NoGo activation states for that response (which in turn reflect prior Go and NoGo learning from positive and negative prediction errors)[2]. Thus, recent work has also explored temporal aspects of choice [64] in a task in which participants make a single response, but in which their response time (RT) is associated with different expected reward values. Despite being a completely different stimulus environment and task context, at the level of Go and NoGo learning results were identical to what we had found in earlier studies: Relative to baseline RT for each participant, PD patients off medication were relatively impaired at Go learning to speed RTs to maximize positive prediction errors, but showed intact NoGo learning to slow RTs to avoid negative prediction errors. Again, medication reversed this bias, with patients showing better speeding but worse slowing. This same pattern of findings was also produced by the BG model (without changing any of its parameters) when presented with precisely the same task reward contingencies, measuring the time it took to facilitate a response [64].

19.4.2   Pharmacological studies in healthy participants

We tested young (college-aged), healthy participants under pharmacological challenge in a repeated measures within-subject design: once on placebo, once on the D2 agonist cabergoline, and once on the D2 antagonist haloperidol [42]. At the low doses used in this study, these drugs exert their effects primarily through presynaptic mechanisms [65], which modulate phasic DA release [66]. Autoreceptor stimulation by D2 agonists *reduces* phasic DA release, while D2 antagonists *increase* phasic DA release in the BG [67–72]. In agreement, while on low doses of haloperidol, participants demonstrated enhanced Go and impaired NoGo learning relative to their own placebo state; cabergoline produced the opposite pattern (Fig. 19.2E) [42]. Further, a consistent pattern of findings was also observed in a different "probabilistic Go/NoGo paradigm" in which only a single stimulus was presented in each trial and participants had to either respond (Go) or withhold their response altogether (NoGo) [42]. Similarly, Pizzagalli and colleagues administered low doses of pramipexole, a D2/D3 agonist, and found converging results in yet a different probabilistic reward learning paradigm [73,74]. Similar to previous accounts [42], the reduced positive reinforcement learning effects were interpreted as resulting from primarily presynaptic reductions in phasic DA. Indeed, when our BG model was presented with the same probabilistic contingencies faced by humans in this paradigm, it exhibited very similar patterns of results [74].

---

[2]This is because the BG output computes relative Go-NoGo activity for each response, and the stronger the difference, the earlier the response will be disinhibited.

19.4.3   Complications and qualifications

Despite these largely convergent results across multiple studies, populations, and pharmacological agents, the state of affairs is not always so straightforward. In particular, in the working memory domain, many studies report that the effects of DA drugs are dependent on participants' baseline working memory span [75–77]. Our previous pharmacological study [42] showed that this baseline dependency applies not only to performance on working memory tasks, but also to the extent to which drugs modulate Go and NoGo probabilistic reinforcement learning. That is, while the above-described effects of cabergoline and haloperidol were significant across all participants, the relative increase in Go learning by haloperidol was observed only in those with low working memory span, whereas the opposite effect of cabergoline was observed only in those with high working memory span. We [42] further reported that a series of otherwise perplexing working memory span-dependent effects of D2 drugs across reinforcement learning, working memory, and attentional shifting domains could all be accounted for by assuming that baseline span was accompanied by differences in the striatal DA system and hence differential sensitivity to D2 drugs. Intriguingly, Cools and colleagues [78] provided direct evidence for this conjecture using positron emission tomography (PET), finding that differences in working memory capacity were accompanied by differences in striatal DA synthesis capacity. More recently, it was shown that individual differences in striatal DA were also predictive of relative learning from positive versus negative prediction errors, and their sensitivity to a D2 drug [79] – largely consistent with the findings and interpretation of Frank and O'Reilly [42]. See below for possible genetic factors that could contribute to these individual difference effects.

Others [80] (see Chapter 12) report data that appear to support a role for DA in Go but not NoGo learning. These investigators administered either L-dopa, which increases presynaptic DA synthesis and is the primary drug used to treat PD, haloperidol, a D2 receptor antagonist, or placebo to healthy participants in a neuroimaging experiment. In one stimulus pairing, participants could either win points or get nothing, whereas in another pairing they could either lose points or get nothing. L-dopa enhanced learning in the win condition, but groups did not differ in the loss condition. The absence of a loss effect is contrary to the prediction of our model, in which DA manipulation should affect NoGo learning. However, note that in this paradigm, reward prediction errors may be computed relative to the learned expected value for each stimulus pairing, such that in the "loss" condition, a null outcome would actually reflect a positive prediction error[3]. The resulting phasic DA burst could drive Go learning to reinforce the response made, allowing the continuing avoidance of the negative outcome. O'Doherty and colleagues [82] present imaging results consistent with this interpretation, showing that avoiding a potentially aversive outcome is associated with activation of the same brain regions associated with positive rewards. Thus, by this account, both "gain" and "loss" conditions in the Pessiglione et al. [80] study could involve some learning from positive prediction errors, which would explain the lack of statistical interaction between conditions (and why the effects of L-dopa in the loss condition were in the same

---

[3]This hypothesis raises an interesting dilemma: learning that a stimulus context has a negative expected value in the first place would require learning from negative prediction errors, so that this learning would have to be at least somewhat spared. However, this learning about particular Pavlovian state values may depend on the "critic." This kind of aversive state learning has been proposed to rely on serotonin signaling rather than dopamine [82], so it is possible that one can learn a negative state value using that system and then, when a loss is avoided, learn from positive DA-mediated prediction errors to drive Go responding in order to continue avoiding the loss.

numerical direction). Alternatively, the single low doses of drugs used in that study make it even more likely that the drug had preferential effects on enhancing phasic DA bursts, but not tonic DA, [48–50], thereby having no detrimental effects on NoGo learning. Finally, relative to haloperidol, L-dopa increased reward learning and brain signals associated with it [80]. Although this may seem at odds with our claim (based on physiological evidence) that low doses of haloperidol actually enhance phasic DA signals – and so should produce similar effects to L-dopa – the haloperidol dose used was quite low (1 mg, compared to 2–5 mg in several other studies), and did not have statistically significant effects relative to placebo.

19.4.4   Genetics

All of these findings between DA-divergent groups raise the question of whether even in healthy, non-medicated individuals, perhaps there are individual differences in learning from positive versus negative decision outcomes. Indeed, although on average healthy participants show roughly equal Go and NoGo learning, individual participants can still perform better on one measure or the other. These subgroups, which preferentially learn from positive or negative feedback, can be reliably distinguished according to reinforcement-related brain potentials using EEG [83,84] and BOLD responses in fMRI [85]. In principle, it is possible that these learning biases arise from a combination of psychological, cultural, and experiential factors. Still, we reasoned that they could (at least in part) stem from genetic differences in BG dopaminergic function (see Chapter 14). We therefore collected DNA from college students and tested them with the probabilistic selection task [86]. Polymorphisms within three genes affecting different aspects of BG and prefrontal DA function were assayed. First, a genetic mutation in DARPP-32 [87], a protein that is highly concentrated in the striatum and is associated with striatal D1-receptor dependent plasticity [88,89], was found to predict relatively better Go learning in the probabilistic selection task (Fig. 19.3A). Conversely, a polymorphism in the DRD2 gene, associated with increased striatal D2 receptor density [90], was strongly predictive of NoGo learning (Fig. 19.3B) ([86]; see also [85] for a similar D2 effect). This genetic dissociation between D1- and D2-mediated learning was further confirmed by a computational analysis in which striatal genes were found to modulate parametric learning rates from positive and negative prediction errors [86]. Moreover, the same genetic effects were replicated in another sample of participants in the context of the temporal decision-making task described above [64,91]. Together with the complementary pharmacological findings, these data provide very suggestive evidence in support of the specific model predictions. Moreover, they are in striking accord with synaptic plasticity studies mentioned above showing D1-dependent effects in Go neurons and D2-effects in NoGo neurons [26].

In addition to the striatal genes, the above genetic study also examined the COMT gene, which regulates prefrontal, but generally not striatal, DA [92–95]. Interestingly, this gene did not affect probabilistic Go or NoGo learning (Fig. 19.3C), but instead modulated participants' tendency to switch stimulus choices following a single instance of negative feedback [86]. This last ability is presumably dependent on participants' ability to hold trial outcomes in working memory in the face of multiple intervening trials until the same stimulus appears again – a function widely agreed to be modulated by prefrontal DA levels [96], and the COMT gene in particular [97]. Moreover, this effect is partially consistent with a modification of our basic BG model, which includes orbitofrontal cortical (OFC) interactions [33] (see below). In this model, OFC represents recent stimulus–reward values in working memory and can override probabilistic associations learned in the BG when task contingencies change rapidly. However, in that model phasic

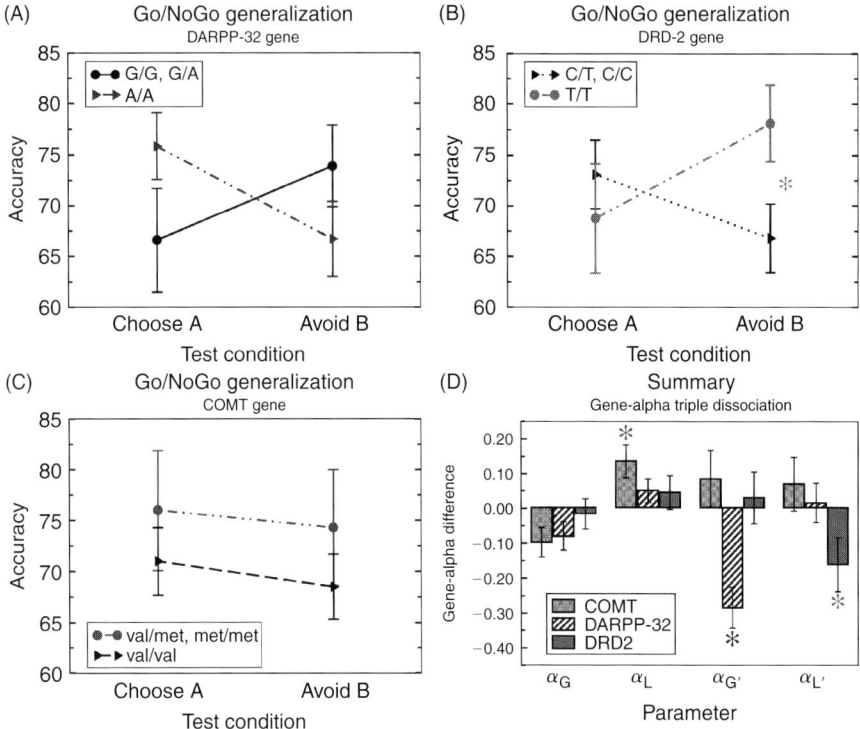

Figure 19.3 Effects of striatal genes (A) DARPP-32 and (B) DRD2 on probabilistic Go and NoGo learning in healthy participants. (C) No effects of COMT were observed. (D) Genetic effects on learning rates derived from mathematical model fits to participant choices. At test DARPP-32 modulated learning rates from probabilistic gains ($\alpha_{G'}$), DRD2 modulated learning rates from probabilistic losses ($\alpha_{L'}$), and COMT modulated learning rates (α_L) associated with rapid trial-by-trial adaptations following negative feedback during training. *Source*: From Frank et al. (2007) [86].

DA bursts potentiate reward information in OFC, whereas DA dips potentiated representations of negative reward values, and the COMT data help to falsify this prediction. Specifically, COMT met allele carriers, who have relatively *elevated* prefrontal DA, were more likely to switch following negative feedback. The reduced efficacy of the COMT enzyme associated with this allele reduces DA clearance from the prefrontal synapse, making them less likely to detect pauses in DA firing. Moreover, it is unlikely in general (irrespective of genetics) that prefrontal cortex (PFC) would be sensitive to DA dips, because unlike striatum, the time constant of DA clearance is quite slow in frontal cortex [98–100]. Thus, future modeling endeavors that include the OFC will refine this mechanism to be more consistent with other biophysical models of prefrontal DA [96,101], in which tonically elevated DA levels support robust maintenance in working memory, and other factors would signal the valence of reward outcomes.

A more recent study [91] investigated the role of these same genes in modulating the speed at which participants made decisions, using the same temporal decision-making paradigm mentioned above [64]. In a large sample of participants, the results largely supported our previous findings. DARPP-32 was again associated with Go learning, measured in this paradigm by the speeding of responses to increase reward. The DRD2 gene controlling D2 receptor density was again associated with NoGo learning, predicting the degree to which participants could slow responses to increase reward. Finally, the COMT gene was not associated with Go/NoGo learning, but rather was predictive of participants' tendency to adapt RTs on a trial-to-trial basis, presumably attempting to discover the most valuable response latencies [91].

This latter result provides novel evidence for the role of PFC function, and individual differences therein, in guiding strategic exploration. Though relatively understudied, the neural mechanisms driving decisions to explore potentially rewarding options, or exploit the best ones currently known, have recently been given more attention [102–105]. Daw and colleagues [104] presented neuroimaging evidence suggesting that anterior PFC might drive strategic exploration. Motivated by theoretical work in reinforcement learning [106,107], we hypothesized that rapid trial-to-trial RT adaptations might reflect a tendency to explore responses in proportion to the relative Bayesian *uncertainty* that those responses might lead to a reward prediction error. In essence, this is a model of exploratory choice based on always trying to outdo oneself by searching for options that might be better than the status quo. Intriguingly, the number of met alleles was strongly predictive of the degree to which participants made exploratory decisions based on Bayesian uncertainty. Below, we contrast this form of guided exploration with an unguided form of exploration which has also been suggested to manage the exploration/exploitation tradeoff [102].

The results of these genetic studies lend support to the basic assertions of the BG model, particularly with respect to D1 and D2 function, and also suggest an important computational role of the PFC in reinforcement learning. This latter finding is a deviation from our *a priori* network models and illustrates a key strength of combining multiple levels of modeling. The COMT gene findings were largely elucidated by abstract computational analysis; they pose a challenge to develop neural models which may further provide insights into the mechanisms responsible for computing, remembering, and using uncertainty representations to drive exploration. Moreover, the abstract level of modeling has also provided a great deal of insight into learning mechanisms, for example, by correlating model variables with signals from functional imaging ([108–110]; see [111] for review).

19.5   Appended models

The basic model described above generated a wealth of predictions for subsequent experiments. However, the modeled BG does not contain all of the details present in the brain. On one hand, this simplification is often a strength of computational modeling efforts in that abstraction of less critical details focuses attention on the core mechanisms that produce a particular behavioral pattern. On the other hand, such abstractions do not allow for insight into the functions of the omitted details. Attempting to strike a balance between these levels of abstraction, structures have been subsequently added onto the basic model to explore their computational contributions to the cognitive roles of the BG. Here we review insights gained by these modifications.

19.5.1   Subthalamic nucleus

Key among the simplifications undertaken to implement the standard model was the omission of the subthalamic nucleus (STN), a BG structure previously considered a part of the indirect pathway [9]. Including this neural structure in the model (Fig. 19.1) in an attempt to account for existing data at both neurophysiological and behavioral levels [31] led to novel predictions regarding the role of the STN, while leaving the functionality of the rest of the BG Go/NoGo system essentially unchanged. Simulation and experimental results suggest that the STN adaptively slows responses when the conflict between them is high, providing valuable time to choose the best option (see also Chapter 18 [112]). In our case, this particular function was not anticipated prior to building the model, exploring its dynamics, and considering their functional relevance in decision making. The kinds of dynamic interactions between multiple BG nuclei required for these effects to occur begin to provide some insights into the seemingly convoluted circuitry of the BG.

Despite previous consideration of the STN as part of the indirect pathway, it is now clear that the STN forms part of a third "hyperdirect" pathway that receives input from frontal cortex and sends excitatory projections directly, and diffusely, to the both segments of the globus pallidus, bypassing the striatum altogether [31,113–116]. At the GPi, these diffuse excitatory projections result in increased inhibition of the thalamus, suppressing all responses, thereby acting as a "Global NoGo" signal. Projections to the GPe comprise a negative feedback circuit, allowing the GPe to detect overall STN activity and to regulate this activity via reciprocal inhibitory projections. These dynamics play out in the following way. First, an initial co-activation of multiple candidate responses in cortex leads to a burst of STN activity via excitatory projections along the hyperdirect pathway (Fig. 19.4A). This burst effectively raises the threshold required for striatal Go activity to disinhibit a response, and therefore delays responding. Finally, feedback inhibition from GPe reduces the initial STN surge; concurrently, striatal Go signals for the best response are now more active, allowing that response to be selected (as evidenced by increased thalamic activation in Fig. 19.4A).

Note that when multiple competing responses are potentially appropriate in cortex, there is greater response *conflict*, and this co-activation of multiple cortical units leads to an exaggerated initial STN surge which slows RT (Fig. 19.4B). Simulations revealed that this surge is adaptive, in that it provides more time for the striatum to resolve reinforcement conflict and to settle on the best response given noisy activity and stochastic activation changes in the different cortical candidate choices. Thus, when the model was faced with a high conflict choice, whereby two responses had similar reinforcement values in the current stimulus context, the inclusion of the STN actually improved its accuracy at selecting the optimal one (Fig. 19.4C) [31]. This result is consistent with rat studies in which STN lesions cause premature responding in choice paradigms [117,118], and is also remarkably compatible with other modeling efforts based on optimal decision-making theories ([112]; see Chapter 18).

A recent study tested this hypothesized role of the STN in humans [45]. In this study, PD patients were tested while under deep brain stimulation (DBS), with their stimulators both on and off in different sessions. DBS is a procedure in which stimulators implanted in the STN reduce the tremor accompanying the disease [119]. Because DBS disrupts STN function (which is normally hyperactive in Parkinson's), testing patients on and off DBS provides an opportunity to test the role of the STN in cognitive function. Patients were compared to age-matched controls and PD patients on and off medication. To assess decision-making ability in high-conflict trials, we analyzed test pairs with similar reinforcement probabilities (e.g., a choice between an 80% and a 70% rewarded stimulus). Notably, all participants except those on DBS exhibited longer reaction times for high conflict decisions than for those with low conflict. In fact, DBS patients on stimulation actually responded *faster* during high-conflict win–win decisions (Fig. 19.4D). When

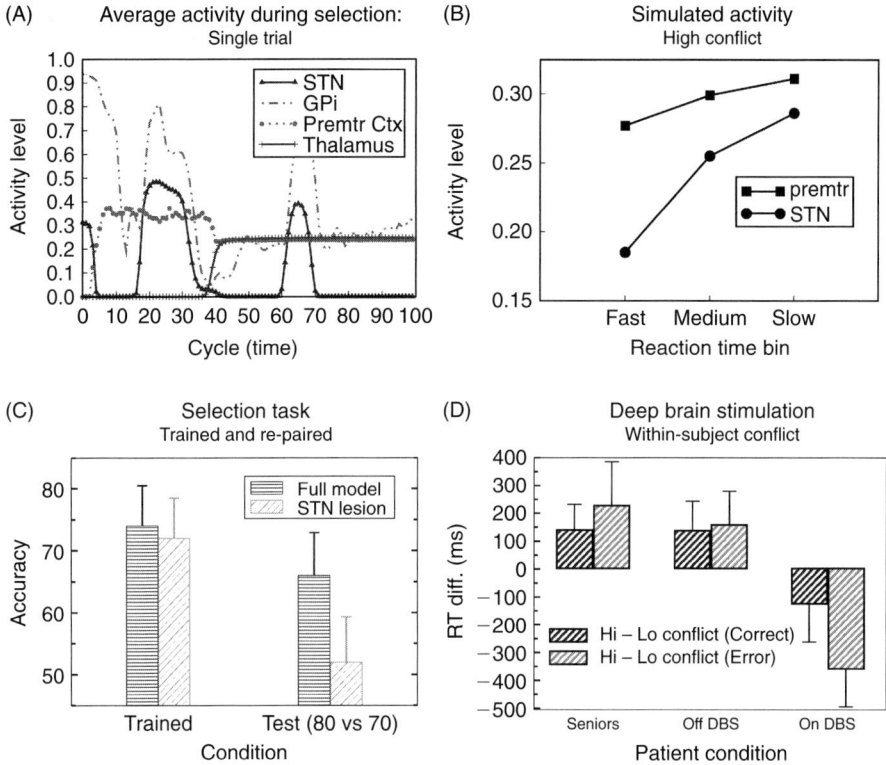

Figure 19.4 (A) Average activity levels across network settling cycles during response selection. Initially, multiple simultaneously active cortical responses excite STN, which sends a "Global NoGo" signal to prevent premature responding by exciting GPi. STN activity then subsides, allowing a response to be facilitated (as seen by increased thalamus activity). (B) During high-conflict trials, increased simulated STN and premotor cortical activity were associated with longer RTs. (C) Model performance in a probabilistic selection task. While not differing from control models at selecting among (trained) low conflict discriminations, STN lesioned networks were selectively impaired at the high-conflict selection of an 80% positively reinforced response when it competed with a 70% response. The STN Global NoGo signal prevents premature responding, which allows the striatum to integrate over all potential responses before selecting one, increasing the likelihood of accurate choice [31]. (D) Behavioral results in Parkinson's patients on and off deep brain stimulation of the STN, confirming model predictions. RT differences are shown for high- relative to low-conflict test trials. Whereas healthy controls, patients on/off medication (not shown), and patients off DBS adaptively slow decision times in high- relative to low-conflict test trials, patients on DBS respond impulsively faster in these trials, particularly when they make suboptimal choices ("errors"). *Source*: Adapted from Frank et al. (2007) [45].

the same patients had their stimulators turned off, they slowed down with conflict just as the other participants had. This pattern of results was mirrored in the model when simulating STN DBS by disrupting the STN with high-frequency stimulation or by lesioning it altogether [45]. Moreover, when DBS patients chose the statistically suboptimal stimulus, their failure to slow down was particularly pronounced, suggesting that intact

STN function is required to slow responses when more time is needed to resolve conflict. Finally, in direct contrast to these DBS effects, medication altered Go versus NoGo learning as described above, but had no effect on conflict-induced slowing. Together these findings reveal a double dissociation of treatment type on two aspects of cognitive decision making in PD: Dopaminergic medication influences positive/negative learning biases but not conflict-induced slowing, whereas DBS influences conflict-induced slowing but not positive/negative learning biases.

Another study showed supporting evidence using neuroimaging. Under high-conflict conditions in a non-reinforcement task, the degree of response slowing was correlated with co-activation of dorsomedial frontal cortex and STN [115], as predicted by the model. No such correlation was observed under low-conflict conditions. In addition, this study showed that the STN activation is predictive of the extent to which participants can inhibit their motor response altogether in a response inhibition task. Such a common role for the STN in conflict-induced slowing and outright response inhibition is currently being modeled, and can provide a mechanistic account of behavioral inhibition via frontosubthalamic interactions.

19.5.2 DA/NE interactions and attention deficit/hyperactivity disorder

A modified version of the basic model was developed to account for behavioral deficits observed in attention deficit/hyperactivity disorder (ADHD) [44,120]. The mechanisms underlying this disorder are heterogeneous, as are the deficits it produces (ADHD is not a unitary disorder, but a cluster of disorder subtypes: inattentive, hyperactive/impulsive, combined) [121]. Recent work implicates both DA and NE in the disorder [122,123], and stimulant medications used to treat it elevate striatal DA levels and frontal DA/NE levels [124]. Regarding DA, predictions from our model (and results from the subsequent experiment) support those summarized above: Stimulant medications enhance Go but not NoGo learning in adult ADHD participants (Fig. 19.2F), and also improved working memory gating [44]. As these effects are not contingent on the model modifications, here we focus on the role of NE in corticostriatal circuits.

Theoretical work [125,126] suggests that noradrenergic neurons in the locus coeruleus (LC) play a role in modulating the tendency to explore the possible actions in a given environment, or to exploit those currently considered valuable. By this view, high tonic LC activity effectively amplifies the effects of intrinsic noise and is accompanied by variable reaction times and random choice behavior that affords the exploration of a statistical environment. Phasic bursting activity, on the other hand, is accompanied by focused attention and exploitation of currently rewarding choices, as well as a tighter distribution of reaction times. This theory was developed by electrophysiological data from monkeys and by computational work that captured the exploration/exploitation tradeoff in the gain of the sigmoidal activation function of simulated neurons (where low gain produces noisy activation, and high gain produces "sharp," target-stimulus locked activation) [126,127].

The BG model was modified to encapsulate these NE functions and to examine how they might interact with the action selection and DA properties of the BG [120]. An LC layer was therefore added which projects to, and receives projections from, the premotor cortex [125]. LC activity modulates premotor activity by dynamically changing the gain of the neural activation function. In the phasic mode, LC neurons fire at low tonic rates but cortical activity induces a phasic LC burst, which reciprocally amplifies the gain of the cortical units that drove the LC response, and thereby enhances activation of those units. Such phasic NE bursts, together with the reinforcement learning functions of the BG, lead to the repeated exploitation of the strongly activated response. Note that it is this *dynamic* nature of the NE signal which affords exploitation. Perpetually high (tonic) NE levels would amplify premotor noise and produce random responses (i.e., reduced accuracy). This modulation system requires that gain be increased precisely at the moment when the correct response is activated.

As mentioned, there is some evidence for dysfunctional noradrenergic processes in ADHD, and some stimulant medications such as atomoxetine act primarily on NE without affecting striatal DA [124]. In a rat model of ADHD, elevated frontal NE levels were observed [128,129]. Thus we posited that some ADHD symptoms might reflect tonically high frontal NE. In the model, high tonic NE effectively amplifies noise in the premotor cortical units, leading to RT variability and more exploratory behavior. In some cases, the model prematurely executed responses that happened to be noisily activated by premotor cortex at the start of the trial (in such cases, the BG had not yet facilitated the reinforced response). In other cases, the premotor cortex and LC activated different responses, slowing the reaction time while resolving the conflict between the competing responses.

A follow-up experiment tested ADHD patients on and off stimulant (DA) medication [44]. In the probabilistic selection task described above, these patients showed an increased tendency to switch responses during the feedback (training) phase, regardless of whether the previous choice was rewarded. Additionally, the extent of switching was highly correlated with RT variability in non-medicated ADHD participants, lending support to the single common mechanism described by the model. Critically, these putative NE measures did not correlate with putative DA measures in the experiment (Go/NoGo learning and working memory updating), suggesting that differences in these neurotransmitter systems independently produce ADHD deficits. While further research that systematically alters NE levels is needed, the computational approach outlined here makes clear predictions about the role of this neurotransmitter in action selection. The suggestion that DA and NE fulfill specific independent roles may help differentiate and treat the varied subtypes of ADHD.

Moreover, the model amendment we used to simulate the NE dysfunction suggests an unguided control mechanism for the exploration/exploitation trade-off. While this mechanism is consistent with those of other bottom-up models of the trade-off [126], it contrasts with our model of top-down *strategic* exploration discussed above [91]. We note that these different accounts do not necessarily require fundamentally different mechanisms [105]. Indeed, top-down control structures might be required to switch bottom-up LC modes and drive exploratory behavior regardless of whether or not the subject engages in strategic exploration. However, simple modulation of bottom-up noise is a poor mechanism for strategizing. Adding noise would level the probabilities of making any choice, whereas under strategic exploration, particular options are explored based on their relative ability to provide new information (e.g., as a function of the uncertainty that they might produce better outcomes). Future research should seek to uncover the degree to which these potential classes of exploration are dependent on overlapping or completely independent mechanisms.

19.5.3 Instructional control

The majority of recent biologically motivated computational work on decision making has focused on learning the value of stimuli by repeatedly experiencing their associated outcomes over trials (for a review, see [130]). However, a body of behavior-analytic and cognitive work suggests that decisions based on experienced outcomes may be treated differently than decisions based on descriptions of outcomes [131,132]. Indeed, some very recent computational cognitive work indicates researchers are attending to this important issue [133,134]. To this end, a modification of the BG model was used to investigate candidate neural mechanisms by which described outcomes might cooperate or compete with experienced outcomes [135].

To elucidate the mechanisms underlying these two routes of decision making, an experimental replication of a behavior-analytic effect known as "rule governance" was utilized [136]. Such a preparation is useful in distinguishing the mechanics of decisions from experience versus those from description because it directly pits them against one another. In a typical rule governance experiment, participants are given inaccurate instructions as to the programmed contingencies they will experience in the task [137]. Intriguingly, this verbal "misinformation" often exerts powerful control over subject choice, despite feedback indicating the inaccuracy of the instructions [132,138].

In the replication of this effect, participants were inaccurately instructed that a specific stimulus in the probabilistic selection task would either be the most probably "correct" or the most probably "incorrect," when in actual fact the instructed stimulus was paired with a statistically better or worse stimulus in contradiction to the instructions [135]. Additionally, the value of the instructed stimuli were near the middle of the distribution, such that roughly half of alternative stimuli in the test phase were reinforced more than the instructed stimulus. Over training, subject choices roughly matched the probabilities of reinforcement for all but the instructed stimulus. On choices featuring the instructed stimulus, participants initially adhered to the instructions, but they began to drift toward probability matching as training progressed. Nevertheless, by the end of the training phase, allocation of responses remained statistically in accordance with the inaccurate instructions rather than with the true probabilities. Interestingly, in the test phase, instructional control reemerged quite strongly. For example, participants instructed to pick a stimulus did so even when it was paired with statistically superior stimuli – including the most positive stimulus of the bunch that had been reinforced 80% of the time during training. This result is striking, given that the instructed stimulus had been reinforced in half as many trials.

In the computational account of this result, a joint PFC/hippocampus (HC) layer was added to the BG model, in which instructions are thought to be represented. Though these brain regions have well-studied neurocomputational properties [96,139], these are abstracted away in this model, due to the focus on their "downstream" effects at the striatum and motor cortex. This simplification honors the rapid, single-trial encoding thought to take place in the HC, and the retrieval and maintenance functions presumed to be housed in the PFC.

The added PFC/HC layer receives stimulus input projections, and also projects to the striatum and motor cortex. Instructions are modeled by giving the model one initial "instructed" trial in which the learning rates along the sensory input to PFC/HC and from PFC/HC to striatum and motor cortex are raised, and the inaccurate response is clamped to the output layer. This trial rapidly increases the likelihood that the model will make the same choice when the stimulus is seen again, just as verbal instructions do in human participants. Learning rates are then returned to their normal level and the model completes the task as usual. This instructed model demonstrates probability matching to all but the instructed stimulus, for which – in accordance with human participants – the model shows a strong preference for instructions which slowly dissipates over time, increasing the number of choices based on experienced contingencies.

An interesting question is whether instructional control biases the reinforcement learning system to learn the incorrect contingencies, or does it simply override the output of the reinforcement learning (RL) system which accurately represents contingencies as usual? The two projections from the PFC/HC layer make differing predictions regarding the mechanism underlying instructional control. These differences are revealed in the test phase. If top-down instructional control is mediated by PFC/HC biasing striatal representations, the striatum shows a preference for the instructed response over the statistically superior response. Conversely, if instructions exert their effects along the PFC/HC to motor cortex projection, the striatum learns that the instructions are incorrect and shows a preference for the statistically superior response – but this preference is "overridden" at the motor cortex.

Subsequent abstract "Q-learning" model fits to individual subject data supported the notion that the striatum is biased to learn the incorrect contingencies rather than being overridden by the PFC/HC [135]. Further, a very recent cognitive model [134] independently investigated a similar effect and came to similar conclusions. Nevertheless, the fate of these two hypotheses awaits biological evidence to discriminate between them.

19.5.4   Orbitofrontal cortex model

The orbitofrontal and ventromedial cortices are commonly implicated decision-making structures [140–142], considered vital in flexible representation of reward value in repeated choice tasks [143,144]. A modification of the basic model sought to integrate this frontal brain structure into the BG model to elucidate its computational role in reinforcement learning [33]. This modification consisted of adding two OFC capacities: the ability to bias striatal representations (in a manner similar to the instructed model) and working memory capacity, which allows the model to hold recent response outcomes "online." In conjunction, these faculties allowed the model to perform well on a number of tasks on which the basic BG model failed (such as rapid reversal learning and a reduced version of the Iowa Gambling Task). Success on these tasks requires flexible weighting of the magnitude aspect of reward structure, such that it can influence decision making above and beyond the influence exerted by contingency probabilities. Current evidence has only partially supported this model [86] – as mentioned above, the precise function of DA in PFC will need to be revisited and subject to further biological constraints and empirical data. However, the two central ideas embedded in the model continue to be well supported. The first mechanism, that OFC supports rapid trial-to-trial adjustments based on changes in stimulus outcome values and is sensitive to working memory-like delays, is consistent with recent lesion data [145,146]. Similarly, the notion that OFC encodes the highest relative reward values is consistent with neuroimaging and electrophysiological data [104,147,148]. Finally, via (admittedly indirect) genetic methods, our data in a temporal decision-making task support the idea that prefrontal magnitude representations (which would be enhanced in met allele carriers) are required to offset the probability bias learned by the BG. Specifically, strong D2 receptor genetic function was associated with a bias to avoid high probability negative prediction errors, despite high-magnitude rewards in the low-probability trials. In contrast, met allele carriers showed greater sensitivity to reward magnitudes, and were able to compensate for this probability bias [91].

19.5.5   Working memory and dorsolateral PFC

Though we have discussed primarily the action selection functions of the BG that respond to decisions with a motor component (i.e., deciding which button to press in an experiment), the BG is also involved in endogenous decisions [4,5]. Among our modeling efforts, we have also investigated the working memory functions of the BG [28], which rely on the identical BG action selection mechanics described above. However, instead of facilitating response selection among a pool of potential actions, the BG serve to choose which contents should be gated into dorsolateral PFC, to be subsequently maintained in working memory. These models build on earlier suggestions that phasic DA signals support gating directly in PFC [27], but assign a critical role to the BG in selective updating and learning. As these modifications are reviewed elsewhere [149,150], we do not cover them at length here. Recent evidence in neuroimaging [151] and in PD patients [152] has supported the role of the BG in gating working memory representations, as well as modulation by DA, suggested by our model [4,28]. Further, in the ADHD study mentioned above, the effects of stimulant medications on relative Go/NoGo learning were correlated with their efficacy in improving working memory gating [44], supporting a common mechanism at the level of the BG.

19.6 Conclusion

Computational neuroscience can be undertaken at a wide range of levels, from the fine-grained details of dendritic geometry and ion channels to the overarching computational goals Bayesian analysis seeks to clarify. The network models reviewed here occupy the middle of this spectrum, and therefore omit many fine-grained details of the biology, and do not attain the elegance and simplicity of some cognitive models. Models at either end of this spectrum, however, are of limited use in elucidating the biological mechanisms by which cognitive processes occur. By focusing our modeling in the middle of this range, we make contact with biology at one end and cognition at the other. Though no approach replaces the need for any other, we have shown how models at this level have made significant progress in understanding the learning and decision-making functions of the BG. Further, by integrating models at various levels of analysis new insights can be gained, informing models at all levels.

References

[1] C.J. Wilson, J.C. Callaway, Coupled oscillator model of the dopaminergic neuron of the substantia nigra, J. Neurophysiol. 83 (2000) 3084.

[2] N.D. Daw, Y. Niv, P. Dayan, Uncertainty-based competition between prefrontal and dorsolateral striatal systems for behavioral control, Nat. Neurosci. 8 (2005) 1704–1711.

[3] K. Gurney, T.J. Prescott, P. Redgrave, A computational model of action selection in the basal ganglia. I. A new functional anatomy, Biol. Cybern. 84 (2001) 401–410.

[4] M.J. Frank, B. Loughry, R.C. O'Reilly, Interactions between the frontal cortex and basal ganglia in working memory: a computational model, Cogn. Affect. Behav. Neurosci. 1 (2001) 137–160.

[5] J.C. Houk, Agents of the mind, Biol. Cybern. 92 (2005) 427–437.

[6] J.W. Mink, The basal ganglia: focused selection and inhibition of competing motor program, Prog. Neurobiol. 50 (1996) 381–425.

[7] G.E. Alexander, M.R. DeLong, P.L. Strick, Parallel organization of functionally segregated circuits linking basal ganglia and cortex, Annu. Rev. Neurosci. 9 (1986) 357–381.

[8] G.E. Alexander, M.D. Crutcher, Functional architecture of basal ganglia cicuits: neural substrates of parallel processing, Trends Neurosci. 13 (1990) 266–271.

[9] R.L. Albin, A.B. Young, J.B. Penney, The functional anatomy of basal ganglia disorders, Trends Neurosci. 12 (1989) 366–375.

[10] F. Sato, P. Lavallée, M. Lévesque, A. Parent, Single-axon tracing study of neurons of the external segment of the globus pallidus in primate, J. Comp. Neurol. 417 (2000) 17–31.

[11] R. Cools, R.A. Barker, B.J. Sahakian, T.W. Robbins, Mechanisms of cognitive set flexibility in
Parkinson's disease, Brain 124 (2001) 2503–2512.

[12] P.R. Montague, P. Dayan, T.J. Sejnowski, A framework for mesencephalic dopamine systems
based on predictive Hebbian learning, J. Neurosci. 16 (1996) 1936–1947.

[13] W. Schultz, Multiple dopamine functions at different time courses, Annu. Rev. Neurosci. 30
(2007) 259–288.

[14] R.C. O'Reilly, M.J. Frank, T.E. Hazy, B. Watz, PVLV: the primary value and learned value
Pavlovian learning algorithm, Behav. Neurosci. 121 (2007) 31–49.

[15] R.S. Sutton, A.G. Barto, Reinforcement Learning: An Introduction, MIT Press, Cambridge,
MA, 1998.

[16] J. O'Doherty, P. Dayan, J. Schultz, R. Deichmann, K. Friston, R.J. Dolan, Dissociable roles of
ventral and dorsal striatum in instrumental conditioning, Science 304 (2004) 452–454.

[17] E. Ince, B.J. Ciliax, A.I. Levey, Differential expression of D and D dopamine and m4 muscarinic
acteylcholine receptor proteins in identified striatonigral neurons, Synapse 27 (1997) 257–366.

[18] O. Aizman, H. Brismar, P. Uhlen, E. Zettergren, A.I. Levet, H. Forssberg, P. Greengard,
A. Aperia, Anatomical and physiological evidence for D1 and D2 dopamine receptor colocalization in neostriatal neurons, Nat. Neurosci. 3 (2000) 226–230.

[19] D.J. Surmeier, J. Ding, M. Day, Z. Wang, W. Shen, D1 and D2 dopamine-receptor modulation of striatal glutamatergic signaling in striatal medium spiny neurons, Trends Neurosci. 30
(2007) 228–235.

[20] J.W. Brown, D. Bullock, S. Grossberg, How laminar frontal cortex and basal ganglia circuits
interact to control planned and reactive saccades, Neural Netw. 17 (2004) 471–510.

[21] M.J. Frank, Dynamic dopamine modulation in the basal ganglia: a neurocomputational
account of cognitive deficits in medicated and non-medicated Parkinsonism, J. Cogn. Neurosci.
17 (2005) 51–72.

[22] J.N. Kerr, J.R. Wickens, Dopamine D-1/D-5 receptor activation is required for long-term
potentiation in the rat neostriatum in vitro, J. Neurophysiol. 85 (2001) 117–124.

[23] P. Calabresi, A. Pisani, D. Centonze, G. Bernardi, Synaptic plasticity and physiological interactions between dopamine and glutamate in the striatum, Neurosci. Biobehav. Rev. 21 (1997)
519–523.

[24] T. Satoh, S. Nakai, T. Sato, M. Kimura, Correlated coding of motivation and outcome of decision by dopamine neurons, J. Neurosci. 23 (2003) 9913–9923.

[25] H.M. Bayer, B. Lau, P.W. Glimcher, Statistics of midbrain dopamine neuron spike trains in the
awake primate, J. Neurophysiol. 98 (2007) 1428–1439.

[26] W. Shen, M. Flajolet, P. Greengard, D.J. Surmeier, Dichotomous dopaminergic control of
striatal synaptic plasticity, Science 321 (2008) 848–851.

[27] T.S. Braver, J.D. Cohen, On the control of control: the role of dopamine in regulating prefrontal function and working memory, in: S. Monsell, J. Driver (Eds.), Control of Cognitive
Processes: Attention and Performance XVIII, MIT Press, Cambridge, MA, 2000, pp. 713–737.

[28] R.C. O'Reilly, M.J. Frank, Making working memory work: a computational model of learning
in the prefrontal cortex and basal ganglia, Neural Comput. 18 (2006) 283–328.

[29] A.J. Gruber, P. Dayan, B.S. Gutkin, S.A. Solla, Dopamine modulation in the basal ganglia locks
the gate to working memory, J. Comput. Neurosci. 20 (2006) 153–166.

[30] R.C. O'Reilly, Y. Munakata, Computational Explorations in Cognitive Neuroscience:
Understanding the Mind by Simulating the Brain, MIT Press, Cambridge, MA, 2000.

[31] M.J. Frank, Hold your horses: a dynamic computational role for the subthalamic nucleus in
decision making, Neural Netw. 19 (2006) 1120–1136.

[32] M.X. Cohen, M.J. Frank, Neurocomputational models of basal ganglia function in learning, memory and choice, Behav. Brain Res., 199 (2009) 141–156.

[33] M.J. Frank, E.D. Claus, Anatomy of a decision: striato-orbitofrontal interactions in reinforcement learning, decision making, and reversal, Psychol. Rev. 113 (2006) 300–326.

[34] M.D. Crutcher, G.E. Alexander, Movement-related neuronal activity selectively coding either direction or muscle pattern in three motor areas of the monkey, J. Neurophysiol. 64 (1990) 151–163.

[35] G.E. Alexander, M.D. Crutcher, Preparation for movement: neural representations of intended direction in three motor areas of the monkey, J. Neurophysiol. 64 (1990) 133–150.

[36] A. Nishi, G.L. Snyder, P. Greengard, Bidirectional regulation of DARPP-32 phosphorylation by dopamine, J. Neurosci. 17 (1997) 8147–8155.

[37] J.N.J. Reynolds, B.I. Hyland, J.R. Wickens, A cellular mechanism of reward-related learning, Nature 412 (2001) 67–69.

[38] J.N. Reynolds, J.R. Wickens, Dopamine-dependent plasticity of corticostriatal synapses, Neural Netw. 15 (2002) 507–521.

[39] D.G. Beiser, S.E. Hua, J.C. Houk, Network models of the basal ganglia, Curr. Opin. Neurobiol. 7 (1997) 185.

[40] F.G. Ashby, J.M. Ennis, b.J. Spiering, A neurobiological theory of automaticity in perceptual categorization, Psychol. Rev. 114 (2007) 632–656.

[41] M.J. Frank, L.C. Seeberger, R.C. O'Reilly, By carrot or by stick: cognitive reinforcement learning in Parkinsonism, Science 306 (2004) 1940–1943.

[42] M.J. Frank, R.C. O'Reilly, A mechanistic account of striatal dopamine function in human cognition: psychopharmacological studies with cabergoline and haloperidol, Behav. Neurosci. 120 (2006) 497–517.

[43] R. Cools, L. Altamirano, M. D'Esposito, Reversal learning in Parkinson's disease depends on medication status and outcome valence, Neuropsychologia 44 (2006) 1663–1673.

[44] M.J. Frank, A. Santamaria, R.C. O'Reilly, E. Willcutt, Testing computational models of dopamine and noradrenaline dysfunction in attention deficit/hyperactivity disorder, Neuropsychopharmacology 32 (2007) 1583–1599.

[45] M.J. Frank, J. Samanta, A.A. Moustafa, S.J. Sherman, Hold your horses: impulsivity, deep brain stimulation and medication in Parkinsonism, Science 318 (2007) 1309–1312.

[46] R.M. Costa, R. Gutierrez, I.E. Araujo, M.R.P. Coelho, A.D. Kloth, R.R. Gainetdinov, M.G. Caron, M.A.L. Nicolelis, S.A. Simon, Dopamine levels modulate the updating of tastant values, Genes Brain Behav. 6 (2007) 314–320.

[47] S.J. Kish, K. Shannak, O. Hornykiewicz, Uneven pattern of dopamine loss in the striatum of patients with idiopathic Parkinson's disease, N. Engl. J. Med. 318 (1988) 876–880.

[48] D.G. Harden, A.A. Grace, Activation of dopamine cell firing by repeated L-DOPA administration to dopamine-depleted rats: its potential role in mediating the therapeutic response to L-DOPA treatment, J. Neurosci. 15 (1995) 6157–6166.

[49] R.M. Wightman, C. Amatore, R.C. Engstrom, P.D. Hale, E.W. Kristensen, W.G. Kuhr, L.J. May, Real-time characterization of dopamine overflow and uptake in the rat striatum, Neuroscience 25 (1988) 513–523.

[50] R.W. Keller, W.G. Kuhr, R.M. Wightman, M.J. Zigmond, The effect of L-dopa on in vivo dopamine release from nigrostriatal bundle neurons, Brain Res. 447 (1988) 191–194.

[51] R. Cools, Dopaminergic modulation of cognitive function-implications for L-DOPA treatment in Parkinson's disease, Neurosci. Biobehav. Rev. 30 (2006) 1–23.

[52] J.A. Molina, M.J. Sáinz-Artiga, A. Fraile, F.J. Jimenez-Jimenez, C. Villanueva, M. Orti-Pareja, F. Bermejo, Pathologic gambling in Parkinson's disease: a behavioral manifestation of pharmacologic treatment?, Mov. Disord. 15 (2000) 869–872.

[53] M.L. Dodd, K.J. Klos, J.H. Bower, Y.E. Geda, K.A. Josephs, J.E. Ahlskog, Pathological gambling caused by drugs used to treat Parkinson disease, Arch. Neurol. 62 (2005) 1377–1381.

[54] W. Shen, X. Tian, M. Day, S. Ulrich, T. Tkatch, N.M. Nathanson, D.J. Surmeier, Cholinergic modulation of Kir2 channels selectively elevates dendritic excitability in striatopallidal neurons, Nat. Neurosci. 10 (2007) 1458–1466.

[55] E. Knapska, L. Kaczmarek, A gene for neuronal plasticity in the mammalian brain: Zif268/Egr-1/NGFI-A/Krox-24/TIS8/ZENK?, Prog. Neurobiol. 74 (2004) 183–211.

[56] A.R. Carta, E. Tronci, A. Pinna, M. Morelli, Different responsiveness of striatonigral and striatopallidal neurons to L-DOPA after a subchronic intermittent L-DOPA treatment, Eur. J. Neurosci. 21 (2005) 1196–1204.

[57] N.D. Volkow, R.C. Gur, G.J. Wang, J.S. Fowler, P.J. Moberg, Y. Ding, R. Hitzemann, G. Smith, J. Logan, Association between decline in brain dopamine activity with age and cognitive and motor impairment in healthy individuals, Am. J. Psychiatry 155 (1998) 344–349.

[58] W.R. Martin, M.R. Palmer, C.S. Patlak, D.B. Calne, Nigrostriatal function in humans studied with positron emission tomography, Ann. Neurol. 26 (1989) 535–542.

[59] C.H.v. Dyck, J.P. Seibyl, R.T. Malison, M. Laruelle, S.S. Zoghbi, R.M. Baldwin, R.B. Innis, Age-related decline in dopamine transporters: analysis of striatal subregions, nonlinear effects, and hemispheric asymmetries, Am. J. Geriatr. Psychiatry 10 (2002) 36–43.

[60] Y. Kraytsberg, E. Kudryavtseva, A.C. McKee, C. Geula, N.W. Kowall, K. Khrapko, Mitochondrial DNA deletions are abundant and cause functional impairment in aged human substantia nigra neurons, Nat. Genet. 38 (2006) 518–520.

[61] V. Kaasinen, J.O. Rinne, Functional imaging studies of dopamine system and cognition in normal aging and Parkinson's disease, Neurosci. Biobehav. Rev. 26 (2002) 785–793.

[62] L. Bäckman, N. Ginovart, R.A. Dixon, T.R. Wahlin, A. Wahlin, C. Halldin, L. Farde, Age-related cognitive deficits mediated by changes in the striatal dopamine system, Am. J. Psychiatry 157 (2000) 635–637.

[63] M.J. Frank, L. Kong, Learning to avoid in older age, Psychol. Aging 23 (2008) 392–398.

[64] A.A. Moustafa, M.X. Cohen, S.J. Sherman, M.J. Frank, A role for dopamine in temporal decision making and reward maximization in Parkinsonism, J. Neurosci. 28 (2008) 12294–12304.

[65] H. Schoemaker, Y. Claustre, D. Fage, et al., Neurochemical characteristics of amisulpiride, an atypical dopamine D2/D3 receptor antagonist with both presynaptic and limbic selectivity, J. Pharmacol. Exp. Ther. 280 (1997) 83–97.

[66] A.A. Grace, Phasic versus tonic dopamine release and the modulation of dopamine system responsivity: a hypothesis for the etiology of schizophrenia, Neuroscience 41 (1991) 1–24.

[67] Y.-C.I. Chen, J.-K. Choi, S.L. Andersen, B.R. Rosen, B.G. Jenkins, Mapping dopamine D2/D3 receptor function using pharmacological magnetic resonance imaging, Psychopharmacology (Berl) 180 (2005) 705–715.

[68] P.A. Garris, E.A. Budygin, P.E.M. Phillips, B.J. Venton, D.L. Robinson, B.P. Bergstrom, G.V. Rebec, R.M. Wightman, A role for presynaptic mechanisms in the actions of nomifensine and haloperidol, Neuroscience 118 (2003) 819–829.

[69] B. Moghaddam, B.S. Bunney, Acute effects of typical and atypical antipsychotic drugs on the release of dopamine from prefrontal cortex, nucleus accumbens, and stiratum in the rat: an in vivo microdialysis study, J. Neurochem. 54 (1990) 1755–1760.

[70] E.A. Pehek, Comparison of effects of haloperidol administration on amphetamine-stimulated dopamine release in the rat medial prefrontal cortex and dorsal striatum, J. Pharmacol. Exp. Ther. 289 (1999) 14–23.

[71] B.H.C. Westerink, Can antipsychotic drugs be classified by their effects on a particular group of dopamine neurons in the brain?, Eur. J. Pharmacol. 455 (2002) 1–18.

[72] Q. Wu, M.E.A. Reith, Q.D. Walker, C.M. Kuhn, F.I. Caroll, P.A. Garris, Concurrent autoreceptor-mediated control of dopamine release and uptake during neurotransmission: an in vivo voltammetric study, J. Neurosci. 22 (2002) 6272–6281.

[73] D.A. Pizzagalli, A.E. Evins, E.C. Schetter, M.J. Frank, P.E. Pajtas, D.L. Santesso, M. Culhane, Single dose of a dopamine agonist impairs reinforcement learning in humans: behavioral evidence from a laboratory-based measure of reward responsiveness, Psychopharmacology (Berl) 196 (2008) 221–232.

[74] D.L. Santesso, A.E. Evins, M.J. Frank, E.C. Schetter, R. Bogdan, D.A. Pizzagalli, Single dose of a dopamine agonist impairs reinforcement learning in humans: Evidence from event-related potentials and computational modeling of striatal-cortical function. Hum. Brain Mapp. (2008)

[75] D.Y. Kimberg, M. D'Esposito, M.J. Farah, Effects of bromocriptine on human subjects depend on working memory capacity, Neuroreport 8 (1997) 3581–3585.

[76] S.E. Gibbs, M. D'Esposito, A functional MRI study of the effects of bromocriptine, a dopamine receptor agonist, on component processes of working memory, Psychopharmacology (Berl) (2005) 1–10.

[77] V.S. Mattay, J.H. Callicott, A. Bertolino, I. Heaton, J.A. Frank, R. Coppola, K.F. Berman, T.E. Goldberg, D. Weinberger, Effects of dextroamphetamine on cognitive performance and cortical activation, Neuroimage 12 (2000) 268–275.

[78] R. Cools, S.E. Gibbs, A. Miyakawa, W. Jagust, M. D'Esposito, Working memory capacity predicts dopamine synthesis capacity in the human striatum, J. Neurosci. 28 (2008) 1208–1212.

[79] R. Cools, M.J. Frank, S.E. Gibbs, A. Miyakawa, W. Jagust, M. D'Esposito, Striatal dopamine predicts outcome-specific reversal learning and its sensitivity to dopaminergic drug administration, J. Neurosci. 29 (2009) 1538–43.

[80] M. Pessiglione, B. Seymour, G. Flandin, R.J. Dolan, C.D. Frith, Dopamine-dependent prediction errors underpin reward-seeking behaviour in humans, Nature 442 (2006) 1042–1045.

[81] P. Dayan, Q.J.M. Huys, Serotonin, inhibition, and negative mood, PLoS Comput. Biol. 4 (2008) e4.

[82] H. Kim, S. Shimojo, J.P. O'Doherty, Is avoiding an aversive outcome rewarding? Neural substrates of avoidance learning in the human brain, PLoS Biol. 4 (2006) e233.

[83] M.J. Frank, B.S. Woroch, T. Curran, Error-related negativity predicts reinforcement learning and conflict biases, Neuron 47 (2005) 495–501.

[84] M.J. Frank, C. D'Lauro, T. Curran, Cross-task individual differences in error processing: neural, electrophysiological and genetic components, Cogn. Affect. Behav. Neurosci. 7 (2007) 297–308.

[85] T.A. Klein, J. Neumann, M. Reuter, J. Hennig, D.Y.v. Cramon, M. Ullsperger, Genetically determined differences in learning from errors, Science 318 (2007) 1642–1645.

[86] M.J. Frank, A.A. Moustafa, H. Haughey, T. Curran, K. Hutchison, Genetic triple dissociation reveals multiple roles for dopamine in reinforcement learning, Proc. Natl. Acad. Sci. USA 104 (2007) 16311–16316.

[87] A. Meyer-Lindenberg, R.E. Straub, B.K. Lipska, et al., Genetic evidence implicating DARPP-32 in human frontostriatal structure, function, and cognition, J. Clin. Invest. 117 (2007) 672–682.

[88] P. Calabresi, P. Gubellini, D. Centonze, B. Picconi, G. Bernardi, K. Chergui, P. Svenningsson, A.A. Fienberg, P. Greengard, Dopamine and cAMP-regulated phosphoprotein 32 kDa controls both striatal long-term depression and long-term potentiation, opposing forms of synaptic plasticity, J. Neurosci. 20 (2000) 8443–8451.

[89] A. Stipanovich, E. Valjent, M. Matamales, et al., A phosphatase cascade by which rewarding stimuli control nucleosomal response, Nature 453 (2008) 879–884.

[90] M. Hirvonen, K. Laakso, J.O. Rinne, T. Pohjalainen, J. Hietala, C957T polymorphism of the dopamine D2 receptor (DRD2) gene affects striatal DRD2 availability in vivo (corrigendum), Mol. Psychiatry 10 (2005) 889.

[91] M.J. Frank, B.B. Doll, J. Oas-Terpstra, F. Moreno, The neurogenetics of exploration and exploitation: prefrontal and striatal depaminergic components. Natr. Neurosci. (In press).

[92] M.F. Egan, T.E. Goldberg, B.S. Kolachana, J.H. Callicott, C.M. Mazzanti, R.E. Straub, D. Goldman, D. Weinberger, Effect of COMT Val met genotype on frontal lobe function and risk for schizophrenia, Proc. Natl. Acad. Sci. USA 98 (2001) 6917–6922.

[93] E.M. Tunbridge, D.M. Bannerman, T. Sharp, P.J. Harrison, Catechol-O-methyltransferase inhibition improves set-shifting performance and elevates stimulated dopamine release in the rat prefrontal cortex, J. Neurosci. 24 (2004) 5331–5335.

[94] M. Slifstein, B. Kolachana, E.H. Simpson, P. Tabares, B. Cheng, M. Duvall, W.G. Frankle, D.R. Weinberger, M. Laruelle, A. Abi-Dargham, COMT genotype predicts cortical-limbic D1 receptor availability measured with [11C]NNC112 and PET, Mol. Psychiatry 13 (2008) 821–827.

[95] J.A. Gogos, M. Morgan, V. Luine, M. Santha, S. Ogawa, D. Pfaff, M. Karayiorgou, Catechol-O-methyltransferase-deficient mice exhibit sexually dimorphic changes in catecholamine levels and behavior, Proc. Natl. Acad. Sci. USA 95 (1998) 9991–9996.

[96] D. Durstewitz, J.K. Seamans, T.J. Sejnowski, Dopamine-mediated stabilization of delay-period activity in a network model of prefrontal cortex, J. Neurophysiol. 83 (2000) 1733–1750.

[97] E.M. Tunbridge, P.J. Harrison, D.R. Weinberger, Catechol-O-methyltransferase, cognition, and psychosis: Val158Met and beyond, Biol. Psychiatry 60 (2006) 141–151.

[98] J.K. Seamans, N. Gorelova, D. Durstewitz, C.R. Yang, Bidirectional dopamine modulation of GABAergic inhibition in prefrontal cortical pyramidal neurons, J. Neurosci. 21 (2001) 3628–3638.

[99] S.J. Cragg, C.J. Hille, S.A. Greenfield, Functional domains in dorsal striatum of the nonhuman primate are defined by the dynamic behavior of dopamine, J. Neurosci. 22 (2002) 5705–5712.

[100] G.W. Arbuthnott, J. Wickens, Space, time and dopamine, Trends Neurosci. 30 (2007) 62–69.

[101] J.K. Seamans, C.R. Yang, The principal features and mechanisms of dopamine modulation in the prefrontal cortex, Prog. Neurobiol. 74 (2004) 1–57.

[102] G. Aston-Jones, J.D. Cohen, An integrative theory of locus coeruleus-norepinephrine function: adaptive gain and optimal performance, Annu. Rev. Neurosci. 28 (2005) 403–450.

[103] A.J. Yu, P. Dayan, Uncertainty, neuromodulation, and attention, Neuron 46 (2005) 681–692.

[104] N.D. Daw, J.P. O'Doherty, P. Dayan, B. Seymour, R.J. Dolan, Cortical substrates for exploratory decisions in humans, Nature 441 (2006) 876–879.

[105] J.D. Cohen, S.M. McClure, A.J. Yu, Should I stay or should I go? How the human brain manages the trade-off between exploitation and exploration, Philos. Trans. R. Soc. Lond. B Biol. Sci. 362 (2007) 933–942.

[106] P. Dayan, T.J. Sejnowski, Exploration bonuses and dual control, Mach. Learn. 25 (1996) 5–22.

[107] L.P. Kaelbling, A.R. Cassandra, J.A. Kurien, Acting under uncertainty: discrete Bayesian models for mobile-robot navigation, in: Proceedings of IEEE/RSJ International Conference on Intelligent Robots and Systems, 1996.

[108] J. Li, S.M. McClure, B. King-Casas, P.R. Montague, Policy adjustment in a dynamic economic game, PLoS ONE 1 (2006) e103.

[109] B.C. Wittmann, N.D. Daw, B. Seymour, R.J. Dolan, Striatal activity underlies novelty-based choice in humans, Neuron 58 (2008) 967–973.

[110] T.E.J. Behrens, M.W. Woolrich, M.E. Walton, M.F.S. Rushworth, Learning the value of information in an uncertain world, Nat. Neurosci. 10 (2007) 1214–1221.

[111] J.P. O'Doherty, A. Hampton, H. Kim, Model-based fMRI and its application to reward learning and decision making, Ann. NY Acad. Sci. 1104 (2007) 35–53.

[112] R. Bogacz, K. Gurney, The basal ganglia and cortex implement optimal decision making between alternative actions, Neural Comput. 19 (2007) 442–477.

[113] A. Nambu, H. Tokuno, I. Hamada, H. Kita, M. Imanishi, T. Akazawa, Y. Ikeuchi, N. Hasegawa, Excitatory cortical inputs to pallidal neurons via the subthalamic nucleus in the monkey, J. Neurophysiol. 84 (2000) 289–300.

[114] A. Parent, L. Hazrati, Functional anatomy of the basal ganglia. II. The place of subthalamic nucleus and external pallidum in basal ganglia circuitry, Brain Res. Rev. 20 (1995) 128–154.

[115] A.R. Aron, T.E. Behrens, S. Smith, M.J. Frank, R.A. Poldrack, Triangulating a cognitive control network using diffusion-weighted magnetic resonance imaging (MRI) and functional MRI, J. Neurosci. 27 (2007) 3743–3752.

[116] M. Isoda, O. Hikosaka, Role for subthalamic nucleus neurons in switching from automatic to controlled eye movement, J. Neurosci. 28 (2008) 7209–7218.

[117] C. Baunez, T. Humby, D.M. Eagle, L.J. Ryan, S.B. Dunnett, T.W. Robbins, Effects of STN lesions on simple vs choice reaction time tasks in the rat: preserved motor readiness, but impaired response selection, Eur. J. Neurosci. 13 (2001) 1609–1616.

[118] C. Baunez, T.W. Robbins, Bilateral lesions of the subthalamic nucleus induce multiple deficits in an attentional task in rats, Eur. J. Neurosci. 9 (1997) 2086–2099.

[119] A.L. Benabid, Deep brain stimulation for Parkinson's disease, Curr. Opin. Neurobiol. 13 (2003) 696–706.

[120] M.J. Frank, A. Scheres, S.J. Sherman, Understanding decision making deficits in neurological conditions: insights from models of natural action selection, Philos. Trans. R. Soc. Lond. B Biol. Sci. 362 (2007) 1641–1654.

[121] APA, Diagnostic and Statistical Manual of Mental Disorders, fourth ed., American Psychiatric Press, Washington, DC, 1994.

[122] T. Sagvolden, E.B. Johansen, H. Aase, V.A. Russell, A dynamic developmental theory of attention-deficit/hyperactivity disorder (ADHD) predominantly hyperactive/impulsive and combined subtypes, Behav. Brain Sci. 28 (2005) 397–419 discussion 419–468.

[123] J. Biederman, T. Spencer, Attention-deficit/hyperactivity disorder (ADHD) as a noradrenergic disorder, Biol. Psychiatry 46 (1999) 1234–1242.

[124] B.K. Madras, G.M. Miller, A.J. Fischman, The dopamine transporter and attention-deficit/hyperactivity disorder, Biol. Psychiatry 57 (2005) 1397–1409.

[125] G. Aston-Jones, J.D. Cohen, An integrative theory of locus coeruleus-norepinephrine function: adaptive gain and optimal performance, Annu. Rev. Neurosci. 28 (2005) 403–450.

[126] S.M. McClure, M.S. Gilzenrat, J.D. Cohen, An exploration-exploitation model based on norepinepherine and dopamine activity, in: Advances in Neural Information Processing Systems 18, 2005.

[127] M. Usher, J.D. Cohen, D. Servan-Schreiber, J. Rajkowski, G. Aston-Jones, The role of locus coeruleus in the regulation of cognitive performance, Science 283 (1999) 549–554.

[128] V.A. Russell, T.M. Wiggins, Increased glutamate-stimulated norepinephrine release from prefrontal cortex slices of spontaneously hypertensive rats, Metab. Brain Dis. 15 (2000) 297–304.

[129] V. Russell, S. Allie, T. Wiggins, Increased noradrenergic activity in prefrontal cortex slices of an animal model for attention-deficit hyperactivity disorder–the spontaneously hypertensive rat, Behav. Brain Res. 117 (2000) 69–74.

[130] A. Rangel, C. Camerer, P.R. Montague, A framework for studying the neurobiology of value-based decision making, Nat. Rev. Neurosci. 9 (2008) 545–556.

[131] S.A. Sloman, The empirical case for two systems of reasoning, Psychol. Bull. 119 (1996) 3–22.

[132] S.C. Hayes (Ed.), Rule-Governed Behavior: Cognition, Contingencies, and Instructional Control, Plenum Press, New York, 1989.

[133] R.K. Jessup, A.J. Bishara, J.R. Busemeyer, Feedback produces divergence from prospect theory in descriptive choice, Psychol. Sci. 10 (2008) 1015–22.

[134] G. Biele, J. Rieskamp, R. Gonzalez, Computational models for the combination of advice and individual learning, Cogn. Sci. in press.

[135] B.B. Doll, W.J. Jacobs, A.G. Sanfey, M.J. Frank, Instructional control of reinforcement learning: a behavioral and neurocomputational investigation, Brain Res., Submitted.

[136] S.C. Hayes, Rule governance: basic behavioral research and applied implications, Curr. Dir. Psychol. Sci. 2 (1993) 193–197.

[137] A. Kaufman, A. Baron, R. Kopp, Some effects of instructions on human operant behavior, Psychon Monogr. Suppl. 1 (1966) 243–250.

[138] M. Galizio, Contingency-shaped and rule-governed behavior: instructional control of human loss avoidance, J. Exp. Anal. Behav. 31 (1979) 53–70.

[139] R.C. O'Reilly, J.W. Rudy, Conjunctive representations in learning and memory: principles of cortical and hippocampal function, Psychol. Rev. 108 (2001) 311–345.

[140] A. Bechara, H. Damasio, D. Tranel, S.W. Anderson, Dissociation of working memory from decision making within the human prefrontal cortex, J. Neurosci. 18 (1998) 428–437.

[141] E.T. Rolls, Convergence of sensory systems in the orbitofrontal cortex in primates and brain design for emotion, Anat. Rec. A Discov. Mol. Cell. Evol. Biol. 281A (2004) 1212–1225.

[142] L. Tremblay, W. Schultz, Reward-related neuronal activity during Go-Nogo task performance in primate orbitofrontal cortex, J. Neurophysiol. 83 (2000) 1864–1876.

[143] Y. Chudasama, T.W. Robbins, Dissociable contributions of the orbitofrontal and infralimbic cortex to Pavlovian autoshaping and discrimination reversal learning: further evidence for the functional heterogeneity of the rodent frontal cortex, J. Neurosci. 23 (2003) 8771–8780.

[144] B. Jones, M. Mishkin, Limbic lesions and the problem of stimulus–reinforcement associations, Exp. Neurol. 36 (1972) 362–377.

[145] P.H. Rudebeck, M.E. Walton, A.N. Smyth, D.M. Bannerman, M.F.S. Rushworth, Separate neural pathways process different decision costs, Nat. Neurosci. 9 (2006) 1161–1168.

[146] H.W. Chase, L. Clark, C.E. Myers, M.A. Gluck, B.J. Sahakian, E.T. Bullmore, T.W. Robbins, The role of the orbitofrontal cortex in human discrimination learning, Neuropsychologia 46 (2008) 1326–1337.

[147] M.R. Roesch, C.R. Olson, Neuronal activity related to reward value and motivation in primate frontal cortex, Science 304 (2004) 307–310.

[148] J.P. O'Doherty, Lights, camembert, action! The role of human orbitofrontal cortex in encoding stimuli, rewards, and choices, Ann. NY Acad. Sci. 1121 (2007) 254–272.

[149] T.E. Hazy, M.J. Frank, R.C. O'Reilly, Banishing the homunculus: making working memory work, Neuroscience 139 (2006) 105–118.

[150] T.E. Hazy, M.J. Frank, R.C. O'Reilly, Towards an executive without a homunculus: computational models of the prefrontal cortex/basal ganglia system, Philos. Trans. R. Soc. Lond. B Biol. Sci. 139 (2007) 105–118.

[151] F. McNab, T. Klingberg, Prefrontal cortex and basal ganglia control access to working memory, Nat. Neurosci. 11 (2008) 103–107.

[152] A.A. Moustafa, S.J. Sherman, M.J. Frank, A dopaminergic basis for working memory, learning, and attentional shifting in Parkinson's disease, Neuropsychologia 46 (2008) 3144–3156.

[153] B.J. Knowlton, J.A. Mangels, L.R. Squire, A neostriatal habit learning system in humans, Science 273 (1996) 1399–1402.

20 Reward-based emotions: affective evaluation of outcomes and regret learning

Giorgio Coricelli[1] and Aldo Rustichini[2]

[1]Cognitive Neuroscience Center, CNRS UMR5229, Lyon 1 University, 67 Bd Pinel 69675 Bron, France
[2]Department of Economics, University of Minnesota, 271 19th Avenue South, Minneapolis, MN 55455

Abstract

This chapter concerns the behavioral effects and the neural substrates of a class of reward-based emotions, which are emotions elicited by rewards and punishers. We describe how outcome evaluation is influenced by the level of responsibility in the process of choice (agency) and by the available information regarding alternative outcomes. The data we report suggest that cognitive context, exemplified by counterfactual thinking (what might have been if a different state of the world had realized) exerts a modulatory influence on the orbitofrontal cortex activation to rewards and punishers. The orbitofrontal cortex is also critically involved in learning in environments where the information about the rewards of the alternative foregone actions is available. These processes are addressed in humans, both in the context of normal and altered brain functions.

Key points

1. The emotions related to experiencing rewards or punishers are not independent from the outcomes that have not occurred. Indeed, it is the counterfactual reasoning between the obtained and unobtained outcomes that determines the quality and intensity of the emotional response.
2. A key behavioral observation is that patients with lesions in the orbitofrontal cortex are unable to experience regret and to anticipate the potential affective consequence of their choices.
3. There exists a neuroanatomical dissociation of regret versus disappointment. The ventral tegmental area and ventral striatum are associated with the reward prediction error models, while regret learning is associated with the orbitofrontal cortex.
4. Negative affective consequences (regret) induce specific mechanisms of cognitive control on subsequent choices.
5. The counterfactual reasoning extends from private to social learning.

This chapter outlines the neural basis of a class of reward-based emotions and their fundamental role in adaptive behavior. We address the following questions: What are the neural underpinnings of reward-based emotions such as disappointment and regret? What are the theoretical implications of incorporating reward-based emotions into the process of choice and into adaptive models of decision making? We discuss scientific literature that uses a fundamentally multidisciplinary approach drawing from economics, psychology, cognitive, and computational neuroscience. Our approach relies on robust behavioral tasks for which the computation underlying optimal responses is established, and we investigate how emotional states affect these optimal responses. In line with recent work on emotion-based decision making we attempt to characterize the brain areas underlying decision processes in individual and social settings and, more specifically, define the functional relationship between "rational" decision making and emotional influences that impact on these decisional processes. Our focus, by way of illustration, is on the contribution of the orbitofrontal cortex (OFC) in both the experience and anticipation of reward-based emotions, such as regret.

20.1 Reward-based emotions: emotions as affective evaluations of outcomes

Emotions may be considered as the affective evaluation of a difference between an expected and a realized reward. For instance, the negative (positive) difference between the realized and the expected reward may elicit disappointment (elation), while regret is elicited by a comparison (counterfactual [1–3]) between the outcome of a choice and the better outcome of a foregone rejected alternatives (what might have been). Regret differs from disappointment in its abstract point of reference: it arises from a discrepancy between the actual outcome and an outcome that would have pertained had an alternative choice been taken. Regret is an emotion characterized by the feeling of responsibility for the negative outcome of our choice [4–6], while disappointment is the emotion related to an unexpected negative outcome independently of the responsibility of the chooser [7,8].

Anticipation of regret induces changing in behavioral strategies [9] and characterizes the learning process in decision-making [10]. Regret results from a decision made and the possibility to compare the obtained outcome with better outcomes of rejected alternatives. The type of feedback information is indeed crucial to determine the emotional response [11] and the decisional process is influenced from the knowledge about the future feedback available. Therefore, the psychological and behavioral impact of outcome (win and losses) is influenced by the amount of feedback information provided to subjects.

One important question is whether regret and disappointment are encoded by specific cerebral regions. Camille et al. [12] studied the relationship between decision making and emotion in normal subjects and in patients with selective lesions to the OFC. The experimental task (Fig. 1) required subjects to choose between two gambles, each having different probabilities and different expected outcomes.

Disappointment could arise when, on a selected gamble, the alternative outcome is more positive than an experienced outcome. Regret was induced by providing information regarding the outcome of the unchosen gamble. When subjects were asked to rate their emotional state after seeing the obtained outcome, normal controls reported emotional responses consistent with counterfactual thinking between obtained and non-obtained outcomes. Thus, a win of $50 when the alternative gamble won $200 induced a strong negative emotion. Conversely the same outcome when confronted with a losing

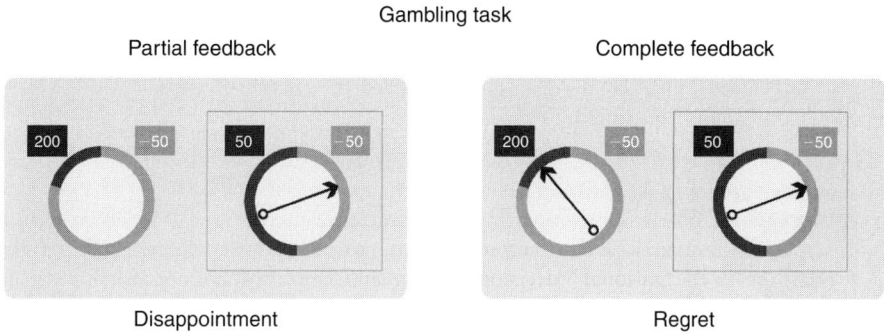

Figure 20.1 The regret gambling task. Subjects choose between two gambles (depicted as two "wheels of fortune"). For instance, if subjects choose the gamble on the left, they might win €200 with 20% probability or lose €50 with 80% probability; if they choose the gamble on the right, they might win or lose €50 with equal probabilities. There are two main contextual conditions in terms of the feedback provided – partial feedback and complete feedback. In partial feedback, only the outcome of the chosen gamble is provided, whereas in the complete feedback condition, both the outcome of the chosen (−50) and the unchosen (+200) gambles are provided. Complete feedback enables the subjects to judge not only the financial consequence of their choice, but also the outcome if they had they selected the other option (regret or relief).

Presumably, for different people, social regret is worse/preferable to material regret

alternative gamble (−$200) created a feeling of relief. After being exposed to a number of trials where they experienced regret, control subjects subsequently begun to choose the gambles with probable outcomes likely to produce minimal regret, indicating that they learnt from their prior emotional experience. Therefore, control subjects chose between risky gambles by a process that involves anticipating regret, thus integrating consideration about future emotional responses to the outcome of their choice.

By contrast, patients with lesions of the OFC did not report regret and did not anticipate negative affective consequences of their choices. They reported being happy when winning and disappointed when losing. Their emotional states were even modulated by the amount of win (+$50 or +$200) or the amount of loss (−$50 or −$200) but not by the value of the outcome in the alternative unchosen gamble. More striking, they persisted in choosing the gamble that normal subjects avoided because more likely to produce regret. Thus, OFC patients are unable to generate outcome evaluation and outcome expectancies, based upon a counterfactual comparison between the value of a chosen and a rejected alternative. Formally, they are unable to generate a specific function, called regret function [4], which represents the counterfactual comparison between the realized outcome and the outcome of the unchosen alternative. Furthermore, the OFC patients are not able to incorporate experienced regret into the process of choice behavior and do not anticipate regret or learn from their regret inducing decisions.

The study by Camille et al. [12] showed that regret generates higher physiological responses and is consistently reported by normal subjects as more intense than disappointment. This was not the case in orbitofrontal patients, demonstrating that distinct neural processes generate these two emotions.

The absence of regret in orbitofrontal patients suggests that these patients fail to grasp this concept of liability for one's own decision that colors the emotion experienced by normal subjects. It is important to highlight the fact that OFC patients are not emotionally

[handwritten margin note: so would they be more likely to go for the material gains option in my task?]

flat or unresponsive. For instance these patients expressed a normal level of disappointment [12] and a higher than normal level of anger in response to unfairness in social situations (unfair offers in an Ultimatum Game) [13]. *Thus, a key behavioral observation is that patients with lesions in the OFC are unable to experience regret and to anticipate the potential affective consequence of their choices.* This result has been confirmed by a recent neuropsychological study that demonstrates the critical role of the OFC in learning from the experience of negative feedback [57].

Coricelli et al. [14] measured brain activity using functional magnetic resonance imaging (fMRI) while subjects participated in the regret gambling task. Increasing regret was correlated with enhanced activity in the medial orbitofrontal region, the dorsal anterior cingulate cortex (ACC), and anterior hippocampus. This hippocampal activity is consistent with the idea that a cognitive-based declarative process of regret is engaged by the task. This supports a modulation of declarative (consciously accessible) memory [15,16] such that after a bad outcome the lesson to be learnt is: "in the future pay more attention to the potential consequences of your choice." Furthermore, Coricelli et al. [14] showed that activity in response to experiencing regret (OFC/ACC/medial temporal cortex) is distinct from activity seen with mere outcome evaluation (ventral striatum) and in disappointment elicited by the mismatch between actual and expected outcome of choice. Indeed, the magnitude of disappointment correlated with enhanced activity in middle temporal gyrus and dorsal brainstem, including periaqueductal gray matter, a region implicated in processing aversive signals such as pain. This suggests distinctive neural substrates in reward processing and the fact that the OFC and medial temporal cortex areas can bias basic dopamine mediated reward responses [17].

OFC activity related with the level of responsibility in the process of choice (agency) and with the available information regarding alternative outcomes (regret) influences basic responses related to reward (monetary wins) and punishers (monetary losses). *Thus, the emotions related to experiencing rewards or punishers are not independent from the alternative outcomes. Indeed, it is the counterfactual reasoning between the obtained and unobtained outcomes that determines the quality and intensity of the emotional response.* Regret and disappointment are elicited by two different counterfactual comparisons characterized by two different levels of personal responsibility for the consequence of one's own choices.

In several studies medial OFC activity reflects reward attainment [18–20], while lateral OFC is often associated with reversal learning, where subjects need to change behavioral strategies that are no longer advantageous [21–24]. This has been interpreted as suggesting that medial OFC may support positive emotions, and lateral OFC may support emotions with negative valence. Nevertheless, other neuroimaging studies [14] highlight a more complex role in reinforcement representations that is also suggested by lesion data [12] (lesions of medial OFC do not impair processing of primary rewards).

OFC has a fundamental role in adaptive behavior. Coricelli et al. [14] reported that across their fMRI experiment subjects became increasingly regret aversive, a cumulative effect reflected in enhanced activity within ventro-medial OFC and amygdale (Fig. 2).

Under these circumstances the same pattern of activity that was expressed with the experience of regret was also expressed just prior to choice, suggesting the same neural circuitry mediates both direct experience of regret and its anticipation. OFC activity related to the effect of experienced emotions in relation to potential behavioral adjustment has been also found in a recent study by Beer et al. [25]. Thus, the OFC and the amygdala contribute to this form of high-level learning based on past emotional experience, in a manner that mirrors the role of these structures in acquisition of value in low-level

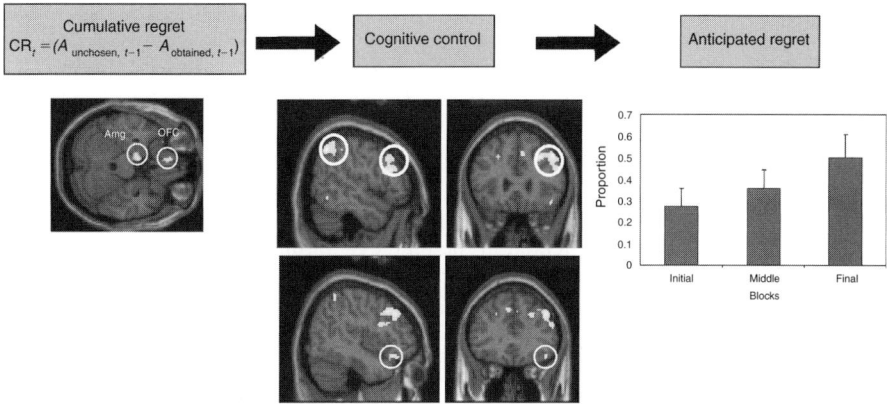

Figure 20.2 The neural basis of the adaptive function of regret [14]. The observed reactivation pattern of the OFC and amygdala (Amg) before subjects made their choices accounts for the behavioral impact (anticipated regret). Across iterations of the experiment, subjects' behavior was more and more in line with a pattern that was explained in terms of regret avoidance, reflecting the "cumulative" (learning) effect of experienced negative outcomes. The process of defining expectancies over possible consequences of the alternative of choice is based on an emotional reinforcement learning account. Cumulative regret (CR) is the difference between the average payoff realized and the average payoff missed (the payoff of the unselected gamble) over time. In other words, the impact of the consequences of rejected choices (regret) is indeed increasingly integrated in the process of choice through experience. Cognitive control activity induced by the experience of regret was observed during choices when the subjects just experienced regret $(t - 1)$. Enhanced activity in the dorsolateral prefrontal cortex (DLPFC), parietal cortex (inferior parietal lobule – IPL), and right OFC is observed.

learning contexts [20]. Indeed, animal [26] and human neuroimaging [27–30] studies assign a fundamental role to the amygdala in classical conditioning experiments, indicating its role in associative learning (acquiring cue outcome association). Schoenbaum et al. [31], recording in the OFC in basolateral amygdala (ABL) lesioned rats, found loss of acquisition of associative information, while the process of outcome anticipation remained intact. This suggests that the basolateral amygdala inputs value-related associative information into the OFC [32]. On the other hand, lesions on the rats' OFC reduced ABL associative encoding ability, showing that OFC itself facilitates learning [33].

Moreover, the affective consequences of choice, such as the experience of regret, can induce specific mechanisms of cognitive control [34]. Coricelli et al. [14] observed enhanced responses in right dorsolateral prefrontal cortex (Fig. 2), right lateral OFC, and inferior parietal lobule during a choice phase after the experience of regret [14], where subsequent choice processes induced reinforcement, or avoidance of, the experienced behavior [35]. Corroborating results from Simon-Thomas et al. [36] show that negative emotions can recruit cognitive-based right hemisphere responses. *Thus, negative affective consequences (regret) induce specific mechanisms of cognitive control on subsequent choices.*

These data suggest a mechanism through which comparing choice outcome with its alternatives, and the associated feeling of responsibility, promotes behavioral flexibility and exploratory strategies in dynamic environments so as to minimize the likelihood of emotionally negative outcomes. In the following section, we show how this evidence from brain studies is related with recent theoretical works in economics. Both theory and neural data show the adaptive role of emotions such as regret.

20.2   Reward-based emotions implement learning

Emotions may be considered as the affective evaluations of a difference between an expected and a realized value. What "value" is depends on the specific choice that is being considered. This general hypothesis assigns to emotions a functional role: learning of the agent is adaptive learning (as opposed to Bayesian learning), and therefore it has to adjust the current value function to a new, updated value function. Emotions keep track of the difference between expected and realized value, and increase or decrease the value depending on the difference.

As we have seen, the difference between the expected and the realized reward of the chosen action may be called disappointment [7,8]. This is a first example of the association between an affective evaluation of the difference between expected and realized value. In current theories of temporal difference (TD) prediction error [37–39], and in current analysis of the dopaminergic implementation of the TD model [40–44], disappointment is the only emotion that is being considered.

Reward prediction error model. The prediction error is a fundamental component in the adaptive learning of optimal actions [45]. In the prediction error model, a value is assigned to every state that the individual faces in his choices. This value is an approximation, and it is updated in every period. The value at the current state is equal to the sum of two terms: the reward at the current state and action plus the continuation value from future state. The prediction error is the difference between what is realized and what is expected. The realized value is the current reward plus the continuation value in the next state, according to the current value function. The expected value is the current value of the current state. The value function is updated by adding a term, typically linear in the difference, to the current value. This process has, under some technical conditions, good properties: the value function converges to the solution of the optimal dynamic programming problem – that is, to the true (under the optimal policy) value function at that state. In this evaluation, the action is the chosen action for the current period. Actions that were available and not chosen are ignored, even if the outcome of those actions is known to the individual.

A model of counterfactual evaluation: regret learning. Regret embodies the painful lesson that things would have been better under a different choice, thus inducing a disposition to behavioral change. People, including those with a deep knowledge of optimal strategies, often try to avoid the likelihood of future regret even when this conflicts with the prescription of decisions based upon rational choice, which predicts that individuals faced with a decision between multiple alternatives under uncertainty will opt for the course of action with maximum expected utility, a function of both the probability and the magnitude of the expected payoff [46]. The theory we adopt makes reference to existing theories of regret as a form of adaptive learning, in the tradition of the Megiddo-Foster-Vohra-Hart-Mas-Colell [47–51] regret-based models. In these theories, learning adjusts the probability of choosing an action depending on the difference between the total rewards that could have been obtained with the choice of that action and the realized rewards. For example, in the Hart-Mas-Colell [49] *regret-matching rule model* the regret for having chosen the action k instead of j is the difference between the total reward obtained if action j had been chosen instead of k in the past, and the total realized value. The probability of choosing an action is determined in every period by adjusting upwards the probability of choosing the action j by an amount proportional to the regret. This type of procedures have optimality properties just as the adjustment process based on prediction error: the Megiddo theorem [47] for the single player case, and the Foster-Vohra-Hart-Mas-Colell theorems for games show that this procedure converges to optimal choices in the single player case and to correlated equilibria in the case of games.

The regret matching rule is adaptive in the sense that leads to flexible behavior (switching to "better" strategies), inducing dynamics similar to reinforcement learning models based on stationary stochastic adjustment, such as the fictitious player. These characteristics of the regret-matching procedure make it reasonably suitable for being implemented in actual ("real") decision making in dynamic settings. For example, in financial decisions, investors often behave using a regret-matching procedure, switching to other investment when they realize that they would have gained more money if they had chosen other investment, and this switching probability is proportional to the amount of missed gains.

Foster and Young [50] propose a similar adaptive procedure, called *regret testing*. This procedure is analogous to aspiration learning models, in which players stochastically change actions if the realized payoff are less than an aspiration level (payoff that the subject hope to achieve). With this rule the players' decision to switch (probabilistically) to other distribution over actions is driven by regret. Regret arises when the payoff from a randomly chosen action is higher than the current aspiration level (realized payoff). Foster and Young prove that the regret testing procedure leads to (arbitrarily close to) Nash equilibrium of the period-by-period behavior in any finite two-person game. Thus, showing how payoff-base rules can approach equilibrium behavior.

In computational neuroscience a similar type of reinforcement learning is called "fictive learning" or counterfactual Q-learning [52,53]. In these models the error signal is a "fictive error" computed as the difference between the obtained reward and the rewards of alternative foregone actions. The function that represents the effect of the foregone actions contributes to the update of values in addition to a standard Q-leaning critic function.

20.3   What should adaptive learning do?

Two problems seem important. The first is that any adaptive procedure to be plausible should have a satisfactory performance from the point of view of the reward: for example, the regret-matching rule leads the choice of an action maximizing expected reward. The fictive learning does not satisfy this condition in an obvious way.

If we do impose some performance criterion, then a second problem arises. Recall that an action has a dual role: it affects the current reward and the transition to the next state. This makes introducing counterfactual thinking into adaptive learning a subtle problem, because we can observe the rewards from other actions, but we cannot observe the transition that would have been produced by them. When an action a out of a set A, say, is chosen, the individual may have available the information on the reward of all the elements in A, and can then compare the reward from a with the reward from the other actions. If the reward from an element in A, b say, different from a is larger, then regret seems natural, and an effective way to use the counterfactual information. It would, however, be deeply wrong, because it would ignore the effect that the actions have on the transition to the next state. Differently from the rewards, the information on where the state would have transited to if b had been chosen is not available to the individual. But if the effect on the transition is ignored, then the relative value of the two actions can be grossly distorted.

For example, suppose that the action b gives a large reward today but makes the state go to a state tomorrow where rewards are very low, while a gives a smaller reward, but also keeps the state in a good position. If a is chosen, the regret we feel by looking at the reward from b would be mistaken, because b free rides on the good effect of a on the state.

We suggest a general theoretical framework to address the general issue of integrating adaptive learning with counterfactual thinking. One important difference between the prediction error model and the counterfactual model is the neural basis of the two: from the existing literature on the topic we know that the ventral tegmental area [41,54] and ventral striatum [43,44] are usually associated with the reward prediction error models, while we propose that the OFC exerts a top-down modulation of the gain of emotions thanks to counterfactual reasoning, after a decision has been made and its consequences can be evaluated. Thus, the feeling of responsibility for the negative result, that is, regret, reinforces the decisional learning process.

20.4   Private and social rewards

Regret is an emotion that is limited to the private sphere: the counterfactual comparison that motivates regret is limited to the set of choices that were available to the individual decision maker. But we live in a society in which many if not most of our choices are not made in isolation: we observe others that make similar choices, and we can observe their outcome as well. The same logic suggesting that using the information on the outcome of the actions we did not choose is useful in improving our future performance also suggests that we should use the information on the outcome of actions that *others* chose. *The counterfactual reasoning extends from private to social learning.* This is Festinger's idea [55], presented in his theory of Social Comparison (1954). In this view, regret has a social correspondent, envy. Just as regret derives from the comparison between what we received from an action, and what we could have received from action that we did not take, so envy may simply derive from the comparison between the outcome from the action we chose and the outcome from an action we did not choose but someone else did.

Emotional evaluation of social rewards is more complex, however, because outcomes that are socially observable also affect the relative ranking of individuals, and so this evaluation is the result of social learning and social ranking. The work by Bault et al. [56] is a way of experimentally separating the two components. The goal of this study was first to directly compare how individuals evaluate the outcome of their decision in private versus social contexts, with the hypothesis that for a given outcome, social context will enhance emotional responses due to social comparison. More important, the study was designed to investigate whether social and private emotions influence monetary decisions in different ways. In Bault et al. [56] participants choose among lotteries, with different levels of risk, and observe the choice that others have made. They are then informed of the monetary outcome of their choice and the choice of others, and have the opportunity in this way to experience regret and envy, or their positive counterparts (relief and gloating). Emotions in the social condition, for the events in which participants made different choices, are stronger than in the single player condition. The second result is that social emotions operate differently from private ones: while regret looms larger than relief, gloating looms larger than envy. The effect in not induced by any social emotion (as opposed to non-social) as shared regret and shared relief received weaker ratings than regret and relief experienced in a non-social context. Thus, envy and gloating matter more because they are socially competitive emotions not just interpersonal ones (Fig. 3).

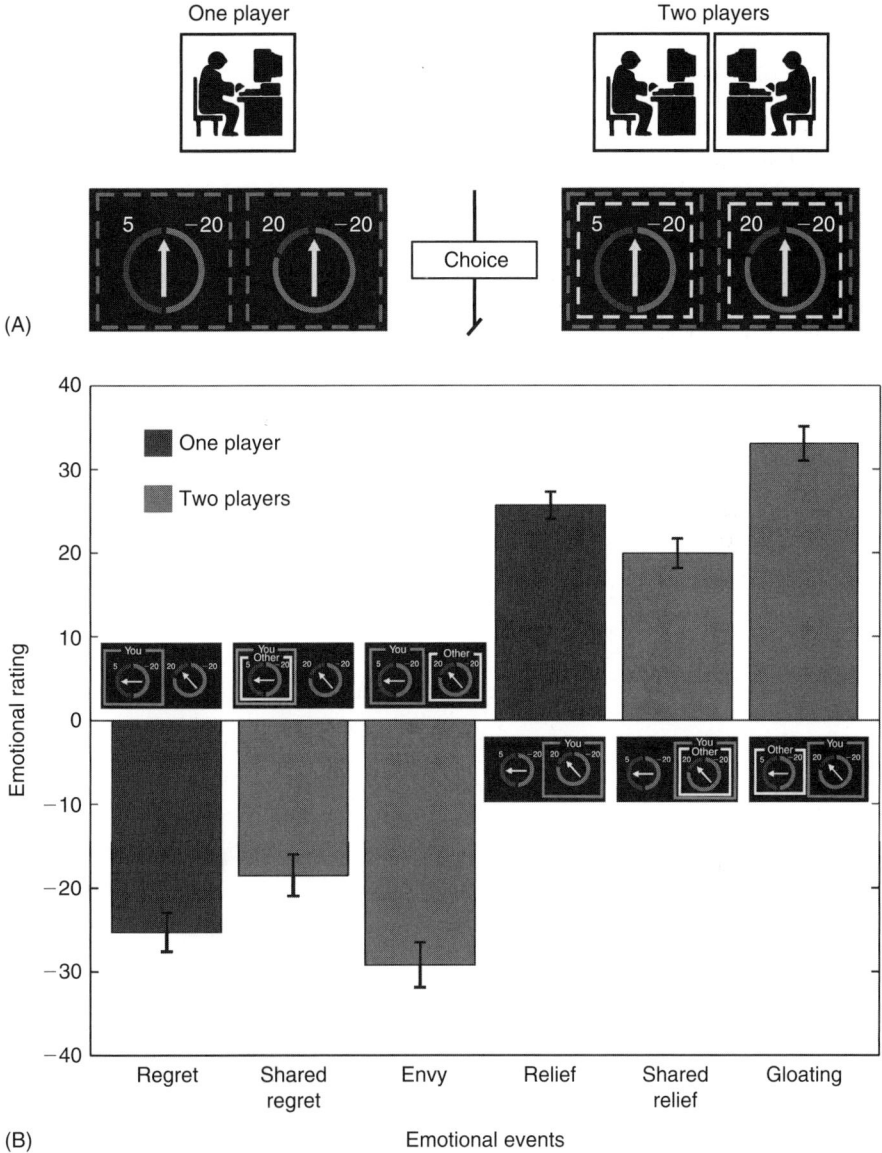

(A)

(B)

Figure 20.3 (A) Typical single (on the left) and two player trial in Bault et al. [56]. Numbers indicated outcomes, and the probabilities were represented by colored sectors of a circle. Each lottery was surrounded with one dotted square in the case of a one player trial or two dotted squares of different colors in the case of a two player trial. (B) Emotional responses: average subjective emotional evaluations for different events. The bars represent the average value (±SEM) of the subjective emotional evaluation given by participants in the different events. The pictures around the horizontal axis show the typical screen display seen by participants in the different events. See Plate 22 of Color Plate section.

When analyzing choice behavior, Bault et al. [56] found an important difference between the private and the social dimensions. In both cases, deviations from expected utility are explained by the effect of the difference between the obtained outcome and the alternative possible outcome. In the private domain, the alternative outcome is that of an action that was not chosen, and aversion to loss (regret) dominates. In the social environment the alternative outcome is that of a choice made by another person, and love of gain (gloating) dominates.

A particularly important issue is the relative attitude to gains and losses in counterfactual evaluations. Regret is a negative affective state; but counterfactual thinking may produce, if the choice was right, an opposite emotion, a positive affective state induced when the outcome of the chosen action is better than the outcome from actions that were not taken. This emotion we may call relief. The general idea described in Prospect Theory (losses loom larger than gains) may be translated in the present context into the conjecture that counterfactual losses (regret) loom larger than counterfactual gains (relief).

Because, as we have just read, social counterfactual thinking has special motivations (because social ranking is added to social learning), the effect might be different in social environments. Indeed, the effect of the social ranking component might be the opposite: because many environments follow the rule winner-takes-all, and being first is much better than being second, while the latter is not much different from being third, gains might loom larger than losses.

The two hypotheses that the attitude to counterfactual gains and losses is similar to that to real gains and losses in private domains, and opposite in social ones is confirmed in Bault et al. [56].

20.5   Conclusions

Experimental and theoretical results demonstrate experimentally an adaptive role of reward-based emotions, such as regret. These emotions also figure prominently in the literature of learning in games. A remarkable result in this literature is that if players in a game minimize regret, the frequency of their choices converges to a correlated equilibrium (i.e., the rational solution) of the game. This has a general implication for our understanding of the role of emotions in decision making and rejects the dual/conflict view of "emotion versus cognition" (rationality) by showing the powerful consequences of full integration between those two components of human decision making. Within this hypothesis, emotions do not necessarily interfere with rational decision making, and on the contrary they may implement it: they are a way of evaluating past outcomes to adjust choices in the future. These are features that are common between the prediction error model and the counterfactual learning. The crucial difference between TD learning and regret learning is the counterfactual difference between the rewards the individual received and those he would have received had he chosen a different action. One important difference between the prediction error model and the counterfactual model is of course the neural basis of the two: from the existing literature on the topic we know that the ventral tegmental area and ventral striatum are usually associated with the prediction error, while counterfactual learning is associated with the OFC.

References

[1]   N.J. Roese, J.M. Olson, What Might Have Been: The Social Psychology of Counterfactual Thinking, Erlbaum, Mahwah, NJ, 1995.

[2] R.M. Byrne, Mental models and counterfactual thoughts about what might have been, Trends Cogn. Sci. 6 (2002) 426–431.

[3] M. Zeelenberg, E. van Dijk, On the comparative nature of the emotion regret, in: D. Mandel, D.J. Hilton, P. Catellani (Eds.), The Psychology of Counterfactual Thinking, Routledge, London, 2004.

[4] D.E. Bell, Regret in decision-making under uncertainty, Oper. Res. 30 (1982) 961–981.

[5] G. Loomes, R. Sugden, Regret theory: an alternative theory of rational choice under uncertainty, Econ. J. 92 (1982) 805–824.

[6] T. Gilovich, V.H. Melvec, The temporal pattern to the experience of regret, J. Pers. Soc. Psychol. 67 (1994) 357–365.

[7] G. Loomes, R. Sugden, Disappointment and dynamic inconsistency in choice under uncertainty, Rev. Econ. Stud. 53 (1986) 271–282.

[8] D.E. Bell, Disappointment in decision making under uncertainty, Oper. Res. 33 (1995) 1–27.

[9] I. Ritov, Probabilities of regret: anticipation of uncertainty resolution in choice, Organ. Behav. Hum. Decis. Process. 66 (1996) 228–236.

[10] M. Zeelenberg, J. Beattie, J. van der Plight, N.K. de Vries, Consequences of regret aversion: effects of expected feedback on risky decision making, Organ. Behav. Hum. Decis. Process. 65 (1996) 148–158.

[11] N.H. Frijda, The Emotions, Cambridge University Press, Cambridge, 1986.

[12] N. Camille, G. Coricelli, J. Sallet, P. Pradat-Diehl, J.R. Duhamel, A. Sirigu, The involvement of the orbitofrontal cortex in the experience of regret, Science 304 (2004) 1167–1170.

[13] M. Koenigs, D. Tranel, Irrational economic decision-making after ventromedial prefrontal damage: evidence from the Ultimatum Game, J. Neurosci. 27 (2007) 951–956.

[14] G. Coricelli, H.D. Critchley, M. Joffily, J.P. O'Doherty, A. Sirigu, R.J. Dolan, Regret and its avoidance: a neuroimaging study of choice behavior, Nat. Neurosci. 8 (2005) 1255–1262.

[15] H. Eichenbaum, Hippocampus: cognitive processes and neural representations that underlie declarative memory, Neuron 44 (2004) 109–120.

[16] S. Steidl, S. Mohi-uddin, A.K. Anderson, Effects of emotional arousal on multiple memory systems: evidence from declarative and procedural learning, Learn. Mem. 13 (2006) 650–658.

[17] B. De Martino, D. Kumaran, B. Seymour, R.J. Dolan, Frames, biases, and rational decision-making in the human brain, Science 313 (2006) 684–687.

[18] E.T. Rolls, The orbitofrontal cortex and reward, Cereb. Cortex 10 (2000) 284–294.

[19] H.C. Breiter, I. Aharon, D. Kahneman, A. Dale, P. Shizgal, Functional imaging of neural responses to expectancy and experience of monetary gains and losses, Neuron 30 (2001) 619–639.

[20] J.A. Gottfried, J. O'Doherty, R.J. Dolan, Encoding predictive reward value in human amygdala and orbitofrontal cortex, Science 301 (2003) 1104–1107.

[21] R. Elliott, R.J. Dolan, C.D. Frith, Dissociable functions in the medial and lateral orbitofrontal cortex: evidence from human neuroimaging studies, Cereb. Cortex 10 (2000) 308–317.

[22] J. O'Doherty, M.L. Kringelbach, E.T. Rolls, J. Hornak, C. Andrews, Abstract reward and punishment representations in the human orbitofrontal cortex, Nat. Neurosci. 4 (2001) 95–102.

[23] L.K. Fellows, M.J. Farah, Ventromedial frontal cortex mediates affective shifting in humans: evidence from a reversal learning paradigm, Brain 126 (2003) 1830–1837.

[24] J. Hornak, J. O'Doherty, J. Bramham, E.T. Rolls, R.G. Morris, P.R. Bullock, C.E. Polkey, Reward-related reversal learning after surgical excisions in orbito-frontal or dorsolateral prefrontal cortex in humans, J. Cogn. Neurosci. 16 (2004) 463–478.

[25] J.S. Beer, R.T. Knight, M. D'Esposito, Controlling the integration of emotion and cognition: the role of frontal cortex in distinguishing helpful from hurtful emotional information, Psychol. Sci. 17 (2006) 448–453.

[26] P. Amorapanth, J.E. LeDoux, K. Nader, Different lateral amygdala outputs mediate reactions and actions elicited by a fear-arousing stimulus, Nat. Neurosci. 3 (2000) 74–79.

[27] C. Buchel, J. Morris, R.J. Dolan, K.J. Friston, Brain systems mediating aversive conditioning: an event-related fMRI study, Neuron 20 (1998) 947–957.

[28] K.S. LaBar, J.C. Gatenby, J.C. Gore, J.E. LeDoux, E.A. Phelps, Human amygdala activation during conditioned fear acquisition and extinction: a mixed-trial fMRI study, Neuron 20 (1998) 937–945.

[29] J.P. O'Doherty, R. Deichmann, H.D. Critchley, R.J. Dolan, Neural responses during anticipation of a primary taste reward, Neuron 33 (2002) 815–826.

[30] K.S. LaBar, R. Cabeza, Cognitive neuroscience of emotional memory, Nat. Rev. Neurosci. 7 (2006) 54–64.

[31] G. Schoenbaum, B. Setlow, M.P. Saddoris, M. Gallagher, Encoding predicted outcome and acquired value in orbitofrontal cortex during cue sampling depends upon input from basolateral amygdala, Neuron 39 (2003) 855–867.

[32] G. Schoenbaum, B. Setlow, S.L. Nugent, M.P. Saddoris, M. Gallagher, Lesions of orbitofrontal cortex and basolateral amygdala complex disrupt acquisition of odor-guided discriminations and reversals, Learn. Mem. 10 (2003) 129–140.

[33] M.P. Saddoris, M. Gallagher, G. Schoenbaum, Rapid associative encoding in basolateral amygdala depends on connections with orbitofrontal cortex, Neuron 46 (2005) 321–331.

[34] T. Yarkoni, J.R. Gray, E.R. Chrastil, D.M. Barch, L. Green, T.S. Braver, Sustained neural activity associated with cognitive control during temporally extended decision making, Brain Res. Cogn. Brain Res. 23 (2005) 71–84.

[35] L. Clark, R. Cools, T.W. Robbins, The neuropsychology of ventral prefrontal cortex: decision-making and reversal learning, Brain Cogn. 55 (2004) 41–53.

[36] E.R. Simon-Thomas, K.O. Role, R.T. Knight, Behavioral and electrophysiological evidence of a right hemisphere bias for the influence of negative emotion on higher cognition, J. Cogn. Neurosci. 17 (2005) 518–529.

[37] P. Dayan, Computational modelling, Curr. Opin. Neurobiol. 4 (1994) 212–217.

[38] W. Schultz, Getting formal with dopamine and reward, Neuron 36 (2002) 241–263.

[39] P.R. Montague, B. King-Casas, J.D. Cohen, Imaging valuation models in human choice, Annu. Rev. Neurosci. 29 (2006) 417–448.

[40] W. Schultz, P. Dayan, P.R. Montague, A neural substrate of prediction and reward, Science 275 (1997) 1593–1599.

[41] W. Schultz, Predictive reward signal of dopamine neurons, J. Neurophysiol. 80 (1998) 1–27.

[42] W. Schultz, L. Tremblay, J.R. Hollerman, Reward prediction in primate basal ganglia and frontal cortex, Neuropharmacology 37 (1998) 421–429.

[43] J.P. O'Doherty, Reward representations and reward-related learning in the human brain: insights from neuroimaging, Curr. Opin. Neurobiol. 14 (2004) 769–776.

[44] B. Seymour, J.P. O'Doherty, P. Dayan, M. Koltzenburg, A.K. Jones, R.J. Dolan, K.J. Friston, R.S. Frackowiak, Temporal difference models describe higher-order learning in humans, Nature 429 (2004) 664–667.

[45] P. Dayan, Y. Niv, Reinforcement learning: the good, the bad and the ugly, Curr. Opin. Neurobiol. 18 (2008) 185–196.

[46] J. Von Neumann, O. Morgenstern, Theory of Games and Economic Behavior, Princeton University Press, Princeton, NJ, 1944.

[47] N. Megiddo, On repeated games with incomplete information played by non-Bayesian players, Int. J. Game Theory 9 (1980) 157–167.

[48] D.P. Foster, R. Vohra, Regret in the on-line decision problem, Game. Econ. Behav. 29 (1999) 7–35.

[49] S. Hart, A. Mas-Colell, A simple adaptive procedure leading to correlated equilibrium, Econometrica 68 (2000) 1127–1150.

[50] D.P. Foster, H.P. Young, Learning, hypothesis testing, and Nash equilibrium, Game. Econ. Behav. 45 (2003) 73–96.

[51] S. Hart, Adaptive heuristics, Econometrica 73 (2005) 1401–1430.
[52] P.R. Montague, B. King-Casas, J.D. Cohen, Imaging valuation models in human choice, Annu. Rev. Neurosci. 29 (2006) 417–448.
[53] T. Lohrenz, K. McCabe, C.F. Camerer, P.R. Montague, Neural signature of fictive learning signals in a sequential investment task, Proc. Natl. Acad. Sci. USA 104 (2007) 9493–9498.
[54] W. Schultz, The phasic reward signal of primate dopamine neurons, Adv. Pharmacol. 42 (1998) 686–690.
[55] L. Festinger, A theory of social comparison processes, Hum. Relat. 7 (1954) 117–140.
[56] N. Bault, G. Coricelli, A. Rustichini, Interdependent utilities: how social ranking affects choice behavior, PLoS ONE 3 (2008) e3477.
[57] E.Z. Wheeler, L.K. Fellows, The human ventromedial frontal lobe is critical for learning from negative feedback, Brain 131 (2008) 1323–1331.

21 Bayesian decision making in two-alternative forced choices

Sophie Deneve[1,2]

[1]Group for Neural Theory, Département d'Etudes Cognitives, Ecole Normale Supérieure, 29, rue d'Ulm, 75005 Paris, France
[2]Groupe de Neuroscience Théorique, Collège de France, 3, rue d'Ulm, 75005 Paris, France

Abstract

In order to make fast and accurate behavioral choices, we need to integrate the noisy sensory input, take into account prior knowledge, and adjust our decision criteria to maximize the expected outcome of our actions. These problems can be formalized in a probabilistic framework: given the sensory input, what decision strategies will result in maximizing the expected reward? In simple two-alternative forced choice tasks, Bayesian decision making is equivalent to a "diffusion" process. However, this apparently simple fact hides a "chicken and eggs" problem: to integrate the sensory input and set the decision threshold, we have to know how reliable the sensory input is. And how can we know that without making a decision and observing the outcome?

In this chapter, we consider a Bayesian decision model that infer both the choice probability and the reliability of the sensory input, within a single trial, and based solely on the responses from a population of sensory neurons. This results in a "modified" diffusion model updating the impact of a sensory spike and the decision threshold online. As a consequence, sensory spikes early in the trial have typically a stronger impact on the final decision, and decisions are made with lower accuracy in harder trials. We show that this Bayesian decision model can account for recent findings in primates trained at a motion discrimination task.

Key points

1. Optimal decisions in two-alternative forced choices (2AFCs) can be separated into an inference stage, computing the probability for each choice, and a decision criteria, setting the time/accuracy trade-off.
2. If the reliability of the sensory input is known, this is equivalent to a diffusion model.
3. Most often, this reliability must be estimated at the same time than the probability of choice. Both can be performed simultaneously by integrating sensory spikes.
4. In difficult tasks, sensory inputs received early should have a stronger impact on the final decisions than later inputs, while decision threshold should collapse over time.
5. The reverse should be true for easy tasks: sensory gain and decision threshold should both increase over the duration of the trial.

Survival requires fast and accurate decisions in an uncertain and continuously changing world. Unfortunately, our sensory input is noisy, ambiguous, and unfolding over time.

The outcome of actions, such as reward or punishment, is also uncertain. As a result, perceptual or motor decisions cannot be predefined, instantaneous responses to sensory stimuli. Instead, sensory evidence needs to be accumulated over time and integrated with prior knowledge and reward predictions. The study of decision making deals with the solutions adopted by living organisms to solve two distinct but related problems: faced with different choices, which one would yield the most desirable outcome ("What to decide?")? In addition, because delaying decision allows more time for collecting information and increases choice accuracy, when should this decision be made ("When to decide?")? Optimal decisions strategies solve this time/accuracy trade-off in order to maximize the amount of rewards collected by units of time, that is, the reward rate.

One of the fundamental question in the study of decision making is whether or not the strategies used by humans or animals are optimal, for example, if these strategies lead to the highest amount of collected reward. Indeed, recent experimental and theoretical results suggest that humans use Bayesian optimal strategies in a wide variety of tasks [1–5]. In simple experimental settings, such as two-alternative forced choice (2AFC) tasks, the optimal decision strategy can be described quantitatively as an integration to threshold [6,7]. In this framework, decision making is divided into two successive stages. First, the inference stage accumulates sensory evidence over time by computing the probabilities that each choice is correct given past sensory observations ("What to decide?"). Second, a decision is made to commit to one of the choice once these probabilities have reached a given criteria ("When to decide?"). This response criterion is critical because it shapes the time/accuracy trade-off and controls the total reward collected by the subject.

In certain context, Bayesian decision making is equivalent to previous decision models such as the diffusion model [7]. In general, however, Bayesian methods lead to non-linear, non-stationary models of integration and decision rules [8–11]. In order to solve a decision problem, a Bayesian integrator needs to constantly adjust its strategy to the statistical structure of the task and the reward. While simple in their formulation, these probabilistic decision problems can have solutions that are quite difficult to analyze mathematically, and are computationally intractable. Simplifying assumptions are required.

On the other hand, a strong advantage of using a Bayesian approach is its adaptability and its capacity to generalize to situations were simpler decision models would not work or would be suboptimal [1,8,12–14]. In this chapter we start from an extremely simple task (i.e., 2AFC task) where Bayesian decision making would be equivalent to the diffusion model, but only if the probability distributions of sensory inputs (i.e., the sensory likelihoods) were known in advance. We then show that when these distributions are not known (which is likely to be true in most realistic decision tasks), enough information can be extracted from the sensory input (in the form of spike trains from sensory neurons) to estimate the precision of the sensory input online and adapt the decision strategy accordingly.

This adaptation has strong consequences on the decision mechanism. This predicts in particular that in hard decision tasks, the sensory input is weighted more strongly early during stimulus presentation. Its influence later decays, implying that the choice is made based on prior knowledge and the first few sensory observations, not the sensory input just preceding the decision. This framework also predict that decision thresholds (i.e., the amount of integrated sensory evidence deemed necessary to commit to a choice) is not fixed but evolve as a function of time and the sensory input: for hard tasks, this threshold collapses, resulting in forcing a decision within a limited time frame. For easy tasks, this threshold increases, that is, decisions are made with higher accuracy at the cost of slightly longer reaction times.

We present simulation implementing a decision task that have proved very influential in the field and whose behavioral and neural basis have been largely unraveled. We compare the Bayesian decision maker with a diffusion model and show that while both models predict similar trends for the mean reaction time and accuracy, the Bayesian model also predict some strong deviations from the diffusion model predictions. These deviations have been observed in behaving monkeys trained at this task [15–18].

21.1 Bayesian decision model

Consider a 2AFC between two possible responses, "A" or "B." This decision needs to be made based on an ongoing, noisy stream of sensory data. Let us suppose that correct choices are rewarded, while incorrect choices are not. How could subjects adjust their decision strategies in order to maximize their total expected reward? As described previously, this problem can be separated into an inference stage and decision criteria.

21.1.1 Inference

The inference stage corresponds to a temporal integration of sensory evidence in order to compute the probability that each of the choice is correct.

The probability of choices can be computed online as the log odd ratio, $L_t = \log(P(A|s_{o \to t})/P(B|s_{o \to t}))$, where $s_{o \to t}$ is the sensory input received up to time t. Inference corresponds to an accumulation of sensory evidence over time

$$\frac{\partial L}{dt} = l(s_t), \qquad (21.1)$$

where $l(s_t) = \log(P(s_t|A)/P(s_t|B))$ is the log likelihood ratio for the sensory input received at time t, and the starting point of integration corresponds to the prior probability of choices $L_o = \log(P(A)/P(B))$. For example, $L_o = \log(2)$ when A is *a priori* twice more likely than B [19].

These suppose of course that probability of sensory inputs given the choices, that is, the likelihoods $P(s_t|A)$ and $P(s_t|B)$, are known. These likelihoods capture the selectivity and variability of sensory responses. Their relative values describe how reliable is the sensory input at time t. Thus, if the likelihood of the sensory input is much larger for choice A than choice B, this input will strongly support choice A against choice B.

As a first illustrative example, we use a toy model of a decision based on the noisy spike train of a single motion-sensitive, direction-selective neuron. In this simple decision task, the two alternative choices are whether the stimulus moves in the preferred direction of this neuron (choice A) or the opposite, anti-preferred direction (choice B). The sensory input s_t corresponds to the spike train of the neuron, that is, a temporal binary stream of 1 or 0 (depending on whether a spike is emitted or not at time t). We suppose that the baseline firing rate q is increased to $q + dq$ in the preferred direction, and decreased to $q - dq$ in the anti-preferred direction. Thus, $q + dq$ and $q - dq$ are respectively the likelihood of a sensory spike given choice A and choice B.

The initial log odds at the starts of the trial is set to $L_o = 0$, indicating that the two stimulus direction occur with the same prior probability. Bayesian inference corresponds in this framework to an integration of input spikes minus a constant negative drift. Each spike instantaneously increases the log odd ratio by a fixed amount $w = \log((q + dq)/(q - dq))$. The temporal evolution of the log odd ratio is then given by:

$$\frac{\partial L_t}{dt} = w(s_t - q), \qquad (21.2)$$

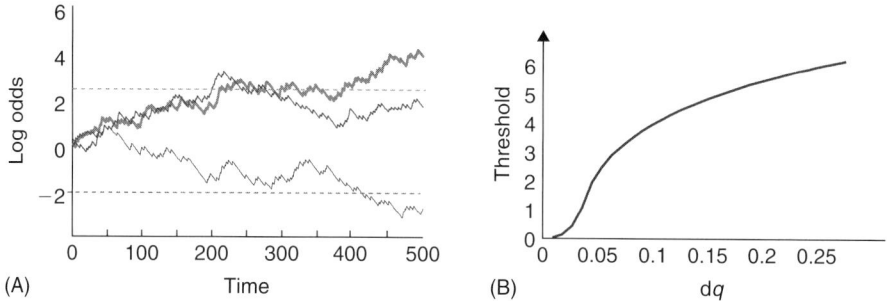

Figure 21.1 "Bayesian" diffusion model. (A) Examples of log odds on three different trails. Thin black line: trials were "choice A" was the correct choice. Thin grey line: trail were "choice B" was correct. Thick grey line: an error trial where choice "A" was made and choice "B" was the correct choice. Dashed line: decision thresholds. (B) Optimal decision threshold as a function of the difference in firing rate expected for the two directions of motion.

where w can be interpreted as the weight given to a sensory spike. The log odds L_t represent the current confidence in choice A versus choice B. It increases on average if the input firing rate is above baseline, and decreases on average if it is below baseline. However, this accumulation is noisy due to the variability in the Poisson spike train of the sensory neuron. Three example trials are plotted in Fig. 21.1A.

21.1.2   Decision criteria

We can distinguish two variants of the 2AFC task leading to two different decision strategies [17]. In "reaction time" tasks, subjects observe the sensory input and are required to respond as soon as they feel ready to do so. In "fixed delay" tasks, subjects observe the sensory input presented for a fixed duration. They indicate their choice only after a "go" signal, and thus cannot control the decision time.

In "fixed delay" tasks, the optimal decision strategy consists simply in measuring the sign of the log odds at the end of stimulus presentation. If the log odds are positive, choice A is more probable than choice B, and vice versa. Going for the most probable choice will maximize the probability of getting rewarded on each trial.

For "reaction time" tasks, the optimal strategy is a little more complicated. The log odd ratio indicates the online probability of making a correct choice if one chooses A versus B. If we decide on option A when the log odd ratio crosses a positive threshold, D and decide on option B when it crosses a negative threshold $-D$ (Fig. 21.1A), the probability of making the correct choice will be given by

$$P_D = \frac{\exp(D)}{1 + \exp(D)}.$$

The decision threshold also controls the duration of the trial, since it takes longer to reach a higher threshold. To optimize the decision strategy, we need to adjust D so as to maximize the total amount of reward collected per unit of time. The optimal threshold depends on the detailed experimental protocol. If, for example, a reward is provided only for correct choices, and each trial is followed by a fixed inter-trial interval T_{iti}, the total reward rate is given by

$$RR_D = \frac{P_D}{RT_D + T_{iti}},$$ (21.3)

where RT_D is the mean reaction time, that is, the time it takes on average for L_t to reach either D or $-D$ [7]. A high threshold increases the reaction time RT_D but also increases the probability of a correct decision P_D. There is a particular threshold for which this reward rate is maximized, setting the optimal time-accuracy trade-off. From this we can compute the optimal threshold as a function of the reliability of the sensory input (see Mathematical appendix). This reliability depends on the selectivity of the sensory cell for motion direction, that is, how large is the difference in firing rate (dq) between the two motion directions. It is contained in the sensory likelihood, and influence the decision time though the sensory weight w.

The optimal boundary maximizing the reward rate increases with the sensory weight. If the input is very reliable, accurate decisions can be made very quickly. Thus, the optimal threshold is high. If, on the other hand, reliabilities and sensory weights are low, reaching high choice accuracy would be very costly in terms of reaction time. In this case, the optimal threshold is small. Below a certain drift rate, waiting to make a decision is not worth the additional gain in accuracy, and the optimal threshold is zero: decisions should be made right away, without waiting for the sensory input, resulting in a random choice with accuracy $P_D = 0.5$ and reaction time $RT_D = 0$. The optimal boundary as a function of dq is plotted on Fig. 21.1B.

21.1.3   Bayesian model and diffusion model

The Bayesian approach contrasts with descriptive models of decision making such as the race model or the diffusion model [7,20,21]. These models were not necessarily derived from principles of optimality. Interestingly, however, these simple decision mechanisms are equivalent to Bayesian optimal decision making in specific contexts. For example, the parameters of a diffusion model can be adjusted to be equivalent to Bayesian optimal decision in 2AFC tasks when the sensory likelihoods are Gaussians [7]. The diffusion model first integrates a noisy signal (analogous to the "inference stage" in the Bayesian framework), and takes a decision when the integrator reaches one of two possible bounds. Variants of diffusion models have been shown to reproduce successful human and animal behavior in 2AFC tasks [7,17,18,22–25].

While they share similar mechanisms with diffusion models, Bayesian decision models (or Bayesian interpretations of the diffusion model) have the advantage of being more constrained by the experimental protocol and the sensory noise. In a diffusion model, the starting point of the integration, the drift rate and the threshold are free parameters that can be adjusted to fit experimental data. In a Bayesian model, these are constrained respectively by the prior probabilities of the choice, the likelihoods of the sensory input, and the reward schedule. These parameters are either constrained by the experimental protocol (such as the prior) or can be estimated separately (such as the sensory reliabilities).

Unfortunately, an important drawback of the Bayesian framework is that the likelihood ratio of the sensory input $l(s_t)$ needs to be known *a priori*. In other words, subjects need to know exactly what sensory signals and noise to expect for each of the choice. Without this knowledge, the weight of the sensory input and the optimal boundary cannot be set. Most past models of decision making did not consider the possibility that the sensory likelihoods could be adjusted online as a function of the sensory input. It was assumed that estimating sensory likelihoods would require a much longer integration time than the decision itself, and thus, that these likelihoods had to be learnt at best over many trials. However, this is not necessarily true, as we demonstrate next.

21.2   Estimating sensory likelihoods on line

Sensory likelihoods are determined not only by the sensory noise, by also by the nature of the decision task. For example, categorization tasks result in very different likelihoods from discrimination tasks. Thus, the likelihoods of the same auditory signals is very different whether the task is to recognize one of two words, "bad" and "dad," or if it is to decide between two possible categories, that is, "adjective" or "noun." In one case, the sensory likelihood corresponds mainly to auditory noise and variability among speakers. In the other case, the likelihoods are strongly dependant on grammar and semantics, since they depend on the probability of encountering words with similar acoustic properties as either "noun" or "adjective."

Most of the decision we make every day are in a unique context that will never be repeated. As a result, it is very unlikely that sensory likelihood could always be derived from past experience. For example, consider the decision of choosing to invest in one of two different stock options. If stock option "A" suddenly rises and stock option "B" falls, this could be due to a higher yield of option "A," or just noise in the stock market. We will never know what to make of this observation without accumulating enough experience of the random fluctuations to expect for option prices. Ideally, we should be able to evaluate these fluctuations at the same time than we accumulate evidence about the best choice. But is it realistic?

There is an equivalent problem in 2AFC tasks. Usually, these protocols inter-mix trials with various levels of difficulties in order to measure psychophysical curves. For example, subjects could be asked to decide between two directions of motion, while varying the level of noise in the motion display [26], or to do a categorization task, while varying the distance between the test stimulus and the category boundary [25]. These protocols imply that the "quality" of the sensory input, that is, the sensory likelihood ratio, is not known at the start of a trial. In our toy model, varying task difficulties could correspond to changes in the background firing rate or the difference in firing rate between the preferred and anti-preferred direction. Any of these changes would affect the sensory weights, drift rate, and optimal boundary for decision making.

For example, let us suppose that the task difficulty in our toy example is varied by controlling the amount of noise in the visual stimulus. This can be done by using motion displays composed of moving dots while varying the portion of dots moving coherently in one direction, the rest of the dots moving in random directions [27]. The proportion of dots moving coherently corresponds to the "motion coherence." Motion coherence of 0.5 for rightward motion means that 50% of the dots move in the rightward direction. These kinds of stimuli have been used intensively to investigate the neural basis of decision making in humans and non-human primates. They cause neural responses in direction-selective sensory neurons (i.e., in the medio-temporal [MT] area) that can roughly be described by a an increase or decrease of the background firing rate by an amount proportional to motion coherence [23,27]. Thus, the firing rate of the sensory neuron is $q + cdq$ for choice A, and $q - cdq$ for choice B, where c is a function of motion coherence (Fig. 21.2A).

The sensory weights and the bounds should be updated accordingly. But how can they be when trials with high and low coherence are randomly intermixed?

There is two possible ways of addressing the problem: one could do a "compromise" between the different possible levels of coherence by using a fixed sensory weight and a fixed threshold. Or one could attempt to estimate the coherence online, adjusting the sensory weight and the bound during the duration of a single trial.

Motion coherence influences the firing rate of sensory neurons, and thus, can be estimated from the sensory input at the same time than the direction of motion. Using the Bayes theorem, we could compute the joint probability of both contrast and choice, $P(A, c|s_{o \to t})$ and $P(B, c|s_{o \to t})$, based on augmented sensory likelihoods (see Mathematical appendix); this is a straightforward extension of the sequential probability ratio method used in Eq. 21.1. The temporal evolution of the estimated coherence and the choice probability are plotted for two motion coherence in Fig. 21.2B. Observe that the coherence estimate evolves on a similar time scale than the choice probability. As a consequence, sensory weights and decision threshold can be adjusted considerably during the duration of a single trial based on the sensory input itself.

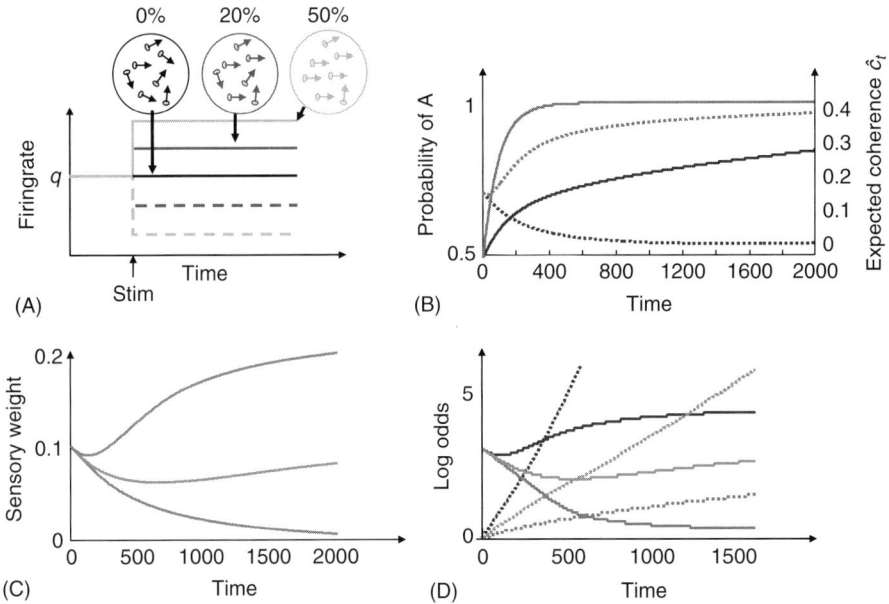

Figure 21.2 Bayesian decision making with varying motion coherence. (A) Modulation of firing rate in response to varying motion coherence. Plain line: stimulus in the preferred direction. Dashed line: simulus in the anti-preferred direction. (B) Outcome of the "full" Bayesian model computing the joint probabilities of all pairs of choices and coherences. Plain line: probability of choice A (averaged over 10,000 trials where A was the correct choice). Dotted line: expected value for motion coherence. Grey: $c = 0.2$. Black: $c = 0.05$. (C) Sensory weights in the simplified Bayesian model (average of 10,000 trials) as a function of time after stimulus presentation. Black: $c = 0.2$. Light grey: $c = 0$ (i.e., sensory input is pure noise). Dark grey: $c = 0.1$. (D) Average temporal evolution of the log odds and the decision threshold in the simplified Bayesian model. Dotted lines: log odds. Plain lines: threshold. Black: $c = 0.2$. Dark grey: $c = 0.05$. Light grey: $c = 0.1$. See Plate 23 of Color Plate section.

Implementing the full Bayesian integration algorithm requires accumulating evidence for all possible combinations of coherence and choice. This is considerably more computationally intensive than a diffusion model, and it is unclear how such mechanisms could be implemented in a neural architecture. Instead, we can considerably simplify the computation and approximate Bayesian optimal decision making by separately estimating the reliability of the sensory input and the choice probability. One way to do this is to use an online estimate of coherence $\bar{c}(t)$ to adjust both the sensory weight and the boundary. This method (see Mathematical appendix) is sub-optimal, but still reaches higher levels of performance than fixed boundaries and sensory weight while requiring only an additional sensory integration.

In this simplified Bayesian model, the evolution of the log odds is gain modulated by the coherence estimate:

$$\frac{\partial L}{dt} = \hat{c}_t w(s_t - q). \tag{21.4}$$

The online estimate $\hat{c}_t$ for coherence can be obtained by measuring the strength of the sensory signal (see Mathematical appendix). It is a function of time and an online measure on the signal over noise ratio in the input, U_t, integrating the sensory evidence gain modulated by the choice probability (see Mathematical appendix).

The sensory weight, that is, the weight given to each new spike for updating the log odds, is multiplied by the contrast estimate. Thus the sensory weight is a dynamic function of time and the integrated sensory signal (Fig. 21.2C). At the start of the trial, the coherence estimate is equal to "average" coherence. As time increases, this estimate converges to its true value. When the "true" motion coherence is higher than average, the sensory weight increases over the duration of the trial. As a result, sensory inputs have a larger impact on the log odds at the end of the trial than at the beginning of trial. If, on the other hand, the true contrast is low, the sensory weight decreases over the duration of the trial. Thus, an input spike has a larger impact on the log odds at the beginning of the trial than at the end.

The decision threshold also needs to be updated online, as it depends on motion coherence. We chose to adjust the online decision threshold D_t to the threshold that would be optimal if the true motion coherence was equal to its current estimate $\hat{c}_t$ (see Mathematical appendix). This "greedy" decision strategy might not optimal in the absolute sense, but it has the advantage of being online. We suspect that any reasonable strategies for choosing the threshold based on past sensory input will result in similar qualitative predictions.

Figure 21.2D represents the average temporal evolution of the log odds and threshold for two levels of (true) motion coherence. Notice that the threshold follows the same trend as the sensory weight: it collapses for hard tasks, but stays constant or increases moderately for easy tasks. The effect of the collapsing bound at low contrast will be to force a decision within a limited time frame if the trial is too difficult. In this case, the cost of waiting longer to make a decision outweighs the benefit of an increase in accuracy. Collapsing bounds have indeed been proposed as an upgrade for diffusion-based decision models with varying levels of sensory input strength.

In particular, Bayesian decision making predicts that a decision is not made at a fixed level of accuracy. Rather, the decision is made with a more permissive threshold (i.e., at a lower degree of confidence in the choice) when the trial is more difficult.

21.3 Prediction in a motion discrimination task

To test the predictions of the model in more details, we focus on noisy motion integration tasks that have been extensively used for studying the neural basis of decision making. The choices are the same as in our toy example, except that the decision is based on the activities of population of neurons rather than a single spike train.

Subjects in these experiments were required to watch a stimulus consisting of randomly moving dots and choose between two opposite direction of motion (direction A or direction B). The level of noise in the motion stimulus is controlled by the "coherence," that is, the proportion of dots moving coherently in direction A or direction B. Motion coherence varied randomly from trial to trial, and thus the subject did not know the coherence at the start of the trial. The subjects indicated their choice by an eye movement in the direction of perceived motion, and were rewarded for correct choices. In a "reaction time" version of this task, the subject responded as soon as ready. In "fixed delay" version of this task, the stimulus is presented for a fixed duration and the subjects respond at the prompt of a "go signal."

Series of experimental studies with macaque monkeys trained at this task showed that at least two brain areas are involved. In particular, the role of the "sensory input" is played (at least in part) by the MT area. The neural responses from MT area are integrated in the lateral intraparietal "LIP" area, a sensorimotor brain area involved in the generation of eye movements. Thus LIP area is a potential candidate for a Bayesian integrator. However, we focus here on the behavioral prediction of a Bayesian decision model based on the sensory input from MT area.

The firing rates of MT cells are modulated by the direction of motion and by motion coherence. MT neurons have a background response to purely noisy visual displays (with zero coherence) and a "preferred" direction of motion, that is, their firing rate will be higher in response to one direction of motion and lower in the opposite direction. To a first approximation, if q_i is the baseline firing of a MT cell, its firing rate is $q_i + cdq_i$ in the preferred direction, and $q_i - cdq_i$ in the anti-preferred direction, where c parameterize motion coherence. To simplify notations, we suppose that the MT population is balanced between the two directions of motions, that is, $\sum_i dq_i = 0$.

As previously, the log odds are computed as a weighted sum of the spikes from the population of MT cells, gain modulated by an online coherence estimate:

$$\frac{\partial L}{dt} = \hat{c}_t \sum_i w_i s_t^i. \tag{21.5}$$

The initial value for the log odds correspond to the prior odds: $L_0 = \log(P(A)/P(B))$.

We compare the predictions from the Bayesian decision model with a diffusion model with fixed sensory weights and a fixed threshold. This diffusion model is similar to a model previously used to account for behavioral and neurophysiological data [17]. The "integrated input" in the diffusion model is:

$$\frac{\partial L^d}{dt} = \bar{c} \sum_i w_i s_t^i. \tag{21.6}$$

The boundary is set at a fixed level $\bar{D}$, and the starting point of integration at a fixed value $\bar{L}_o$. For easier comparison with the Bayesian decision model, $\bar{D}$ and $\bar{L}_o$ were adjusted in order to achieve the same mean reaction time and the same average effects of priors on choice probability than the Bayesian model.

As in our toy example, sensory weights and decision threshold evolve dynamically during the trial (not shown, but similar to Fig. 21.2C and 21.2D). The weight of sensory evidence decreases and the threshold collapses for low coherence trials, sensory weights, and threshold increase for high coherence trials.

Results from the simulations are presented separately for "reaction time" and "fixed delay" tasks. To investigate the effect of priors, we also performed two distinct "experiment." In "experiment 1," the two direction of motion were presented with equal probability ($L_o = 0$) and in "experiment 2," direction A is presented more often than direction B ($L_o = 0.6$).

21.3.1 Reaction time task

Psychophysical curves and reaction times as a function of motion coherence are plotted in Fig. 21.3.

While the psychophysical curves are similar for the diffusion model and the Bayesian model (Fig. 21.3A and 21.3B), the mean reaction times (Fig. 21.3C and 21.3D) and reaction time distribution (Fig. 21.3E and 21.3F) are very different. Reaction times are shorter at low coherence and larger at high coherence than expected from a diffusion model (Fig. 21.3C and 21.3D). This is mainly because for low coherence trials, the online estimate of coherence tends to decrease the decision threshold, thus shortening the reaction

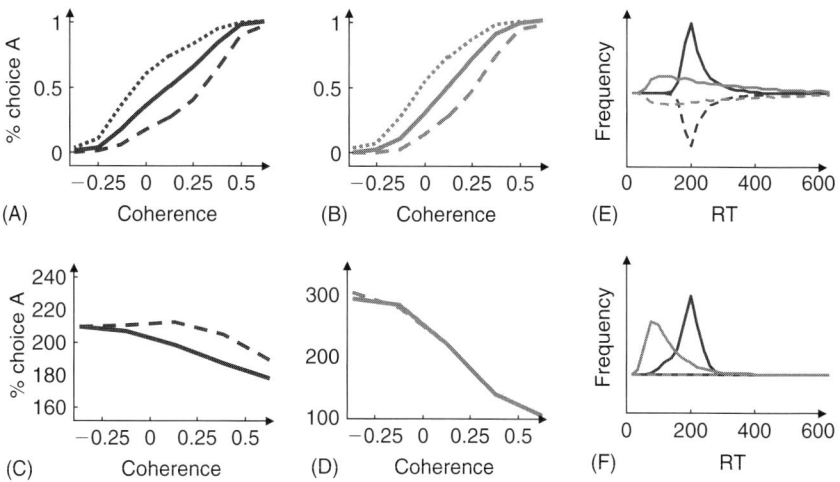

Figure 21.3 Bayesian and "diffusion" decision model in the "reaction time" task. (A) Proportion of choice as a function of motion coherence for the Bayesian model. Positive coherence corresponds to stimuli moving in direction A, negative coherence to stimuli moving in the opposite direction. Plain line: two choices equiprobable ($L_o = 0$), dashed line: B more probable ($L_o = -0.6$), dotted line: A more probable ($L_o = 0.6$). (B) Same as in (A), for the diffusion model. (C) Reaction time as a function of motion coherence for the Bayesian model. Plain line: correct trial. Dashed line: error trials. (D) Same as in (C) for the diffusion model. (E) Reaction time distribution for low coherence trials ($c = 0.05$). Black: Bayesian model. Grey: diffusion model. Plain: correct trials. Dashed: error trials. Error trials are represented upside down for clarity. (F) Same as in (E) for high coherence trials ($c = 0.3$).

time, while the reverse is true at high coherence. As a consequence, the animal spends less time on difficult trials (that are not worth the wait), and more time on easy trials (were a little extra-time results in a large increase in accuracy) than would be predicted by a diffusion model. The effect of the collapsing bound is particularly visible in the reaction time distribution (Fig. 21.3E and 21.3F).

While the reaction time distributions for a diffusion model are very asymmetrical, with a fast rise and a long tail toward large reaction times, the reaction time distribution predicted by the Bayesian model are almost symmetrical. The decision threshold is initially high, resulting in an absence of very short reaction time. The collapsing bound also prevents very long reaction times, which explains why the reaction time distributions of the Bayesian model do not have a long tails. This occurs at all motion coherence even if, on average, the threshold does not collapse at high coherence: long trials correspond to "bad trials" trials where the quality of the sensory input was low (because the decision threshold was not crossed early). In these trials, the estimated motion coherence is also low (even if true motion coherence is high). The bound collapses, resulting is a shortening of the duration of these "bad trials," which would have formed the tail of the *RT* distribution in a diffusion model.

For the same reason, the Bayesian model predicts longer reaction time for error trials than for correct trials (Fig. 21.3C). A diffusion model would predict the same reaction time for correct and error trials (Fig. 21.3D). This is another consequence of the correlation between the length of the trial and the estimated coherence. In trials where the quality of the sensory input is low (due to sensory noise), the threshold collapses and is usually crossed at a lower value of accuracy. These "bad trials" have both longer reaction times and lower accuracy.

The benefit of using a Bayesian decision model is particularly strong when it comes to incorporating prior knowledge with the sensory evidence. By estimating motion coherence, the Bayesian integrator can adjust the contribution of the sensory evidence compare to the prior. The diffusion model, on the other hand, overestimates the quality of the sensory input at low coherence and underestimates it at high coherence. As a result, the overall effect of the prior (as implemented by a bias in the starting point of integration) is too weak at low coherence, too high at high coherence, and decays over time even when the sensory input is completely uninformative (see Section 21.3.2).

As a result, the effect of the prior in a Bayesian decision model is much more than a higher or lower starting point for sensory integration. Rather, the prior has a non-linear and complex effect on the dynamics of the sensory weight and decision threshold, resulting in an influence of the prior that appears to act in part as additional "sensory evidence." This is illustrated in Fig. 21.4A and 21.4B. While the diffusion model (Fig. 21.4A) starts integration at a level set by the prior, but later behaves as a simple integrator regardless of the prior, the Bayesian model (Fig. 21.4B) will see the apparent influence of the prior amplify during the trial. The combined effect mimics some of the consequence of a change in drift rate, as if the priors were a "pseudo" motion signal.

21.3.2 Fixed delay tasks

During fixed delay tasks, subjects see the stimulus for a fixed duration and are required to respond only after presentation of a "go" signal. Thus, in this case, there is no time/accuracy trade-off and no need for a dynamic decision threshold. Instead, the decision is taken according to the sign of the log odd ratio at the end of stimulus presentation.

In a diffusion model, all sensory inputs are taken equally into account, regardless of whether they occur at the beginning or at the end of stimulus presentation. By contrast, the Bayesian decision model re-weight the sensory evidence as a function of the estimated motion coherence, and thus, sensory inputs do not all contributes equally to the final decision depending on their timing. This is illustrated in Fig. 21.4. In this figure, we plotted the average sensory input ($\langle \sum_i w_i s_t^i \rangle$) at different times during stimulus presentation, conditioned on the fact that the final choice was A. We consider only trials with zero coherence, that is, in this case the decision is driven by random fluctuations in the sensory input. In this case, "choice A" is made as often as choice B. The curves are a result of averaging from 20,000 trials, the stimulus was presented for 2000 ms and decision was made at $t = 2000$ ms. Only trials with $L_{2000} > 0$ (choice A) were kept for averaging. For a diffusion model (grey line), the curves is flat and slightly above zero. This is because positive inputs tend to increase the probability that the final log odds will be positive, and the final choice will be "A." In a diffusion model, the order of arrival of these inputs does not matter. In contrast, the Bayesian decision model (black line) gives more confidence to inputs presented early in the trial. This is because the initial coherence estimate is actually larger that the real motion coherence (here, zero) resulting in the first "noisy" inputs being taken into account much more than later inputs. The decision-triggered average of the input thus decays over time.

A non-intuitive consequence of estimating motion coherence online is actually to decrease the apparent temporal window of integration for the Bayesian decision model. For low coherence trial, the initial input will influence the final decision much more than

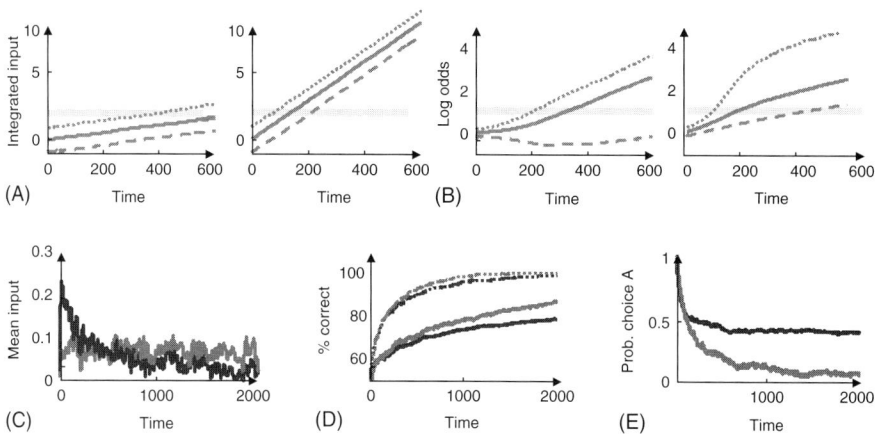

Figure 21.4 Bayesian decision model and diffusion model in the "fixed delay" task. (A) Average integrated input (L_t) as a function of time in the diffusion model. Left panel: low coherence ($c = 0.05$). Right panel: medium coherence ($c = 0.2$). Plain line: equiprobable choice ($L_o = 0$). Dotted line: $L_o = 0.6$. Dashed line: $L_o = -0.6$. Thick horizontal line: decision threshold. (B) Same as in (A), but plotting the average log odds divided by the decision threshold (i.e., L_t/D_t) for the Bayesian diffusion model. (C) Choice-averaged input as a function of time in the trial. Black line: average input for all trials leading to choice A in the Bayesian model. Grey line: same thing for the diffusion model. (D) Percent of correct choices as a function of the duration of stimulus presentation. Same color code as in (C). Plain: $c = 0.05$. Dotted: $c = 0.1$. (E) Probability of choosing A in zero coherence trial with prior $L_o = 0.6$, as a function of the duration of stimulus presentation. Same color code as in (C). See Plate 24 of Color Plate section.

it should. Later in the trial, the influence of the input decays, but can never completely overcome the initial bias produced by early sensory noise. As a consequence, integration is initially fast and later slows considerably, to a point where the decision accuracy do not appear to benefit much from longer stimulus presentation (Fig. 21.4D). This does not happen in a diffusion model, where each sensory input is equally weighted at all time. For very long stimulus presentation, the diffusion model performs paradoxically better than a Bayesian model (Fig. 21.4D, blue lines). This sub-optimally is a consequence of the approximation used in the simplified Bayesian model: coherence is estimated separately from motion direction, rather than computing the full joint probability distribution over all coherences and choices. The full Bayesian model computing the probabilities of all pairs of choice and coherence does not have this limitation.

Finally, the diffusion model and the Bayesian model behave very differently in the presence of priors for long stimulus presentations. This is illustrated in Fig. 21.4E. For zero coherence trial, the influence of the prior is very strong for short stimulus presentation, but decays for longer stimulus presentation, even when the stimulus is pure noise. This decay is not a desirable feature: because the sensory input is completely uninformative, the influence of prior information about the choice should stay strong regardless of the length of stimulus presentation (the optimal strategy would be to always respond in the direction most probable according to the prior). Unfortunately, this decay cannot be completely prevented if one does not know initially that the coherence is zero. By dynamically reweighing sensory evidence, the Bayesian decision model prevents this "washing away" of prior information by noise. Once enough sensory information has been collected to bring the coherence estimate to zero, it stops integrating and relies on the prior. The diffusion model, on the other hand, keeps accumulating "noise" and forgets the prior.

21.3.3 Comparison of model predictions with experimental results

The Bayesian model predicts significant deviation from the prediction of a diffusion model when the precision of the sensory input (or the task difficulty) is varied randomly from trial to trial. Some of these predictions qualitatively fit results than have been reported previously. These results concern mainly monkeys trained at the motion discrimination task presented previously. Human behavior in the same task seems to obey the prediction of a diffusion model more closely [7]. We report qualitative similarities, not quantitative fit. Experimental evidence for the Bayesian model predictions that are not easily predicted by the diffusion model are listed below, together with the corresponding figure and relevant reference:

- Reaction times slower for error trials than correct trials in Fig. 21.3C [17].
- Quasi-symmetrical reaction time distribution in Fig. 21.3E and 21.3F [28].
- Effect of prior resembling a pseudo "motion" signal in Fig. 21.4B [18].
- Stronger influence of sensory signals early in the trial than later in the trial in Fig. 21.4C [29].
- Limited integration time, saturation of performance with longer stimulus presentation in Fig. 21.4D [29].

In addition, a strong prediction of the Bayesian model is that the effect of prior will not "wash away" for longer presentation time when the motion coherence is zero (Fig. 21.4E), but will "wash away" when coherence is higher. To our knowledge, this prediction has not been tested experimentally.

21.4 Conclusion

21.4.1 Comparison with other models

Our model is not the first variant of a diffusion model that accounts for the observed animal behavior in the motion discrimination task. Other models of decision making have focused on proposing a biologically plausible neural basis for decision mechanisms. They did not consider that the drift rate of a diffusion process or the bound could be adjusted online as a function of the sensory input. However, they share similar mechanisms with Bayesian decision model, such as a decision thresholds that collapses over time or, equivalently, an urgency signal that increases over time [28]. The "integration to bound" model [29] considers that sensory integration takes place as in a diffusion model, but only until the integrated evidence reaches a fixed bound. No further integration is performed after that. This accounts for the stronger weight of sensory evidence at the beginning of the trial and the saturation of performance for longer stimulus duration. Recurrent network models used two competing population of neurons receiving evidence for each direction of motion [30–32]. These networks slowly converge to a stable state with one population more active than the other, resulting in a decision. Integration takes place as the sensory input progressively brings the network state towards one or the other basin of attraction. As the network gets closer to one of the stable state, it loses its sensitivity to the input, resulting in a stronger impact of sensory input at the start of the trial, and also something that could be considered as a "collapsing bound."

   We propose an alternative explanation for the phenomena captured by these models. According to our framework, these non-linearities are signatures of an ongoing estimate for the sensory likelihoods. In other words, they are a consequence of optimal decision making in the presence of uncertainty about the quality of the sensory input. However, the Bayesian makes predictions that are notably different from previous models for trials were motion coherence is not zero. It predicts constant or slightly increasing thresholds, increasing sensory weights and vanishing priors for high coherence trials. This suggests a simple way to test our theory experimentally.

21.4.2 Why does human behavior fit better the prediction of a diffusion model?

Reaction time distributions of humans in decision tasks are often very well fitted by a diffusion model, even in the motion discrimination task described previously [7]. This suggests that the subjects do not adjust the sensory likelihoods online in these experiments. There are two possible reasons for this apparent discrepancy between animal and human behavior: the quality of the sensory signal might be readily available from the stimulus itself, without requiring a long integration of sensory evidence. For example, the contrast of a visual stimulus is a direct predictor of its reliability in a difficult orientation discrimination task. If sensory likelihoods can readily be inferred from the in the initial sensory input or from an independent cue, the "coherence" estimate can be set from the start and will not be adjusted online. In addition, human subject, who are less experienced in the task than overtrained animals, might not be able to exploit the widely different quality of sensory signal available from to trials to trials.

   While the importance of reweighing sensory evidence might be minor in well controlled, repeated 2AFCs tasks, dynamic reweighing of sensory evidence is likely to play an important role in the "one shot" decision we have to perform everyday. Interestingly, this apparently complex mechanism might have a straightforward and ubiquitous neural basis in the form of sensory adaptation. Bayesian decision making predicts that sensory weights tend to decay over time in "difficult" tasks. By studying the average dynamic of Eq. 21.6, we can show that when motion coherence is around zero,

$$\hat{c}_t \approx \frac{1}{1 + c\bar{l}t}. \tag{21.7}$$

Such hyperbolic decay in sensory weights could be implemented by adaptation processes occurring at many different time-scales in the central nervous system [33]. In our framework, the role of such sensory adaptation would be to insure that meaningless sensory noise is not taken into account by later processing stages. Stimuli present for a long time would see their "weight" decrease, unless they are "rescued" by feedback signals indicating that these inputs are relevant to the current perceptual decision.

21A   Mathematical appendix

We can express all the sensory information received up to time t as an unfolding history of sensory inputs, $s_{0 \to t} = \{s_0, s_{dt}, \ldots, s_{t-dt}\}$ where s_t is the sensory input received between time t and $t + dt$. The inference stage can be performed by a linear integration of log likelihoods ratio using the Bayes rule. The log odds for choices A and B is computed recurrently as:

$$L_t = \log\left(\frac{P(A|s_{0 \to t})}{P(B|s_{0 \to t})}\right) = L_o + L_{t-dt} + l(s_t).$$

By taking the limit for small temporal steps dt, we get Eq. 21.1.

Derivation for the log odd ratio differential equations when the sensory input is Poisson distributed spike train (equations 2, 3, and 8 can be found in Deneve [9].

Equation 21.3 and the expression for the reaction time as a function of the diffusion rate are derived from standard results from diffusion models [7,21]. We replaced the "Poisson noise" in spike counts by a white Gaussian noise with variance equal to the mean, using the law of large numbers. To compute the optimal threshold, we approximated the mean first passage time (i.e., reaction time) as $RT_D \approx (D/\bar{l}) \tanh(D)$, where $\bar{l} = 4(dq^2/q)$ is the average log-likelihood ratio of the sensory input, or, equivalently, the average slope of L_t. In analogy with diffusion models, $\bar{l}$ corresponds to the "drift rate."

21A.1   Full Bayesian model

Let suppose that motion coherence is picked randomly from trial to trial among five possible values, that is, $c \in [0, 0.05, 0.1, 0.2, 0.5]$. Let us call x the unknown direction of motion, with $x = 1$ for direction A and $x = 0$ for direction B. To implement the "full" Bayesian model computing the joint probability of all choices and coherence $P_t(x, c) = P(x, c|s_{0 \to t})$ (used in Fig. 21.2B) we use the sensory likelihoods $\frac{1}{dt}P(s_t = 1|x, c) = q + (2x - 1)c\,dq$ to derive the following recurrent equation:

$$P_t(x, c) = \frac{1}{Z}P_{t-dt}(x, c)(q + c\,dq)^{xs_t}(q - c\,dq)^{(1-x)s_t}(1 - (q + c\,dq)dt)^{x(1-s_t)}$$
$$(1 - (q - c\,dq)dt)^{(1-x)(1-s_t)},$$

where Z is a normalization term. An estimate of contrast can be obtained by computing the expected value $\hat{c}_t = \sum_c c(P(A, c|s_{o \to t}) + P(B, c|s_{o \to t}))$, while the probability for choice A is given by marginalizing over all possible coherence $P(A|s_{o \to t}) = \sum_c P(A, c|s_{o \to t})$.

21A.2   Simplified Bayesian model

To derive expression 21.4 and 21.5 for the simplified Bayesian model, we use a method inspired from an online version of the "expectation maximization" algorithm [11]. The problem is to estimate both the "hidden state" x and the "parameter" c from the sensory observation $s_{o \to t}$. At each time step, we perform an "expectation stage" corresponding to updating the log odds L_t (Eq. 21.5) using the current parameter estimate. This provides us with an estimate of the direction of motion $\hat{x}_t = P_t = (e^{L_t}/1 + e^{L_t})$. We then perform a maximization stage by replacing the unknown direction of motion by its estimate in the expression of the sensory likelihoods:

$$P(s_t|c)\big|_{\hat{x}_t} = (q + c\,dq)^{\hat{x}_t s_t}(q + c\,dq)^{(1-\hat{x}_t)s_t}(1 - (q + c\,dq)dt)^{\hat{x}_t(1-s_t)}(1 - (q - c\,dq)dt)^{(1-\hat{x}_t)(1-s_t)}.$$

Using this method, we can compute $L_t^c = \log((P(s_t|c)\big|_{\hat{x}_t})/(P(s_t|c = 0)\big|_{\hat{x}_t}))$:

$$\frac{\partial L^c}{dt} = P_t \log\left(\frac{q + c\,dq}{q - c\,dq}\right)(s_t - q) + s_t \log\left(1 - \frac{c\,dq}{q}\right) + c\,dq.$$

Exploiting $dq \ll q$, we do a Taylor expansion on the order 2 in $\frac{dq}{q}$, and obtain:

$$\frac{\partial L^c}{dt} = c(2P_t - 1)\frac{dq}{q}(s_t - q) + c^2 \frac{dq^2}{q^2}s_t.$$

And thus, $L_t^c = \frac{c}{2}U_t - \frac{c^2}{4}V_t$, where U and V are initialized at zero and evolve as

$$\frac{\partial U}{dt} = (P - 0.5)w(s_t - q)$$

and

$$\frac{\partial V}{dt} = w^2 s_t.$$

To complete the maximization stage, we need to find the new parameter estimate $\hat{c}_t$ maximizing the likelihood of the sensory input. However, rather than taking the true max, which would result in a very noise estimate, we use a soft-max to select the coherence estimate:

$$\hat{c}(t) = \sum_c c\frac{e^{2L^c}}{\sum_c e^{2L_c}}.$$

The extension to a population of motion-selective neurons is straightforward. The coherence estimate can be computed as $L_t^c = \frac{c}{2}U_t - \frac{c^2}{4}V_t$ with

$$\frac{\partial U}{dt} = \frac{\exp(L_t) - 1}{\exp(L_t) + 1}\sum_i w_i s_t^i$$

and

$$\frac{\partial V}{dt} = \sum_i w_i^2 s_t^i.$$

For all practical purposes, we found we could replace V_t by its average over trial $\overline{lt}$ where $l = 4\sum_i dq_i^2/q_i$ is the average slope of the log odds, or the drift rate in a diffusion model. Neural correlates of elapsed time have been reported in LIP area [34].

An optimal threshold is estimated numerically as follows. We compute what would be the optimal threshold if motion coherence was known and equal to each of the coherence used in the experiment. The threshold as a function of the contrast estimate is then obtained by interpolating the optimal boundary between these values. Thus, if the coherence estimate is 0.07 the boundary is chosen by interpolating linearly between the optimal threshold for $c = 0.05$ and $c = 0.1$.

References

[1] K. Doya, Metalearning and neuromodulation, Neural Netw. 15 (4–6) (2002) 495–506.
[2] D.C. Knill, A. Pouget, The Bayesian brain: the role of uncertainty in neural coding and computation, Trends Neurosci. 27 (12) (2004) 712–719.
[3] L.P. Sugrue, G.S. Corrado, W.T. Newsome, Matching behavior and the representation of value in the parietal cortex, Science 304 (5678) (2004) 1782–1787.
[4] N.D. Daw, J.P. O'Doherty, P. Dayan, B. Seymour, R.J. Dolan, Cortical substrates for exploratory decisions in humans, Nature 441 (7095) (2006) 876–879.
[5] D.M. Wolpert, Probabilistic models in human sensorimotor control, Hum. Mov. Sci. 26 (4) (2007) 511–524.
[6] J.I. Gold, M.N. Shadlen, Banburismus and the brain: decoding the relationship between sensory stimuli, decisions, and reward, Neuron 36 (2) (2002) 299–308.
[7] R. Ratcliff, G. McKoon, The diffusion decision model: theory and data for two-choice decision tasks, Neural Comput. 20 (4) (2008) 873–922.
[8] T.E. Behrens, M.W. Woolrich, M.E. Walton, M.F. Rushworth, Learning the value of information in an uncertain world, Nat. Neurosci. 10 (9) (2007) 1214–1221.
[9] S. Deneve, Bayesian spiking neurons I: inference, Neural Comput. 20 (1) (2008) 91–117.
[10] S. Deneve, Bayesian spiking neurons II: learning, Neural Comput. 20 (1) (2008) 118–145.
[11] G. Mongillo, S. Deneve, Online learning with hidden Markov models, Neural Comput. 20 (7) (2008) 1706–1716.
[12] A.J. Yu, P. Dayan, Uncertainty, neuromodulation, and attention, Neuron 46 (4) (2005) 681–692.
[13] M.E. Walton, P.L. Croxson, T.E. Behrens, S.W. Kennerley, M.F. Rushworth, Adaptive decision making and value in the anterior cingulate cortex, Neuroimage 36 (Suppl. 2) (2007) T142–T154.
[14] L. Whiteley, M. Sahani, Implicit knowledge of visual uncertainty guides decisions with asymmetric outcomes, J. Vis. 8 (3) (2008) 1–15.

[15] M.N. Shadlen, K.H. Britten, W.T. Newsome, J.A. Movshon, A computational analysis of the relationship between neuronal and behavioral responses to visual motion, J. Neurosci. 16 (4) (1996) 1486–1510.

[16] J.I. Gold, M.N. Shadlen, The influence of behavioral context on the representation of a perceptual decision in developing oculomotor commands, J. Neurosci. 23 (2) (2003) 632–651.

[17] M.E. Mazurek, J.D. Roitman, J. Ditterich, M.N. Shadlen, A role for neural integrators in perceptual decision making, Cereb. Cortex 13 (11) (2003) 1257–1269.

[18] J. Palmer, M.K. McKinley, M. Mazurek, M.N. Shadlen, Effect of prior probability on choice and response time in a motion discrimination task, J. Vis. 5 (8) (2005) 235.

[19] J.I. Gold, C.T. Law, P. Connolly, S. Bennur, The relative influences of priors and sensory evidence on an oculomotor decision variable during perceptual learning, J. Neurophysiol. (2008) 2653–2668.

[20] D.R.J. Laming, Information Theory and Choice Reaction Time, Academic Press, New York, 1968.

[21] S.W. Link, The Wave Theory of Difference and Similarity, Erlbaum, Hillsdale, NJ, 1992.

[22] T. Ferguson, Mathematical Statistics: A Decision Theoretic Approach, Academic Press, New York, 1967.

[23] W.T. Newsome, K.H. Britten, J.A. Movshon, Neural correlates of a perceptual decision, Nature 341 (1989) 52–54.

[24] A.L. Yuille, H.H. Bulthoff, Bayesian decision theory and psychophysics, in: D.C. Knill, W. Richards (Eds.), Perception as Bayesian Inference, Cambridge University Press, New York, 1996.

[25] R. Ratcliff, A. Cherian, M. Segraves, A comparison of macaque behavior and superior colliculus neuronal activity to predictions from models of two-choice decisions, J. Neurophysiol. 90 (3) (2003) 1392–1407.

[26] M.N. Shadlen, W.T. Newsome, The variable discharge of cortical neurons: implications for connectivity, computation, and information coding, J. Neurosci. 18 (10) (1998) 3870–3896.

[27] K.H. Britten, M.N. Shadlen, W.T. Newsome, J.A. Movshon, The analysis of visual motion: a comparison of neuronal and psychophysical performance, J. Neurosci. 12 (12) (1992) 4745–4765.

[28] J. Ditterich, Computational approaches to visual decision making, Novartis Found. Symp. 270 (2006) 114–126 discussion 126–128, 164–169.

[29] R. Kiani, T.D. Hanks, M.N. Shadlen, Bounded integration in parietal cortex underlies decisions even when viewing duration is dictated by the environment, J. Neurosci. 28 (12) (2008) 3017–3029.

[30] X.J. Wang, Probabilistic decision making by slow reverberation in cortical circuits, Neuron 36 (5) (2002) 955–968.

[31] K.F. Wong, X.J. Wang, A recurrent network mechanism of time integration in perceptual decisions, J. Neurosci. 26 (4) (2006) 1314–1328.

[32] X.J. Wang, Decision making in recurrent neuronal circuits, Neuron 60 (2) (2008) 215–234.

[33] S. Fusi, P.J. Drew, L.F. Abbott, Cascade models of synaptically stored memories, Neuron 45 (4) (2005) 599–611.

[34] M.I. Leon, M.N. Shadlen, Representation of time by neurons in the posterior parietal cortex of the macaque, Neuron 38 (2) (2003) 317–327.

22 Predicting risk in a multiple stimulus-reward environment

Mathieu d'Acremont[1], Manfred Gilli[2] and Peter Bossaerts[1]

[1]Laboratory for Decision-Making under Uncertainty, Ecole Polytechnique Fédérale de Lausanne, Odyssea, Station 5, CH-1015 Lausanne, Switzerland
[2]Department of Econometrics, University of Geneva, Uni Mail, CH-1205 Geneva, Switzerland

Abstract

There is no doubt that humans are sensitive to risk when making decisions. Recently, neurobiological evidence has emerged of risk prediction along the lines of simple reinforcement learning. This evidence, however, is limited to one-step-ahead risk, namely, the uncertainty involved in the next forecast or reward. This is puzzling, because it would appear that multistep prediction risk is more relevant. Multiple stimuli may all predict the same future reward or a sequence of future rewards, and only the risk of the total reward is relevant. It is known (and the neurobiological basis of it is well understood) that subjects are indeed interested in predicting the total reward (sum of the discounted future rewards), and that learning of the expected total reward accords with the temporal differencing algorithm. Here, we posit that subjects should analogously be interested in predicting the risk of the total reward, not just the one-step-ahead risk. Using a simple example, we illustrate what this means, and how the risk of the total reward is related to one-step-ahead risks. We propose an algorithm that the brain may be employing to nevertheless learn total risk on the basis of learning of one-step-ahead forecasting risks. Simulations illustrate how our proposed algorithm leads to successful learning of total risk. Our analysis explains why activation correlating with one-step-ahead risk prediction errors emerged recently in a task with multiple stimuli and a single reward. We also discuss how temporal discounting may induce "ramping" of total risk, suggesting an explanation for a recently documented phenomenon in risk-related firing of dopaminergic neurons.

Key points

1. Reinforcement learning in an environment where multiple stimuli and rewards are experienced through time.
2. Learning algorithm to estimate the total risk carried by future rewards.
3. Mathematical formula to calculate total risk based on one-step-ahead risk.
4. Simulation to test the learning algorithm performance.
5. Risk temporal discounting.

22.1 Introduction

The simplest strategy for decision making under uncertainty is to select the option with the highest expected reward. However, a multitude of behavioral data documents that humans and animals are sensitive to risk as well [1,2]. Usually, subjects forego expected return when risk is deemed too high; at other times, subjects show a tendency to seek risk.

Recent neurobiological evidence suggests that certain brain regions are specialized in tracking risk (see Chapter 2 and 6). For instance, single neuron recordings during a visual gambling task with two male rhesus macaques [3] showed that neurons in the parietal cortex had a higher activity when the monkey selected the risky versus the sure option. In humans, the parietal cortex as well as other regions like the anterior cingulate cortex, the insula, the inferior frontal gyrus, the orbitofrontal cortex, or the striatum have been related to risk encoding [4–10]. For a review, see [11].

Risk needs to be distinguished from ambiguity. In economics and cognitive neuroscience, ambiguity refers to conditions in which outcome probabilities are incomplete or unknown. Under ambiguity, decision making has been related to neural response in the amygdala, the orbitofrontal cortex, the inferior frontal gyrus, and the insula [12,13]. From a Bayesian perspective, the distinction between ambiguity and risk is artificial; among others, ambiguity involves risk, because outcomes are uncertain even when one conditions on an estimate of the probabilities [14]. This may explain the partial overlap of brain activation for decision making under ambiguity and risk.

In many circumstances, expected reward and risk are unknown and, hence, need to be learned. Reinforcement learning has long been associated with learning of expected rewards [15]. Complex extensions of simple reinforcement learning such as temporal difference (TD) learning have been proposed for situations where there are multiple stimuli and rewards; in those cases, the object to be learned is the expected total reward, namely, the expected value of the sum of discounted future rewards (see Chapter 10). The TD learning algorithm has been shown to be consistent with neural activity of the dopaminergic system [16].

The literature on incorporation of risk assessment in learning of discounted future rewards is far less extensive. There are two branches in this literature. First, there are models that directly adjust for risk in learning of total reward by applying a nonlinear (strictly concave) transformation to individual rewards [17] or to the reward prediction error [18]. Note that there is no role for risk learning[1]. In contrast, other authors propose a model of reward risk learning based on simple reinforcement learning, on the grounds that risk is separately encoded in the brain (as discussed previously), which presupposes that it be learned separately from expected reward as well [20].

In fact, transforming rewards through some strictly concave function is inspired by expected utility theory [21]. In this theory of choice under uncertainty, the curvature of the utility function explains risk attitudes, with strict concavity corresponding to risk aversion. Expected utility theory is the dominant approach to modeling choice under uncertainty in the fields of economics. But in finance, the mean-variance model is favored [22], whereby expected (total) reward is separately represented from reward risk, and one is traded off against the other. This approach presents a number of advantages over expected utility (for a review, see [23]), but in particular situations it may lead to dominated

[1]Closely related is an approach whereby one adjusts rewards with a risk penalty obtained from some model of the evolution of risk like GARCH (Generalized Autoregressive Conditional Heteroskedasticity [19]); again, this approach is silent about risk learning.

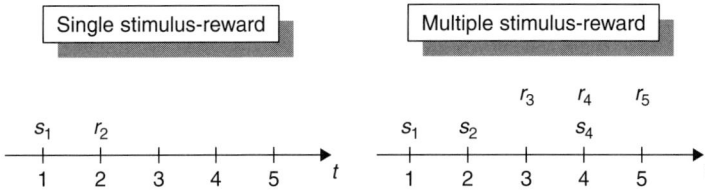

Figure 22.1 Trial organization of single stimulus-reward (left) and multiple-stimuli, multiple-rewards (right) environment.

choices, and it relies on representation of risk in terms of variance (although higher moments are sometimes considered as well).

The separate encoding of risk indicates that the human and nonhuman primate brain may be implementing the mean-variance approach to evaluate choice under uncertainty. The activations are consistent with reward variance as a metric of risk [5,8,10]. Higher moments may also be encoded, but this possibility has not yet been probed systematically. The relatively modest amount of risk in usual experiments may preclude detecting activation that correlates with higher moments.

In simple situations, it is known how reinforcement learning (the Rescorla–Wagner rule) can be used to learn risk [20]. Figure 22.1 (left) illustrates how the Rescorla–Wagner rule operates when there is a single stimulus that predicts a single subsequent stochastic reward. Two types of prediction errors are computed: a reward and risk prediction error. The reward prediction error is the difference between the predicted and the experienced reward. The predicted reward is updated after each trial, based on the reward prediction error and a learning rate. After a sufficient number of trials, and provided the learning rate is reduced appropriately, the predicted reward converges to the expected value of the reward. The risk prediction error is defined as the difference between the predicted and the realized risk. The realized risk is the squared reward prediction error; the predicted risk equals its expectation and, hence, the outcome variance. The predicted risk is updated after each trial based on the risk prediction error and a learning rate. After sufficient number of trials and with a correctly declining learning rate, the predicted risk converges to the expected value of the realized risk, that is, the true outcome variance.

In a recent fMRI study [24], this novel algorithm was applied to uncover the neural signatures of reward and risk prediction errors while subjects played several versions of the Iowa Gambling Task [25] (for a description of the ABCD version, see Chapter 13). In the task, subjects chose repetitively from four decks of cards, and each selection was immediately followed by a stochastic payoff. Expected reward and risk differed among the decks, and subjects were free to choose among the four decks. Payoff probabilities are unknown, so expected value and variance need to be learned through experience. Results showed that the reward prediction error was correlated with the Blood Oxygen Level Dependent (BOLD) response in the striatum, while the risk prediction error correlated with the BOLD response in the inferior frontal gyrus and insula.

Correlation between activation in the insula and risk prediction error has been documented elsewhere [26]. In this study, a card was drawn from a deck of ten (numbered from 1 to 10), without replacement, followed several seconds later by a second card. Subjects bet one dollar on whether the second card would be lower than the first card. In contrast with [24], reward probability was unambiguous, implicitly revealed through the numbers on the cards. So, risk and reward prediction errors emerged without a need for reinforcement. Decision making was also imperative because subjects had no control over the card selected.

For the purpose of the present study, the paradigm in [26] differed in another important respect: it involved two consecutive stimuli that together predicted a single reward. As such, it was a specific case of a multiple-stimuli, multiple-rewards environment like the one depicted in Fig. 22.1 (right). Evidently, the risk prediction error encoded in the human brain referred only to forecasting one-step-ahead. Specifically:

1. Upon display of the first stimulus, it measured the difference between the risk expected at the beginning of the trial and the risk realized after the stimulus presentation.
2. Upon display of the final outcome (reward), a second risk prediction error emerged, measuring the difference between the risk expected before the outcome and the risk realized after the outcome.

As such, it seems that this evidence points to representation in the human brain only of what time series statisticians call the *one-step-ahead risk prediction errors*.

The findings are puzzling in one important respect. In the context of multiple stimuli and multiple rewards the decision maker is not really interested in one-step-ahead risk, but in the risk of predicting the *total* reward (the sum of the discounted future rewards). Why, then, would the brain care to encode one-step-ahead prediction risk errors?

There exist more realistic examples of multiple-stimuli, multiple-rewards environments, such as blackjack (or "twenty-one"). In this game between a player and a dealer, the player initially receives two cards and is asked whether to take additional cards. That is, the player has the choice to "hit" (take another card) or "sit" (to not take another card). For the player to win, the sum of her cards must be above that of the dealer's, but not greater than 21. In blackjack, each time the player draws a card, she has to update the one-step-ahead as well as the total risk.

This paper provides a mathematical rationale for the encoding of one-step-ahead prediction risks. It does so by exploring how TD learning could be implemented to learn risk in a multiple-stimuli, multiple-rewards setting. To fix ideas, the paper will illustrate total reward risk learning in a simple, but generic example, which we shall call the Multistep Risk Example.

The remainder of the paper is organized as follows. We first introduce the Multistep Risk Example. Subsequently, we introduce formulae for expected total reward and total reward risk for this example. Particular attention is paid to how total reward risk relates to one-step-ahead prediction risks. The relationship turns out to be extremely simple. The paper then proposes how TD learning could be used to learn total reward risk. It is shown that TD learning is an effective way to learn one-step-ahead prediction risks, and from estimates of the latter, total reward prediction risk can be learned. Simulations illustrate how the proposed learning algorithm works. We demonstrate how it provides one potential explanation for the "ramping" in neural encoding of risk [1]. The paper finishes with a discussion of some tangential issues.

22.2 Models

22.2.1 The Multistep Risk Example

To facilitate the study of reinforcement learning of risk in a multiple-stimuli, multiple-rewards environment, we use a generic example, the Multistep Risk Example (Fig. 22.2). In the example, only risk is manipulated; expected reward and expected total reward remain zero at all times. The example is of the imperative type: the subject will be presented consecutively with pairs of two lotteries (gambles), but has no choice; the lotteries that will determine the final total reward are picked at random without the subject having any control over it.

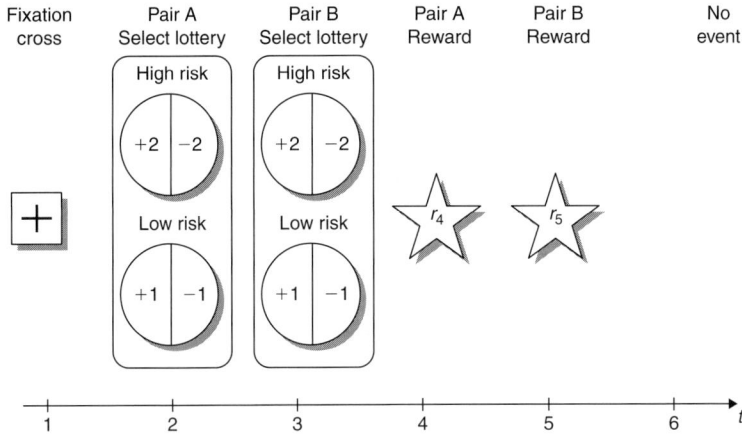

Figure 22.2 The Multistep Risk Example.

The trial begins at time $t = 1$ (one can imagine that the subject is presented with a fixation cross). At $t = 2$, a first pair of lotteries is presented. The pair consists of a high risk and a low risk lottery. One of these two lotteries is selected at random. At $t = 3$, a second pair of lotteries is presented with again a high risk and a low risk lottery. One of the two lotteries is picked. At $t = 4$, the first selected lottery is played and the reward r_4 is revealed. At $t = 5$, the second lottery is played and the reward r_5 is revealed. The trial ends at $t = 6$.

Our subject is obviously interested in the *total* reward, that is, the sum of r_4 and r_5. In fact, the subject should be interested in the *discounted* sum, since rewards occurring later in time are usually valued less. Until all the rewards are revealed, the total reward remains stochastic. When using mean-variance analysis, the subject is supposed to evaluate the desirability of all the outcomes by means of the expected value of the total reward and its risk; we measure the latter in terms of the variance (of the total reward).

The central feature of our example is that risk changes over time when a lottery is selected and whenever a lottery is played. For instance, the variance of the total reward increases if the most risky lottery is selected at $t = 2$ but it decreases after the first lottery is played.

Theoretical values of expected reward and risk

Let I_t refer to the information available at time t. Define the discounted total reward at time t:

$$R_t = \sum_{\tau=t+1}^{T} \gamma^{\tau-t-1} r_\tau,\qquad(22.1)$$

where T is the number of time steps in the trial, γ is the temporal discounting factor, and r_τ denotes the reward at time τ.

The *expected value* of the total reward at time t and given I_t is:

$$V_t = E(R_t | I_t).\qquad(22.2)$$

In our example, this expected value V_t is insensitive to information before $t = 4$; it always equals 0.

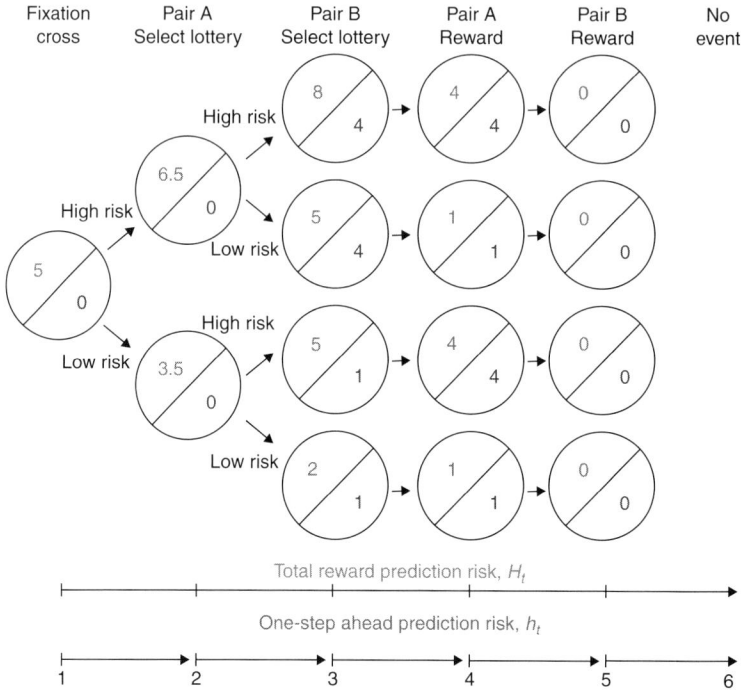

Figure 22.3 Theoretical values of one-step-ahead and total reward risk.

Define the risk of the total reward at time t conditional on I_t as:

$$H_t = Var(R_t|I_t). \tag{22.3}$$

As an illustration, consider the total reward risk at $t = 2$ knowing that the high risk lottery was selected. Temporarily ignore discounting, that is, set $\gamma = 1$. The possible values of the total reward from $t = 2$ onwards can be $R_2 \in \{+3, +1, -1, -3\}$, if the low risk lottery is selected at $t = 3$, or $R_2 \in \{+4, 0, 0, -4\}$, if the high risk lottery is selected instead. All outcomes are equally likely. The variance of R_2 is, therefore, $H_2 = 6.5$. This computation can be made at each time step and for each lottery. Figure 22.3 displays the results, in red.

By comparing the sum of the actually obtained reward and the future discounted expected value of the total reward with the past expectation of the total reward, one generates the *TD reward error*. Specifically, at $t + 1$, the TD error equals:

$$\delta_{t+1} = r_{t+1} + \gamma V_{t+1} - V_t. \tag{22.4}$$

Going back to our numerical example, TD errors are always zero before any reward is delivered (i.e., for $t < 4$). At $t = 4$ or $t = 5$, the TD error is generically different from 0. For instance, if the reward at $t = 4$ r_4 equals -1, then $\delta_4 = -1$.

The *one-step-ahead prediction risk* at time t conditional on I_t, is defined as follows:

$$h_t = Var[\delta_{t+1}|I_t] = E[\delta_{t+1}^2|I_t]. \tag{22.5}$$

As such, the one-step-ahead prediction risk is the variance of the TD error, conditional to I_t. One can write this differently, as follows:

$$h_t = Var[r_{t+1} + \gamma V_{t+1}|I_t].$$ (22.6)

To illustrate, let's imagine that the high risk lottery was selected at $t = 2$ and the low risk lottery was selected at $t = 3$. Rewards at $t = 4$ can be $r_4 \in \{+2, -2\}$. Hence, looking forward from time 3 on, all possible time-4 TD errors are: $\delta_4 \in \{+2, -2\}$. These values occur with equal likelihood. Hence, the variance of the TD error, or the one-step-ahead prediction risk, equals $h_3 = 4$. Contrast this with the risk (variance) of the total reward, which in this case would be $H_3 = 5$. In Fig. 22.3, the one-step-ahead risks are indicated in blue.

The important message is that the *one-step-ahead and total reward risks do not coincide*.

One wonders, however, whether one-step-ahead and total reward risks are not somehow related. Indeed, they are. In Box 22.1, we prove the following relationship:

$$H_t = \sum_{\tau=t}^{T-1} \gamma^{2(\tau-t)} E[h_\tau | I_t].$$ (22.7)

This result states that the risk of the total (discounted) reward is the discounted sum of the expected one-step-ahead prediction risks.

Referring again to our illustration, let us calculate the total reward risk as of $t = 2$, in case the high risk lottery was selected at $t = 1$. From the one-step-ahead prediction risks for $t \geq 2$ displayed in Fig. 22.3, and using Eq. 22.7, we conclude: $H_2 = \frac{0}{1} + \frac{4+4}{2} + \frac{4+1}{2} = 6.5$.

This is the same result one obtains when directly calculating the variance of the total reward R_2 (Fig. 22.3, red entry in top circle at $t = 2$).

It is possible to write the risk of the total reward H_t as a recursive function involving the immediate one-step-ahead prediction risk (for proof, see Box 22.1):

$$H_t = h_t + \gamma^2 E(H_{t+1}|I_t).$$ (22.8)

Box 22.1 Mathematical Proof

We demonstrate here that total risk is a function of one-step-ahead risk. Let the TD error be:

$$\delta_{t+1} = r_{t+1} + \gamma V_{t+1} - V_t.$$ (22.9)

Putting r on the left side, we get:

$$r_{t+1} = \delta_{t+1} - \gamma V_{t+1} + V_t,$$
$$r_{t+2} = \delta_{t+2} - \gamma V_{t+2} + V_{t+1},$$
$$r_{t+3} = \delta_{t+3} - \gamma V_{t+3} + V_{t+2},$$

...

$$r_T = \delta_T - \gamma V_T + V_{T-1}.$$

The discounted total reward at time t is:

$$R_t = \sum_{\tau=1}^{T-t} \gamma^{\tau-1} r_{t+\tau} = \gamma^0 r_{t+1} + \gamma^1 r_{t+2} + \gamma^2 r_{t+3} \ldots + \gamma^{T-t-1} r_T. \qquad (22.10)$$

Now consider:

$$\gamma^0 r_{t+1} = \gamma^0 \delta_{t+1} - \underline{\gamma^1 V_{t+1}} + \gamma^0 V_t,$$

$$\gamma^1 r_{t+2} = \gamma^1 \delta_{t+2} - \underline{\gamma^2 V_{t+2}} + \underline{\gamma^1 V_{t+1}},$$

$$\gamma^2 r_{t+3} = \gamma^2 \delta_{t+3} - \underline{\gamma^3 V_{t+3}} + \underline{\gamma^2 V_{t+2}},$$

$$\ldots$$

$$\gamma^{T-t-1} r_T = \gamma^{T-t-1} \delta_T - \gamma^{T-t} V_T + \underline{\gamma^{T-t-1} V_{T-1}}.$$

When summed, the underlined elements cancel out. Because no reward can be expected after the last trial, $V_T = 0$. So, the discounted sum of reward is:

$$R_t = \gamma^0 \delta_{t+1} + \gamma^1 \delta_{t+2} + \gamma^2 \delta_{t+3} \ldots + \gamma^{T-t-1} \delta_T + \gamma^0 V_t. \qquad (22.11)$$

The total risk at time t knowing I_t equals:

$$H_t = Var(R_t | I_t) = Var(\gamma^0 \delta_{t+1} + \gamma^1 \delta_{t+2} + \gamma^2 \delta_{t+3} \ldots + \gamma^{T-t-1} \delta_T + \gamma^0 V_t | I_t). (22.12)$$

At time t, V_t is known and becomes a fixed variable. Thus it can be ignored in the calculation of the variance. We write the H_t as a sum of variance and covariance:

$$H_t = \sum_{\tau=1}^{T-t} Var(\gamma^{\tau-1} \delta_{t+\tau} | I_t) + 2 \sum_{i=1}^{T-t-1} \sum_{j=i+1}^{T-t} Cov(\gamma^{i-1} \delta_{t+i}, \gamma^{j-1} \delta_{t+j} | I_t). \qquad (22.13)$$

The covariance can be simplified to:

$$Cov(\gamma^{i-1} \delta_{t+i}, \gamma^{j-1} \delta_{t+j} | I_t) = \gamma^{i+j-2} E(\delta_{t+i} \delta_{t+j} | I_t), i < j \qquad (22.14)$$

because $E(\delta_{t+k}) = 0$ for any k.

Now apply the law of iterated expectations:

$$\begin{aligned} E(\delta_{t+i} \delta_{t+j} | I_t) &= E(E(\delta_{t+i} \delta_{t+j} | I_{t+i}) | I_t) \\ &= E(\delta_{t+i} E(\delta_{t+j} | I_{t+i}) | I_t) \\ &= 0, i < j \end{aligned} \qquad (22.15)$$

because at time $t + i$, δ_{t+i} becomes a fixed variable and can be moved out of the inner expected value. Thus it appears that there is no covariance between the TD errors δ. As a consequence, the total reward variance simplifies to:

$$H_t = \sum_{\tau=1}^{T-t} Var(\gamma^{\tau-1} \delta_{t+\tau} | I_t) = \sum_{\tau=1}^{T-t} \gamma^{2(\tau-1)} E(\delta_{t+\tau}^2 | I_t). \qquad (22.16)$$

The one-step-ahead risk h_t is defined as:

$$h_t = E[\delta_{t+1}^2|I_t].$$
(22.17)

By using the law of iterated expectations, one can write H_t as a function of h_t:

$$H_t = \sum_{\tau=1}^{T-t} \gamma^{2(\tau-1)} E(E(\delta_{t+\tau}^2|I_{t+\tau-1})|I_t) = \sum_{\tau=1}^{T-t} \gamma^{2(\tau-1)} E(h_{t+\tau-1}|I_t)$$

$$= \sum_{\tau=0}^{T-t-1} \gamma^{2\tau} E(h_{t+\tau}|I_t).$$
(22.18)

H_t can be written in a recursive way. To do so we apply the law of iterated and total expectations:

$$H_t = h_t + \sum_{\tau=1}^{T-t-1} \gamma^{2\tau} E(h_{t+\tau}|I_t) = h_t + \sum_{\tau=1}^{T-t-1} \gamma^{2\tau} E(E(h_{t+\tau}|I_{t+1})|I_t)$$

$$= h_t + E(\sum_{\tau=1}^{T-t-1} \gamma^{2\tau} E(h_{t+\tau}|I_{t+1})|I_t) = h_t + E(\sum_{\tau=0}^{T-t-2} \gamma^{2(\tau+1)} E(h_{t+\tau+1}|I_{t+1})|I_t)$$

$$= h_t + \gamma^2 E(\sum_{\tau=0}^{T-t-2} \gamma^{2\tau} E(h_{t+\tau+1}|I_{t+1})|I_t) = h_t + \gamma^2 E(H_{t+1}|I_t)$$
(22.19)

We exploited this recursive form in the simulations that we will report on later. To see how this works in our illustrative example, note that $H_2 = 0 + \frac{8+5}{2} = 6.5$, which again is the value originally computed with Formula 22.7.

22.3 Learning

We here propose a learning algorithm with which to learn the risk of the total reward. It consists of two steps: (i) a simple reinforcement-learning based algorithm to update one-step-ahead prediction risks; (ii) application of our Formula 22.7 to update the total reward risk.

We represent I_t with a state vector $\vec{s}_t$ that summarizes what happened in the past (which gamble was picked, etc.). Information in $\vec{s}_t$ is represented with a tapped delay line, a vector composed of 0s and 1s (see Box 22.2 for details). Let $\hat{h}_t$ denote the

---

Box 22.2   Tapped Delay Line Representation

Tapped delay line is a usual way to represent information in TD learning. Stimuli are numbered $s = 1, 2, ..., S$ where S is the total number of stimuli. For instance, we can set $s = 1$ for the fixation cross, $s = 2, 3$ for the low and high risk lottery of the first pair, and $s = 4, 5$ for the low and high risk lotteries of the second pair. Hence $S = 5$. Each stimuli s is represented by a time dependent Boolean vector $\vec{s}_{st}$ of size T. All elements in $\vec{s}_{st}$ are equals to 0, except if the stimuli was presented at time t or before. The element number e in $\vec{s}_{st}$ is set to 1 with $e = t - \tau + 1$. τ indicates the time when the stimuli was presented. For instance, consider the sequence (1) fixation cross and (2) high risk lottery. The fixation cross $s = 1$ was presented at $\tau = 1$, so at $t = 2$ we have:

$$\vec{s}_{1,2} = [0,1,0,0,0]'.$$

The low risk lottery of the first pair was not presented, so we have:

$$\vec{s}_{2,2} = [0,0,0,0,0]'.$$

The high risk lottery of the first pair was presented at $\tau = 2$, so we have:

$$\vec{s}_{3,2} = [1,0,0,0,0]',$$

The low risk lottery of the second pair was not yet presented, so we have:

$$\vec{s}_{4,2} = [0,0,0,0,0]',$$

and so on until the last stimuli is reached ($s = S$).

The tapped delay line representation of all stimuli at time t is:

$$\vec{s}_t = [\vec{s}'_{1t}, \vec{s}'_{2t}, \ldots \vec{s}'_{st}, \ldots \vec{s}'_{St}]'.$$

estimate of the one-step-ahead risk h_t. In our learning algorithm, $\hat{h}_t$ is a function of the state of the world $\vec{s}_t$ and a weight vector $\vec{w}_{risk}$:

$$\hat{h}_t = \vec{w}'_{risk}\vec{s}_t. \tag{22.20}$$

Consider the prediction error for the one-step-ahead risk h_t:

$$\xi_{t+1} = \delta^2_{t+1} - \hat{h}_t. \tag{22.21}$$

The prediction error serves to compute an updating vector $\vec{\Theta}_t$,

$$\vec{\Theta}_t = \beta\xi_{t+1}\vec{s}_t, \tag{22.22}$$

where β is the learning rate for risk. Intuitively, we can explain the latter formula by saying that only stimuli presented before or at time t will receive the credit (debit) of a positive (negative) prediction error.

At the end of the trial, the weight vector $\vec{w}_{risk}$ is updated by summing all the updating vectors:

$$\vec{w}_{risk} = \vec{w}_{risk} + \sum_{t=1}^{T-1}\vec{\Theta}_t. \tag{22.23}$$

After a sufficient number of trials, by the law of large numbers, $\hat{h}_t$ will exhibit the usual convergence properties of reinforcement learning algorithms.

Thus the first step (i) on how to learn one-step-ahead prediction risks is solved. For the second step (ii), we rely on a crucial feature of the algorithm, namely: the weight vector $\vec{w}_{risk}$ can be used to compute one-step-ahead risks at any time and for all contingencies within the same trial (see Formula 22.20). For instance, at time $t = 2$ in the Multistep Risk Example, it is possible to compute the one-step-ahead risk *when* the low risk lottery is selected at time $t = 3$. Likewise, it is possible to compute the one-step-ahead risk *when* the high risk lottery is selected at time $t = 3$. As a consequence, it is feasible to estimate the expected value of all possible one-step-ahead risks at $t = 3$, and also $t = 4$, and so forth. It becomes straightforward to use Formula 22.7 (or its recursive version Formula 22.8) to compute the total reward risk H_t. (In our simulations, we used the recursive formula, because it is more efficient from a programming point of view.)

The prediction error ξ_{t+1} is key to reinforcement learning of one-step-ahead risk. But notice that it depends on the TD error δ_{t+1} used to update the expected value of the total reward. This effectively means that the same error that allows one to update the expected total reward can also generate an update of the total reward risk. In other words, our proposed algorithm will use information parsimoniously.

22.4.1   One-step-ahead risk algorithm

Separate algorithms for the one-step-ahead and total risks were written in Matlab. For the one-step-ahead algorithm, the value V_t is computed by multiplying a weight vector for reward with the tapped delay line at time t, $V_t = \vec{w}'_{rew}\vec{s}_t$. In the same way, the one-step-ahead risk h_t is computed by multiplying a weight vector for risk with the tapped delay line, $h_t = \vec{w}'_{risk}\vec{s}_t$. The weight vector for reward and risk are updated through trials with Algorithm 22.1. (see supplementary material online).

22.4.2   Total risk algorithm

The number of different states that can be experienced at time k is denoted n_k with $k = 1$, ..., T. T is the number of time steps in trials. In the Multistep Risk Example, $n_1 = 1$ (fixation cross), n_2, $n_3 = 2$ (low/high risk lottery), and n_4, n_5, $n_6 = 1$ (non-stimuli). Stimuli within each time step can be identified with an index $i \in \{1,2, ... n_k\}$. In the paradigm, the index of the low risk lotteries is arbitrarily set to $i = 1$ and the index of the high risk lotteries set to $i = 2$. The fixation cross and the absence of stimuli have index $= 1$. The vector of information $\bar{I}_t$ contains the index of the stimuli experienced until time t. For example, if the sequence of events was (1) fixation cross, (2) high risk lottery, (3) low risk lottery, and (4) no stimulus, then the information available at time 4 is $\bar{I}_4 = \{1,2,1,1\}$. It is easy to build a tapped delay line based on $\bar{I}_t$.

To compute the total risk, we use a recursive function ComputeH (Algorithm 22.2, see supplementary material online). The function takes as argument the information available at time t and returns the total risk, $H_t = \text{ComputeH}(\bar{I}_t)$. The function looks at the number of possible stimuli in the next time step. For instance, after the fixation cross (parent), there are two possible stimuli (children): the low and high risk lottery. The function is then applied on each child (who becomes the parents in the next time step). When the total reward risk H_{t+1} of all parent's children has been computed, the mean $\bar{H}_{t+1}$ of these value is calculated. The one-step-ahead risk of the parent h_t is computed using the risk weights. Adding h_t to the discounted $\bar{H}_{t+1}$ gives the total reward risk H_t of the parent. The recursive call of the function ends when the last time step T is reached (parents with no children).

22.5 Results

22.5.1 One-step-ahead prediction risk and total reward risk

We performed simulations to illustrate that our reinforcement learning algorithm can make accurate predictions in the Multistep Risk Example. Estimation of h_t and H_t were done with 1000 iterations. The reward and risk learning rates α and β were both set to 0.01. The parameter γ was set to 1, so there was no discounting.

Results of the simulations are reported in Fig. 22.4. Results are close to the theoretical values displayed in Fig. 22.3. Thus, it can be concluded that TD learning successfully predicts one-step-ahead as well as total risk. Notice that before $t = 3$, the one-step-ahead risk prediction are not exactly equal to zero. This is due to sampling variability induced by the non-zero and constant reward learning rate α.

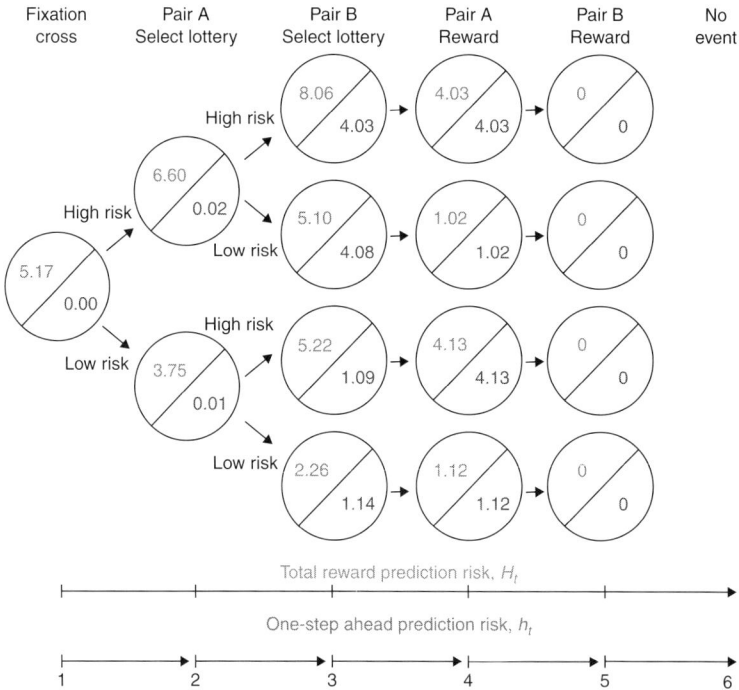

Figure 22.4 One-step-ahead and total reward risk as estimated by TD learning.

22.5.2 Temporal discounting

In the simulations described in the previous section, there was no discounting, that is, $\gamma = 1$. It is interesting to study the impact of discounting ($\gamma < 1$) on total reward risk. The formula tying total reward risk with one-step-ahead risks (Eq. 22.7) provides insights. Imagine a situation where there is a single stimulus at $t = 1$ and reward is realized at $t = T$. In that case, there is one-step-ahead prediction risk only at $t = T - 1$. As a result, according to Eq. 22.7, total reward risk will *grow over time* till $t = T - 1$ and then drop to zero.

The fact that total reward risk increases in this case may provide an explanation for a recently described phenomenon in firing of midbrain dopaminergic neurons in monkeys [1]. The experimental setup was as described previously: an initial stimulus predicted a stochastic reward at some future time. Sustained firing of some dopaminergic neurons during the anticipation interval appeared to be correlated with total reward risk (which changed with the displayed stimulus). Curiously, the firing was not constant over the interval between display of the stimulus and realization of reward. The firing could best be described as "ramping" up (see Fig. 2.4B, Chapter 2).

The specifics of the experiment were as follows. Trials started with the presentation of one of five different stimuli. Each stimulus was associated with a particular reward probability: 0, .25, .50, .75, or 1. Stimuli where presented during 2s. Rewards were delivered when the stimuli disappeared (i.e., no trace conditioning). Inter-stimulus interval varied randomly. The (two) monkeys completed each 18,750 trials on average.

After extensive training, the authors showed how activity of a sub-population of dopaminergic neurons increased progressively as the delivery of an uncertain reward approached, a phenomenon they referred to as "ramping effect." The ramping effect was maximum when the probability was .50 that is, when the reward variance was maximum.

We can easily illustrate ramping with a simulation. The setup is similar to the classical condition task where ramping was first observed [1]. At the beginning of a trial, one of five different stimuli can occur. Each stimulus is associated with a different reward probability. The reward is either 0 or 1 and is delivered 10 time steps after the stimuli ($T = 10$). Risk and reward learning rates are set to 0.01. The number of iterations is set to 18,750, the number of trials processed by each monkey in the original study [1]. We set the discounting factor equal to .90, a number usually proposed in the literature.

The simulation generates estimates of one-step-ahead risks at $t = 9$ (one step before reward is delivered, and hence, uncertainty is realized) equal to 0, 0.19, 0.25, 0.20 and 0, for probabilities equal to 0, .25, .50, .75 and 1, respectively. These estimates are close to the true one-step-ahead risks, which are 0, 0.19, 0.25, 0.19 and 0, respectively. The one-step-ahead prediction risks converge to zero for $t < 9$, as expected.

As concerns the total reward risks for $t = 1, ..., 9$, without discounting they would equal the one-step-ahead prediction risk at $t = 9$. Consequently, the total reward risk is constant between $t = 1$ and $t = 9$. With discounting, however, the total reward risk increases with time. This is illustrated in Fig. 22.5, which is based on the values of one-step-ahead prediction risks we recorded by the end of our simulations. The curve in the figure reproduces the ramping effect observed in actual firing of some dopaminergic neurons.

If our interpretation of the ramping phenomenon is right, one can also conclude that dopaminergic neurons encode *total risk*, not one-step-ahead risk. Indeed, ramping is a property of total risk (Fig. 22.5).

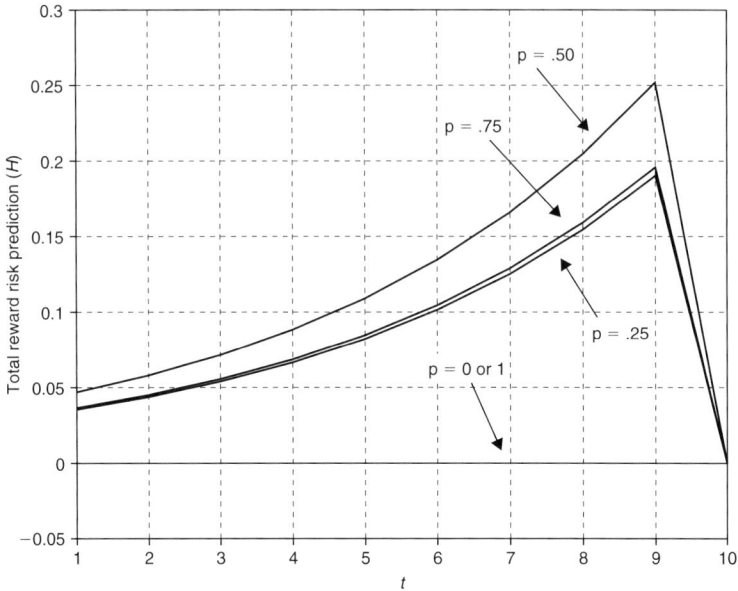

Figure 22.5 Total reward risk for different reward probabilities as estimated by TD learning. Stimuli are presented at $t = 1$ and reward are delivered at $t = 10$.

22.6 Discussion

Our mathematical analysis of reward prediction risk was prompted by recent discoveries that specific cortical regions correlated with errors in the estimation of one-step-ahead prediction risks [24,26]. To find a teaching signal for the prediction of risk one step in the future seems paradoxical because one would expect the brain to be involved in learning total reward risk, in analogy with encoding of errors in expected value of *total reward*. The paradox can be resolved when one realizes that one-step-ahead prediction risks can be viewed as the building blocks of total reward risk—the link is provided through the formula in Eq. 22.7—so that learning of one-step-ahead prediction risks automatically leads to learning of total reward risk.

As a by-product of our analysis, we showed that temporal discounting offers a plausible explanation of risk-related "ramping" in the firing of dopaminergic neurons in the monkey midbrain [1]. The ramping effect is consistent with the increase of mathematical total risk over the course of the trial. This suggests that the dopaminergic neurons may be encoding *total reward risk*, in contrast with activation in anterior insula or inferior frontal gyrus, which correlates with the error in estimating one-step-ahead risks [24–26].

However, it is not known how the evidence of "ramping" of firing of dopaminergic neurons applies to the human brain. While fMRI analysis of striatal dopamine projection areas of the human brain has uncovered sustained activation correlating with risk [4,10], the time resolution of fMRI does not allow us to discern whether this activation increases progressively over time, as is the case with the firing of dopaminergic neurons. It should be added that an alternative explanation has been advanced for the ramping phenomenon, based on experimental design, asymmetric firing of dopamine neurons, and back-propagation of learning signals in the TD learning algorithm [27]. The explanation has been challenged, however, for various reasons [28].

In addition to human striatum, risk and uncertainty in general activate a number of other brain regions, such as anterior cingulate cortex [29–31], and orbitofrontal cortex [8]. The sustained nature of these activations suggests that they reflect total reward risk. It has yet to be determined whether activations concerning total reward risk are consistent with one-step-ahead prediction risk. That is, do the different types of activation satisfy the restriction implicit in Eq. 22.7? Further research is needed.

References

[1] C. Fiorillo, P. Tobler, W. Schultz, Discrete coding of reward probability and uncertainty by dopamine neurons, Science 299 (2003) 1898–1902.

[2] J.C. Cox, G.W. Harrison, Risk Aversion in Experiments: an introduction, Emerald Group Publishing Limited, Bingley, UK, 2008 Research in experimental economics.

[3] A. McCoy, M. Platt, Risk-sensitive neurons in macaque posterior cingulate cortex, Nat. Neurosci. 8 (2005) 1220–1227.

[4] J. Dreher, P. Kohn, K. Berman, Neural coding of distinct statistical properties of reward information in humans, Cereb. Cortex 16 (2006) 561–573.

[5] S. Huettel, A. Song, G. McCarthy, Decisions under uncertainty: probabilistic context influences activation of prefrontal and parietal cortices, J. Neurosci. 25 (2005) 3304–3311.

[6] C. Kuhnen, B. Knutson, The neural basis of financial risk taking, Neuron 47 (2005) 763–770.

[7] E. Rolls, C. McCabe, J. Redoute, Expected value, reward outcome, and temporal difference error representations in a probabilistic decision task, Cereb. Cortex 18 (2008) 652–663.

[8] P. Tobler, J. O'Doherty, R. Dolan, W. Schultz, Reward value coding distinct from risk attitude-related uncertainty coding in human reward systems, J. Neurophysiol. 97 (2007) 1621–1632.

[9] M. Paulus, C. Rogalsky, A. Simmons, J. Feinstein, M. Stein, Increased activation in the right insula during risk-taking decision making is related to harm avoidance and neuroticism, Neuroimage 19 (2003) 1439–1448.

[10] K. Preuschoff, P. Bossaerts, S. Quartz, Neural differentiation of expected reward and risk in human subcortical structures, Neuron 51 (2006) 381–390.

[11] B. Knutson, P. Bossaerts, Neural antecedents of financial decisions, J. Neurosci. 27 (2007) 8174–8177.

[12] S. Huettel, C. Stowe, E. Gordon, B. Warner, M. Platt, Neural signatures of economic preferences for risk and ambiguity, Neuron 49 (2006) 765–775.

[13] M. Hsu, M. Bhatt, R. Adolphs, D. Tranel, C. Camerer, Neural systems responding to degrees of uncertainty in human decision-making, Science 310 (2005) 1680–1683.

[14] C. Rode, L. Cosmides, W. Hell, J. Tooby, When and why do people avoid unknown probabilities in decisions under uncertainty? Testing some predictions from optimal foraging theory, Cognition 72 (1999) 269–304.

[15] R. Sutton, A. Barto, Reinforcement Learning: An Introduction, MIT Press, Cambridge, MA, 1998.

[16] W. Schultz, P. Dayan, P. Montague, A neural substrate of prediction and reward, Science 275 (1997) 1593–1599.

[17] R. Howard, J. Matheson, Risk-sensitive Markov decision processes, Manag. Sci. 18 (1972) 356–369.

[18] O. Mihatsch, R. Neuneier, Risk-sensitive reinforcement learning, Mach. Learn. 49 (2002) 267–290.

[19] J. Li, C. Laiwan, Reward adjusted reinforcement learning for risk-averse asset allocation, in Proc. International Joint Conference on Neural Networks, 2006.

[20] K. Preuschoff, P. Bossaerts, Adding prediction risk to the theory of reward learning, Ann. NY Acad. Sci. 1104 (2007) 135–146.

[21] J. Von Neumann, O. Morgenstern, Theory of Games and Economic Behavior, Princeton University Press, Princeton, NJ, 1947.

[22] H. Markovitz, Portfolio selection, J. Finance 7 (1952) 77–91.

[23] M, d'Acremont, P. Bossaerts, Neurobiological studies of risk assessment: a comparison of expected utility and mean-variance approaches, Cogn. Affect. Behav. Neurosci. 8 (2008) 363–374.

[24] M. d'Acremont, Z.L. Lu, X. Li, M. Van der Linden, A. Bechara, Neural correlates of risk prediction error during reinforcement learning in humans, Neuroimage (in press).

[25] A. Bechara, A. Damasio, H. Damasio, S. Anderson, Insensitivity to future consequences following damage to human prefrontal cortex, Cognition 50 (1994) 7–15.

[26] K. Preuschoff, P. Bossaerts, Human insula activation reflects risk prediction errors as well as risk, J. Neurosci. 28 (2008) 2745–2752.

[27] Y. Niv, M. Duff, P. Dayan, Dopamine, uncertainty and TD learning, Behav. Brain Funct. 1 (2005) 1–9.

[28] P. Tobler, C. Fiorillo, W. Schultz, Adaptive coding of reward value by dopamine neurons, Science 307 (2005) 1642–1645.

[29] J. Brown, T. Braver, Learned predictions of error likelihood in the anterior cingulate cortex, Science 307 (2005) 1118–1121.

[30] J. Brown, T. Braver, Risk prediction and aversion by anterior cingulate cortex, Cogn. Affect. Behav. Neurosci. 7 (2007) 266–277.

[31] T. Behrens, M. Woolrich, M. Walton, M. Rushworth, Learning the value of information in an uncertain world, Nat. Neurosci. 10 (2007) 1214–1221.

Index

Plate Section

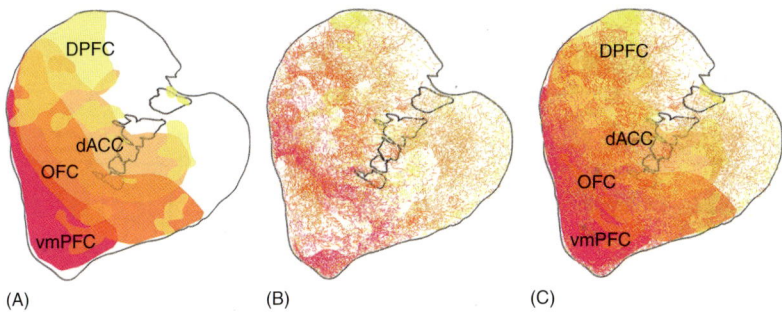

Plate 1 Schematics demonstrating convergence of cortical projections from different reward-related regions and dorsal prefrontal areas. (A) Convergence between focal projections from different prefrontal regions. (B) Distribution of diffuse fibers from different prefrontal regions. (C) Combination of focal and the diffuse fibers. ACC, dorsal anterior cingulate cortex; DPFC, dorsal lateral prefrontal cortex; OFC, orbital prefrontal cortex; vmPFC, ventral medial prefrontal cortex. Red, inputs from vmPFC; dark orange, inputs from OFC; light orange, inputs from dACC; yellow, inputs from DPFC.

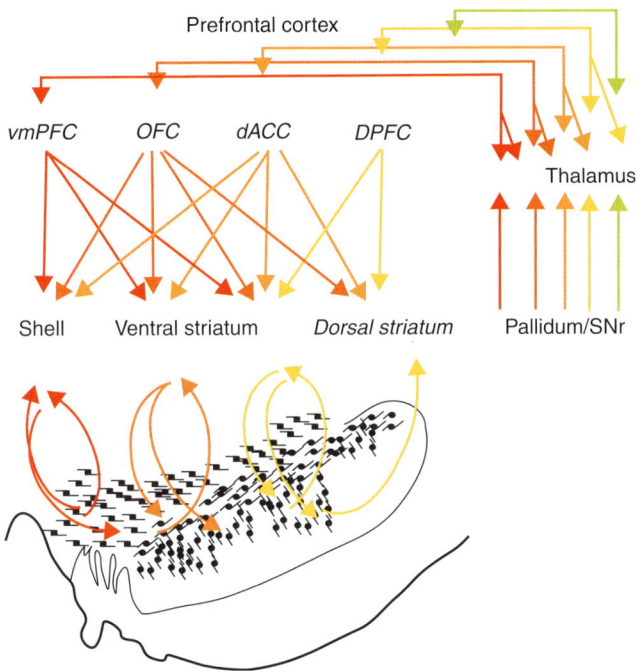

Plate 2 Three networks of integration through cortico-BG pathways. (1) Fibers from different prefrontal areas converge within subregions of the striatum. (2) Through the organization of striato-nigro-striatal (SNS) projections, the ventral striatum can influence the dorsal striatum [5]. Midbrain projections from the shell target both the VTA and ventromedial SNc. Projections from the VTA to the shell form a "closed," reciprocal loop, but also project more laterally to impact on DA cells projecting the rest of the ventral striatum, forming the first part of a feed-forward loop (or spiral). The spiral continues through the SNS projections, through which the ventral striatum impacts on cognitive and motor striatal areas via the midbrain DA cells. (3) The non-reciprocal cortico-thalamic projection carries information from reward-related regions, through cognitive and motor controls. dACC, dorsal anterior cingulate cortex; DPFC, dorsal prefrontal cortex; OFC, orbital prefrontal cortex; vmPFC, ventral medial prefrontal cortex. Red, vmPFC pathways; dark orange, OFC pathways; light orange, dACC pathways; yellow, DPFC pathways; green, output to motor control areas.

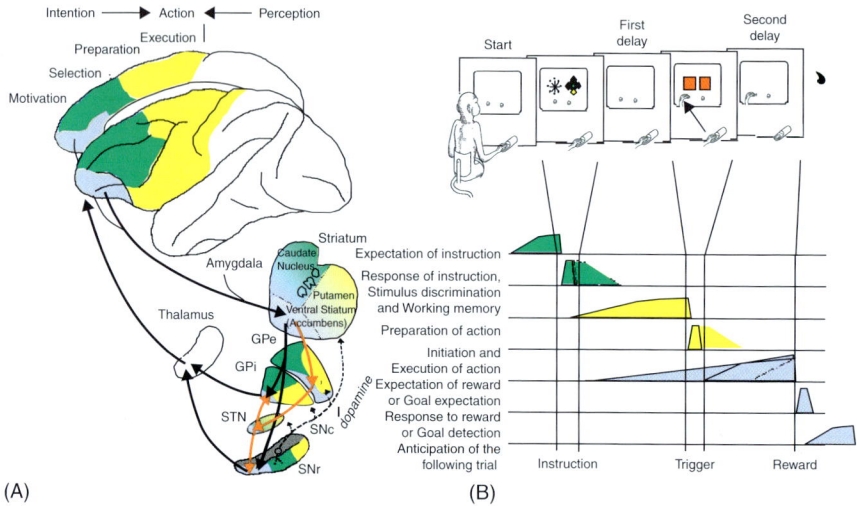

Plate 3 Schematic representation of the anatomical circuits of the striatum (A) and a schematic overview of the main forms of activity (B) that could be observed in the striatum when monkeys perform a delayed response and reward task. The colors purple, green, and yellow delineate territories and activities that reflect motivation, cognitive, and motor processes, respectively. Inside the striatum the territories have been characterized based on anatomical and electrophysiological investigations, whereas the territories inside the two segments of the globus pallidus (internal GPi and external GPe) as well as the substantia nigra pars reticulata (SNr) are based only on anatomical investigation. Return projections to cortex are illustrated only for the limbic circuit that is presumed to be dedicated to motivation processes. The direct and indirect pathways from the ventral striatum to the output structure of basal ganglia are indicated in black and red arrows, respectively. In order not to overload the picture, some basal ganglia projections are not illustrated. All type of neuronal activities illustrated in B could be found in the striatum with a gradient that respects the striatal territories illustrated in A.

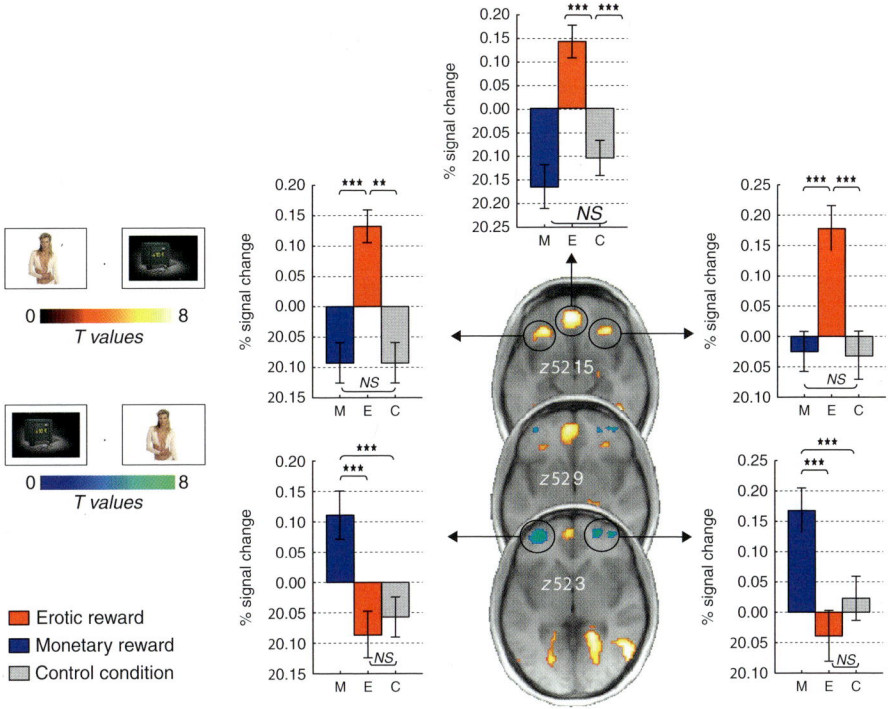

Functional divisions in the orbitofrontal cortex according to reward nature
(primary *vs* secondary reinforcers)

Plate 4 Antero-posterior dissociation within the orbitofrontal cortex according to reward nature. The anterior orbitofrontal cortex codes secondary reward (money) while the posterior and medial orbitofrontal cortex code primary reward (erotic stimuli). Brain regions specifically activated by monetary rewards outcomes are shown in blue-green, and those specifically activated by erotic rewards are shown in red-yellow. Mean percent signal change shows an interaction between reward type and orbitofrontal cortex (OFC) region in both the left and right sides of the brain. Functional maps are overlaid on axial slices of an average anatomical scan of all subjects and are significant at $P < 0.05$ family-wise error (FWE) corrected for multiple comparisons. Asterisks in the bar graphs denote significance of paired comparisons (***$P < 0.001$; **$P < 0.01$; NS, non-significant). Error bars indicate standard error to the mean (SEM) [28].

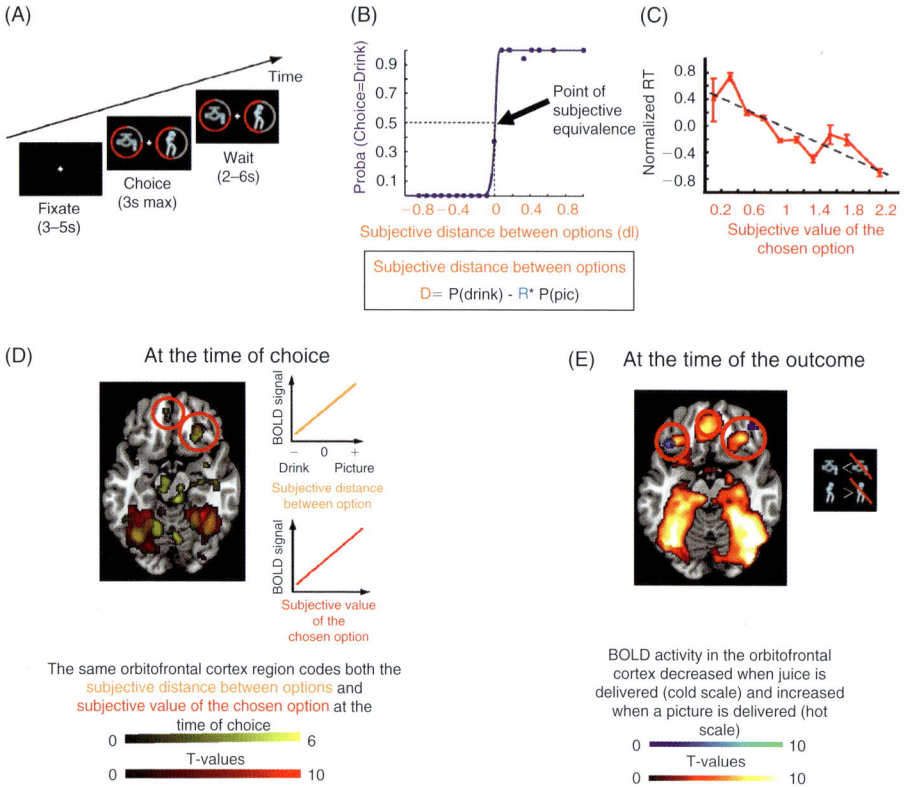

Plate 5 (A) Design of the experiment. Participants were asked to freely make motivated choices between two types of rewards with varying reward probability. For example, the offer consisted in a choice between an option rewarded 75% of the time by fruit juice and by an option rewarded 50% of the time by an erotic picture. The red part of the circle around each symbol indicates the reward probability. After a waiting period lasting 2-6 seconds, participants were probabilistically rewarded with juice or by viewing an erotic picture. (B) Estimation of the preference of each participant for drinking fruit juice over viewing erotic pictures was expressed as an equivalent offer by fitting a logistic model of the probability of choice that included the probability of being rewarded by a drink, by a picture and by the trial number. The preference was computed as the ratio of the betas for the picture and the drink. The subjective distance between options was computed for each offer as the difference between the subjective value of the drink option and the subjective value of the picture option. (C) Response times decreased as the subjective value of the chosen option increased. (D) At the time of choice, the same orbitofrontal regions coding the subjective distance (yellow scale) between options also coded the subjective value of the chosen option (red). (E) At the time of the outcome, the error prediction signal varied in the same direction as the subjective difference between options: it decreased at the time of reward when juice was delivered compared to when it was not delivered (cold scale), and it increased when a picture was delivered compared to when is was not viewed (hot scale).

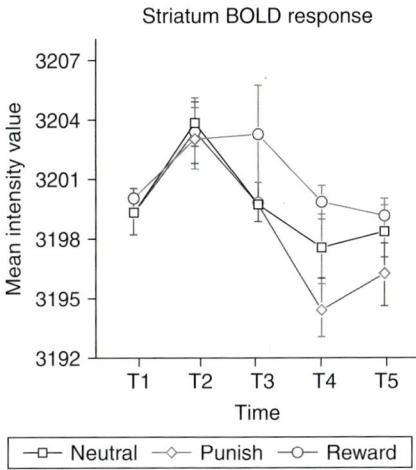

Striatum BOLD response

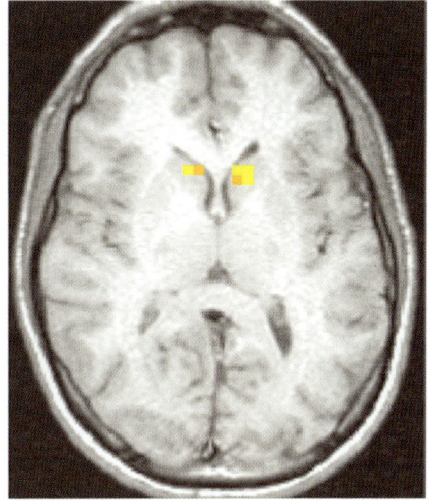

(A)

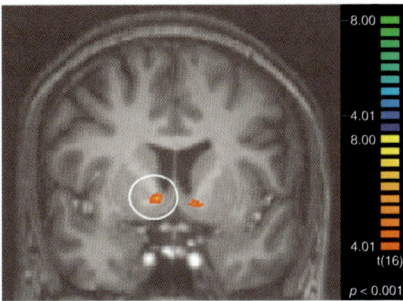

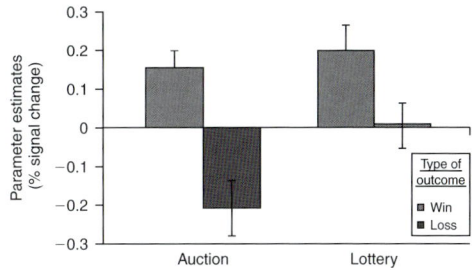

(B)

Plate 6 (A) Differential responses to reward and punishment in the striatum. Figure depicts activation in dorsal striatum and hemodynamic response graph with reward, neutral, and punish responses. A typical trial was 15 s and each time point (e.g., T1) represents 3-s bins. Differential responses are observed at T3 and T4 6–9 s after delivery of outcome. (B) BOLD signals in the ventral caudate nucleus during the outcome phase of an auction or lottery game. No differences between auction and lottery games were observed when the outcome was positive ("wins"). Instead, a negative outcome ("losses") during the competitive environment of an auction lead to a greater decrease in signals in the striatum compared to lottery games, which correlated with overbidding behavior. *Source*: For A, adapted from Delgado et al. (2000) [49] with permission; for B, adapted from Delgado et al. (2008) [115] with permission.

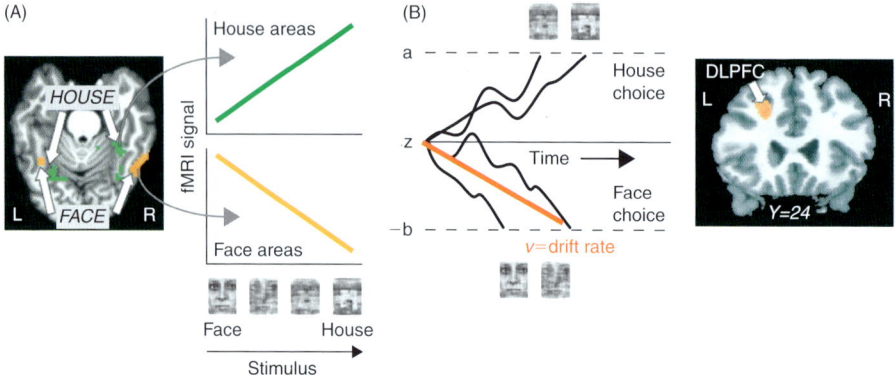

Plate 7 Representation and integration of sensory evidence during perceptual decision making in humans. (A) Using fMRI, Heekeren et al. [5] identified face- and house-selective regions (orange and green clusters, respectively) that are thought to represent the sensory evidence required to make a face-house discrimination. Specifically, they found a greater response in face-selective areas to clear images of faces than to noisy images of faces. Conversely, house-selective areas showed a greater response to clear images of houses than to noisy images of house. The orange and green lines illustrate this point in a cartoon-like fashion. (B) Decision making in higher-level brain regions is thought to involve an integration of sensory evidence over time. The diffusion model for simple decision making [27,28] assumes that decisions are made by continuously accumulating sensory information until one of two response criteria (a or b) is reached as illustrated graphically in this panel. Moment-to-moment fluctuations in the sample path reflect noise in the decision process. The accumulation rate, termed drift rate (v) in the model, reflects the quality of the available sensory evidence. For example, clear images of faces/houses contain more sensory evidence than noisy images, and therefore have a higher drift rate. Heekeren et al. [5] showed that such computations are carried out in the DLPFC.

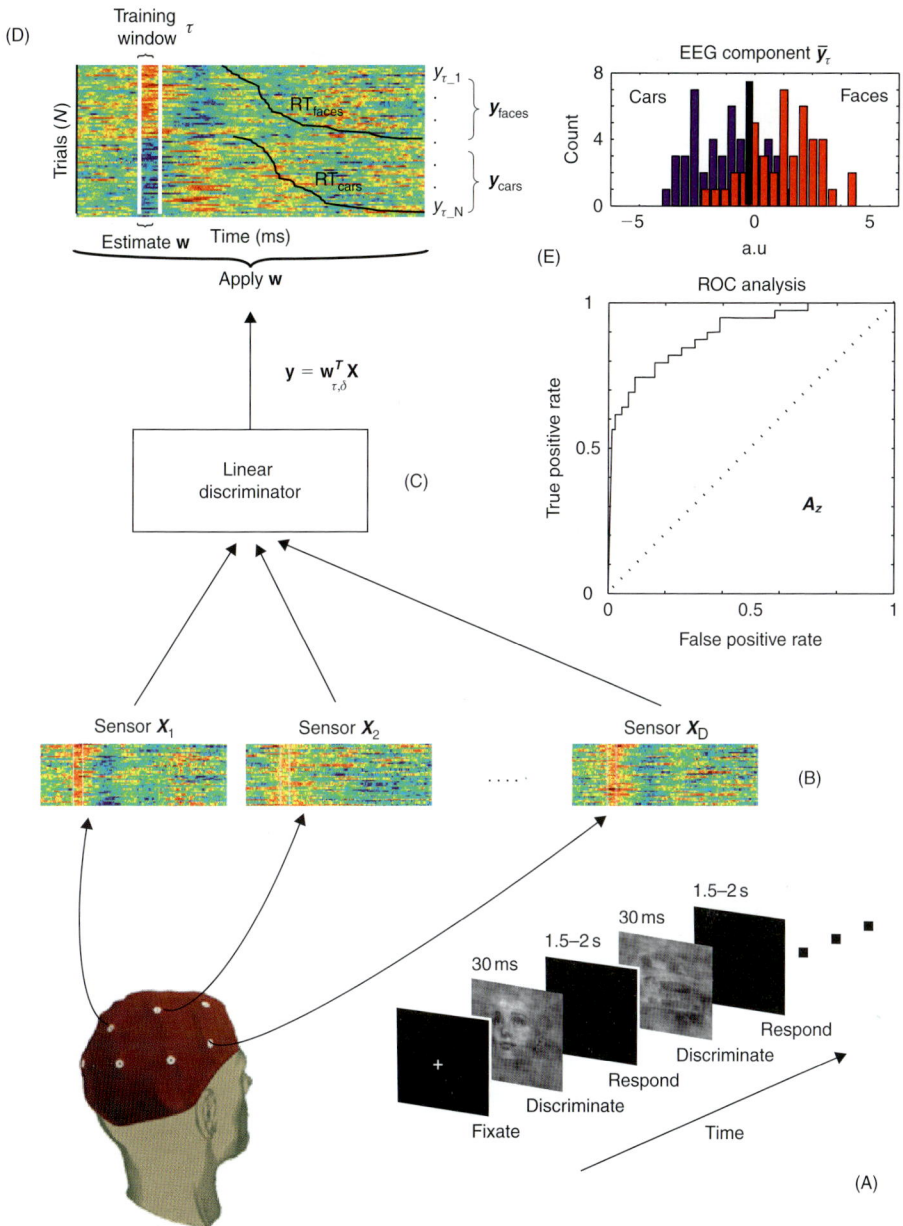

Plate 8 Summary of the single-trial EEG linear discrimination approach. (A) Subjects are discriminating between two classes of images while EEG is simultaneously recorded from D sensors. (B) EEG trials are locked to stimulus onset and a time window is defined with a latency, τ, relative to the stimulus and a width, δ (typically 50 ms wide). (C) EEG data from each sensor ($\mathbf{X}_1 \rightarrow {}_D$) and each window are used to train a linear classifier (i.e., estimate spatial filters $\mathbf{w}_{\tau,\delta}$), to discriminate labeled trials (here, faces versus cars). (D) The linear classifier, through application of $\mathbf{w}_{\tau,\delta}$ on the D sensors, collapses the D–dimensional EEG space into a 1–dimensional discriminating component

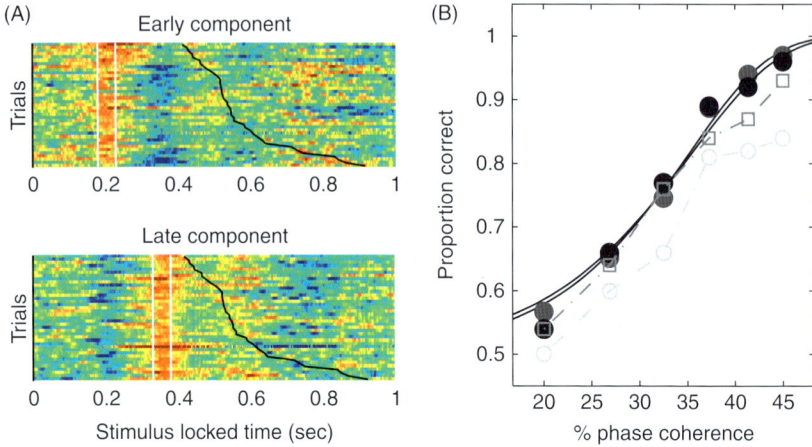

Plate 9 Single-trial EEG components correlate with decision accuracy on a face versus car discrimination task. (A) Discriminant component maps for the early ($\approx$170 ms) and late ($\approx$300 ms) decision accuracy components identified by [9]. All trials are aligned to the onset of visual stimulation (time 0 ms) and sorted by RT (black sigmoidal curves). Unlike the discriminant component maps in Fig. 8.3 only half the trials are represented here. Specifically, each row of these maps represents the output of the linear discriminator for a single face trial with the mean of all car trials subtracted (i.e., $\mathbf{y}_{face\_i} - \bar{\mathbf{y}}_{cars}$). (B) Comparison of one subject's psychometric function (gray solid line) with neurometric functions obtained from the early component (light-gray dotted line), the late component (dark-gray dotted line), and a combination of the two (black solid line). Note that integrating data across both time windows helped produce a neurometric function that was statistically indistinguishable from its corresponding psychometric curve. In addition, the neurometric function from the late component alone was a better match to the psychophysical data than that of the early one.

Plate 8 (Continued)

space $\mathbf{y}$. Compared to individual sensors this 1–dimensional projection is considered a better estimator of the underlying neural activity, as it usually carries a higher SNR and reduces interference from other sources. To visualize the profile of the discriminating component across trials (indexed by $i = 1 \rightarrow N$), the classifier, trained only on EEG within each of the selected windows, is applied across all time points to construct the component map seen here. Trials of class 1 (i.e., faces) are mapped to positive $\mathbf{y}$–values (red), whereas those of class 2 (i.e., cars) to negative ones (blue). In this example the sigmoidal curves represent the subject's reaction time profile for each of the two image classes. (E) The discriminating components are validated using a ROC analysis based on a leave-one-out procedure. Specifically, left-out single-trial discriminating components, averaged within the training window (i.e., $\bar{\mathbf{y}}_{\tau\_i}$), are used to generate discriminator output distributions for each of the two classes. The area under the ROC curve, also known as an A_z value, is used to quantify the degree of separation between the two distributions and can be used to establish a relationship between behavioral and neuronal responses as in [15,144].

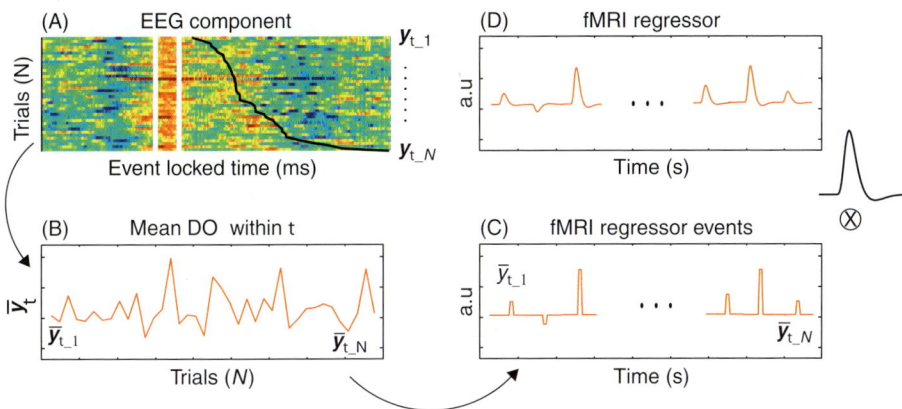

Plate 10 Graphical representation of how single-trial EEG can be used to construct fMRI regressors. The discriminator output (DO) can be used to derive as many fMRI regressors as there are temporally distinct EEG components. The onset time and duration of each of the regressor events are determined by the onset time (τ) and duration (δ) of the EEG components as identified by the single-trial EEG analysis (as in Fig. 8.3). More important, the amplitude of each regressor event will be based on the output of the linear discriminator $\mathbf{y}_\tau$ as defined in Eq. 8.2.

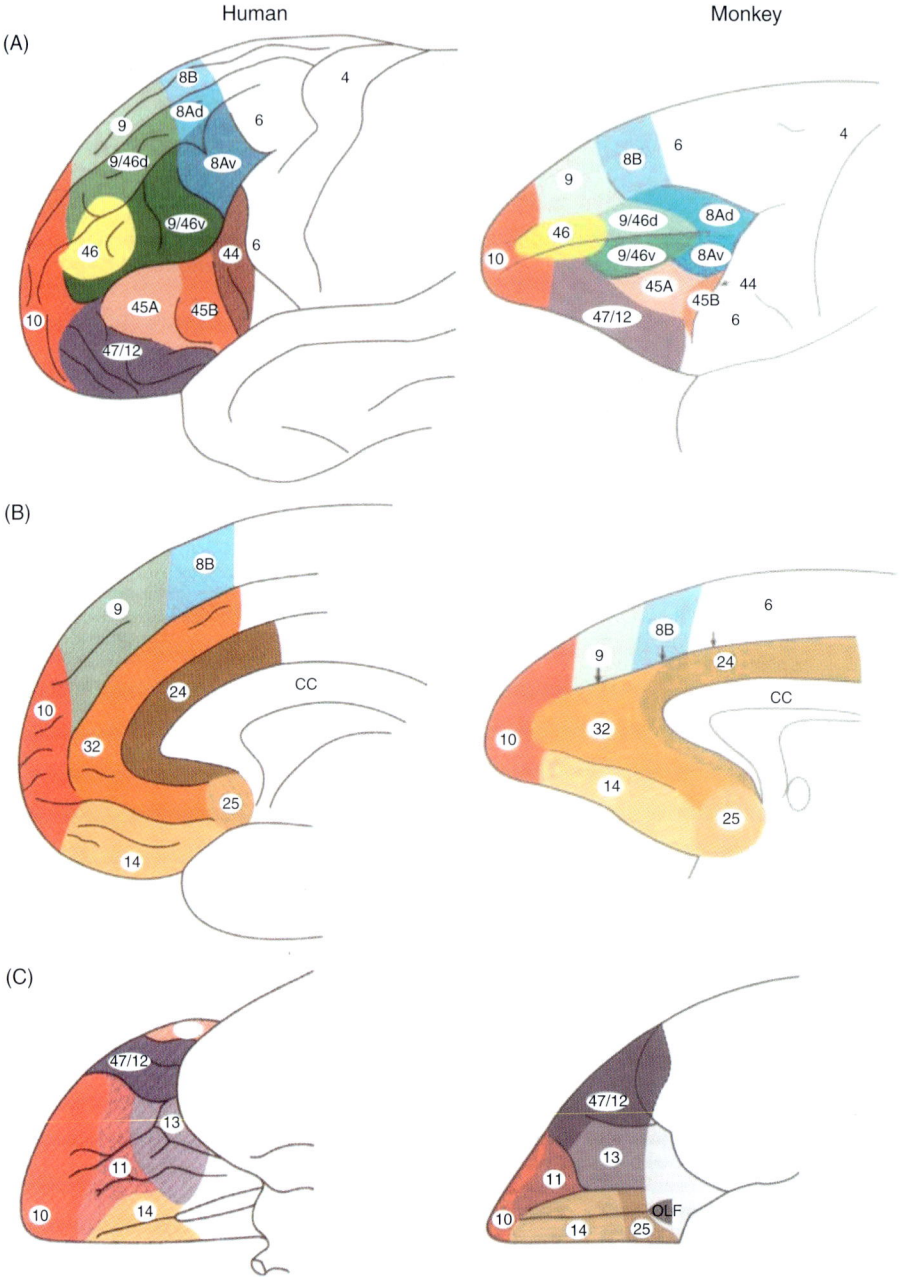

Plate 11 Comparative cytoarchitectonic map of the lateral (A), medial (B), and orbital (C) surfaces of the human and macaque monkey frontal cortex by Petrides and Pandya [17].

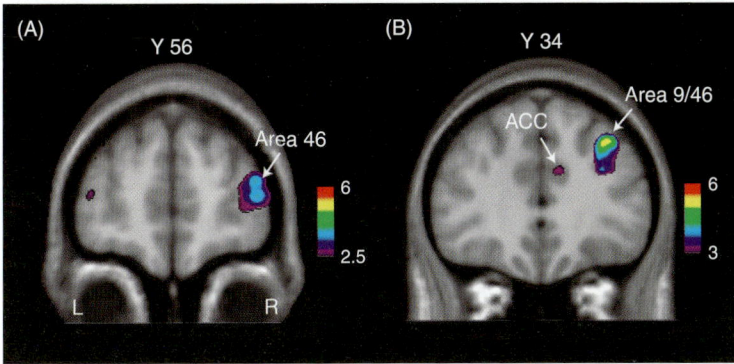

Plate 12 Results from the search minus repetition period comparison during the period of presentation of the stimuli (A) and the period of presentation of the feedback (B). The increased activity in the mid-dorsolateral prefrontal cortex and the anterior cingulate cortex (ACC) are represented on coronal sections. The Y value refers to the anteroposterior level in the Montreal Neurological Institute standard stereotaxic space. The color scale indicates the range for the t-statistic. L and R, left and right hemisphere.

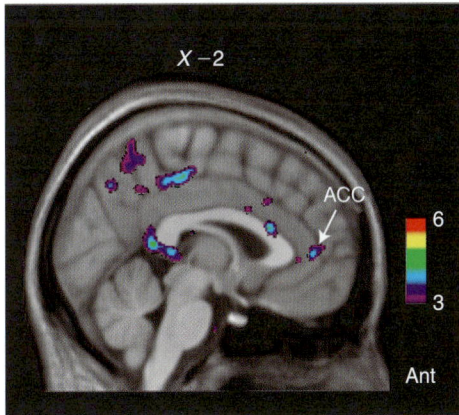

Plate 13 Results from the comparison of the decision intertrial interval minus the search period intertrial interval. Increased activity peak in the ACC is represented on a sagittal section. The X value corresponds to the mediolateral level in the Montreal Neurological Institute standard stereotaxic space. The color scale indicates the range for the t-statistic. Ant, anterior; ACC, anterior cingulate cortex.

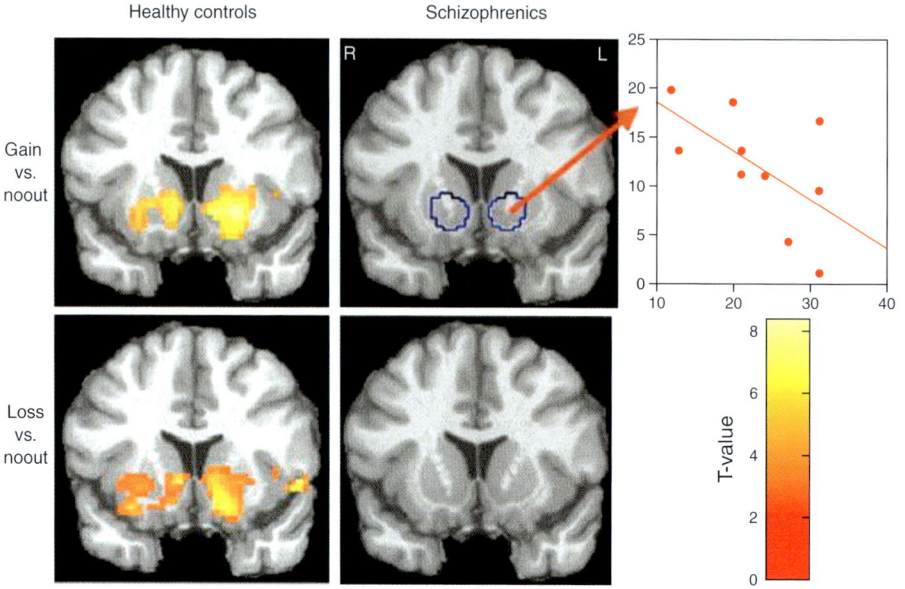

Plate 14 Ventral striatal activations in controls and patients performing a reward-processing task. As can be seen, there is reduced ventral striatal response in patients. The graph shows that the degree of reduction across patients is predictive of negative symptoms. *Source*: Taken from Juckel et al. (2006) [64].

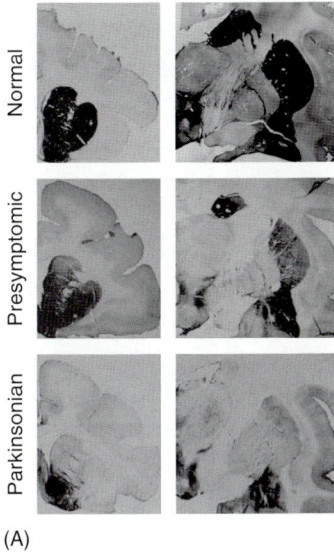

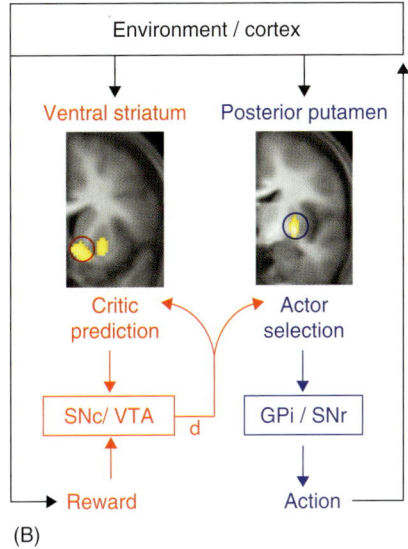

Plate 15 Summary of main anatomo-functional concepts underlying the effects of dopamine depletion on reward-seeking behavior. (A) Pattern of dopamine fibers degeneration, as revealed by tyrosine hydroxylase immuno-staining [36]. Successive stages of MPTP-induced parkinsonism are shown from top to bottom. Pictures were taken over frontal sections passing through the anterior (lefthand panels) and posterior (righthand panels) striatum. Note the relative preservation of ventral regions at every stage. (B) Schematic illustration of an actor–critic architecture tentatively implemented in fronto-striatal circuits. Brain images and activations were taken from a functional neuroimaging study in humans [64]. In this model, the posterior putamen plays the role of the actor, selecting an action through focal disinhibition of basal ganglia outputs (via GPi/SNr). The ventral striatum plays the role of the critic, generating a reward prediction based on the contextual information conveyed by cortical inputs. Midbrain dopamine neurons (in the SNc/VTA) compute the difference (δ) between the actual reward coming from the environment and the reward predicted by the critic. Dopamine release would thus be commensurate with reward prediction error and serve as a teaching signal tuning the efficacy of fronto-striatal synapses. In the ventral striatum it would improve reward prediction, while in the dorsal striatum it would improve action selection. As learning progresses, striatal activities would go less correlated, allowing the various fronto-striatal channels to encode different dimensions (such as reward prediction and action selection) of the behavioral response to the environmental context.

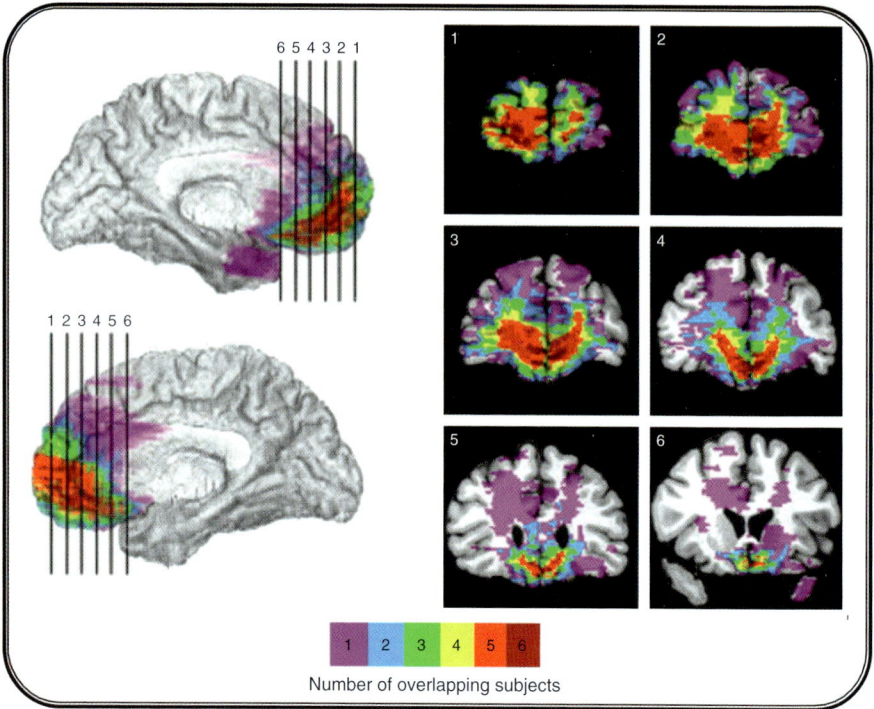

Plate 16 Lesion overlap of VMPC patients. Lesions of six VMPC patients displayed in mesial views and coronal slices. The color bar indicates the number of overlapping lesions at each voxel. This lesion overlap map is typical of bilateral VMPC lesion groups used in studies at the University of Iowa. *Source*: Adapted from Koenigs et al. (2007) [12].

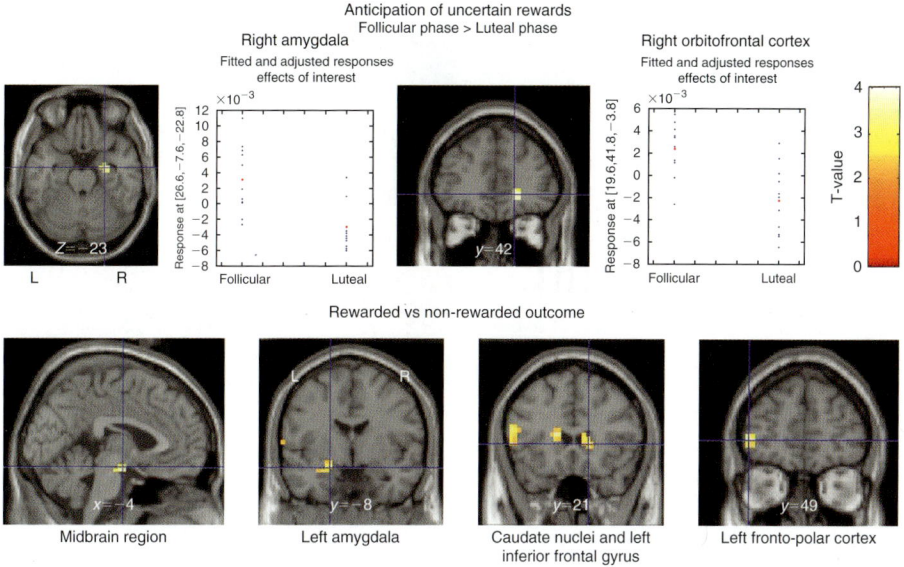

Anticipation of uncertain rewards
Follicular phase > Luteal phase

Right amygdala

Right orbitofrontal cortex

Rewarded vs non-rewarded outcome

Midbrain region | Left amygdala | Caudate nuclei and left inferior frontal gyrus | Left fronto-polar cortex

Plate 17 Cross-menstrual cycle phase differences in blood oxygen level-dependent (BOLD) response during reward anticipation and at the time of reward delivery. *Top.* During reward anticipation, higher BOLD responses were observed in the follicular phase than in the luteal phase in the right amygdala and orbitofrontal cortex. To the right of each map are shown distributions of BOLD signal response for each woman. *Bottom.* Cross-menstrual cycle phase differences in BOLD response at the time of reward outcome. Greater BOLD response during the follicular phase than during the luteal phase in midbrain, left amygdala, heads of the caudate nuclei, left inferior frontal gyrus, and left fronto-polar cortex [13].

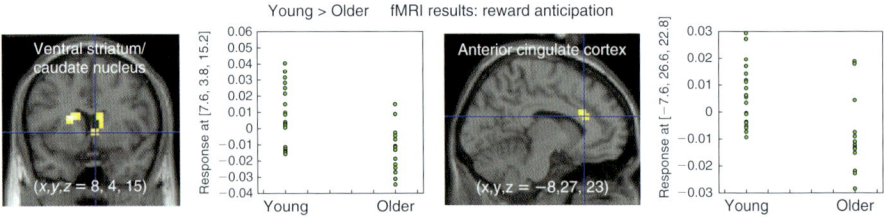

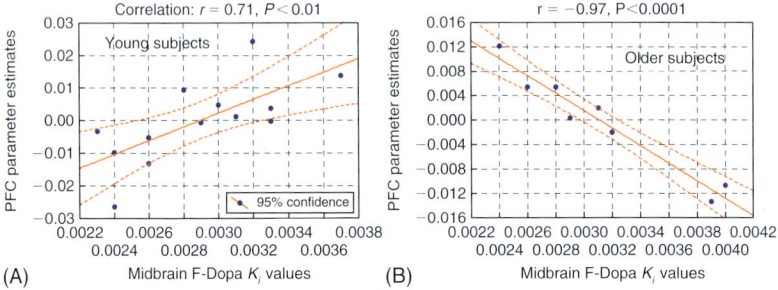

Plate 18 *Top.* Between-group comparison during reward anticipation, showing higher ventral striatum and anterior cingulate cortex activation in young subjects. The graphs show parameter estimates in these two brain regions in young and old subjects. *Bottom.* Relationship between midbrain dopamine uptake (K_i) and lateral prefrontal blood oxygen level-dependent (BOLD) signal in young and old adults during reward anticipation. Significant positive correlation of midbrain K_i with BOLD change during reward anticipation in young subjects ($x,y,z = 42, 46, 19$; Spearman's $r = 0.71$, $P < 0.01$; regression line with 95% confidence bands) (A) and significant negative correlation of midbrain K_i with BOLD change in older subjects ($x,y,z = -23, 30, 15$; $r = -0.97$, $P < 0.0001$) (B). A similar relationship was also observed at the time of reward delivery [152].

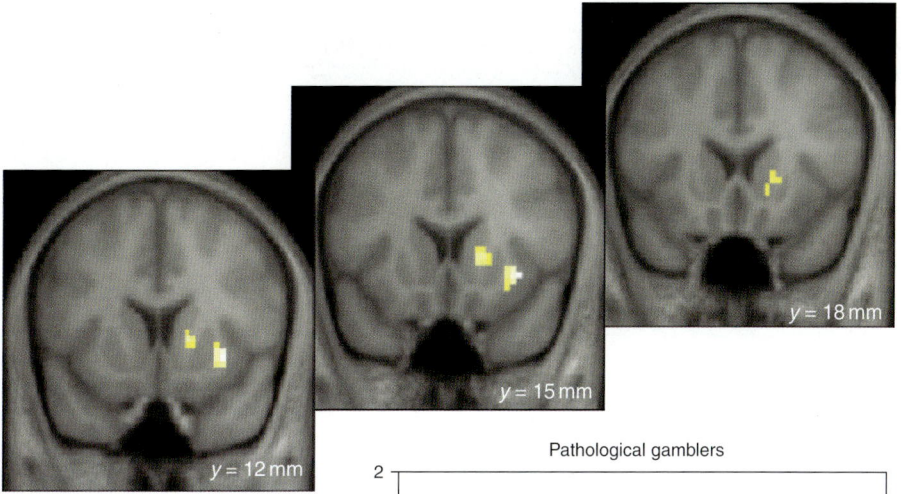

(A)

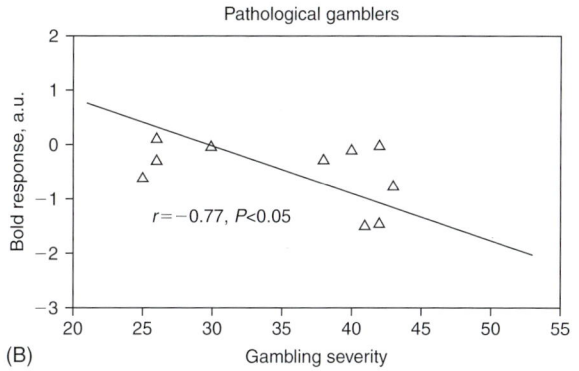

(B)

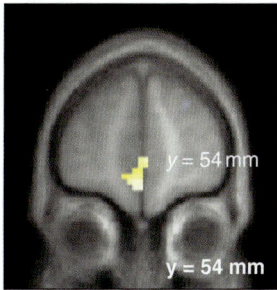

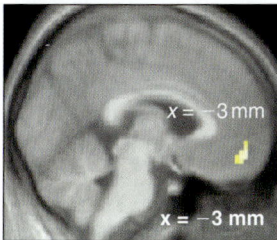

(C)

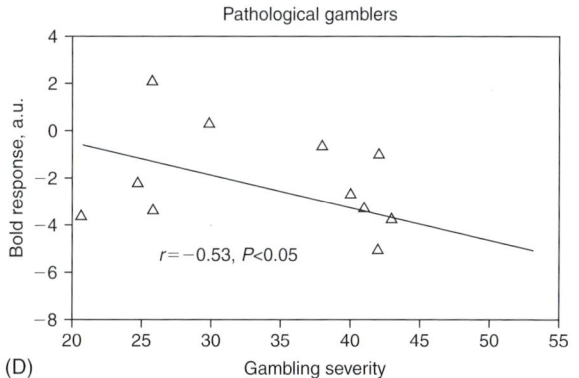

(D)

Plate 19 Differences in activation between the controls and the pathological gamblers. (A) Lower activation in the right ventral striatum of pathological gamblers compared with controls at $P < 0.001$ masked with the contrast winning > losing at $P < 0.001$. Activity within this area was negatively correlated with gambling severity of individual pathological gamblers (B). (C) Pathological gamblers also showed less activation in the ventromedial prefrontal cortex. Again, activation was negatively correlated with gambling severity (D). The y axes in B and D represent parameter estimates from the single-subject analysis and are directly related to BOLD signal change.

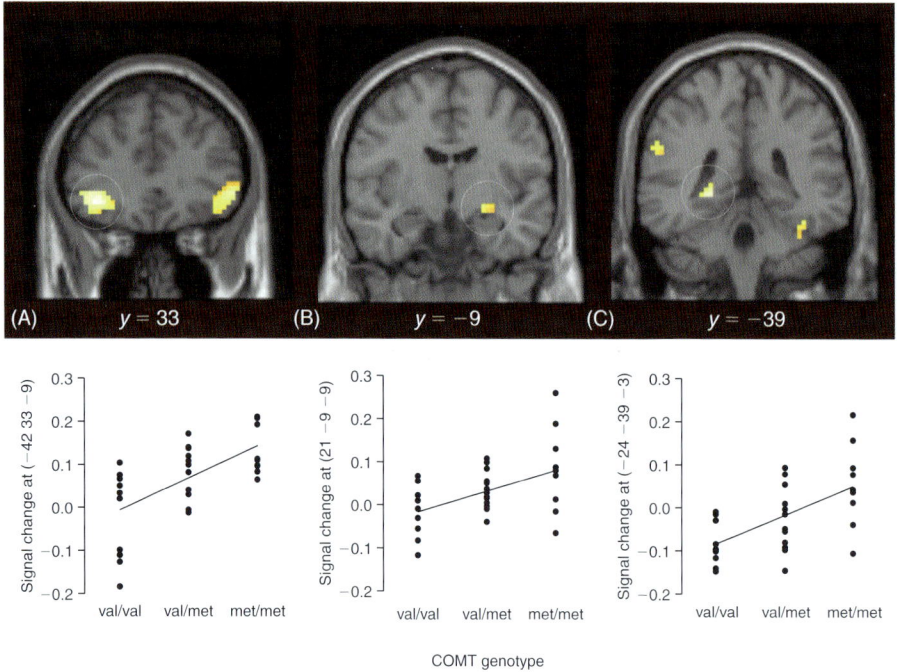

Plate 20 Correlation between COMT met[158] allele dosage (0 = val/val, 1 = val/met or 2 = met/met) and activation by aversive stimuli of the (A) ventrolateral PFC, (B) right amygdala, and (C) left dorsal hippocampus. In the upper row, statistical maps are shown ($P < 0.05$ *corrected* for volume of mask, cluster size ≥ 10 voxels). In the lower row, neural responses of individuals are shown as related to COMT genotype, showing an allele-dose dependent effect with heterozygotes having intermediate effects. Individual BOLD responses were extracted from the voxel with the highest T value inside the cluster circled on the left. *Source*: Modified from Smolka et al. (2005) [39].

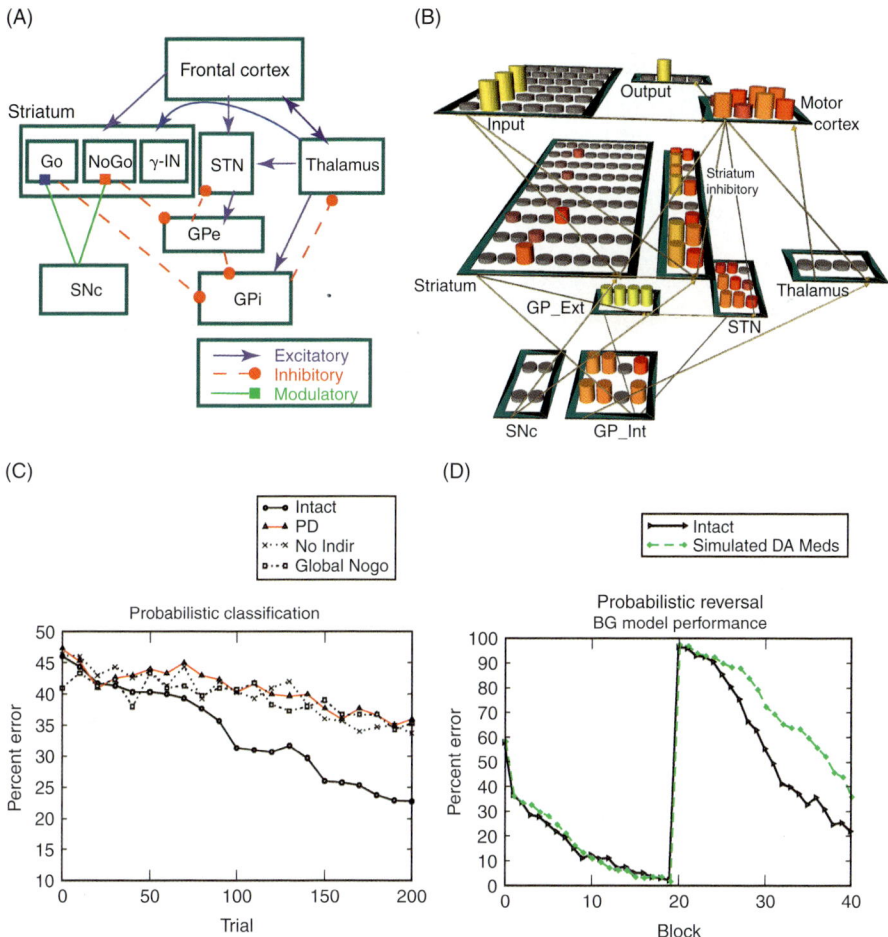

(A)

(B)

(C)

(D)

Plate 21 (A) Functional anatomy of the BG circuit. In addition to the classic "direct" and "indirect" pathways from striatum to BG output nuclei originating in striatonigral (Go) and striatopallidal (NoGo) cells, respectively, this updated architecture features focused projections from NoGo units to GPe and strong top-down projections from cortex to thalamus. Further, the STN is incorporated as part of a hyperdirect pathway, receiving inputs from frontal cortex and projecting directly to both GPe and GPi. (B) Neural network model of this circuit, with four different responses represented by four columns of motor units, four columns each of Go and NoGo units within striatum, and corresponding columns within GPi, GPe, and thalamus. In this updated model, fast-spiking GABA-ergic interneurons (γ-IN) regulate striatal activity via inhibitory projections. (C) Probabilistic learning, simulating the challenging probabilistic classification "weather prediction" task. Models with simulated PD were impaired at learning to resolve complex probabilistic discriminations [153], as were models without the indirect NoGo pathway, or with only nonspecific "Global" NoGo representations. (D) Model probabilistic reversal learning. Simulated medication, via partial blockade of DA dips, led to selectively impaired reversal, as seen in medicated patients [11].

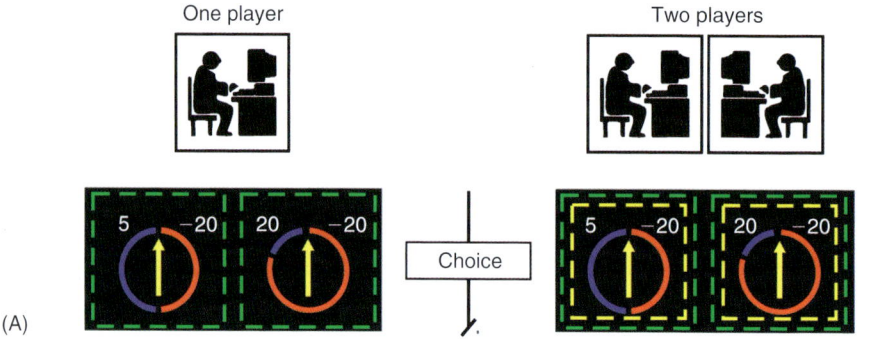

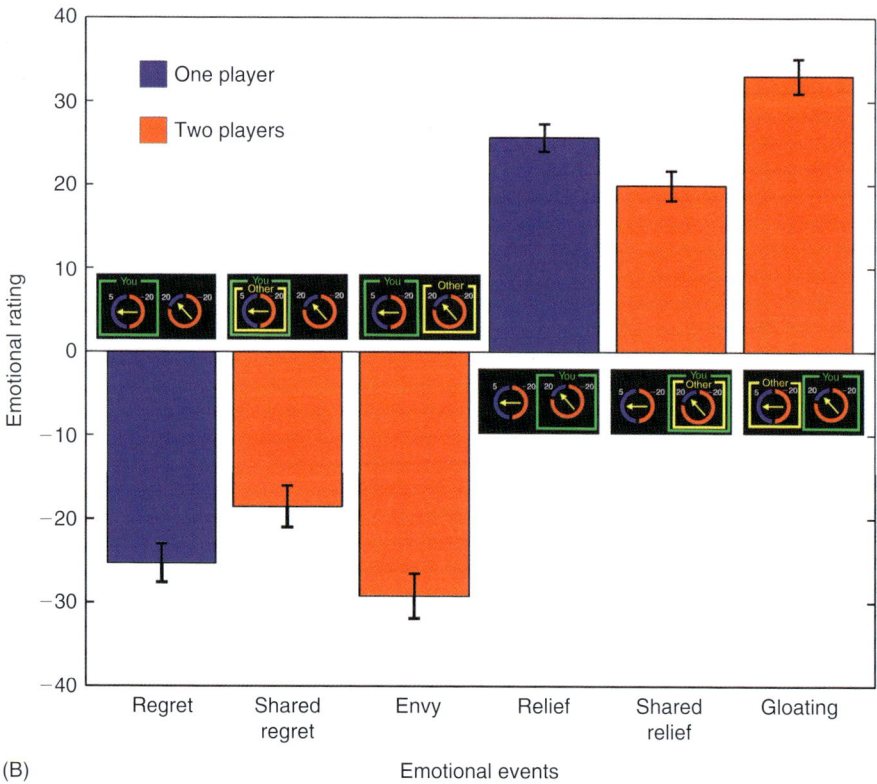

Plate 22 (A) Typical single (on the left) and two player trial in Bault et al. [56]. Numbers indicated outcomes, and the probabilities were represented by colored sectors of a circle. Each lottery was surrounded with one dotted square in the case of a one player trial or two dotted squares of different colors in the case of a two player trial. (B) Emotional responses: average subjective emotional evaluations for different events. The bars represent the average value (±SEM) of the subjective emotional evaluation given by participants in the different events. The pictures around the horizontal axis show the typical screen display seen by participants in the different events.

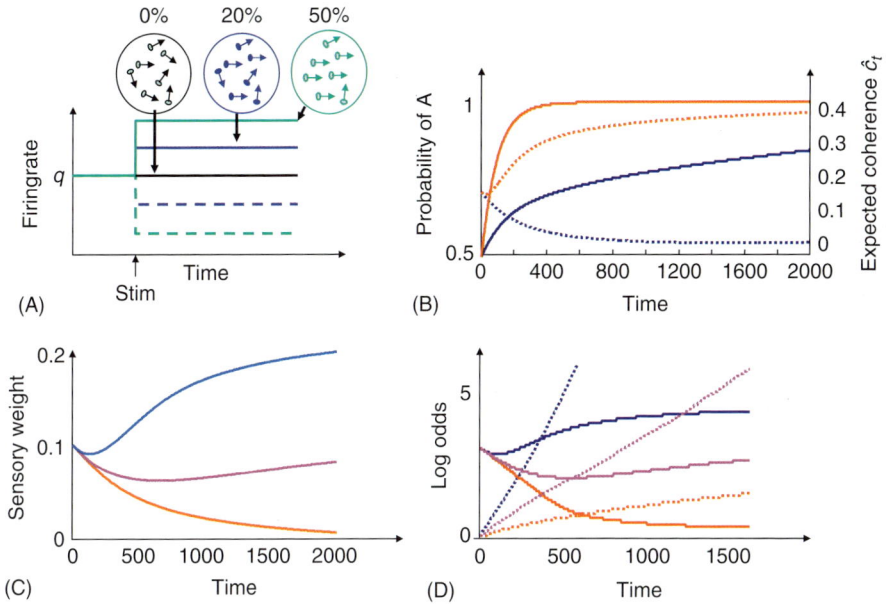

(A) (B) (C) (D)

Plate 23 Bayesian decision making with varying motion coherence. (A) Modulation of firing rate in response to varying motion coherence. Plain line: stimulus in the preferred direction. Dashed line: simulus in the anti-preferred direction. (B) Outcome of the "full" Bayesian model computing the joint probabilities of all pairs of choices and coherences. Plain line: probability of choice A (averaged over 10,000 trials where A was the correct choice). Dotted line: expected value for motion coherence. Red: $c = 0.2$. Blue: $c = 0.05$. (C) Sensory weights in the simplified Bayesian model (average of 10,000 trials) as a function of time after stimulus presentation. Blue: $c = 0.2$. Red: $c = 0$ (i.e., sensory input is pure noise). Magenta: $c = 0.1$. (D) Average temporal evolution of the log odds and the decision threshold in the simplified Bayesian model. Dotted lines: log odds. Plain lines: threshold. Blue: $c = 0.2$. Red: $c = 0.05$. Magenta: $c = 0.1$.

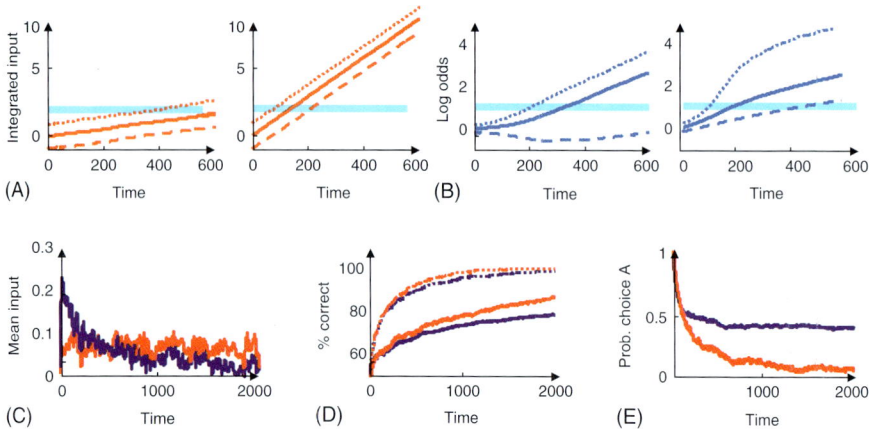

Plate 24 Bayesian decision model and diffusion model in the "fixed delay" task. (A) Average integrated input ($\bar{L}_t$) as a function of time in the diffusion model. Left panel: low coherence ($c = 0.05$). Right panel: medium coherence ($c = 0.2$). Plain line: equiprobable choice ($L_o = 0$). Dotted line: $L_o = 0.6$. Dashed line: $L_o = -0.6$. Thick horizontal line: decision threshold. (B) Same as in (A), but plotting the average log odds divided by the decision threshold (i.e., L_t/D_t) for the Bayesian diffusion model. (C) Choice-averaged input as a function of time in the trial. Blue: average input for all trials leading to choice A in the Bayesian model. Red: same thing for the diffusion model. (D) Percent of correct choices as a function of the duration of stimulus presentation. Same color code as in (C). Plain: $c = 0.05$. Dotted: $c = 0.1$. (E) Probability of choosing A in zero coherence trial with prior $L_o = 0.6$, as a function of the duration of stimulus presentation. Same color code as in (C).